# Human Anatomy

AN ILLUSTRATED COLOUR TEXT

*Commissioning Editor:* Timothy Horne
*Development Editor:* Hannah Kenner
*Project Manager:* Nancy Arnott
*Design Direction:* Erik Bigland
*Illustration Manager:* Bruce Hogarth

# Human Anatomy

## A Clinically-Orientated Approach

AN ILLUSTRATED COLOUR TEXT

**S. Jacob** MBBS MS (Anatomy)
Senior Lecturer
University of Sheffield;
Member of the Court of Examiners
Royal College of Surgeons of England, London;
Visiting Professor St George's University
Grenada, West Indies

*Dissections by*
**David J. Hinchliffe**

*Photography by*
**Mick A. Turton**

*Illustrated by*
**Amanda Williams**

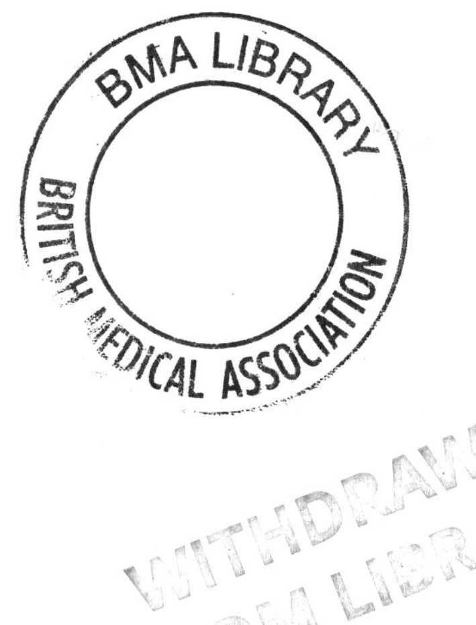




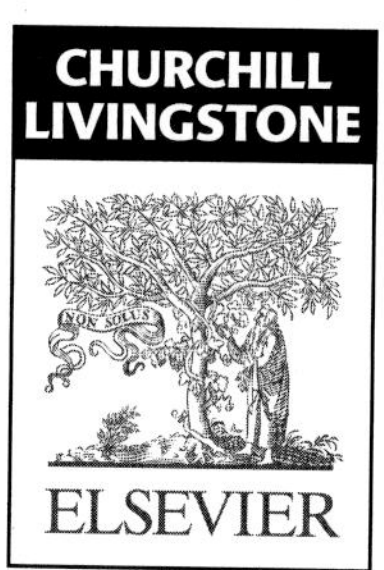


EDINBURGH LONDON NEW YORK OXFORD PHILADELPHIA ST LOUIS SYDNEY TORONTO 2007

CHURCHILL
LIVINGSTONE
ELSEVIER



This book was originally published as *Atlas of Human Anatomy*
ISBN 0-443-05364-2 in 2002
This edition 2007

ISBN-13: 978-0-443-10373-5

**British Library Cataloguing in Publication Data**
A catalogue record for this book is available from the British Library

**Library of Congress Cataloging in Publication Data**
A catalog record for this book is available from the Library of Congress

**Note**
Neither the Publisher nor the Author assume any responsibility for any loss or injury and/or damage to persons or property arising out of or related to any use of the material contained in this book. It is the responsibility of the treating practitioner, relying on independent expertise and knowledge of the patient, to determine the best treatment and method of application for the patient.
**The Publisher**



The publisher's policy is to use **paper manufactured from sustainable forests**

Printed in China

# Preface

Human gross anatomy is one of the most important subjects in the study of Medicine and Allied Health Sciences. Dissection of the cadavers is the best means of studying gross anatomy. However, this is often difficult because of limitations of facilities, the short time available in the curriculum and the growing scarcity of cadavers for dissection. By using a combination of fully labelled photographs of dissections, radiological anatomy, and drawings along with a comprehensive descriptive text this book aims to provide the student with a real understanding of the anatomy of the human body. This illustrated colour text of human anatomy contains illustrations of surface anatomy, osteology, dissections, radiological, CT and MRI images and line artwork. There are nearly 480 illustrations. The background text, concise but comprehensive, describes the most important features of each area with special emphasis on clinical relevance and application. Features of anatomy that are of clinical importance are indicated with an ✪ icon in the text. Clinical anatomy is further emphasised by clinical boxes relevant to each area of description. Each clinical box illustrates the value of anatomy in medical practice. The book has about 85 such clinical boxes.

Organised on a regional basis this human anatomy book contains illustrations and description of the upper limb, thorax, abdomen and pelvis, vertebral column and spinal cord, lower limb and head and neck. Each chapter starts with a relevant account of surface anatomy and osteology.

In planning this book I took into account the time constraint affecting most modern Anatomy courses as well as the wide variety of teaching methodology used. It is hoped that the book will act as a useful companion for those who learn anatomy by dissection or by using prosections and plastinated specimens.

The level of details contained in the book is more than adequate for most undergraduate medical and dental courses. This illustrated text may also be useful for students of Biological, Biomedical and Allied Health Sciences where human anatomy is part of the curriculum. Surgeons in training can use this for a rapid review of anatomy while preparing for postgraduate examinations.

Anatomy is a descriptive subject. In the past a medical student was expected to master all the detailed accounts of the subject. I do appreciate the fact that there are medical curricula which still demand a lot of factual details which can be quite daunting to a student who is doing the subject for the first time. Having been in the front line of medical undergraduate and postgraduate teaching for nearly 40 years I have a good idea as to what is humanly possible during the time available and what is essential for the practice of medicine. Students can no longer afford to master the voluminous details in traditional textbooks, nor should they try to learn anything other than what is essential for clinical practice.

A forerunner of this book was published as *Atlas of Human Anatomy* in 2002 by Churchill Livingstone. It was received well by students world over and had translations into Portuguese, Spanish, Greek and Chinese, besides the original English edition.

I would like to express my gratitude to many co-workers and friends who gave me invaluable help and encouragement towards the production of this book. I am greatly indebted to David Hinchliffe for producing the excellent dissections and to Mick Turton for his exceptional expertise in photography. This work would not have been possible without their dedicated efforts and unswerving enthusiasm. Jill Revill, Caroline Couldwell, Andy Fitzgerald and Malcolm Hinchliffe also deserve credit for facilitating this work. Professor Rachel Koshi and the late Dr Thomas Koshi (Christian Medical College, Vellore) provided many of the radiographs. The MRI and CT scans were obtained from Dr Matthew Bull, Consultant, Northern General Hospital, Sheffield. Dr Sujatha Varkey, Consultant Radiologist, Rotherham District General Hospital provided the mammogram and the renal ultrasound scan. I am grateful to them all.

Finally my sincere thanks to Hannah Kenner, Nancy Arnott and the Elsevier production team for the expertise and care with which they made possible the preparation of this book, and to Timothy Horne of Elsevier for entrusting me with this project.

Sheffield 2007 S. Jacob

# Contents

# Chapter 1
# **What is anatomy?**

Anatomy is the study of the structure of the body. The word anatomy is derived from the Greek word *anat'ome* which means to cut up. The Latin equivalent of this is *dissecare* from which the word dissection is derived. Of all the basic science courses offered to students of medicine, dentistry and allied health sciences there is none more directly related to their professional practice than gross anatomy and its application.

The arrangement of structures in the body is very complex. The first task in the study of anatomy is the

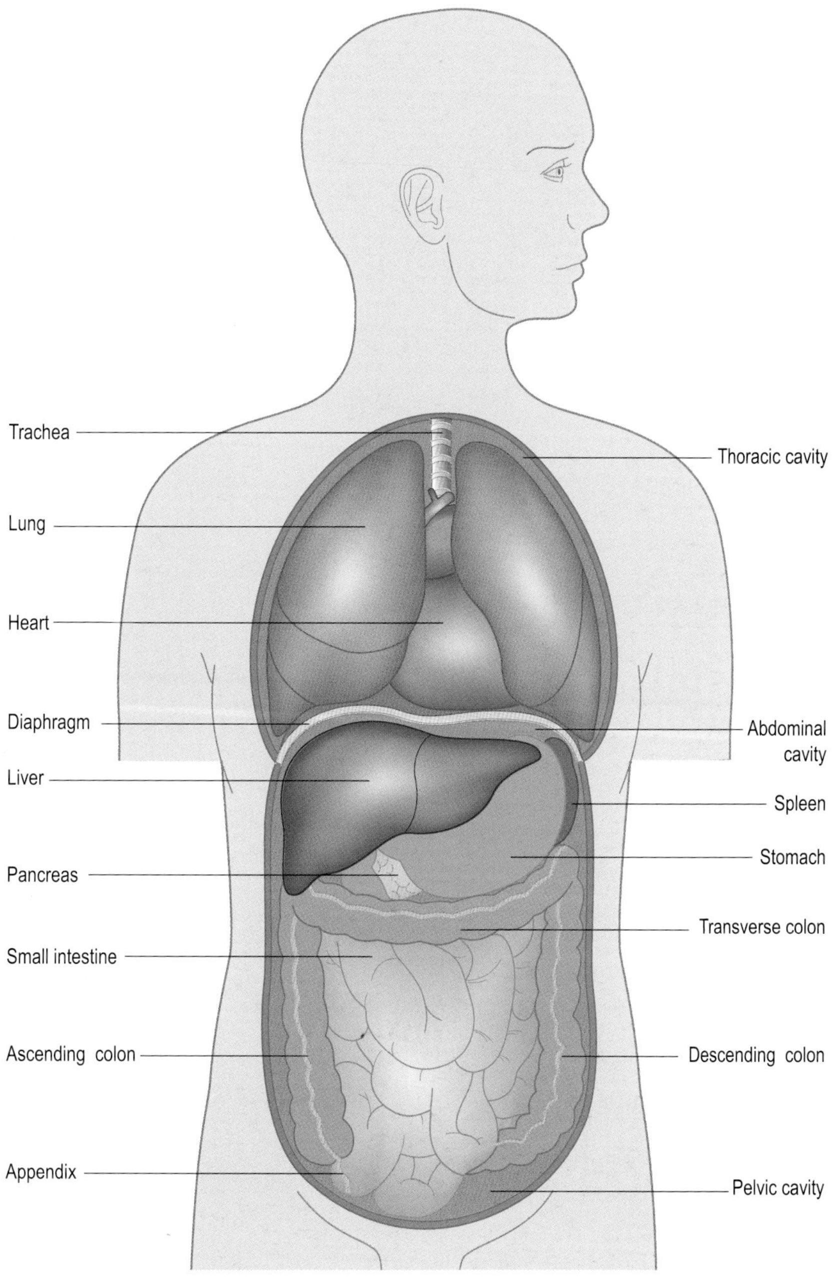


Fig. 1.1 The internal organs within the various cavities of the body – anterior view.

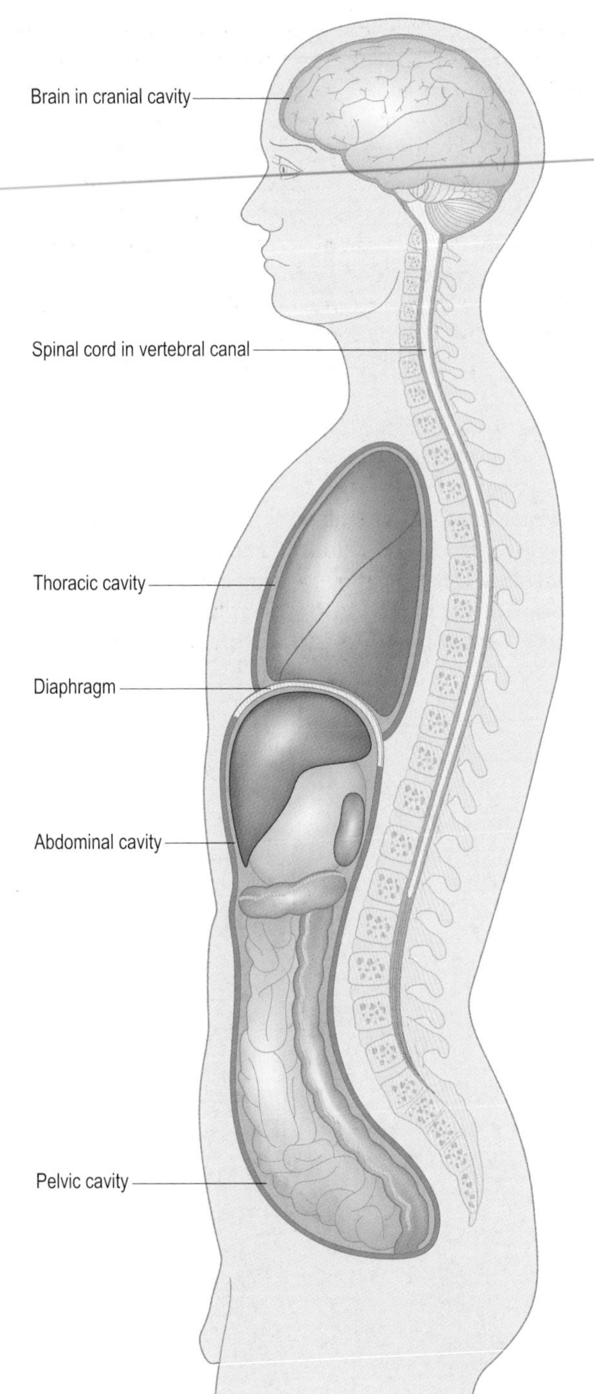


Fig. 1.2 Internal organs within the various cavities of the body – lateral view.

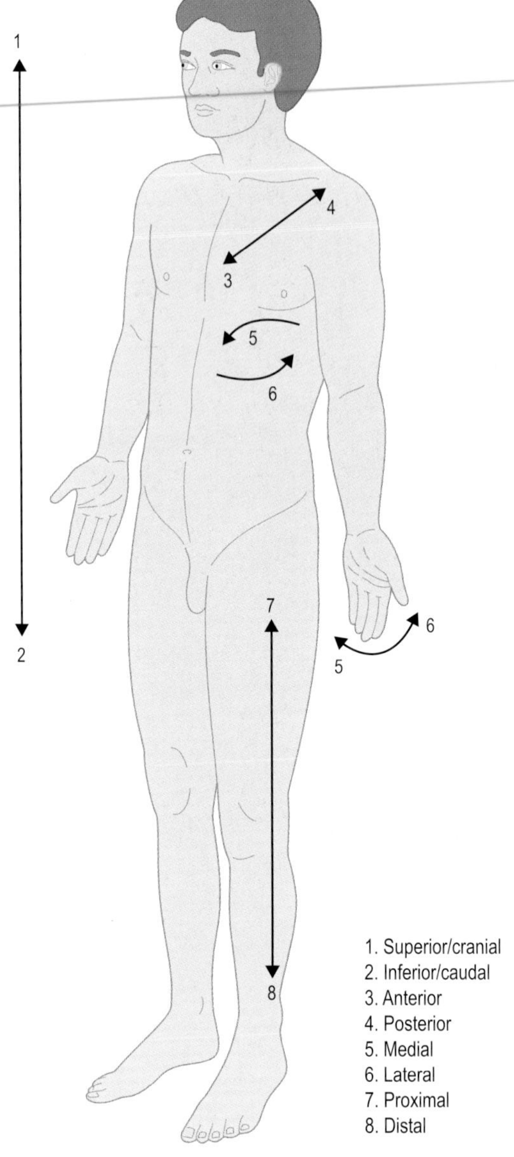


Fig. 1.3 Commonly used positional and directional terms when the body is in standard anatomical position.

visualisation of the different structures, appreciating especially the way they are packaged in the body and their relationship to one another. Study of dissection illustrations along with that of diagnostic images such as plain radiographs, angiograms, CT and MRI scans play a major role in achieving this goal. Surface anatomy is the art of projecting on to the surface the underlying structures. Many definitive elements of the living body can be easily identified on the surface. Ignorance of this part of anatomy will be a serious handicap during the physical examination of a patient.

The main divisions of the body are the head, neck, thorax, abdomen and the upper and lower limbs (Figs 1.1, 1.2). The internal organs are located within the various cavities of the body. The cranial cavity contains the brain and the vertebral canal in the vertebral column contains the spinal cord. The right and left lungs and the heart are in the thoracic cavity. Each lung is surrounded by the pleural cavity and the heart by the pericardial cavity. The thoracic cavity is separated from the abdominal cavity by the dome-shaped diaphragm, which is a sheet of muscle. The abdominal cavity is further divided into the abdominal cavity proper, which contains the liver, stomach, small intestine, parts of the large intestine, pancreas, spleen and kidneys, and the pelvic cavity, which has the sigmoid colon, rectum, urinary bladder and parts of the reproductive system.

Anatomy has a highly specialised vocabulary, most of them derived from Greek or Latin. It is the language of medicine. Communications between health professionals can be severely hampered without the accurate use of anatomical nomenclature.

The anatomical position, about which the anatomical relations of structures are described, is that in which the

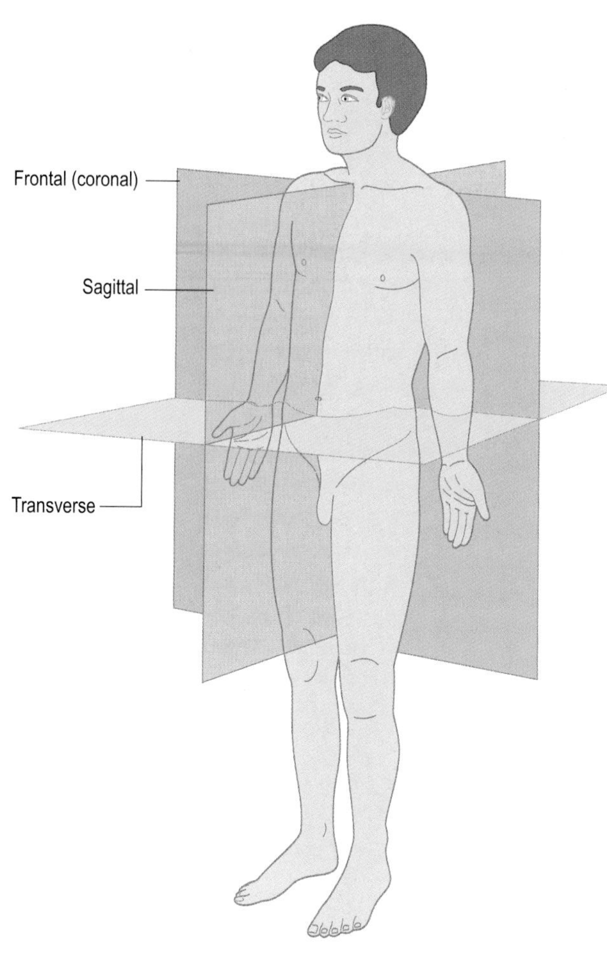


Fig. 1.4 Body planes.

person stands erect, arms by the sides, palms of the hands facing forwards (Fig. 1.3). Structures in front are termed anterior and those behind, posterior. Structures above are superior and those below, inferior. Structures nearer the midline of the body are medial and those away from the midline, lateral. Structures nearer to the surface are superficial and those further from the surface are deep. In the limbs, the term proximal is used to describe structures nearer to the trunk and distal for those away from the trunk. A sagittal plane passes vertically anteroposteriorly through the body and the coronal plane is at right angles to the sagittal plane. A plane that passes at right angles to both the coronal and sagittal plane dividing the body into cross sections is the transverse or horizontal plane (Fig. 1.4).

Movement in the coronal plane away from the midsagittal plane is called abduction, return towards the midsagittal plane is adduction. Bending of any part in the sagittal plane is flexion and straightening is extension. Rotation occurs around a vertical axis. It may be medial rotation, towards the midline, or lateral, away from it.

# Chapter 2
# Upper Limb



## Introduction

The human upper limb, which is primarily used for grasping and manipulating objects, consists of the following five regions (Fig. 2.1):

- shoulder
- axilla
- arm
- forearm
- hand.

The shoulder has a wide range of mobility by virtue of the movements of the humerus, the clavicle and the scapula. The axilla or the armpit is the space between the chest wall and the upper part of the arm and contains the principal nerves and vessels. The bone of the arm, the region between the shoulder and the elbow, is the humerus (Fig. 2.2). In the arm the muscles are arranged in two compartments, flexors anteriorly and extensors posteriorly. A similar arrangement is seen in the forearm as well. The forearm is the region between the elbow and the wrist. The radius and the ulna of the forearm articulate with the humerus at the elbow joint and with each other at the superior and inferior radioulnar joints. Pronation and supination to rotate the forearm and hand for grasping and manipulating objects occur at the radioulnar joints; flexion and extension of the forearm take place at the elbow joint.

The wrist containing the carpal bones connects the forearm and hand. The skeleton of the hand is formed by the five metacarpal bones and that of the fingers by the phalanges. The anterior aspect of the hand is the palm of the hand. The hand can act as a tactile organ as the skin of the palm has a rich sensory innervation. The hand is for grasping objects. In the precision grip, as in holding a pen, the thumb is in the opposed position where the pulp of the thumb faces the pulp of the index finger. The thumb is of great functional value in all grips, especially in the precision grip. In a power grip, as in holding a hammer, the wrist is kept extended and the powerful long flexors of the digits contract to make the fingers flex to hold the handle (Fig. 2.3). The thumb reinforces the grip. All grips and manipulations rely on normal mobility of all the fingers. A single immobile finger can make the whole hand clumsy.

## Surface anatomy and bones of the shoulder and pectoral regions

The clavicle, which is subcutaneous, is palpable throughout and its movements during the movements of the upper limb can be felt by holding it between finger and thumb. The jugular notch (suprasternal notch) is felt between the prominent medial ends of the clavicles. The clavicular and sternal heads of the sternocleidomastoid muscle are visible (Fig. 2.4). The pulsation of the subclavian artery is felt on deep palpation against the first rib in the supraclavicular region just lateral to the clavicular head of the muscle. More posteriorly in the root of the neck the upper lateral border of the trapezius is visible. The muscle can be felt contracting by elevating the shoulder against resistance. The pectoralis major muscle, as it bridges across the chest wall and arm, forms the anterior wall of the axilla. Its lower border is the anterior axillary fold. The muscle can be felt contracting when the abducted arm is adducted against resistance. The clavicular and the sternocostal heads of the muscle may be visible in a muscular person. Below and lateral to the pectoralis major the digitations of the serratus anterior may be seen (Fig. 2.4).

The acromion of the scapula (Fig. 2.5) forms the highest bony point of the shoulder region. This point is used to measure the length of the upper limb. The coracoid process of the scapula is felt on deep palpation below the clavicle at its junction between the lateral third and the medial two-thirds. The muscle covering the whole of the shoulder region and giving it its rounded contour is the deltoid. The cephalic vein, a superficial vein of the upper limb, lies subcutaneously in the deltopectoral triangle, which is the gap between the deltoid and the pectoralis major.

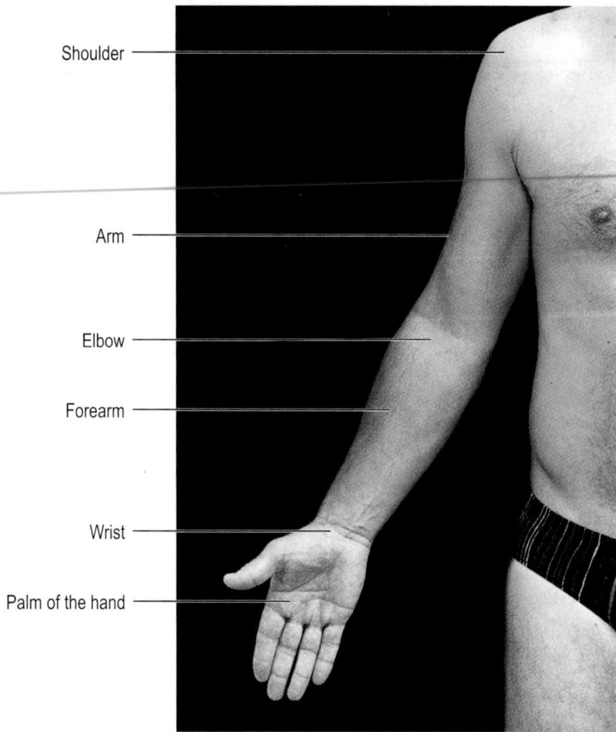


Fig. 2.1 Regions of the upper limb.

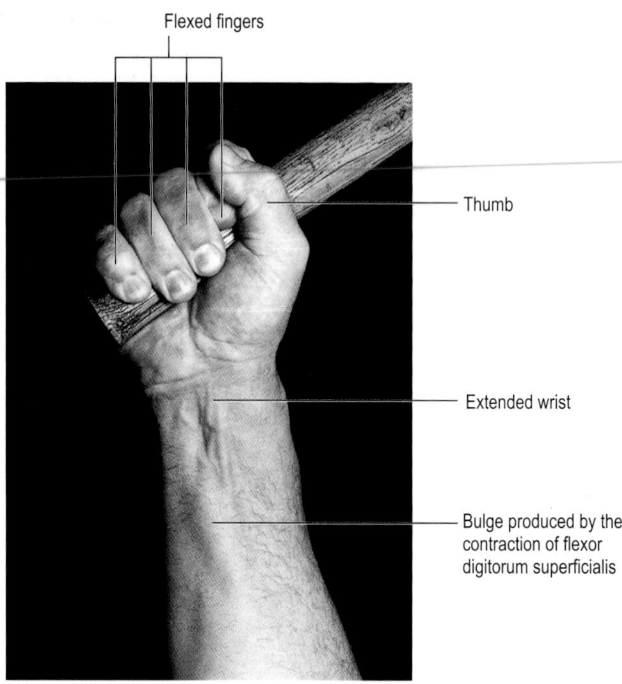


Fig. 2.3 Power grip.

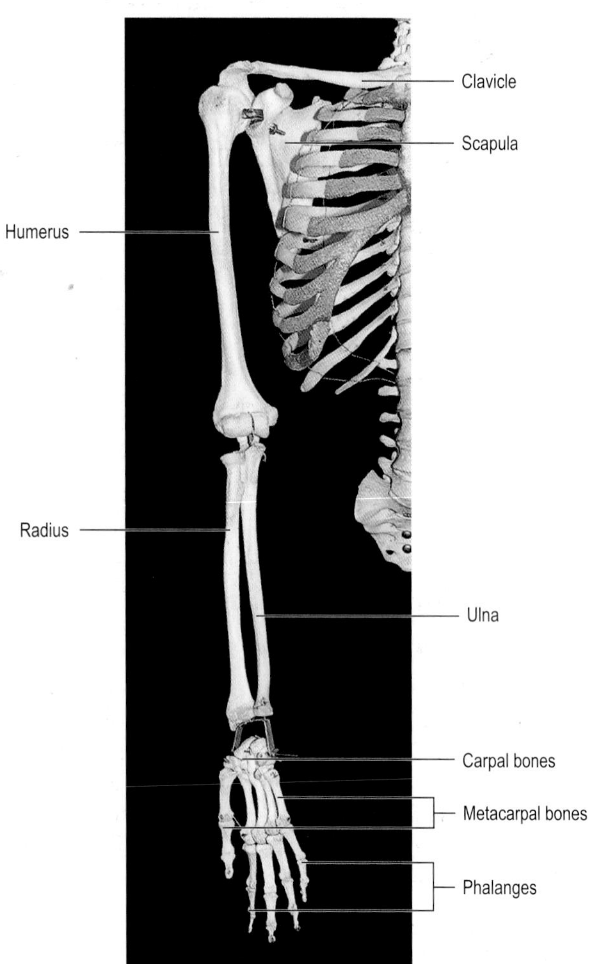


Fig. 2.2 Bones of the upper limb.

**Pectoralis major**

This large muscle connects the upper part of the chest wall to the upper extremity (Fig. 2.6).

*Origin* Medial third of the clavicle (clavicular head) and the sternum and costal cartilages (sternocostal head).

*Insertion* Lateral lip of the bicipital groove on the shaft of the humerus.

*Nerve supply* Lateral and medial pectoral nerves.

*Action* The sternocostal fibres adduct and medially rotate the humerus at the shoulder joint. The clavicular fibres flex the humerus. If the upper limb is abducted and fixed the muscle can move the ribs and act as an accessory muscle of respiration.

*Test* ✪ For clavicular head – abduct the arm to 90° and ask the patient to push the arm forward (flex) against resistance. For sternocostal head – abduct the arm to 60° and adduct it against resistance. The contracting heads can be seen and felt.

**Pectoralis minor**

This lies deep to the pectoralis major (Fig. 2.7).

*Origin* Third to fifth (often second to fourth) ribs.

*Insertion* The coracoid process of the scapula.

*Nerve supply* Medial pectoral nerve.

*Action* Draws the scapula (hence the arm) forwards – protraction of shoulder. It can also depress the shoulder.

**Serratus anterior**

*Origin* By a series of digitations from the upper eight ribs.

*Insertion* The costal surface of the scapula along its medial border. The muscle forming the medial wall of the axilla lies between the scapula and the chest wall before reaching its insertion.

*Nerve supply* Long thoracic nerve from the roots of the brachial plexus (Clinical box 2.1; see Fig. 2.36).

*Action* Protraction (forward movement) of the scapula as in pushing, punching and fencing.

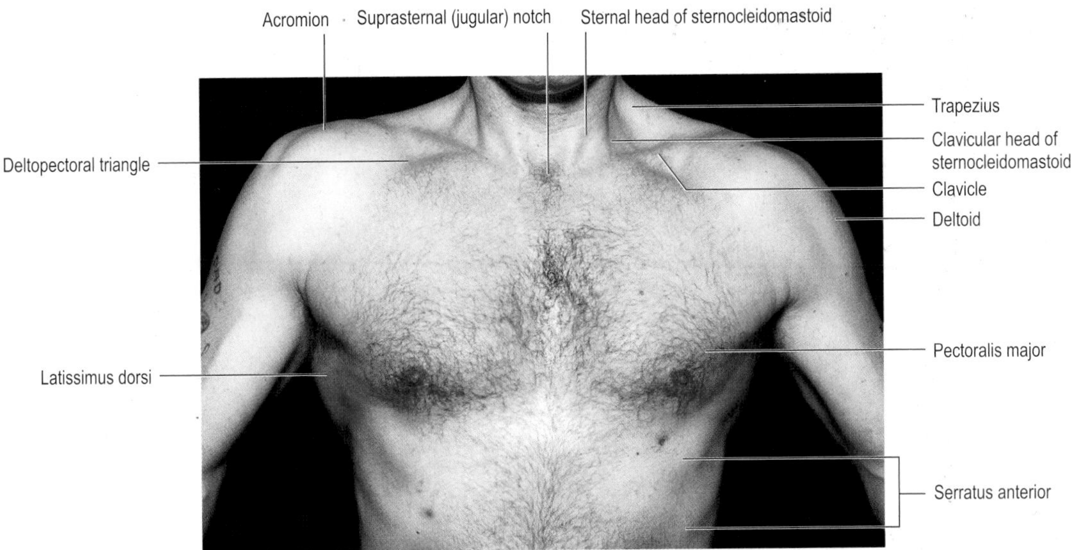


Fig. 2.4 Surface anatomy of the shoulder and pectoral region.

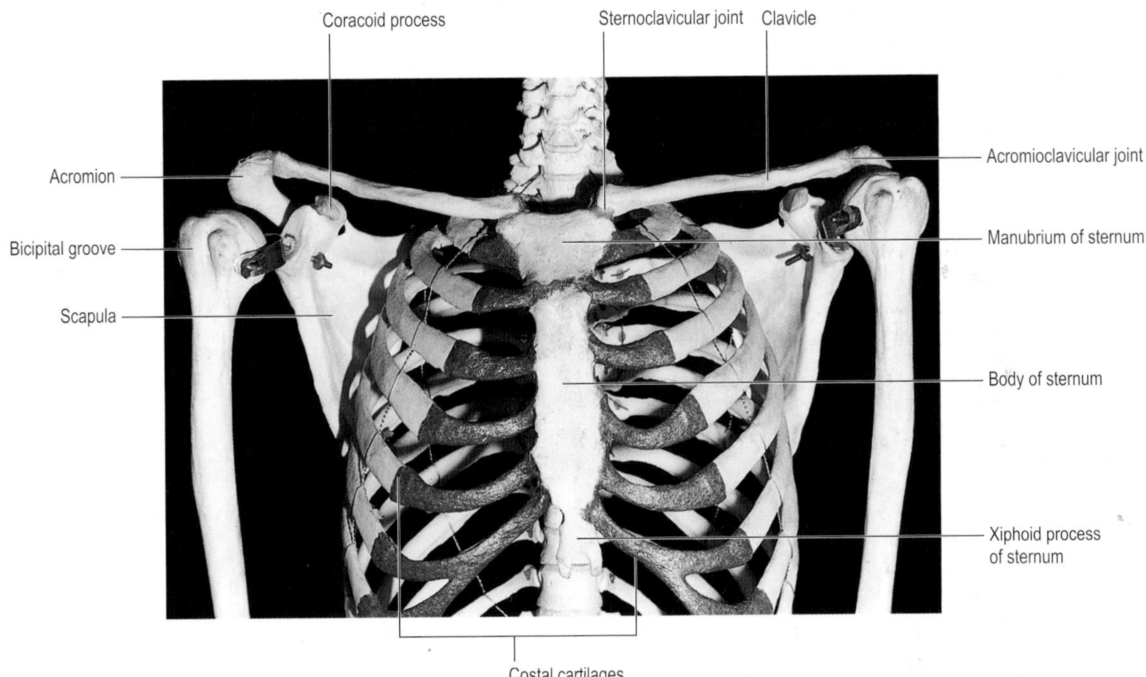


Fig. 2.5 Bones of the pectoral and shoulder regions.

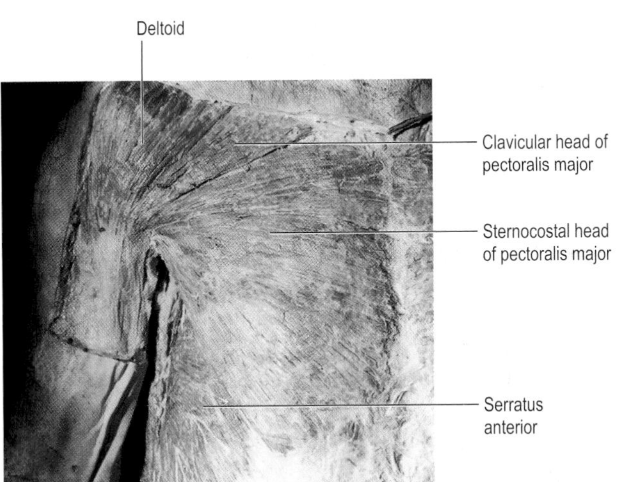


Fig. 2.6 Pectoralis major, deltoid and serratus anterior.

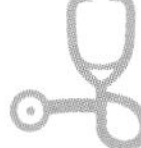

*Clinical box 2.1*

**Winging of the scapula**

The long thoracic nerve supplying the serratus anterior lies on the surface of the muscle on the medial wall of the axilla and is vulnerable in surgical procedures such as 'axillary clearance' of lymph nodes for the treatment of carcinoma of the breast (p. 228). Nerve damage causes 'winging' of the scapula where its medial border is seen more raised and prominent.

## The skeleton viewed from the back

Figure 2.8 illustrates the skeleton as viewed from the back. The most prominent point in the midline on the occipital bone is the external occipital protuberance from which the

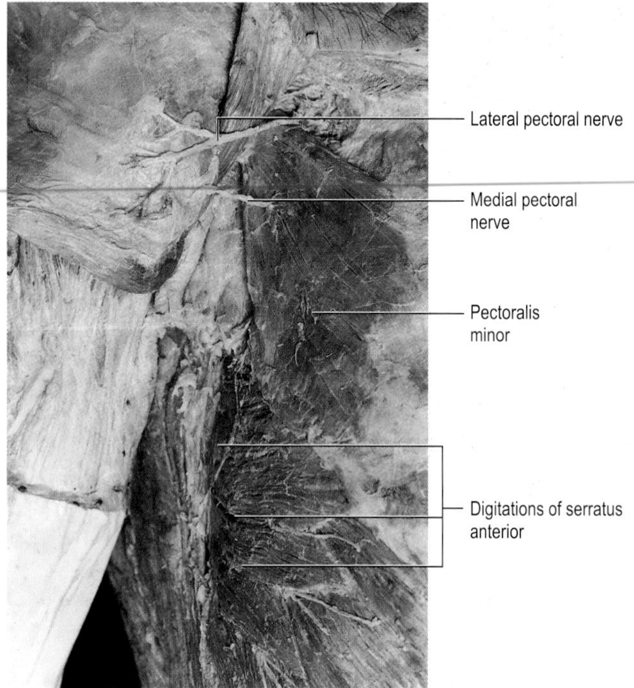


Fig. 2.7 Pectoralis minor.

superior nuchal line, a transverse ridge, extends laterally. The vertebral column consists of seven cervical, twelve thoracic and five lumbar vertebrae, and the sacrum. The upper border of the hip bone, the iliac crest, forms the border between the back of the trunk and the gluteal region of the lower limb. The spinous processes of the vertebrae to which the latissimus dorsi and the trapezius muscles are attached project backwards in the midline. The scapula whose concave costal surface lies against the convex rib cage has a projection backwards, the spine of the scapula. When the arm is by the side of the trunk the medial end of the spine, known as the root of the spine of the scapula, lies at the level of the third rib.

## Surface anatomy of the back

Figure 2.9 illustrates the surface anatomy of the back. Surface features of the trapezius and the latissimus dorsi can be examined at the back. The superolateral border of the trapezius is seen and felt in the lower part of the neck. This can be made more prominent by raising the point of the shoulder against resistance. The spinous processes of the vertebrae are palpable in the midline. They can be made more prominent by bending the trunk forward. The lateral border of the latissimus dorsi is visible as the posterior axillary fold. The muscle can be palpated here by adducting the abducted arm against resistance. The medial border, the inferior angle and the spine of the scapula and the acromion are also seen. As the scapula contributes to the movement of the shoulder, the mobility of the shoulder joint (glenohumeral joint) is assessed by immobilising the scapula by holding on to it at the back.

## Superficial muscles of the back

### Trapezius

This triangular muscle (muscles on the two sides together has the form of a trapezium) covers the back of the neck and most of the back of the trunk and connects the trunk to the upper extremity (Fig. 2.10). It contributes to the wide range of movements at the shoulder.

Fibres of the trapezius take origin from the external occipital protuberance and the superior nuchal line,

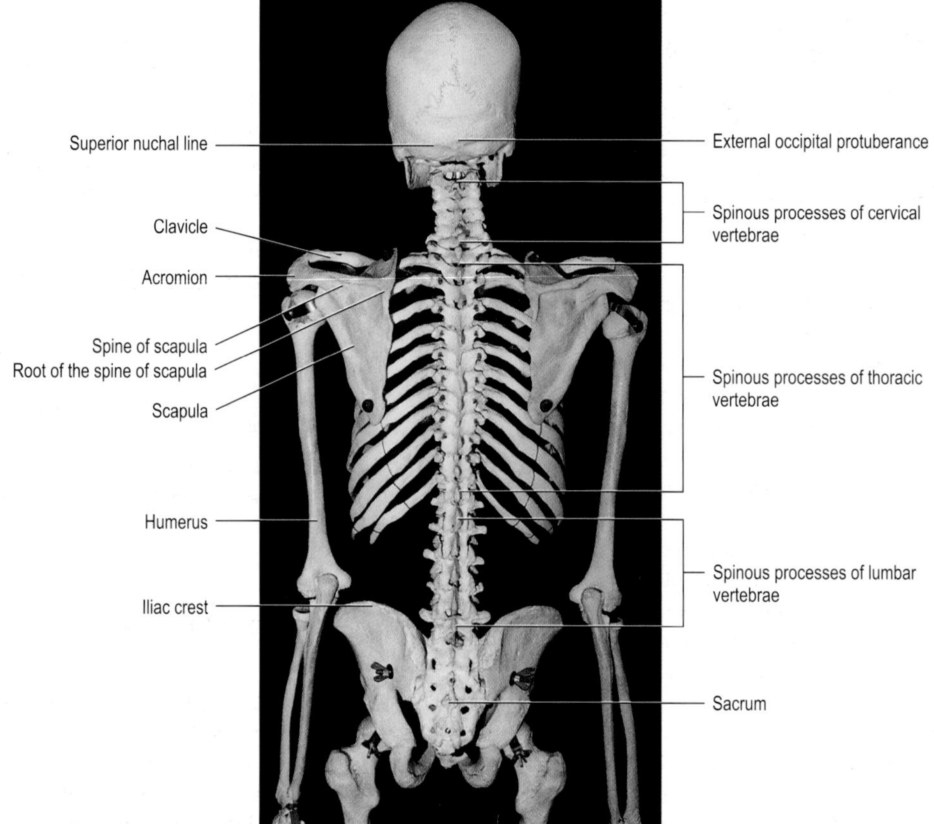


Fig. 2.8 The skeleton viewed from the back.

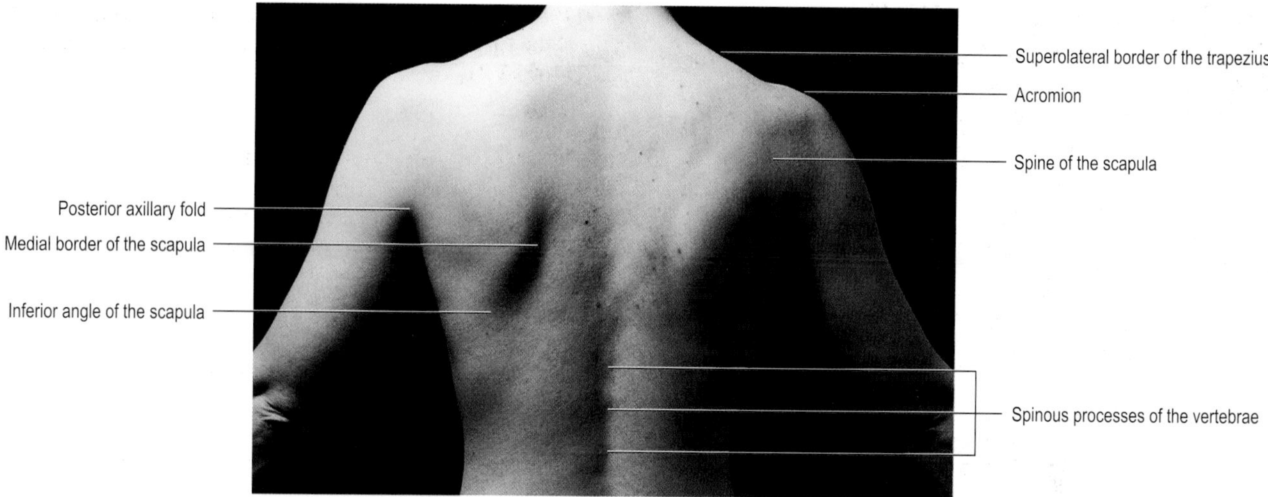


Fig. 2.9 Surface anatomy of the back.

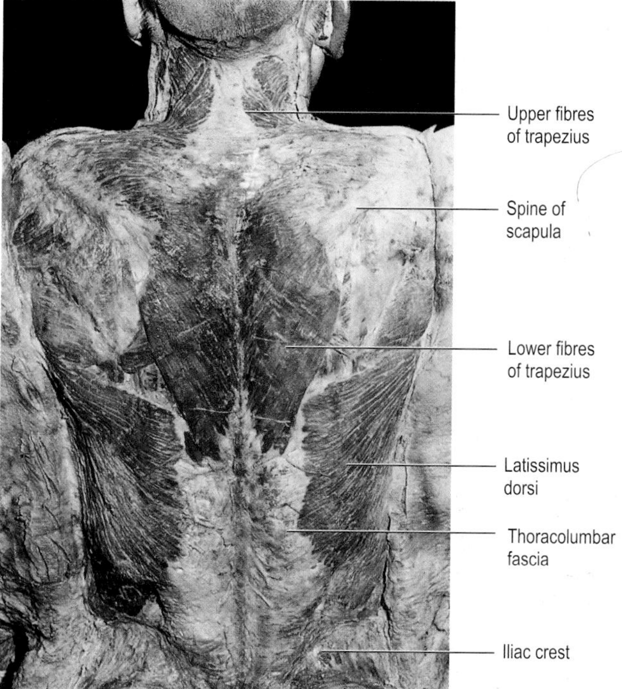


Fig. 2.10 Superficial muscles of the back.

ligamentum nuchae – fibroelastic tissue connecting the muscle to the spines of the cervical vertebrae, spinous processes of seventh cervical to twelfth thoracic vertebrae.

The upper fibres of the muscle are inserted to the lateral third of the clavicle, the middle fibres to the acromion, and the lower fibres to the spine of the scapula.

*Nerve supply* Spinal part of the accessory nerve.

*Actions* Assisted by the lower fibres of the serratus anterior the trapezius rotates the scapula so that the glenoid fossa faces upwards. This action is important for raising the arm above the level of the shoulder. The shoulder is elevated by the upper fibres (as in shrugging the shoulder). All fibres of the muscle help to retract the scapula. See Clinical box 2.2.

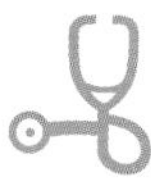

*Clinical box 2.2*

**Accessory nerve damage**

The accessory nerve supplying the trapezius can be easily damaged because of its superficial position in the posterior triangle (p. 189). This may happen during a careless biopsy (removal for histological examination) of lymph nodes in this region. The trapezius muscle will be paralysed resulting in inability to lift the arm above the level of the shoulder. The muscle can be tested by asking the patient to shrug the shoulder against resistance. The upper part of the muscle can be seen and felt as contracting on the side of the neck.

### Latissimus dorsi

This large superficial muscle is seen in the lower half of the back (Fig. 2.10). It wraps around the chest wall and as it comes to be inserted in the bicipital groove of the humerus, contributes to the posterior axillary fold.

*Nerve supply* The thoracodorsal nerve (C6, 7, 8) from the posterior cord of the brachial plexus. It is vulnerable in operations on the axilla.

*Actions* Extension, medial rotation and adduction of the shoulder (as in scratching the opposite scapular region). The muscle is used as a myocutaneous flap in reconstructive breast surgery.

*Test* Abduct the arm and adduct it against resistance. The muscle can be felt contracting in the posterior fold of the axilla.

## Structures deep to the trapezius

The levator scapulae and the two rhomboids lying deep to the trapezius are inserted on the medial border of the scapula (Fig. 2.11)

## Bones of the shoulder girdle

### Clavicle

The clavicle (Figs 2.12, 2.13) holds the upper limb away from the trunk and allows it to have a wide range of movements in the shoulder region. It is subcutaneous throughout and is easily palpable. It has two curves, the lateral third being concave forward and the medial two-thirds convex forward. Medially the clavicle articulates with the sternum at the

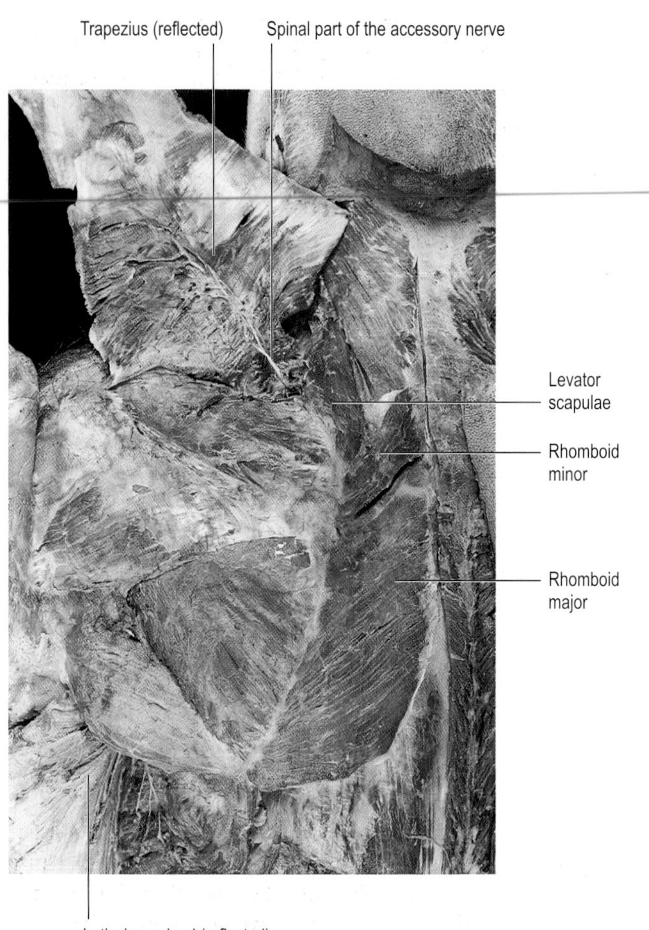


Fig. 2.11 Structures deep to the trapezius.

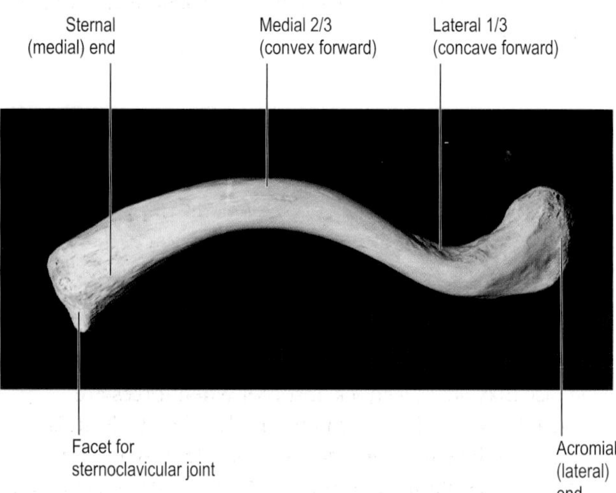


Fig. 2.12 Right clavicle viewed from above.

sternoclavicular joint and laterally with the acromion of the scapula at the acromioclavicular joint. The lateral end of the clavicle is held firmly on to the coracoid process by the strong coracoclavicular ligament attached to the conoid tubercle and the trapezoid ridge. Through this ligament the scapula, and hence the upper limb, is held suspended from the clavicle. Four major muscles of the shoulder region are attached to the clavicle, medially the pectoralis major and the clavicular head of the sternocleidomastoid and laterally the deltoid and the trapezius. The small subclavius muscle arising from the first rib is attached to the groove on the under surface. See Clinical box 2.3.

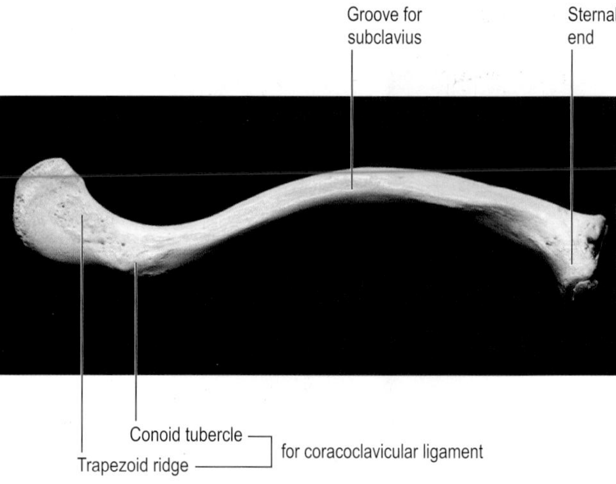


Fig. 2.13 Right clavicle viewed from below.

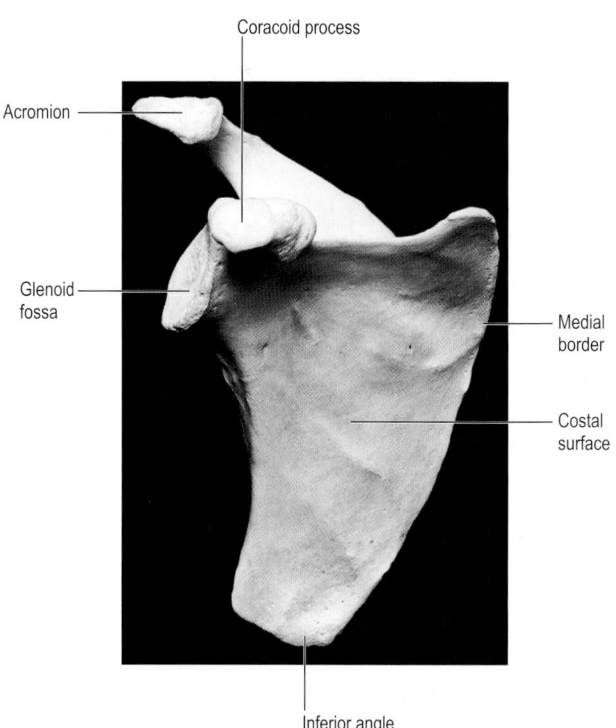


Fig. 2.14 Scapula anterior aspect.

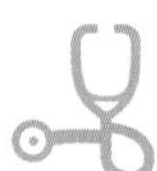

*Clinical box 2.3*

**Fracture of clavicle**

A fall on the shoulder or on the outstretched hand may break the clavicle. The middle of the shaft is the weakest point and is the commonest site of clavicular fractures. After a fracture the lateral fragment of the clavicle may get displaced downwards due to the weight of the upper limb. A fall on the outstretched hand can fracture the clavicle as the body weight is then transmitted through the clavicle to the sternum.

## Scapula – anterior aspect

The scapula (Fig. 2.14), whose mobility is essential to facilitate the wide range of movements of the shoulder, is rarely fractured as the bone is almost completely encased in muscles. From the anterior aspect of the scapula (the costal

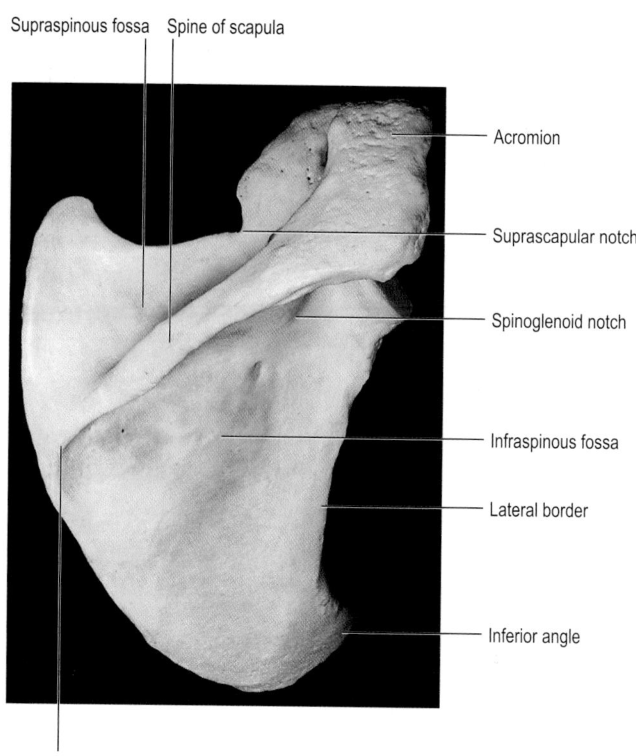


Fig. 2.15 Scapula posterior aspect.

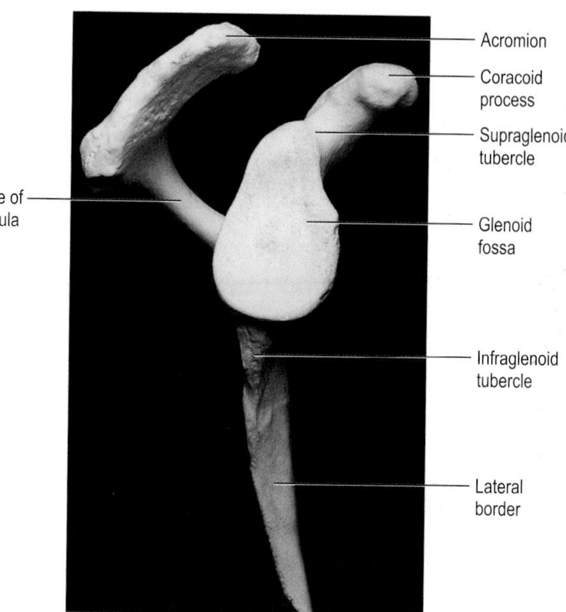


Fig. 2.16 Lateral view of scapula.

surface) which covers the thoracic cage the subscapularis muscle originates. The surface is marked by ridges for the attachment of fibrous septae of this multipennate muscle. The serratus anterior muscle which moves the scapula forward (protraction of scapula) is inserted on the medial margin on the costal surface. The glenoid fossa, seen at the lateral aspect in the upper part, faces forward as well as laterally. Above this is the acromion which is the uppermost bony point in the shoulder region. The coracoid process projecting anteriorly receives the attachments of three muscles, i.e. short head of biceps, coracobrachialis and the pectoralis minor. The coracoclavicular and the coracoacromial ligaments are also attached to the coracoid process.

### Scapula – posterior aspect

As seen in Figure 2.15 the lateral end of the spine projects forwards as the acromion. The medial end of the spine, the root of the spine, lies at the level of the spinous process of the third thoracic vertebra. The spine of scapula and the acromion are subcutaneous and are palpable. The trapezius and the deltoid are attached to the spine of the scapula and the acromion. The teres minor arises from the lateral border of the scapula, and the teres major from the inferior angle. The upper border of the scapula has the suprascapular notch near the root of the coracoid process. This lodges the suprascapular nerve. The notch is bridged by the supraspinous ligament which separates the suprascapular artery from the nerve, the nerve being deep to the artery. The nerve and the artery, after supplying the supraspinatus, enter the infraspinous fossa by passing through the spinoglenoid notch to supply the infraspinatus muscle.

### Scapula – lateral aspect

Figure 2.16 shows the glenoid fossa, the coracoid process and the acromion more fully. The shallow glenoid fossa or the glenoid cavity articulates with the head of humerus. Its upper end has the supraglenoid tubercle for the long head of the biceps. The infraglenoid tubercle is below its lower border. The glenoid fossa is lined by articular cartilage and is slightly deepened by the fibrocartilagenous glenoid labrum attached to its margins. The capsule of the shoulder joint is attached to the labrum and the surrounding bone. The origin of the long head of the biceps from the supraglenoid tubercle is within the capsule of the joint whereas the long head of the triceps arising from the infraglenoid tubercle is extracapsular.

## Joints of the shoulder girdle

### Sternoclavicular joint

This is a synovial joint between the medial end of the clavicle, the manubrium sternum and the first costal cartilage (Fig. 2.17). The joint is atypical in that unlike most synovial joints the articular cartilage covering the articular surfaces is fibrocartilage and not hyaline. Besides, the cavity is separated into two by a fibrocartilagenous articular disc. The disc may act as a shock absorber when forces are transmitted to the joint through the clavicle. The joint is surrounded by strong ligaments which stabilise it. The clavicle moves like a 'see-saw'. Elevation of the shoulder end (lateral end) of the clavicle makes the sternal end move downwards. Protraction (forward movement) of the shoulder end makes the sternal end move backwards.

### Acromioclavicular joint

This is a synovial joint between the lateral end of the clavicle and the medial border of the acromion. The sloping surfaces of the two bones, as seen in Figure 2.18, make the articulation weak. The clavicle will override the acromion when the joint is subluxated or dislocated. Like the sternoclavicular joint the articular surfaces are covered by fibrocartilage. There is also an incomplete fibrocartilagenous intra-articular disc. The gap between the two bones, as seen in the radiograph (Fig. 2.18), is mostly occupied by the disc.

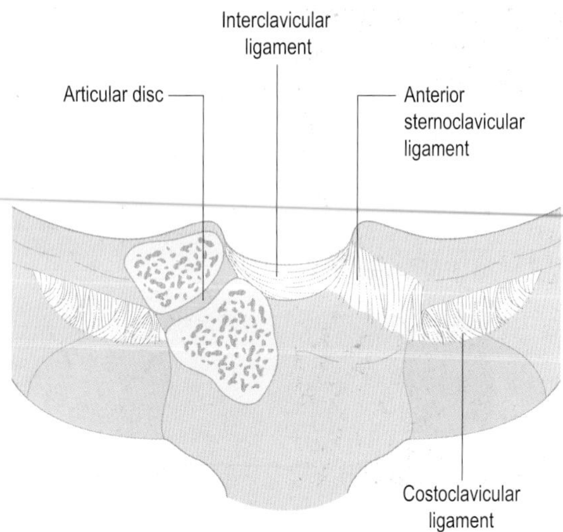


Fig. 2.17 The sternoclavicular joint. The right-hand side shows the interior.

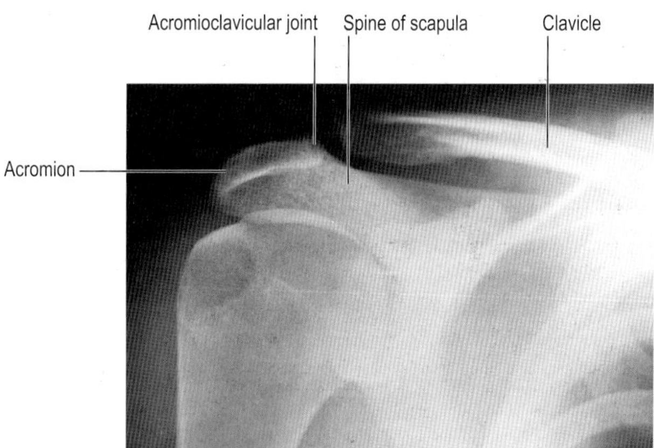


Fig. 2.18 Radiograph of the acromioclavicular joint.

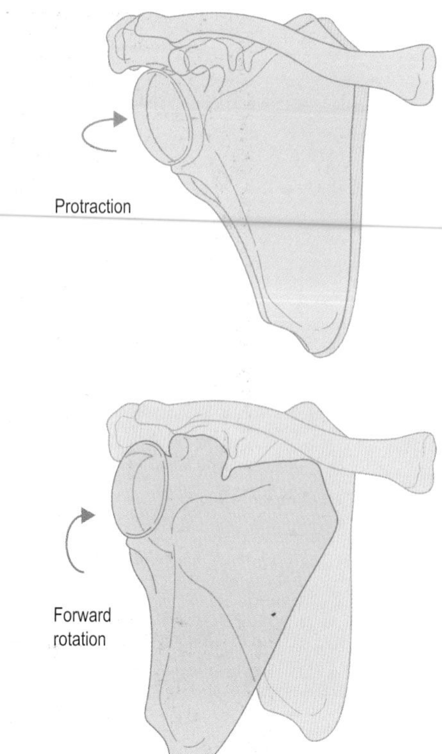


Fig. 2.19 Movements of the shoulder girdle.

## Movements of the pectoral girdle (scapula and clavicle)

Movements of the scapula make the coracoclavicular ligament taut and from then on the clavicle and the scapula move as a single unit at the sternoclavicular joint. Following are the movements of the shoulder girdle (Fig. 2.19):

| Movements | Muscles |
|---|---|
| Protraction — scapula moves forward hugging the chest wall | Serratus anterior<br>Pectoralis minor |
| Retraction — as in bracing the shoulder backwards | Trapezius<br>Rhomboids |
| Elevation (shrugging the shoulder) | Trapezius (upper fibres)<br>Levator scapulae |
| Depression | Serratus anterior<br>Pectoralis minor |
| Forward rotation of the scapula making the glenoid face upwards — a mechanism to increase the range of abduction of the shoulder | Trapezius<br>Lower fibres of the serratus anterior |

## The shoulder joint

The shoulder joint is completely surrounded by the massive deltoid muscle. Deep to the deltoid lies the supraspinatus,

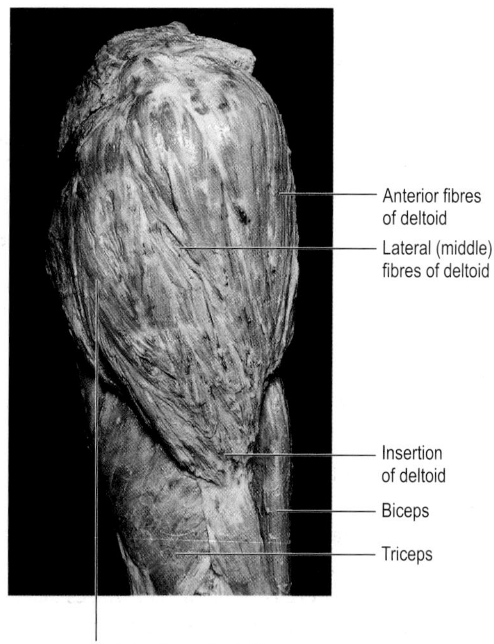


Fig. 2.20 Deltoid lateral view.

infraspinatus and teres minor and subscapularis, the four muscles connecting the various aspects of the scapula to the humerus. These reinforce the capsule of the shoulder joint and are collectively known as the rotator cuff muscles or SITS.

### Deltoid

See Figure 2.20.

*Origin* Lateral third of the clavicle, acromion and the spine of the scapula.

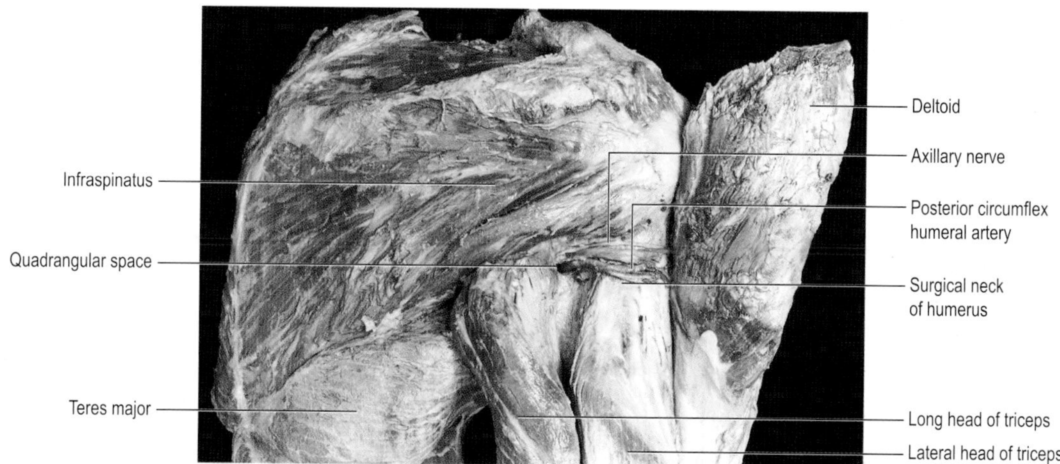


Fig. 2.21 Structures deep to the deltoid aspect.

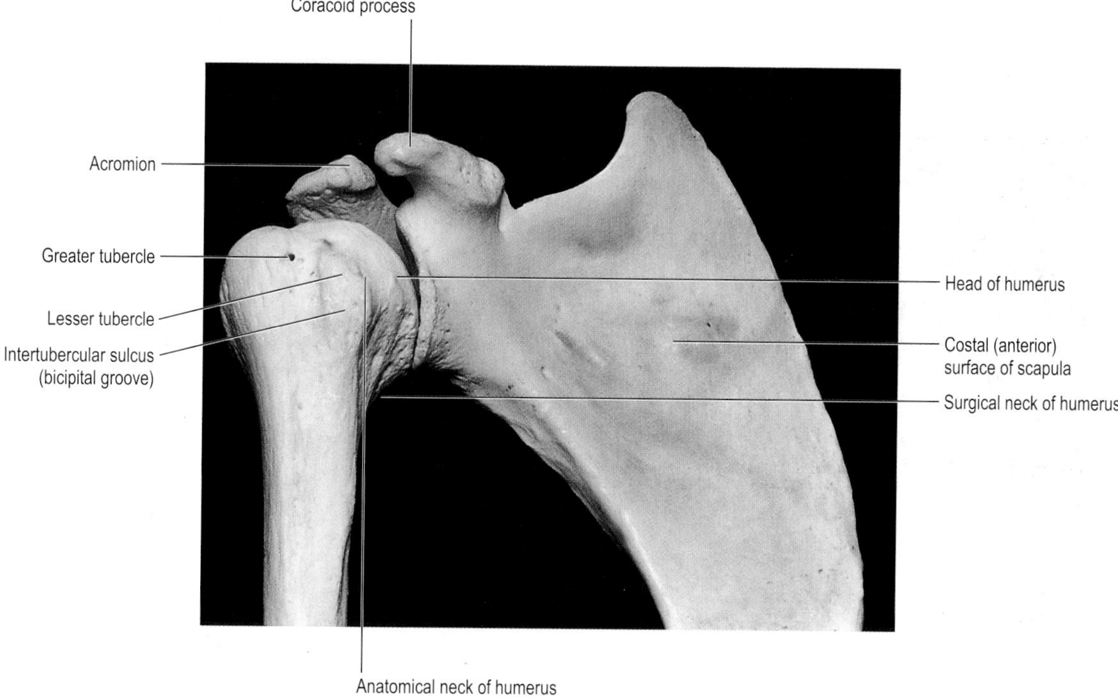


Fig. 2.22 Scapula and the upper end of the humerus – anterior view.

*Insertion* Deltoid tuberosity at the middle of the shaft of the humerus.

*Action* Anterior fibres help pectoralis major to flex the shoulder. Lateral fibres combine with the supraspinatus to abduct the shoulder, whereas the posterior fibres along with the latissimus dorsi and teres major extend the joint.

*Test* Hold the arm in the abducted position against resistance. Inability to do so suggests paralysis of the muscle.

*Nerve supply* Axillary nerve, a branch of the posterior cord of the brachial plexus, passes through the quadrangular space winding round the surgical neck of the humerus to enter the muscle (Fig. 2.21).

## Scapula and the upper end of humerus

The upper end of humerus shows the spherical head which articulates with the glenoid fossa and the greater and lesser tubercles which receive muscle attachments (Fig. 2.22). The area of the head of humerus is about four times larger than that of the shallow glenoid fossa, making the shoulder joint unstable but very mobile. The capsule of the joint is attached to the anatomical neck of humerus except in the lower part where it extends on to the surgical neck. The upper part of the greater tubercle receives the attachment of the supraspinatus. The subscapularis is inserted to the lesser tubercle. The intertubercular sulcus or the bicipital groove lodges the tendon of the long head of biceps arising from the supraglenoid tubercle. Three muscles are inserted in the region of the intertubercular sulcus; the pectoralis major to its lateral lip, teres major to the medial lip and the latissimus dorsi to its floor.

## Subscapularis and the anterior aspect of shoulder joint

Figure 2.23 shows the subscapularis arising from the costal surface of scapula, its insertion to the lesser tubercle of the humerus as well as the anterior aspect of the capsule of the shoulder joint. The short head of biceps and the coracobrachialis, both arising from the coracoid process are also related to the anterior aspect of the shoulder joint and cover the insertion of the subscapularis.

## Supraspinatus and the superior aspect of shoulder joint

The supraspinatus (Fig. 2.24) arising from the supraspinous fossa of scapula is related to the superior aspect of shoulder.

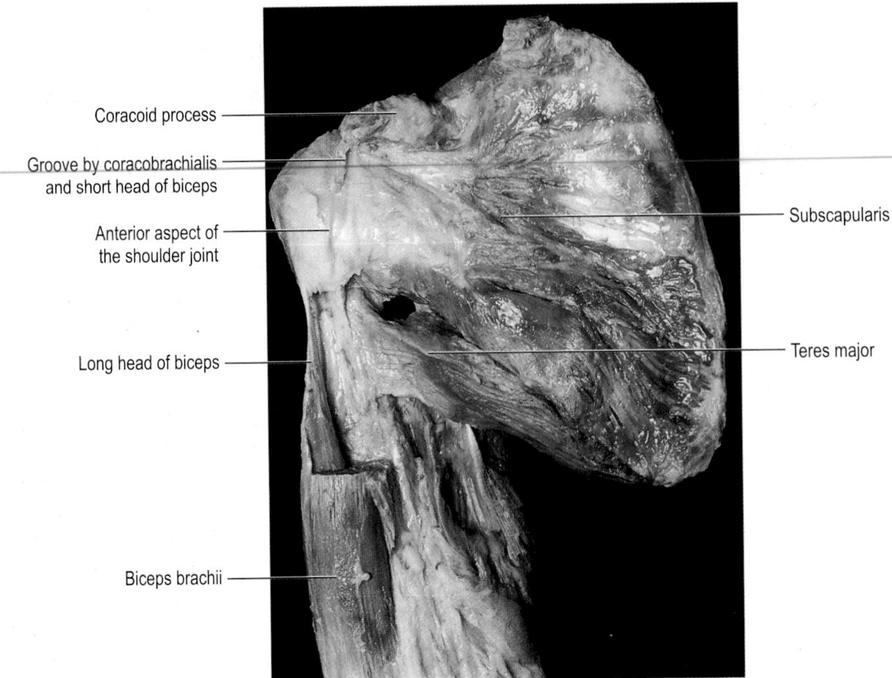


Fig. 2.23 Subscapularis and the anterior aspect of the shoulder joint.

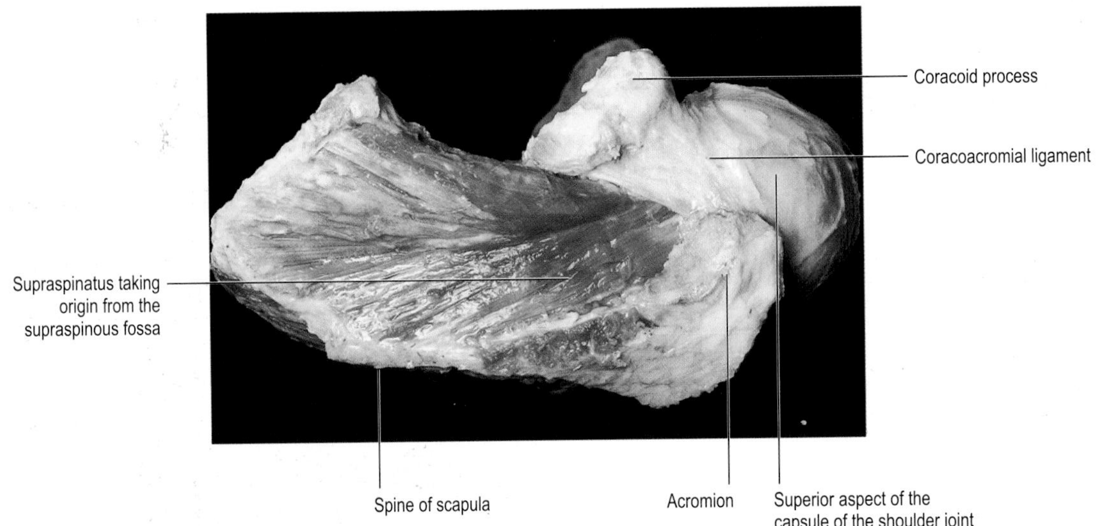


Fig. 2.24 Supraspinatus and the superior aspect of the shoulder joint.

The tendon of the muscle passes deep to the coracoacromial ligament to gain insertion to the greater tubercle and the superior aspect of the capsule of the shoulder joint. It is supplied by the suprascapular nerve. Besides stabilising the shoulder joint by reinforcing the capsule it assists the deltoid in abduction. The supraspinatus initiates abduction which is then continued by the deltoid. Together the two muscles abduct the shoulder up to about 120°. The subacromial bursa which is continuous with the subdeltoid bursa separates the tendon of the supraspinatus from the coracoacromial ligament. See Clinical box 2.4.

### Infraspinatus and the posterior aspect of shoulder joint

The features of the posterior aspect of the scapula and the upper end of the humerus are shown in Figure 2.25. The tendon of the infraspinatus arising from the infraspinous fossa lies across the posterior aspect of the shoulder joint to

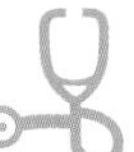

*Clinical box 2.4*

**Supraspinatus tendinitis**

Degenerative disorders causing supraspinatus tendinitis can lead on to subacromial bursitis, both conditions producing pain during abduction of the shoulder. Pain is worse as the arm traverses the arc between 60° and 120° (painful arc) when the impingement is maximal. This 'painful arc syndrome' can also be produced by osteoarthritis of the acromioclavicular joint, the formation of osteophytes or bony ridges on the anterior edge of the acromion and/or by inflammation of the subacromial bursa.

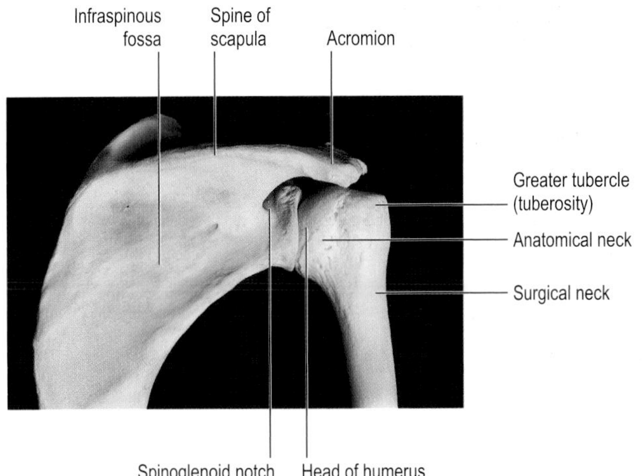


Fig. 2.25 Scapula and the upper end of humerus – posterior aspect.

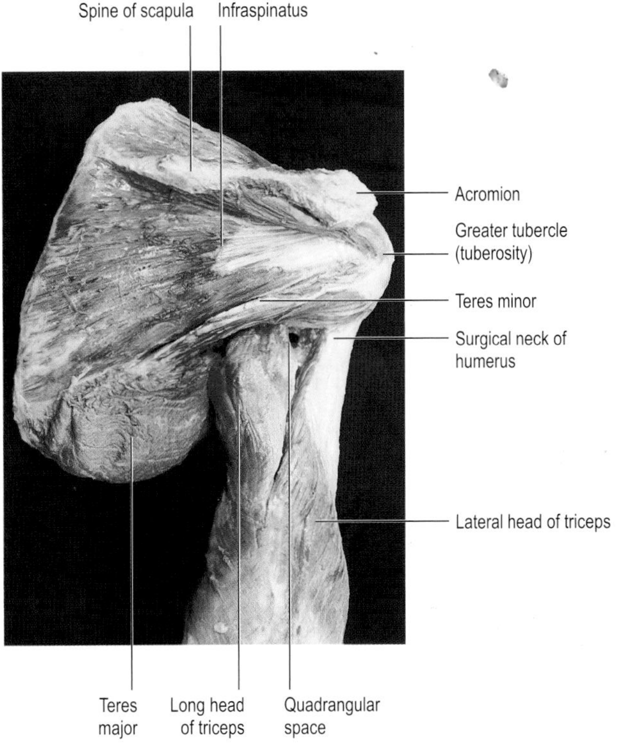


Fig. 2.26 Infraspinatus and the posterior aspect of the shoulder joint.

reach the posterior surface of the greater tubercle for its insertion (Fig. 2.26). The teres minor which is inserted on the greater tubercle below the infraspinatus arises from the lateral border of the scapula. The tendons of these two muscles along with those of the supraspinatus and the subscapularis fuse with the capsule of the shoulder joint. The rotator cuff thus formed by these four muscles is the main factor stabilising the shoulder joint. See Clinical box 2.5.

### The interior of the shoulder joint

The shoulder joint is a synovial joint of the ball and socket type where the head of the humerus articulates with the glenoid fossa of the scapula (Fig. 2.27). The area of the rounded head of the humerus is about four times larger than that of the shallow glenoid fossa. The humeral head and glenoid fossa are lined by articular cartilage (hyaline) and additionally the labrum glenoidale (fibrocartilage) forms a ring around the margin of the glenoid fossa (Fig. 2.27).

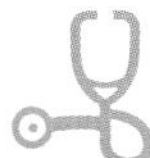

*Clinical box 2.5*

**Surgical exposure of the shoulder joint**

The surgical exposure to the anterior aspect of the shoulder can be done through the deltopectoral groove leading to detachment of the tip of the coracoid process with coracobrachialis and short head of the biceps. This will expose the anterior surface of the capsule covered by the subscapularis. The long head of biceps emerging from the capsule of the shoulder joint and the teres major inserting to the medial lip of the bicipital groove are also seen (Fig. 2.23).

For surgical exposure via a posterior approach the deltoid is detached to expose the infraspinatus and teres minor. These are cut to expose the capsule. Care is taken not to damage the branches of the axillary nerve and the accompanying posterior circumflex humeral artery which emerges through the quadrangular space to supply the deltoid. The space is bounded by the surgical neck of the humerus laterally, the long head of the triceps medially, teres minor above and teres major below (also see Fig. 2.21).

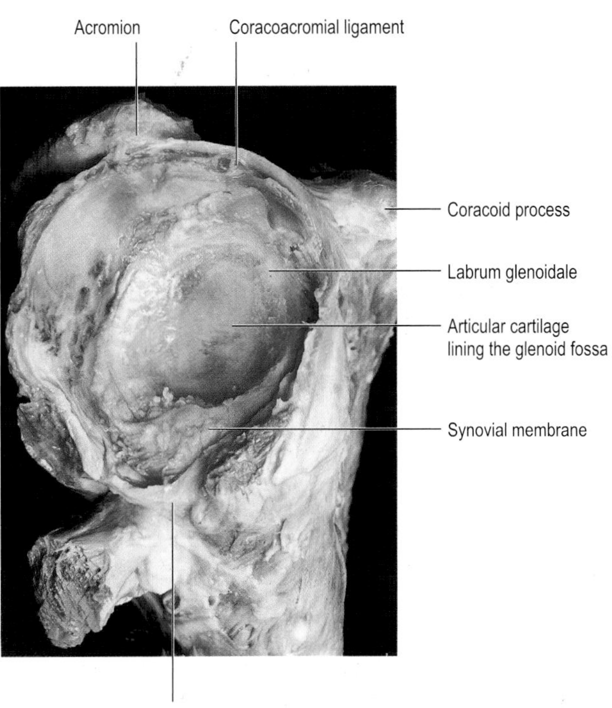


Fig. 2.27 Interior of the right shoulder joint – medial aspect.

The fibrous capsule is attached to the scapula beyond the labrum and to the humerus around its anatomical neck, except inferiorly, where its attachment is lower, into the surgical neck. The capsule is thin and loose, facilitating mobility at the expense of stability (Fig. 2.28).

The inner surface of the fibrous capsule and all intracapsular structures except the articular cartilage are lined by the synovial membrane. It herniates through the hole in the capsule to communicate with the subscapularis bursa. It may also communicate with the infraspinatus bursa. It forms a sleeve around the tendon of the long head of biceps which traverses the joint. A radiograph of the shoulder joint is shown in Figure 2.29.

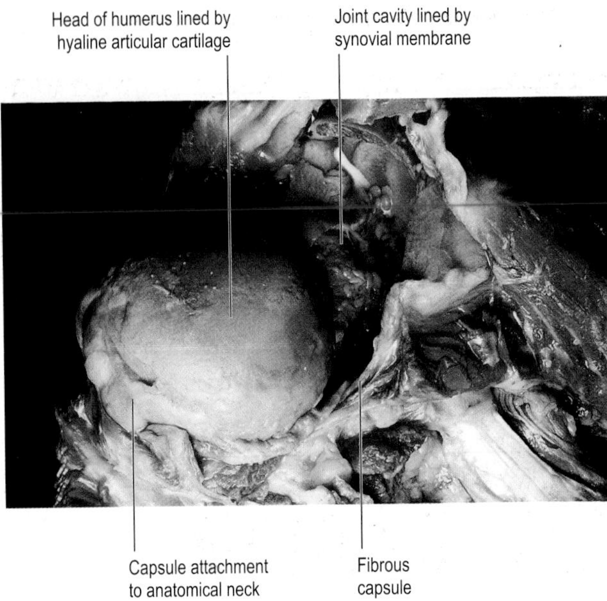


Fig. 2.28 Interior of the shoulder joint.

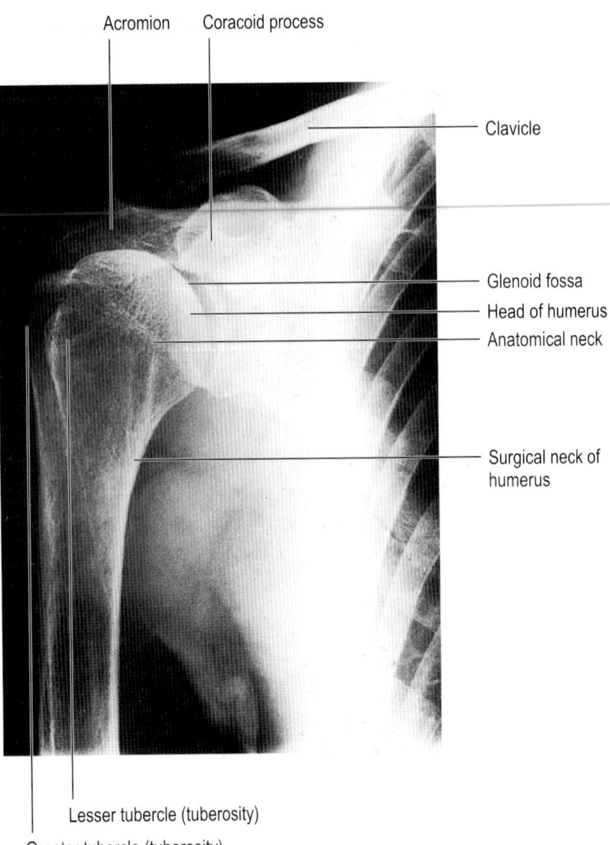


Fig. 2.29 Radiograph of the anteroposterior view of the shoulder.

### Movements of the shoulder joint

| Movement | Muscles |
|---|---|
| Abduction | Supraspinatus<br>Deltoid (lateral part) |
| Adduction | Pectoralis major (sternocostal head)<br>Teres major<br>Latissimus dorsi |
| Flexion | Pectoralis major (clavicular head)<br>Deltoid (anterior fibres) |
| Extension | Teres major<br>Deltoid (posterior fibres)<br>Latissimus dorsi |
| Medial rotation | Pectoralis major, teres major, subscapularis<br>Deltoid (anterior), latissimus dorsi |
| Lateral rotation | Infraspinatus, teres minor, deltoid (posterior) |

The wide-ranging movements of the shoulder are allowed by complex mechanisms. All the movements of the shoulder joint are accompanied by movements of the shoulder girdle. The first 30° of abduction mostly takes place in the shoulder joint. Subsequently the shoulder joint and the shoulder girdle move simultaneously. For every 15° of abduction 10° takes place in the shoulder joint and 5° in the shoulder girdle. The movement of the shoulder girdle is achieved by the contraction of the trapezius and the lower fibres of the serratus anterior facilitating forward rotation of the scapula to make the glenoid face upwards. If this is prevented (as in trapezius paralysis) the arm cannot be raised much above the level of the shoulder. The latter part of abduction of the shoulder is also accompanied by a lateral rotation of the humerus. See Clinical box 2.6.

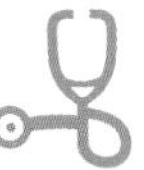

*Clinical box 2.6*

**Dislocation of the shoulder joint**

The wide range of movements at the shoulder is achieved at the expense of its stability. It is the most commonly dislocated major joint. As its inferior aspect is not reinforced by muscle, in violent abduction the head of the humerus tears that part of the capsule and dislocates to lie in the subglenoid region, from where it gets displaced anteriorly to lie in the subcoracoid position. Hence the condition is known as anterior or subcoracoid dislocation. The axillary nerve which lies close to the inferior aspect of the joint may be damaged in this injury (Clinical Box 2.8 p. 20).

## Axilla

The axilla (Figs 2.30, 2.31) is the space between the trunk and the upper arm. It is pyramidal in shape and its boundaries are:

- anterior wall – pectoralis major and the pectoralis minor muscles
- posterior wall – subscapularis, teres major and the latissimus dorsi muscles
- lateral wall – upper end of the humerus with the biceps brachii and the coracobrachialis muscles
- medial wall – the serratus anterior muscle covering the ribs and intercostal spaces
- apex – formed by the first rib medially with the clavicle in front and the scapula behind (it is the channel of communication between the posterior triangle and the axilla)
- base – skin and deep fascia extending between the chest wall and the arm.

The walls of the axilla are illustrated in Figs 2.30 and 2.31.

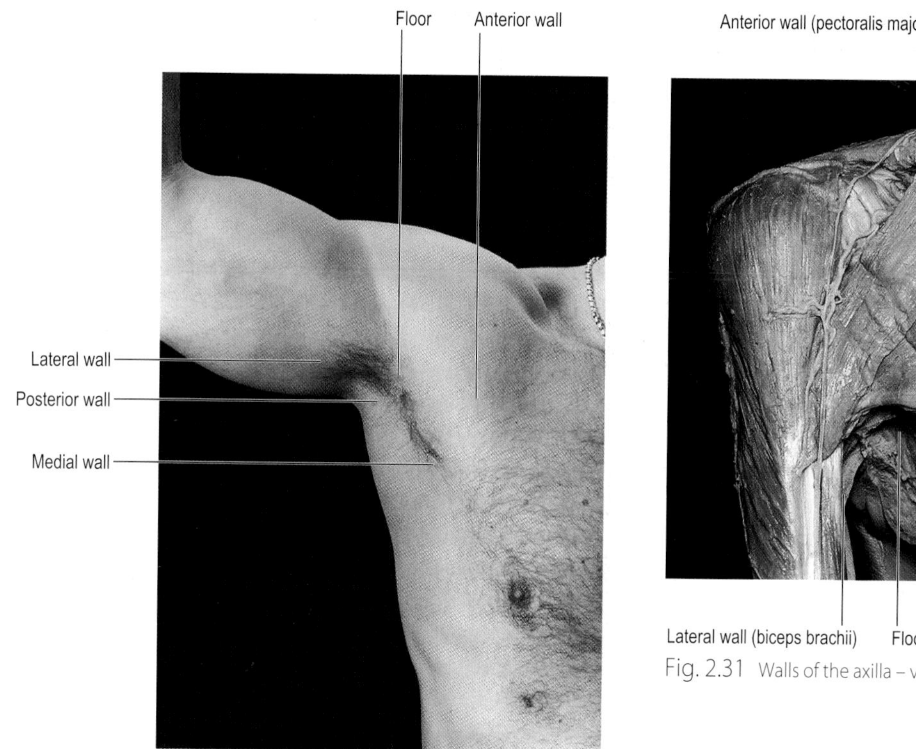


Fig. 2.30 Walls of the axilla – surface anatomy.

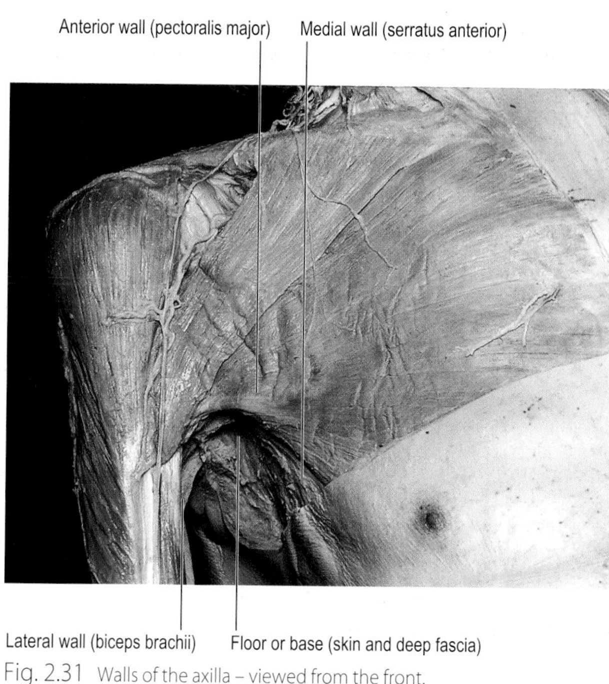


Fig. 2.31 Walls of the axilla – viewed from the front.



Fig. 2.32 The structures related to the axillary artery.

The axilla contains:

- fat and lymph nodes
- axillary artery and vein
- brachial plexus.

## Axillary artery

The axillary artery (Fig. 2.32) is a continuation of the subclavian artery and it extends from the outer border of the first rib to the lower border of the teres major, from where it continues as the brachial artery. For descriptive purposes it can be divided into three parts by the pectoralis minor. The part above the muscle is the first part, the part underneath is the second with the part below being the third part. The three cords of the brachial plexus are arranged around the second part of the artery.

The axillary vein is medial to the artery separated from it for most of its course by the medial cord and its branches. Branches of the axillary artery are:

- First part
  - superior thoracic artery

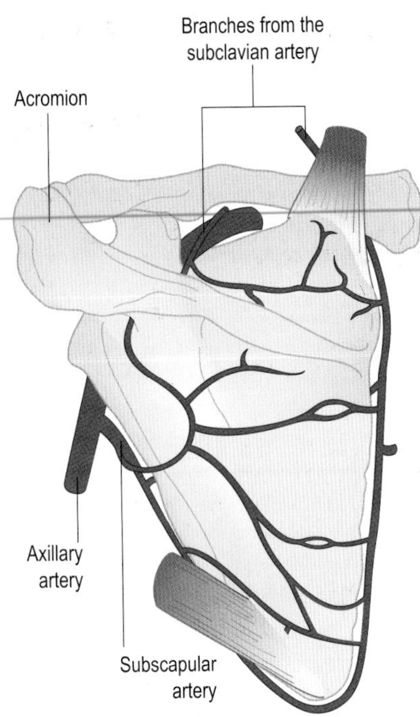


Fig. 2.33 Arterial anastomoses over the scapula.

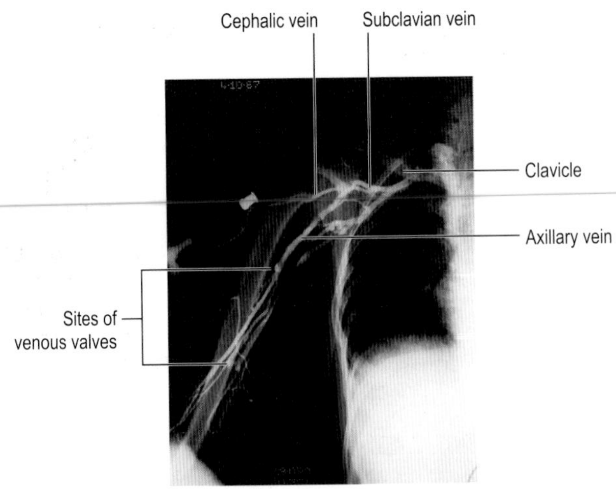


Fig. 2.34 Axillary venogram.

- Second part
  - acromiothoracic
  - lateral thoracic
- Third part
  - posterior circumflex humeral
  - anterior circumflex humeral
  - subscapular.

✪ Branches of the axillary artery anastomose with those of the subclavian around the scapula (Fig. 2.33), which may be an important collateral channel in case of obstruction to the distal part of the subclavian artery.

### Surface marking of the artery

Draw a line from the middle of the clavicle to the groove behind the coracobrachialis. Pulsation of the artery can be felt by deep palpation of the axilla after abducting the arm.

### ✪ Surgical exposure

The first part of the artery lies deep to the clavicular head of the pectoralis major and can be exposed by splitting the muscle fibre and incising the clavipectoral fascia which connects the upper border of the pectoralis minor to the clavicle.

## Axillary vein

This vein commences at the lower border of the teres major as a continuation of the basilic vein and it continues into the neck as the subclavian vein in front of the scalenus anterior muscle. The venae comitantes of the brachial artery join it near its commencement. As seen in Figure 2.34, the cephalic vein drains into it in its upper part. The lateral thoracic vein, which is a tributary of the axillary vein, is connected to the tributaries of the great saphenous vein of the lower limb. These connecting veins on the side of the chest wall enlarge in inferior vena caval obstruction.

## Brachial plexus

The brachial plexus, branches of which innervate the upper limb, is illustrated in Figure 2.35. The nerves and vessels of the axilla are shown in Figure 2.36. The brachial plexus is described as having:

### Roots

Anterior rami of C5–T1 spinal nerves.

### Trunks

The upper trunk formed of roots from C5 and C6, the middle trunk by C7 and the lower trunk by union of roots from C8 and T1.

### Divisions

Each trunk divides into anterior and posterior divisions.

### Cords

The anterior divisions of upper and middle trunks join to form the lateral cord, the anterior division of the lower trunk continues as the medial cord and the posterior divisions of all the three trunks join together to form the posterior cord.

### Branches

- Medial cord:
  - ulnar nerve
  - medial pectoral nerve
  - medial root of the median nerve
  - medial cutaneous nerve of the forearm
  - medial cutaneous nerve of the arm
- Lateral cord:
  - lateral pectoral nerve
  - lateral root of the median nerve
  - musculocutaneous nerve
- Posterior cord (see Fig. 2.37):
  - subscapular nerves
  - axillary nerve
  - thoracodorsal nerve
  - radial nerve.

The clinical importance of the brachial plexus is outlined in Clinical boxes 2.7, 2.8 and 2.9.

## Lymph nodes of the axilla

The lymph nodes in the axilla (Fig. 2.39) are of tremendous clinical importance as they drain the mammary gland (p. 228). There are about 20–30 lymph nodes scattered in the fibro-fatty tissue.

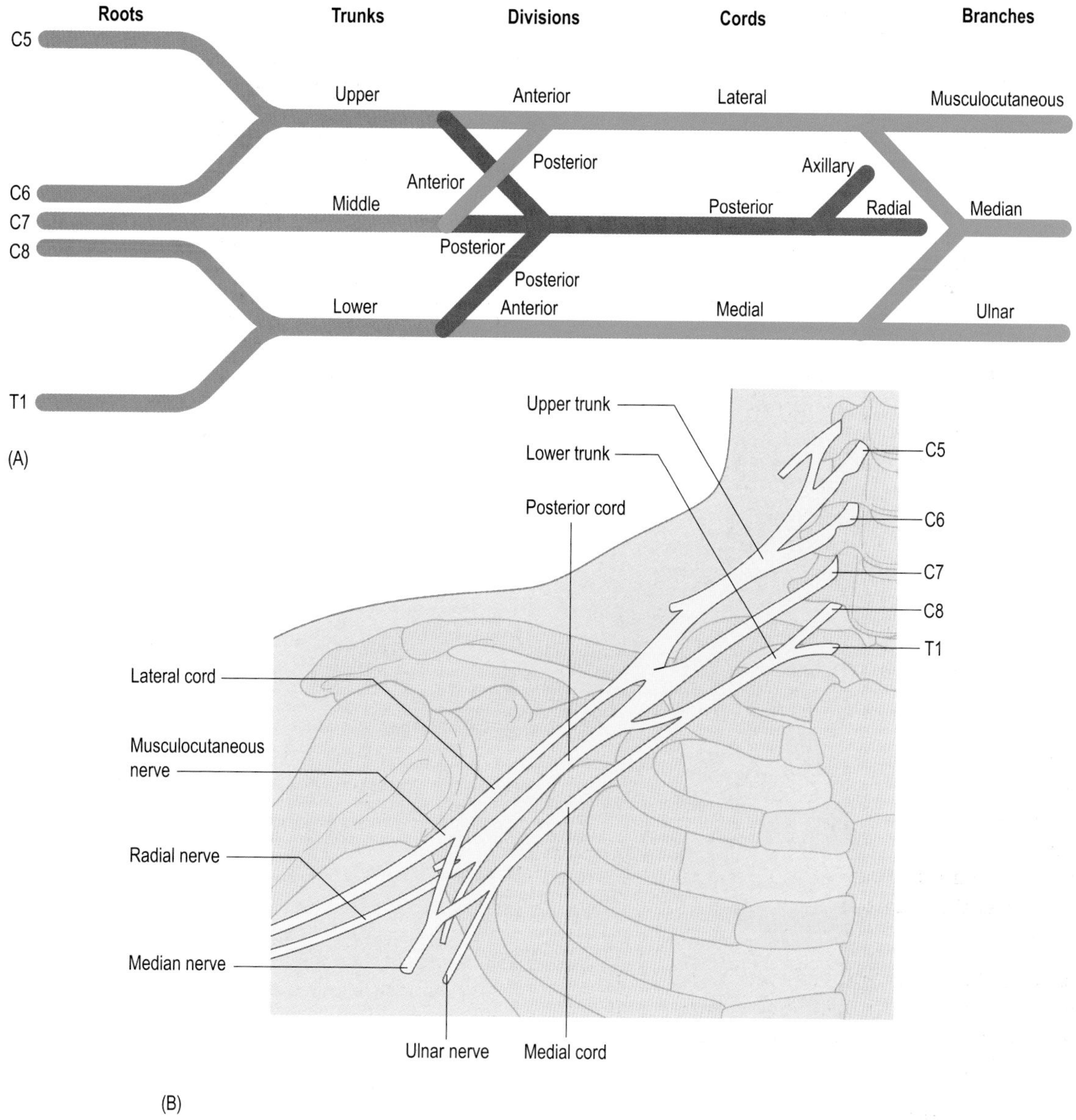

Roots
Trunks
Divisions
Cords
Branches
C5
Upper
Anterior
Lateral
Musculocutaneous
Posterior
Axillary
Anterior
C6
Middle
C7
Posterior
Radial
Median
C8
Posterior
Posterior
Lower
Anterior
Medial
Ulnar
T1
(A)
Upper trunk
Lower trunk
Posterior cord
C5
C6
C7
C8
T1
Lateral cord
Musculocutaneous nerve
Radial nerve
Median nerve
Ulnar nerve
Medial cord
(B)

Fig. 2.35 (A) Simplified schematic of the brachial plexus. (B) The brachial plexus.

Trunks of the brachial plexus
Subclavian artery
Scalenus anterior
Subclavian vein
Lateral root of median nerve
Medial root of median nerve
Musculocutaneous nerve
Median nerve
Axillary artery
Axillary vein
Thoracodorsal nerve
Intercostobrachial nerve
Latissimus dorsi
Long thoracic nerve
Serratus anterior

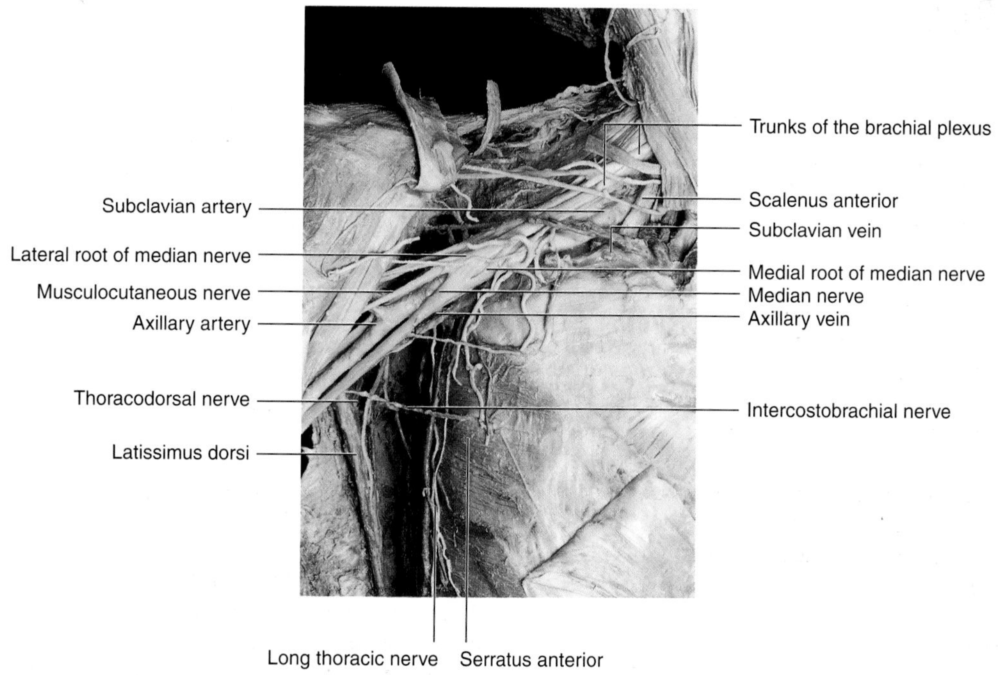

Fig. 2.36 Nerves and vessels of the axilla.

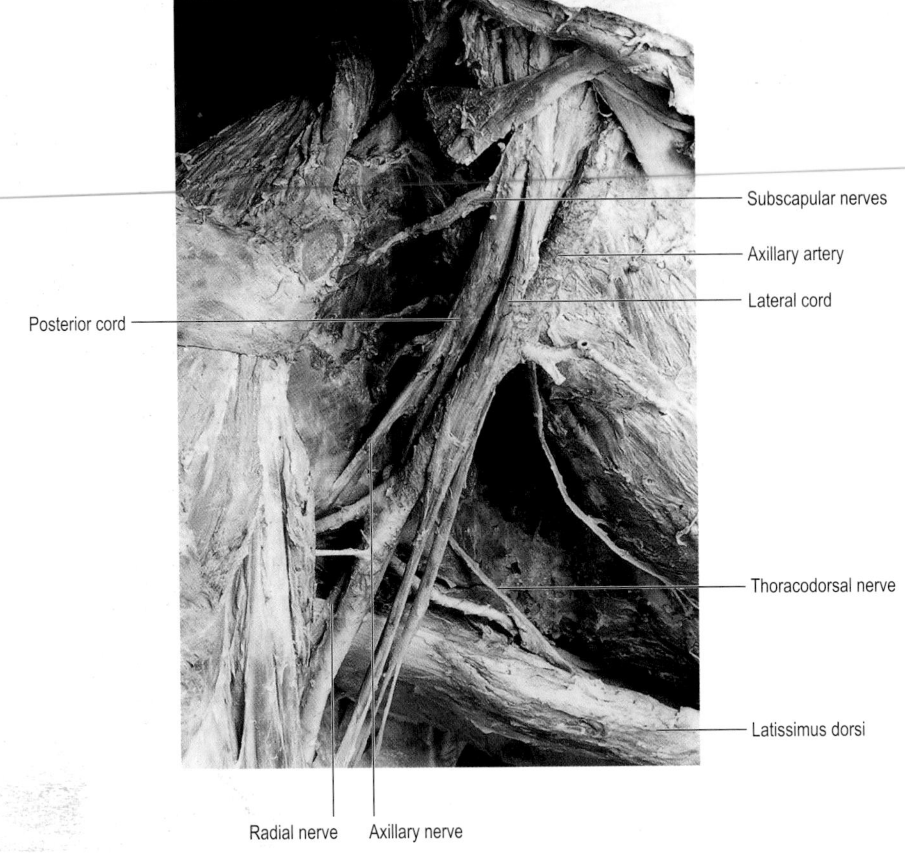


Fig. 2.37 Posterior cord branches (axillary artery and the lateral and medial cords are displaced medially).

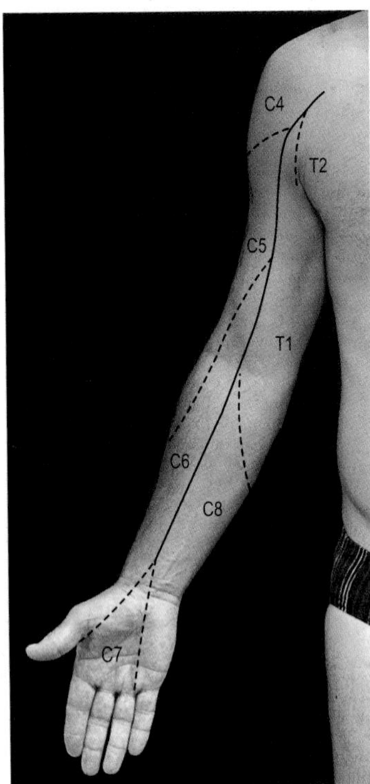


Fig. 2.38 Dermatomes of the upper limb. Continuous line represents the axial line across which there is no overlap. However there is considerable overlap across the interrupted lines which demarcate adjoining dermatomes.

- Anterior or pectoral group: lies along the lateral thoracic artery at the lower border of the pectoralis minor.
- Posterior or subscapular group: lies along the posterior wall of the axilla in its posterior part related to the subscapular artery.

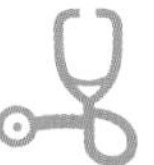

*Clinical box 2.7*

**Nerves vulnerable in axillary clearance**

The intercostobrachial nerve, which is a branch of the second intercostal nerve, supplies a small area of skin of the medial aspect of the arm. This is the only nerve supplying the upper limb without passing through the brachial plexus. This nerve and the long thoracic nerve and the thoracodorsal nerve supplying the latissimus dorsi are vulnerable in 'axillary clearance', a surgical dissection to remove the axillary lymph nodes, in the treatment of carcinoma of the breast.

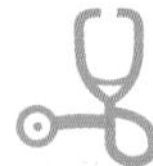

*Clinical box 2.8*

**Nerve vulnerable in shoulder dislocation**

The axillary nerve leaves the axilla winding round the surgical neck of the humerus, passing below the shoulder joint. It is accompanied by the posterior circumflex humeral branch of the axillary artery (see Fig. 2.21). The nerve can be damaged in dislocation of the shoulder as well as in fracture of the surgical neck of the humerus. Damage to the axillary nerve will cause atrophy of the deltoid and flattening of the contour of the shoulder. In shoulder dislocation the skin over the region of insertion of the deltoid ('regimental badge area') is tested for sensation as the cutaneous nerve supply here is solely derived from the axillary nerve.

## *Clinical box 2.9*

### Segmental innervation of the upper limb

Knowledge of the dermatomes (segmental innervation of the skin) and myotomes (segmental innervation of muscles) are important for testing for nerve root compression and assessing the level of spinal cord injuries (Fig. 2.38). The dermatomes of the upper segments of the brachial plexus (C5, C6) are on the lateral aspect, the lower segments (C8, T1) on the medial aspect and C7 in the middle. There is considerable overlap across adjoining dermatomes. However there is no overlap across the axial line as it separates discontinuous segments.

The pattern of the myotomes is more complex. There is a proximal to distal gradient as the C5 supplies the shoulder and T1 the intrinsic muscles of the hand. The flexors of the elbow are by C5 and C6, whereas C7 and C8 supply the extensors (triceps). The biceps tendon jerk therefore tests C5, C6 segments and the triceps jerk C7, C8.

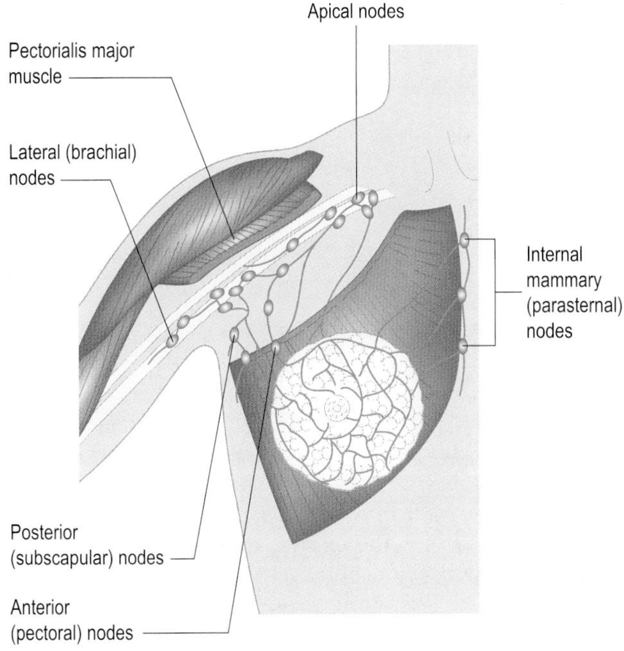


Fig. 2.39 The axillary lymph nodes and the lymphatic drainage of the breast.

- Lateral group: lies on the lateral wall of the axilla along the axillary vein.
- Central group: lies in the fat of the axilla and receives afferent vessels from the above groups.
- Apical group: lies in the apex of the axilla. The apical nodes are also connected to the supraclavicular or lower deep cervical lymph nodes (of the neck).

Axillary lymph nodes can also be grouped in terms of the levels at which they lie. This is more useful in staging the spread of malignancy from the breast. Level I nodes lie lateral to the lower border of the pectoralis minor, level II nodes lie behind the muscle, whereas level III are medial to it.

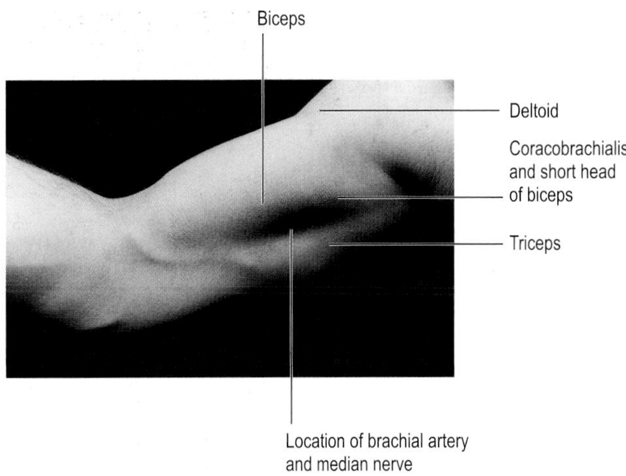


Fig. 2.40 Surface anatomy of the front of arm.

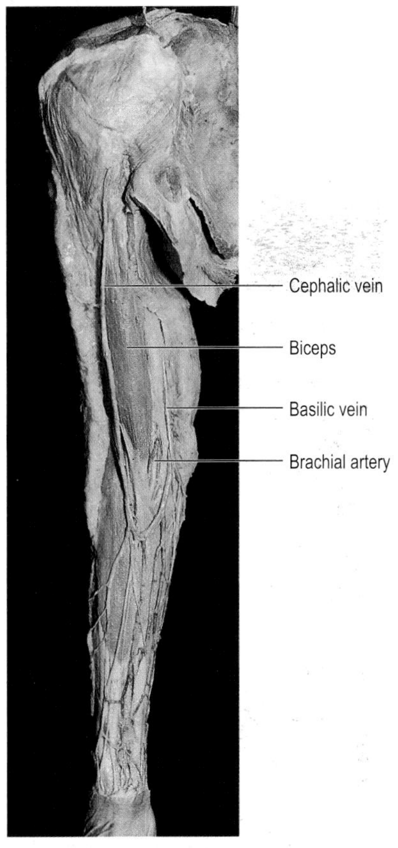


Fig. 2.41 Superficial veins of the arm.

## Anterior aspect of the arm

See Clinical box 2.10.

### The superficial veins of the arm

The upper limb is drained by two sets of veins, superficial and deep. The superficial veins (Fig. 2.41) lie superficial to the deep fascia and are clinically important as they are frequently used for cannulation. The deep veins accompany the arteries as venae comitantes until the middle of the arm where the axillary vein is formed. The cephalic and the basilic are the two major superficial veins. Both are formed in the dorsal venous arch at the back of the hand. In the arm the cephalic vein lies on the lateral border of the biceps and

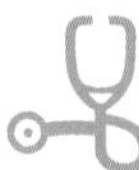

## Clinical box 2.10

**Surface anatomy of the front of arm**

The medial border of the biceps is known as the danger zone of the arm as it is related to the brachial artery and its venae comitantes and the median nerve (Fig. 2.40). Surgical exposure of the humerus is preferably done by incisions along the lateral border of the muscle to avoid cutting the artery and the nerve. Brachial artery pulsation is felt by palpating the artery against the humerus. The upper part of the medial border of the biceps has the coracobrachialis along with its short head. The musculocutaneous nerve enters the coracobrachialis at this level and can be blocked by intramuscular injection of local anaesthetic agents in this area. The median nerve along with the axillary artery lies in the groove behind the coracobrachialis. Laterally the prominent deltoid is easily visible and it can be seen tapering to its insertion on the deltoid tuberosity at the middle of the humerus.

ascends to the shoulder region to reach the deltopectoral groove where it pierces the deep fascia to join the axillary vein. The basilic vein lies along the medial border of the biceps up to the middle of the arm where it pierces the deep fascia to join the venae comitantes of the brachial artery to become the axillary vein.

### Biceps brachii

See Figure 2.42.

*Origin*

- Short head – coracoid process.
- Long head – supraglenoid tubercle of the scapula. The tendon of the long head, lined by synovial sheath, passes through the shoulder joint to enter the bicipital groove of the upper part of the humerus.

*Insertion* Tendon of biceps – posterior aspect of the radial tuberosity (p. 27). In the cubital fossa the tendon gives off a medial expansion, the bicipital aponeurosis, which merges with the deep fascia to be inserted to the subcutaneous border of the upper end of the ulna.

*Action* The biceps is a powerful flexor of the elbow and a supinator of the forearm. The tendon of the long head may contribute to the stability of the shoulder as it runs over the head of the humerus. It is a weak flexor of the shoulder.

*Test* Flex the supinated forearm against resistance, the biceps can be seen and felt as contracting.

#### ✪ Rupture of the long head of biceps

This can happen spontaneously, often while lifting a heavy weight. The patient will have a painful arm. If the forearm is flexed the detached head will be visible as a prominent lump in the lower part of the arm.

### Brachialis

Brachialis (Fig. 2.43) takes origin from the anterior surface of the lower half of the humerus. It covers the anterior surface of the elbow joint before getting inserted to the coronoid process of the ulna. The muscle is supplied by the musculocutaneous nerve. The lateral half is also supplied by the radial nerve. The radial nerve emerges between its lower part and the brachioradialis. It is a flexor of the elbow joint.

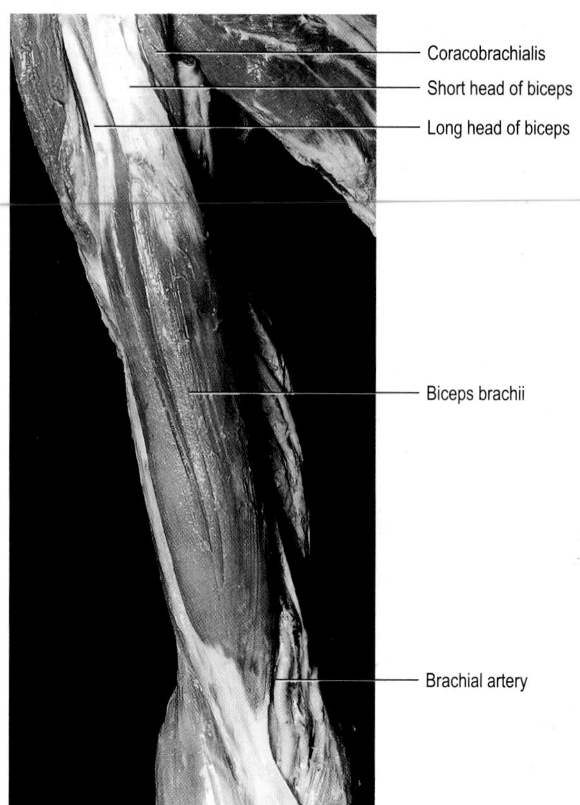


Fig. 2.42 Biceps brachii.

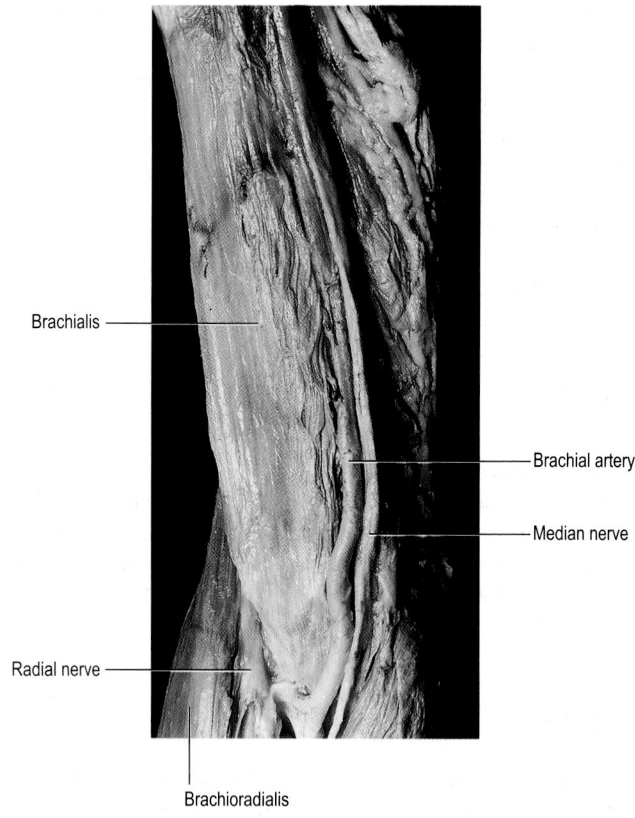


Fig. 2.43 Brachialis (after removal of biceps).

### Nerves and vessels of the front of arm

The nerves and vessels in the anterior aspect of the arm can be seen in Figure 2.44.

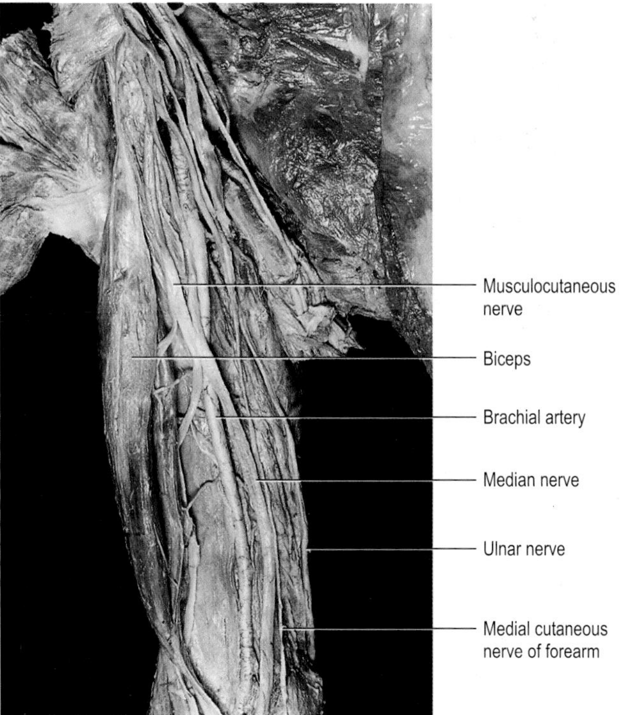


Fig. 2.44 Nerves and vessels of the front of arm (biceps is displaced laterally).

### Brachial artery

The brachial artery, which is the continuation of the axillary artery, terminates in the cubital fossa by dividing into the radial and ulnar arteries. The profunda brachii accompanying the radial nerve is one of its major branches.

✪ The lower part of the brachial artery can be damaged in supracondylar fractures of the humerus especially in children. Intense spasm of the artery may lead to Volkmann's ischaemic contracture (ischaemic damage and fibrosis of the forearm muscles).

### The musculocutaneous nerve (C5, 6, 7)

This is a branch of the lateral cord of the brachial plexus. The nerve, after supplying the coracobrachialis, biceps and brachialis, continues as the lateral cutaneous nerve of the forearm.

### Median nerve

This nerve is formed by contributions from the lateral and medial cords. In the upper part the nerve is lateral to the brachial artery but crosses anterior to the artery to its medial side at the middle of the arm as it descends. It gives off no branch in the arm.

## Posterior compartment of the arm

The posterior compartment of the arm contains the triceps muscle through which runs the radial nerve accompanied by the profunda brachii artery. The ulnar nerve lies in the lower part closely behind the medial epicondyle.

### Triceps

The origins of the triceps (Figs 2.45, 2.46) are as follows:

- long head from the infraglenoid tubercle of the scapula
- lateral head from the back of the humerus above the groove for the radial nerve

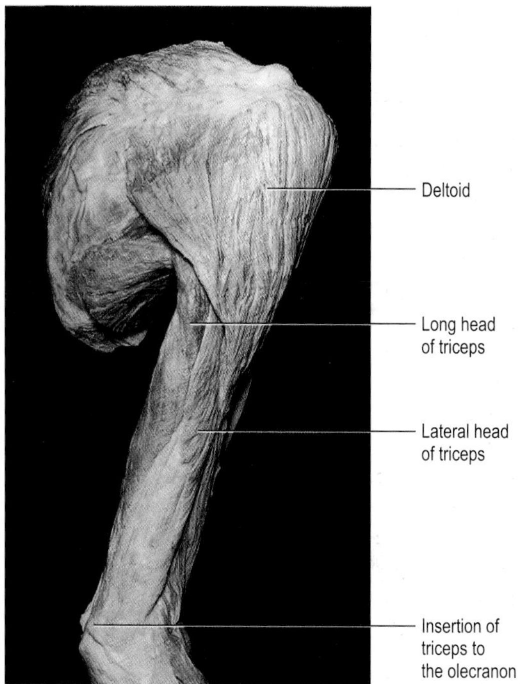


Fig. 2.45 The triceps and the deltoid viewed from the back.

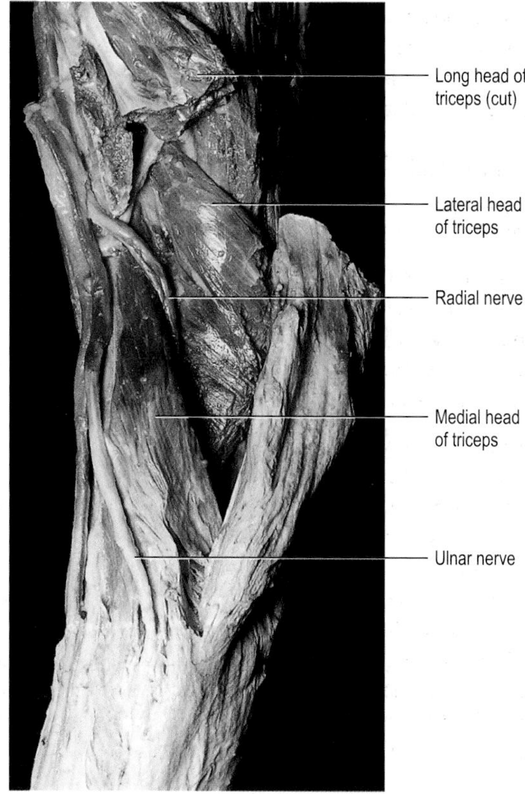


Fig. 2.46 The triceps viewed from the medial aspect.

- medial head from the back of the humerus below the groove for the radial nerve.

The muscle has a tendon lower down which is inserted to the upper surface of the olecranon of the ulna.

### Nerve supply

The long and medial heads of the triceps are supplied by branches from the radial nerve given off in the axilla

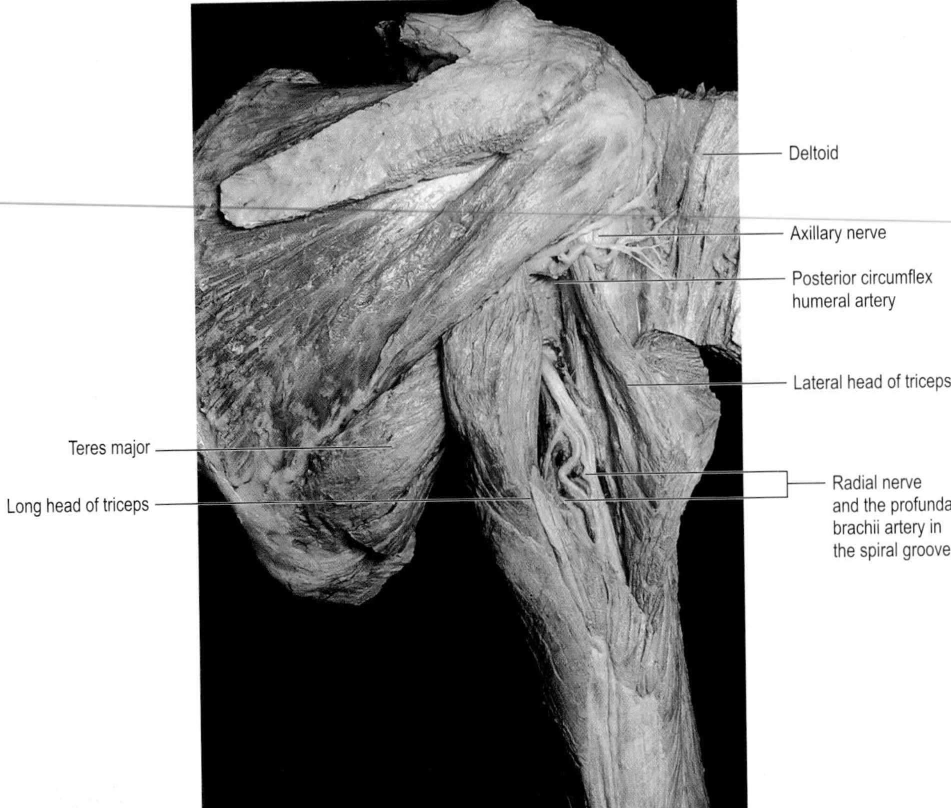


Fig. 2.47 Nerves and vessels in the posterior aspect of arm.

(Fig. 2.47). A branch to the lateral head and an additional branch to the medial head are given off from the radial nerve in the spiral (radial) groove of the humerus.

✪ Fractures of the middle of the shaft of the humerus damaging the radial nerve will not paralyse the triceps as it is supplied by branches given off in the axilla.

### Radial nerve

The radial nerve, which is almost the continuation of the posterior cord, passes obliquely down from medial to lateral closely related to the posterior surface of the shaft of the humerus lying in the groove for the radial nerve (spiral groove). The nerve then pierces the lateral intermuscular septum to enter the anterior compartment where it lies between the brachialis and brachioradialis. Just above the elbow the radial nerve gives off branches to the brachioradialis, extensor carpi radialis longus and lateral half of the brachialis. In front of the lateral epicondyle it divides into its two terminal branches, the superficial radial branch and the deep branch, also known as the posterior interosseous nerve. See Clinical box 2.11.

✪ *Surface marking of the radial nerve*

This can be marked by drawing a line from the junction of the posterior wall of the axilla and arm obliquely downwards along the back of the arm to the junction of the lower and middle third of its lateral surface and from there to the front of the lateral epicondyle. It can be blocked by local anaesthetic agents by inserting the needle medial to the brachioradialis (see p. 26) to hit the lateral epicondyle. Injection of the drug after withdrawing the needle slightly will block the nerve as it lies in front of the lateral epicondyle.

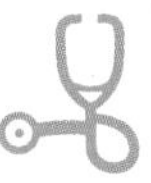

*Clinical box 2.11*

**Wrist drop**

Paralysis of the radial nerve above the elbow will paralyse all the extensors of the wrist. The flexors of the wrist will overact and the wrist will adopt a flexed position, a condition known as wrist drop. Gripping with the hand is impossible in the flexed position of the wrist.

### Ulnar nerve

This nerve from the medial cord of the brachial plexus as it descends pierces the medial intermuscular septum to enter the posterior compartment. At the elbow the nerve lies in the groove behind the medial epicondyle where it is palpable. It gives off no branch in the arm. See Clinical box 2.12.

## Anatomy of the forearm

### The cubital fossa

The cubital fossa is a triangular area in front of the elbow and contains the brachial artery, median nerve, radial nerve as well as superficial veins. Superficial veins here are often used for intravenous injections. Such injections can inadvertently be made into the brachial artery or the median nerve which are closely related to the veins, resulting in disastrous consequences.

### Surface anatomy

Superficial veins (Fig. 2.48) are made visible by compressing the arm and occluding the venous return. The tendon of the

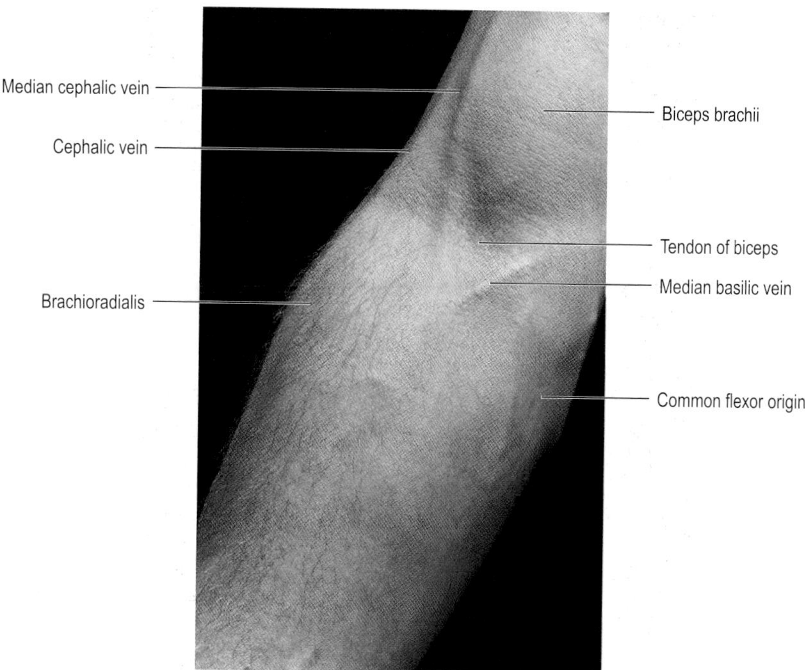


Fig. 2.48 Cubital fossa – surface anatomy.

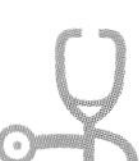

## Clinical box 2.12

### Nerves closely related to the humerus

Three nerves are closely related to the humerus and hence are vulnerable. The axillary nerve accompanied by the posterior circumflex humeral artery, related to the surgical neck of the humerus (Fig. 2.21), can be damaged by a fracture of the surgical neck or by dislocation of the shoulder joint. The radial nerve and the accompanying profunda brachii, lying in the spiral groove (Fig. 2.47), may be damaged in fractures of the middle of the shaft of the humerus. The ulnar nerve lying behind the medial epicondyle (Fig. 2.95) can be lacerated by a fracture of the epicondyle or compressed against the bone by external pressure.

biceps is easily felt in the middle of the fossa as it reaches its insertion on the radial tuberosity. The bicipital aponeurosis which separates the superficial veins from the brachial artery and the median nerve is palpated by flexing and supinating the forearm against resistance.

Pulsation of the brachial artery is felt medial to the biceps tendon. The median nerve lies medial to the artery. The brachioradialis is visible and can be felt contracting if the forearm is flexed against resistance in the midprone position. Similarly the pronator teres forming the medial boundary of the fossa is made prominent by pronating the forearm against resistance. The lateral and medial epicondyles of the humerus are felt easily at the lower end of the humerus. The radial nerve is located deeply in the cubital fossa in front of the lateral epicondyle, a site often used to induce local anaesthesia.

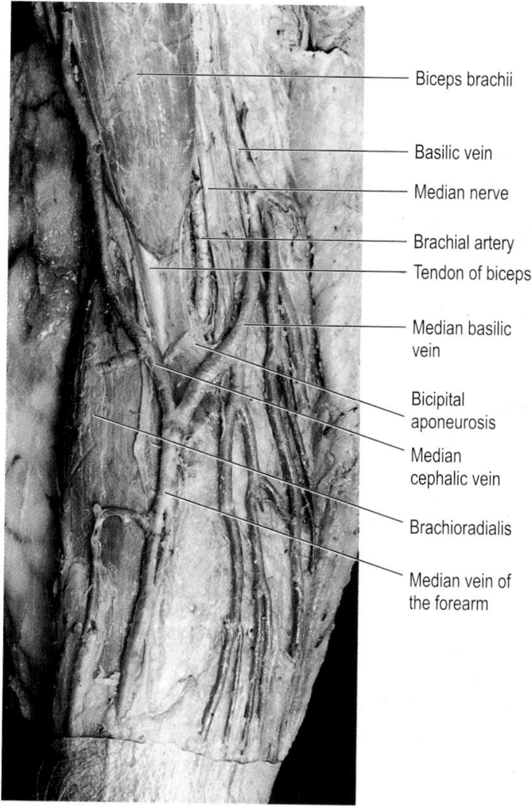


Fig. 2.49 Superficial dissection of the cubital fossa.

### Superficial veins of the cubital fossa

The arrangement of the superficial veins in the cubital fossa is variable. In the dissection shown (Fig. 2.49) a median vein of the forearm gives off the median cephalic and median basilic ('M' arrangement). Alternatively a large median cubital vein may run obliquely upwards from the cephalic vein to join the basilic vein ('H' arrangement). The dissection also shows the brachial artery and the median nerve medial to the tendon of biceps being separated from the vein by the bicipital aponeurosis.

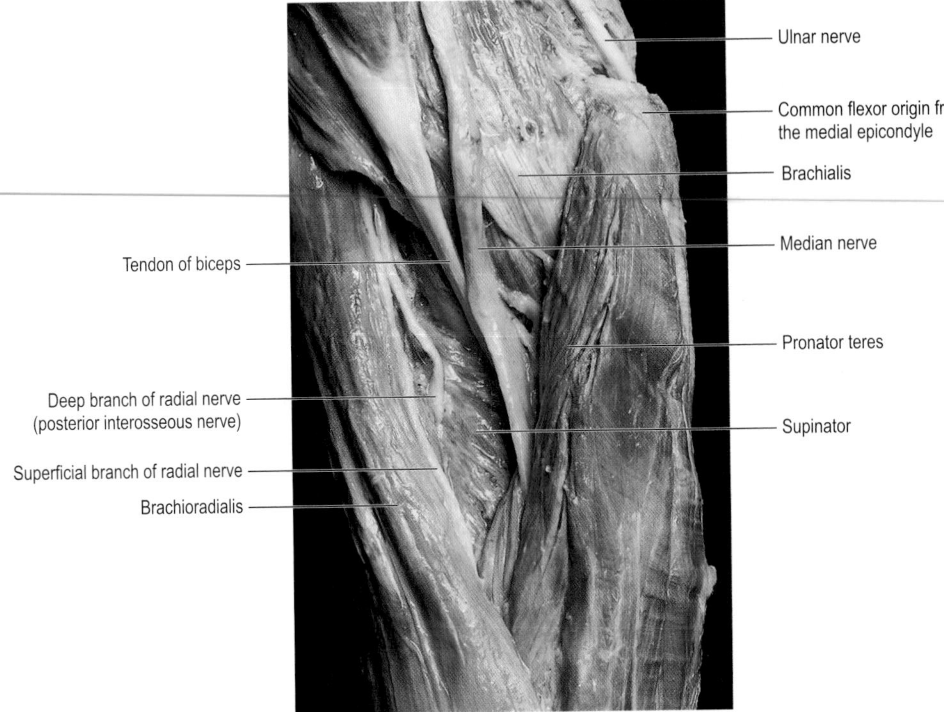


Fig. 2.50 Boundaries and floor of the cubital fossa.

### Boundaries and floor of the cubital fossa

A dissection where most of the contents except the median and the radial nerves are removed is shown in Fig. 2.50. The structures forming the boundaries and floor of the cubital fossa are:

- lateral boundary – the brachioradialis
- medial boundary – the pronator teres
- roof – deep fascia reinforced by the bicipital aponeurosis
- floor – mostly brachialis, supinator laterally.

### Contents of the cubital fossa

From lateral to medial are the tendon of the biceps, brachial artery and the median nerve (Fig. 2.51). The brachial artery divides into the radial and ulnar arteries in the middle of the cubital fossa. Deep to the brachioradialis in the lateral part of the fossa the radial nerve divides into its superficial (cutaneous) branch and the posterior interosseous nerve, the latter then passes through the supinator which clasps the upper end of the radius.

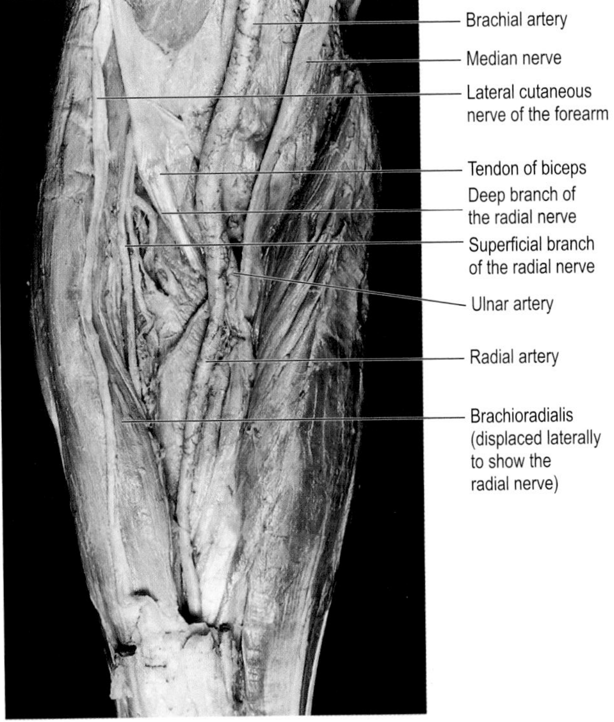


Fig. 2.51 Contents of the cubital fossa.

### Division of the brachial artery

The brachial artery normally divides into its two terminal branches, the radial and ulnar arteries, in the cubital fossa. However this division can be at a higher level and in this case one of the branches, often the radial, can be superficial in the cubital fossa and can be mistaken for a vein. The angiogram (Fig. 2.52) shows the high origin of the radial artery, the other branch being a common trunk for the ulnar and common interosseous arteries, the latter a major branch of the ulnar in the forearm. There are rich anastomoses around the elbow between ulnar, radial and common interosseous branches as seen in the angiogram.

## Lower end of the humerus and the radius and ulna

These are illustrated in Figures 2.53, 2.54 and 2.55. The upper end of the radius has a palpable head which articulates with the capitulum and it can be felt to rotate during pronation and supination of the forearm below the lateral epicondyle of the humerus. The annular ligament runs around the head. The supinator wraps around the neck and the proximal shaft. Within the supinator the posterior interosseous nerve (deep branch of radial nerve) winding around the neck is vulnerable. The radial (bicipital) tuberosity receives the insertion of the tendon of biceps. At the upper end of the ulna the coronoid

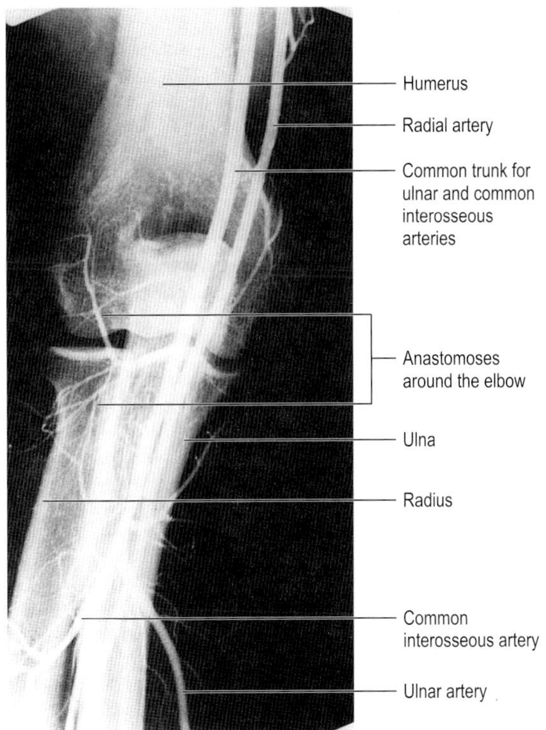


Fig. 2.52 High division of the brachial artery (angiogram).

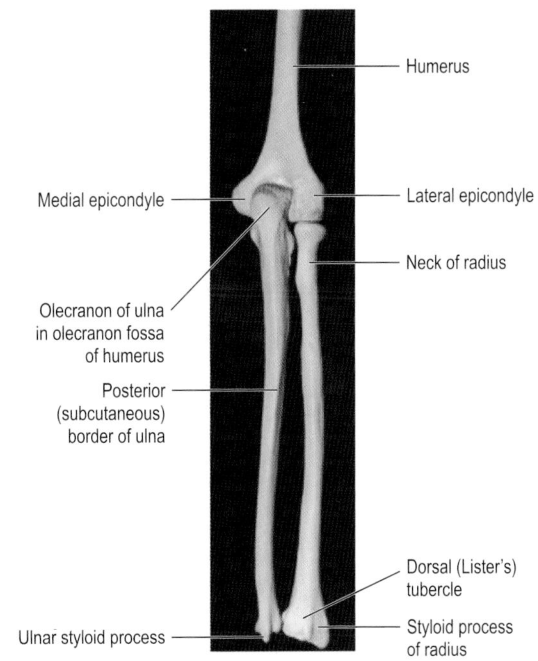


Fig. 2.54 Lower end of humerus and radius and ulna – posterior aspect.

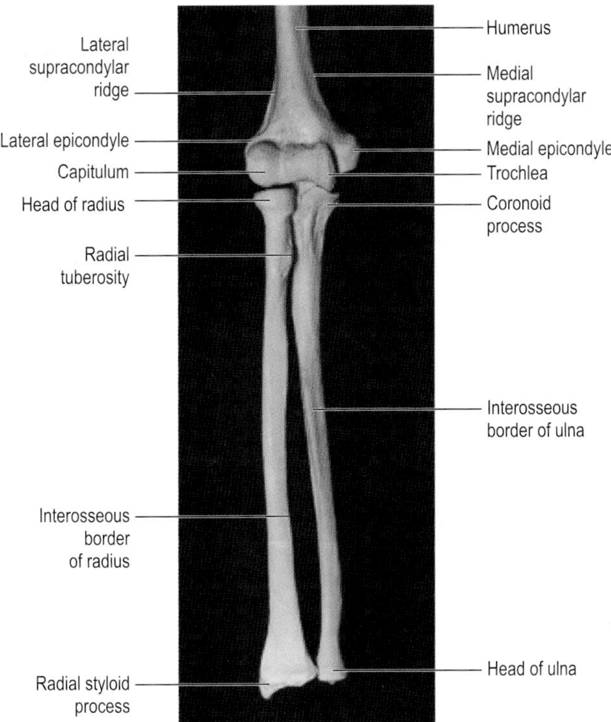


Fig. 2.53 Lower end of humerus and the radius and ulna – anterior aspect.

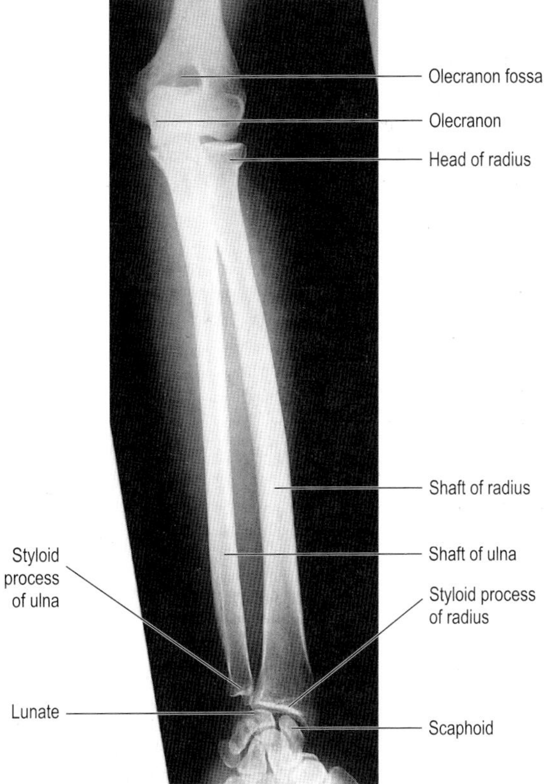


Fig. 2.55 Radiograph of the lower end of humerus and the radius and ulna.

process projects anteriorly. Between this and the olecranon lies the trochlear notch for articulation with the trochlea of the lower end of humerus. The shaft of the radius which is convex laterally receives the insertion of the pronator teres in its middle. The interosseous membrane connecting the radius and ulna is attached to the medial borders of the two bones and it separates the anterior (flexor) and posterior (extensor) compartments of the forearm.

The deep muscles of the flexor and extensor compartments arise from interosseous membrane as well as the shafts of the two forearm bones. The expanded lower end of the radius articulates with the scaphoid and lunate at the wrist joint. The grooves in its posterior aspect hold the extensor tendons crossing the wrist. The tendon of the extensor pollicis longus lies in the groove medial to the Lister's (dorsal) tubercle of the radius. The ulna does not articulate with any carpal bone. The head of the ulna is covered by a fibrocartilagenous disc connecting the radius and ulna and forming a part of the inferior radioulnar joint (Fig. 2.56). The shaft of ulna has a subcutaneous posterior border which gives attachment to an aponeurosis from which the flexor digitorum profundus, flexor carpi ulnaris and the extensor carpi ulnaris take origin. Surgical exposure of the ulna is usually done by incising along this border. Both radius and ulna have styloid processes. The styloid of the former is at a lower level compared with that of the latter.

### Skeleton of the hand

The skeleton of the hand (Figs 2.56, 2.57) consists of eight carpal bones, five metacarpal bones and the phalanges of the fingers. The carpal bones are arranged in two rows. The proximal row from lateral to medial contains the scaphoid, lunate and triquetral with the pisiform articulating with the triquetral. The distal row has the trapezium, trapezoid, capitate and hamate. The metacarpal bones have expanded bases proximally and rounded heads at their distal ends. The first metacarpal is shorter and thicker than the others. Proximally it articulates with the trapezium to form the versatile carpometacarpal joint of the thumb. The thumb has only two phalanges, proximal and distal, whereas each of the remaining four fingers has a proximal, middle and distal phalanx. See Clinical box 2.13.

## Muscles of the front of the forearm

The flexor compartment of the forearm has the muscles arranged in two groups, the superficial group containing five muscles and the deep three muscles. The bulkier flexor compartment muscles act to make the grip powerful.

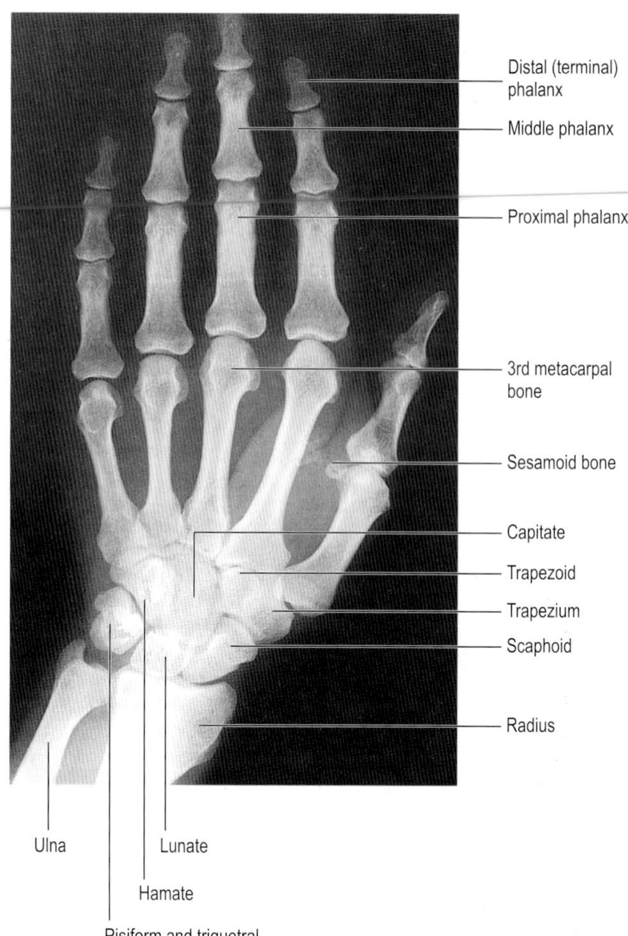


Fig. 2.56 Radiograph of the hand.

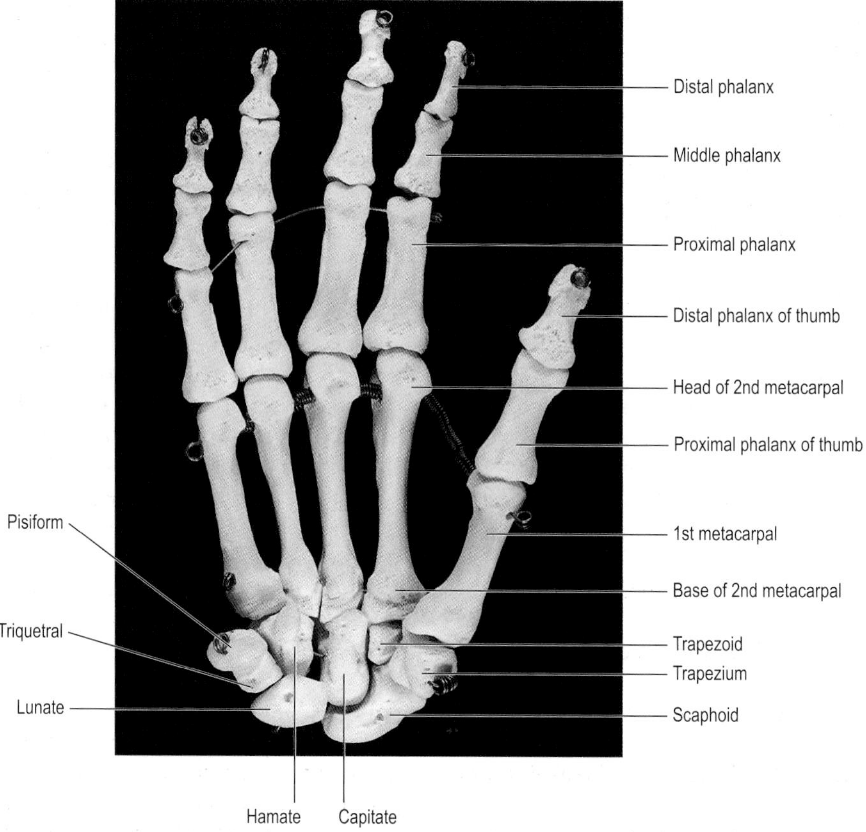


Fig. 2.57 Skeleton of the hand (also see Fig. 2.56).

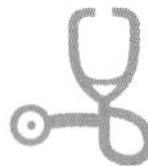

## Clinical box 2.13

### Injuries to the carpal bones

Fracture of the scaphoid and dislocation of the lunate are common injuries sustained by the carpal bones. The scaphoid fractures through its waist (middle portion). The artery to the bone usually enters its distal half and hence when it fractures the proximal half will be without blood supply and may undergo avascular necrosis. A fall on the hand may dislocate the lunate bone or may dislocate the whole carpus backwards with the lunate remaining stationary (perilunar dislocation). These injuries tear the soft tissue and produce avascular necrosis of the bone and may also damage the median nerve.

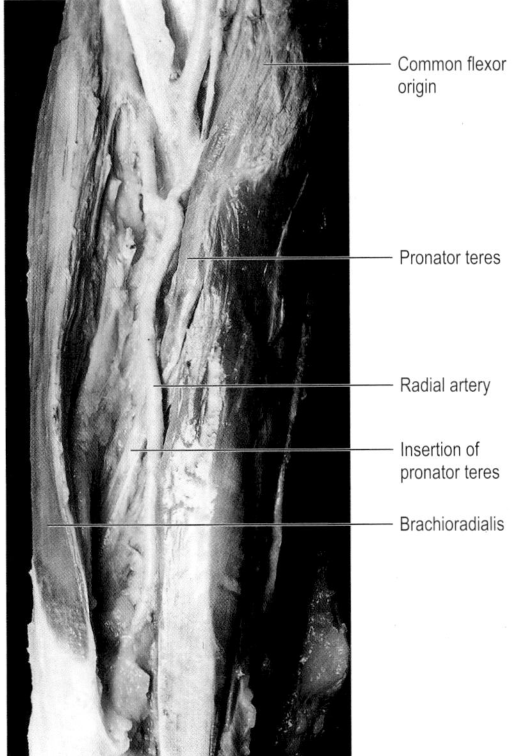


Fig. 2.58 Common flexor origin, pronator teres.

## The superficial muscles

All the superficial muscles of the front of forearm (Figs 2.58, 2.59) take origin from the anterior surface of the medial epicondyle – the common flexor origin. There are additional attachments to the forearm bones as well as the deep fascia.

### Pronator teres

*Origin* The superficial head from the medial epicondyle, the deep head from the ulna (Fig. 2.58).

*Insertion* On the lateral surface of the middle of the shaft of the radius.

*Nerve supply* The first muscular branch of the median nerve (C6, C7).

*Action* It is a pronator of the forearm and a weak flexor of the elbow.

*Test* Pronate the forearm against resistance and feel the muscle at the medial border of the cubital fossa.

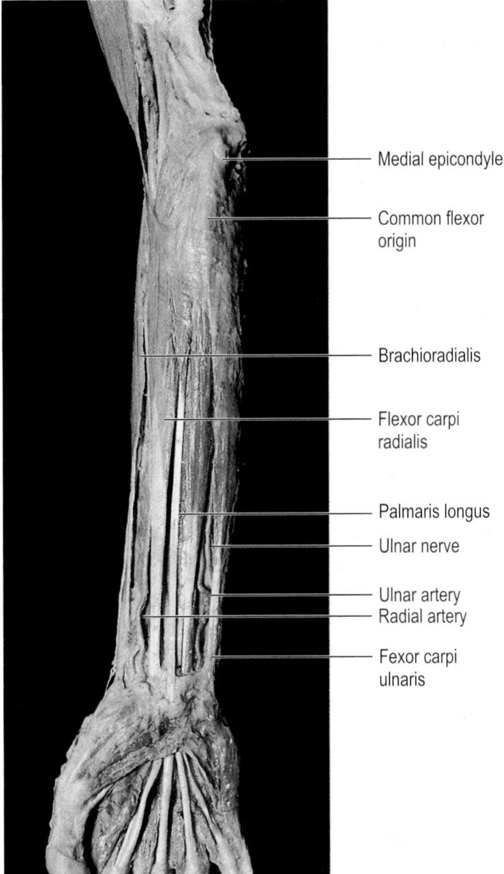


Fig. 2.59 Superficial muscles of the front of forearm – flexor carpi radialis, palmaris longus.

### Brachioradialis

The brachioradialis, a muscle supplied by the radial nerve, lies along the lateral border of the forearm.

*Origin* Lateral supracondylar ridge of the humerus.

*Insertion* On the base of the styloid process of the radius.

*Nerve supply* By a branch of the radial nerve, given off above the elbow.

*Action* It is a powerful flexor of the elbow when the forearm is in the midprone position. The muscle can be seen and felt if this action is produced against resistance.

### Flexor carpi radialis

The tendon of flexor carpi radialis, enclosed in a synovial sheath, passes through the carpal tunnel to lie in the groove on the trapezium before inserting to the bases of the second and third metacarpals. In the region of the wrist the radial artery lies lateral to the tendon and the median nerve with the overlying palmaris longus medial to it.

*Nerve supply* Median nerve (C6, C7).

*Action* Flexes the wrist as well as abducts it (radial deviation).

*Test* Flex the wrist against resistance. The tendon of the flexor carpi radialis can be seen and felt at the lateral aspect of the front of the wrist.

### Palmaris longus

The long flat tendon of the muscle passes in front of the flexor retinaculum to merge with the palmar aponeurosis. Just above the wrist the tendon covers the median nerve. This muscle supplied by the median nerve may be absent in about 13% of arms.

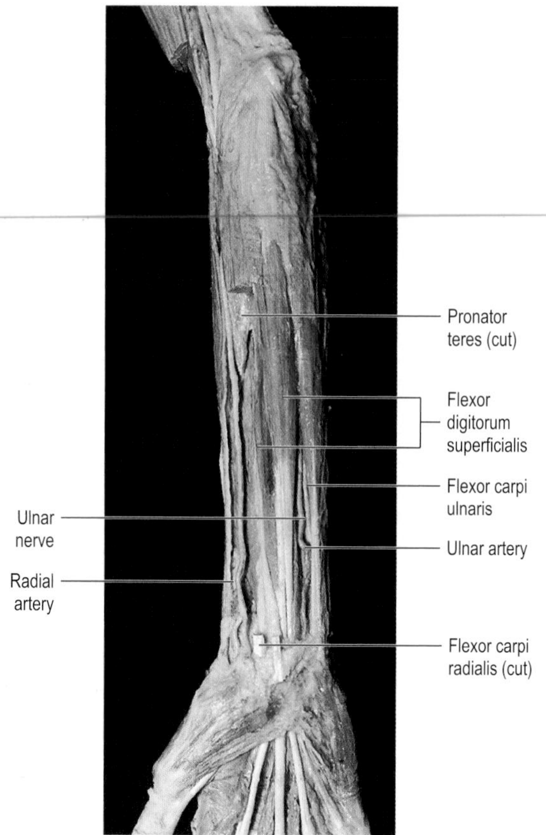


Fig. 2.60 Flexor digitorum superficialis, flexor carpi ulnaris.

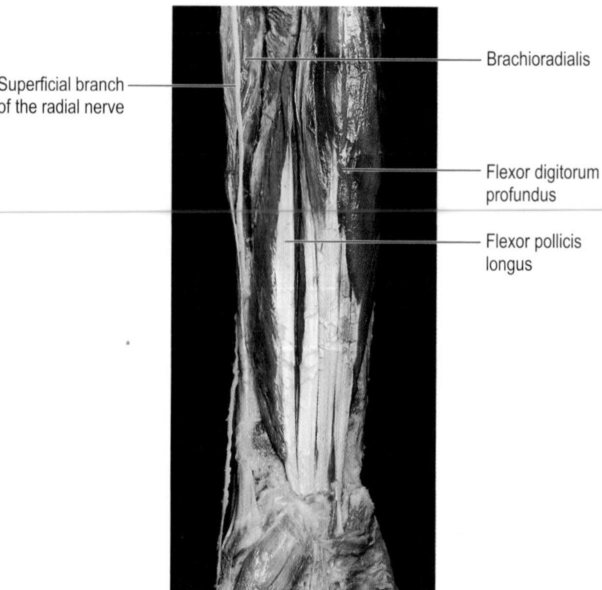


Fig. 2.61 Flexor digitorum profundus, flexor pollicis longus after removal of superficial muscles.

### Flexor digitorum superficialis

This muscle (Fig. 2.60) has four tendons which traverse the palm to be inserted to the middle phalanx of the digits. In the forearm the muscle has the median nerve adherent to its deep surface where it can be easily mistaken for a tendon during exploration.

*Nerve supply* Median nerve (C7, C8).

*Action* It is a flexor of the proximal interphalangeal joints and its continued action may flex the metacarpophalangeal joints and the wrist joint. It contracts to make a power grip.

*Test* Flex the fingers at the proximal interphalangeal joints against resistance while the distal interphalangeal joints are held extended (to prevent the action of flexor digitorum profundus).

### Flexor carpi ulnaris

At the wrist the tendon of the flexor carpi ulnaris lies medial to the ulnar artery and nerve and can be palpated at the wrist. It is inserted to the pisiform, hamate and fifth metacarpal bone.

*Nerve supply* Ulnar nerve.

*Action* It flexes as well as adducts (ulnar deviation) the wrist.

*Test* It can be tested by adducting the little finger or by flexing the wrist against resistance.

## Deep muscles

### Flexor digitorum profundus

This muscle (Fig. 2.61) taking origin mostly from the anterior surface of the ulna and the interosseous membrane, has four tendons which pass through the carpal tunnel enclosed in the same synovial sheath as the tendons of the superficialis – the ulnar bursa. In the palm the tendons proceed towards their insertion on the base of the terminal phalanx.

*Nerve supply* The muscle is supplied by the anterior interosseous branch of the median nerve as well as the ulnar nerve (through C8, T1 fibres), the lateral half of the muscle by the former and the medial the latter.

*Action* It is the only flexor of the distal interphalangeal joints and its continued action will flex the proximal interphalangeal, metacarpophalangeal and wrist joints. The power of digital flexion is maximum when the wrist is extended. Along with the superficialis this muscle makes the power grip.

*Test* Flex the distal phalanx against resistance with the middle and proximal phalanges held extended.

### Flexor pollicis longus

This muscle (Fig. 2.61), the long flexor of the thumb (pollex), is the only flexor of its interphalangeal joint. It takes origin from the anterior surface of the radius and the interosseous membrane and its tendon passes through the carpal tunnel ensheathed by the radial bursa (synovial sheath). It is inserted to the base of the distal phalanx of the thumb.

*Nerve supply* By the anterior interosseous branch of the median nerve (C8, T1).

*Action* This muscle primarily is a flexor of the interphalangeal joint of the thumb but it can also flex the metacarpophalangeal joint and the carpometacarpal joint of the thumb, as well as the wrist joint.

*Test* Hold the proximal phalanx of the thumb steady and flex the distal phalanx.

### Pronator quadratus

This quadrangular muscle (Fig. 2.62) arises from the distal end of the shaft of the ulna and is inserted to the anterior surface of the lower fourth of the radius. It is supplied by the anterior interosseous nerve (C7, C8). It is a pronator of the forearm and it also helps to hold the radius and ulna together when the hand is weight-bearing. See Clinical box 2.14.

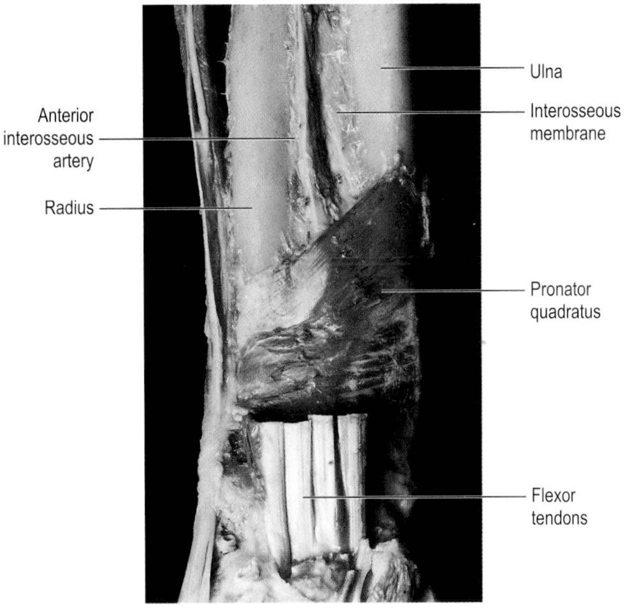


Fig. 2.62 Pronator quadratus, interosseous membrane.

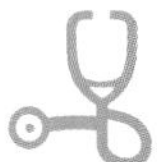

## Clinical box 2.14

### Space of Parona

This is a fascial space of surgical importance. It is anterior to the pronator quadratus and extends upwards up to the oblique line of attachment of the flexor digitorum superficialis to the radius. Into the space of Parona protrude the synovial sheaths of the flexor tendons and infection can extend into it when the sheaths are affected. Drainage is facilitated by incisions on either side of the flexor tendons.

## Arteries and nerves of the forearm

The division of brachial artery into radial and ulnar arteries (Figs 2.63, 2.64) is seen in the cubital fossa, and the latter is seen going deep to the pronator teres. As it descends the ulnar artery lies on the flexor digitorum profundus and is accompanied by the ulnar nerve on its medial side (Fig. 2.63). The artery and the nerve are under cover of the flexor carpi ulnaris, except at the lower end where they lie lateral to the tendon of the muscle. The nerve and the artery enter the palm passing superficial to the flexor retinaculum. In the forearm the ulnar artery gives off the common interosseous artery, which in turn divides into anterior and posterior interosseous branches. The radial artery as it descends lies on the supinator, the insertion of the pronator teres, radial origin of the flexor digitorum superficialis, flexor pollicis longus and the pronator quadratus (i.e. all the muscles attached to the anterior aspect of the shaft of the radius). Distally it winds round the radius deep to the tendons of the abductor pollicis longus and extensor pollicis brevis to reach the anatomical snuff box. In the upper part the artery is covered by the brachioradialis. In the lower part of the forearm it is more superficial and its pulsation can easily be felt lateral to the tendon of the flexor carpi radialis. An angiogram of the radial and ulnar arteries is shown in Figure 2.64.

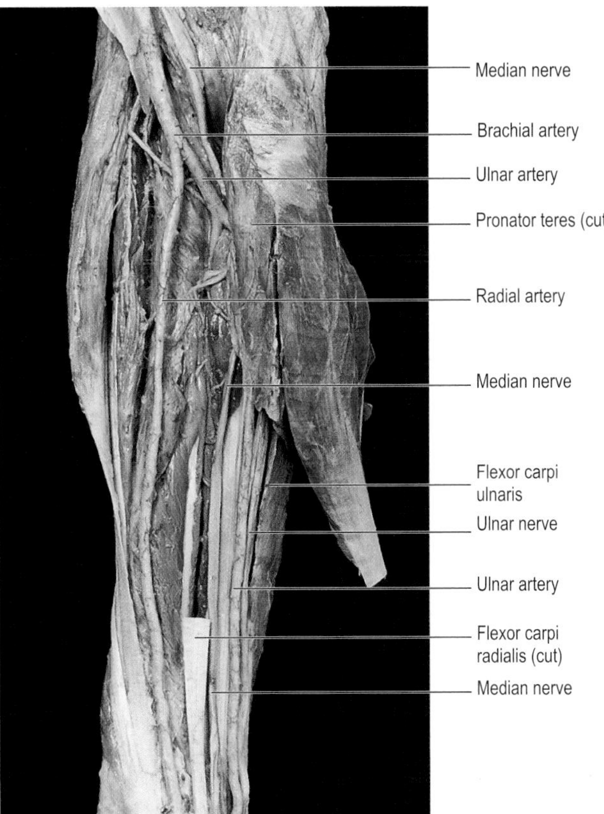


Fig. 2.63 Arteries and nerves in the front of the forearm.

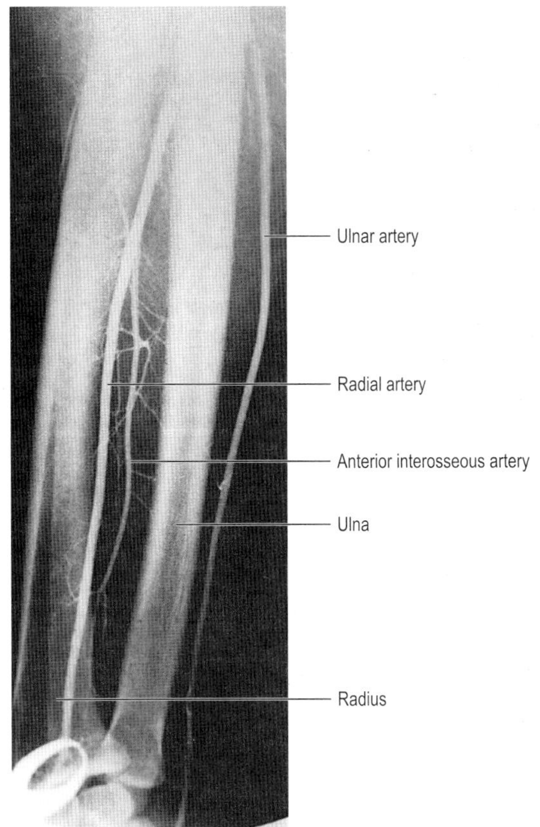


Fig. 2.64 Radial and ulnar arteries (angiogram).

The median nerve leaves the cubital fossa by passing between the two heads of the pronator teres. At the distal aspect of the forearm the nerve lies medial to the tendon of the flexor carpi radialis, almost covered by the tendon of the palmaris longus. It then passes through the carpal tunnel to enter the palm. The anterior interosseous branch supplying the flexor pollicis longus, flexor digitorum profundus and the pronator quadratus is given off as the nerve passes in between the two heads of the pronator teres. Branches to the superficial flexors in the forearm are given off earlier. The median nerve and its anterior interosseous branch together supply all the muscles in the front of the forearm except flexor carpi ulnaris and the medial half of the profundus, which are supplied by the ulnar nerve. The ulnar nerve enters the forearm by passing in between the two heads of the flexor carpi ulnaris. As it descends it lies medial to the ulnar artery.

## Palm of the hand

The skin of the palm is adherent to the underlying connective tissue. The fixity will prevent the skin from slipping over objects whilst gripping. The flexure creases (lines of the palm) and papillary ridges also improve the grip. There is an abundance of sweat glands on the palm. The cutaneous innervation of the palm and digits are through the median and ulnar nerves. The palm is supplied by the palmar branches of the nerves. The digital branches of the median nerve supply the skin of the lateral three and a half fingers and that of the ulnar nerve the medial one and a half fingers.

The proximal limit of the flexor retinaculum is in level with the distal skin wrist crease. The tubercle of the scaphoid and the pisiform are palpable at this level. The trapezium and the hook of the hamate are felt deep to the overlying thenar and hypothenar muscles. Tenderness can be elicited by pressing the ulnar nerve against the hook of the hamate. See Clinical box 2.15.

### Flexor retinaculum and the carpal tunnel

The flexor retinaculum (Figs 2.67, 2.68) is a thickening of the deep fascia bridging the concavity across the anterior surfaces of the carpal bones to prevent 'bow stringing' of the flexor tendons passing deep to it. It is attached to the scaphoid and trapezium laterally and to the pisiform and hook of the hamate medially. The carpal tunnel is the space

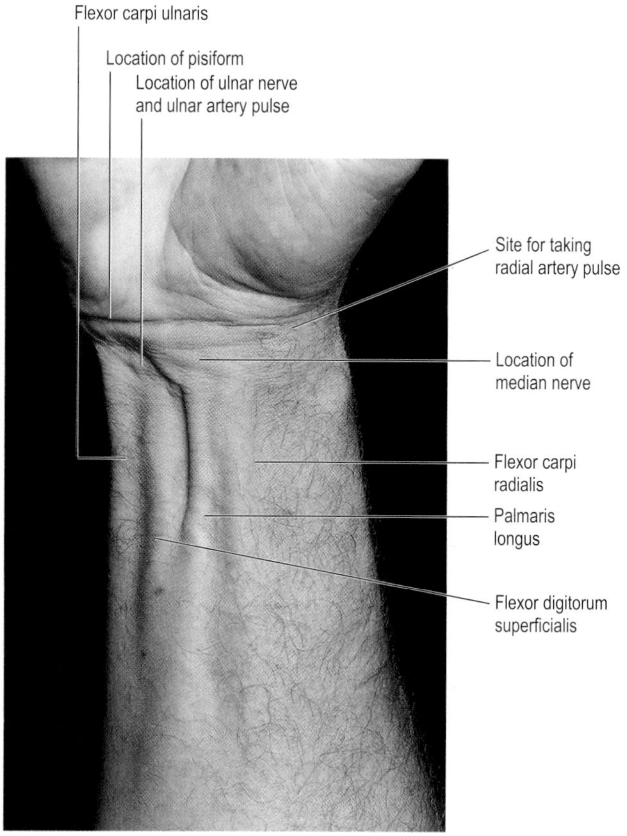


Fig. 2.65 Surface anatomy of the wrist.

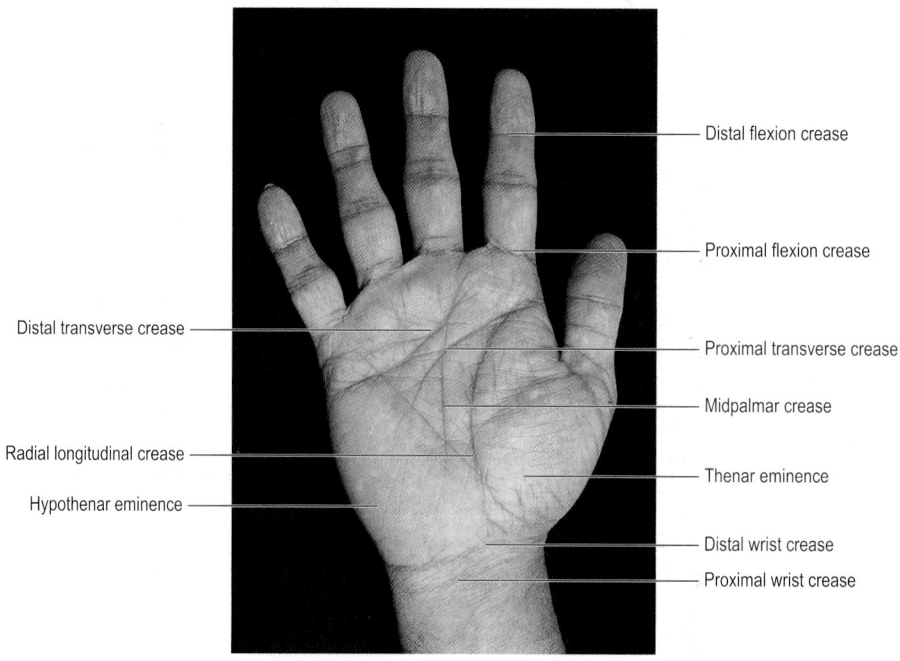


Fig. 2.66 Surface anatomy of the hand.

between the flexor retinaculum and the anterior concavity of the carpal bones. The thenar and hypothenar muscles take origin from the flexor retinaculum. See Clinical boxes 2.16 and 2.17.

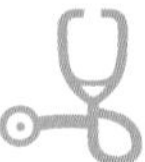

## *Clinical box 2.15*

### Surface anatomy of the wrist and hand

On flexing the wrist the flexor carpi radialis, the palmaris longus, the flexor digitorum superficialis as well as the flexor carpi ulnaris can be seen and felt. The radial artery pulsation is felt lateral to the flexor carpi radialis (Fig. 2.65). This is the usual site for arterial cannulation. The surface marking of the radial artery is along a line connecting a point medial to the tendon of the biceps to the point where its pulsation is felt. The proximal wrist crease is at the level of the wrist joint (Fig. 2.66).

The pulsation of the ulnar artery can be felt at the distal end of the forearm lateral to the tendon of the flexor carpi ulnaris. It can be exposed in the lower part of the forearm by displacing the flexor carpi ulnaris and by safeguarding the ulnar nerve.

The median nerve is located between the flexor carpi radialis and the palmaris longus and the ulnar nerve and artery lateral to the flexor carpi ulnaris.

A slash across the wrist is likely to cut the following structures from medial to lateral:

- the ulnar nerve
- the ulnar artery
- palmaris longus tendon
- median nerve
- tendon of flexor carpi radialis
- radial artery.

### The palmar aponeurosis

The palmar aponeurosis (Fig. 2.69) lies immediately deep to the subcutaneous tissue of the palm. It extends distally from the flexor retinaculum and divides into four slips, one to each finger, to be attached to the fibrous flexor sheath. ✪ The palmar aponeurosis is clinically important as it can be affected by Dupuytren's contracture in its medial part. In

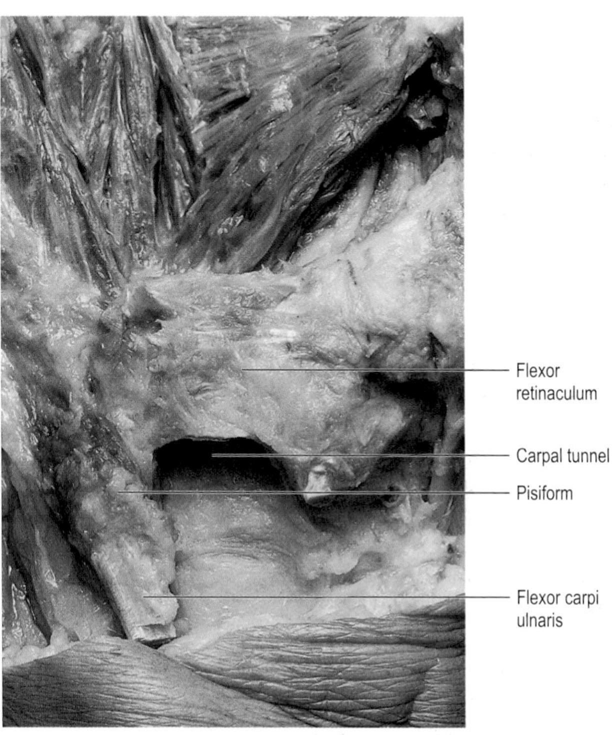


Fig. 2.67 Flexor retinaculum and the carpal tunnel (after removal of most of the related structures).

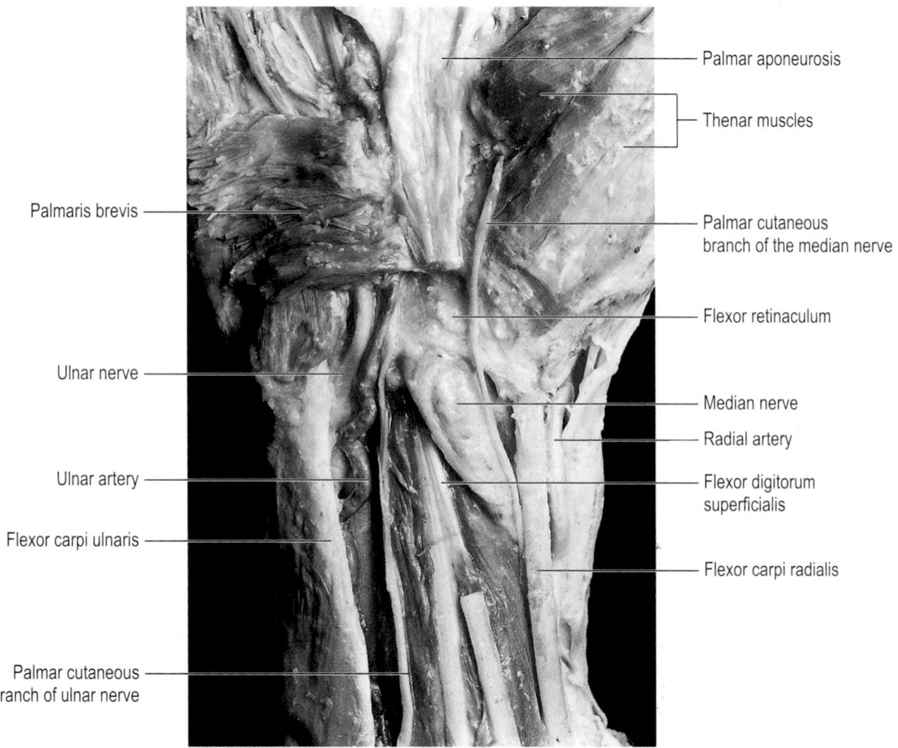


Fig. 2.68 Flexor retinaculum and carpal tunnel with related structures.

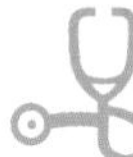

## *Clinical box 2.16*

### Carpal tunnel syndrome

The carpal tunnel is packed with the flexor tendons entering the hand. The median nerve goes through the tunnel. The nerve can be compressed by swelling of the tendons or by arthritis affecting the joints of the carpal bones increasing pressure in the tunnel. The condition is known as carpal tunnel syndrome, which manifests as pain and diminished sensation on the skin along the distribution of the median nerve to the digits as well as weakness of the thenar muscles. The palmar cutaneous branch of the median nerve supplying skin over the thenar eminence lies superficial to the retinaculum and hence is not affected in carpal tunnel syndrome. Surgical treatment of the condition is incising the flexor retinaculum in line with the flexed ring finger. The site is chosen to avoid cutting the median nerve and its palmar cutaneous branch.

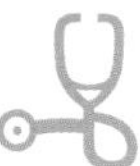

## *Clinical box 2.17*

### Ulnar nerve and the Flexor retinaculum

The ulnar nerve as well as the ulnar artery lie superficial to the flexor retinaculum, the nerve being medial to the artery. The ulnar nerve along with the artery is covered by a band of fibrous tissue forming the Guyon's canal (Fig. 2.70) as it passes over the flexor retinaculum. The ulnar nerve may become compressed as it lies in the Guyon's canal. It is not that easily blocked by local anaesthetic agents at the flexor retinaculum because of its fibrous covering.

this condition the aponeurosis undergoes fibrosis to produce flexion deformity of the medial two fingers.

The subcutaneous palmaris brevis muscle which stretches across the hypothenar muscles is supplied by the superficial branch of the ulnar nerve. Its contraction may steady the grip on the ulnar side of the palm.

### Superficial and deep palmar arches

Deep to the palmar aponeurosis lies the superficial palmar arch (Figs 2.70–2.72), the arterial arcade formed by the ulnar artery with a small contribution from the radial artery. This contribution may be missing and hence the arch incomplete (Fig. 2.70).

The arch gives off four digital branches. The first three run distally to the webs of the fingers where they divide to supply the adjacent fingers. The fourth digital branch supplies the medial surface of the little finger. The digital arteries are accompanied by the digital branches of the ulnar and the median nerves.

The deep palmar arch lies deep to the flexor tendons and is usually complete. It runs across the palm about 1 cm proximal to the superficial arch. See Clinical box 2.18.

### The median and the ulnar nerves

The ulnar nerve (Fig. 2.73) divides into a superficial and a deep branch as it leaves the flexor retinaculum. The

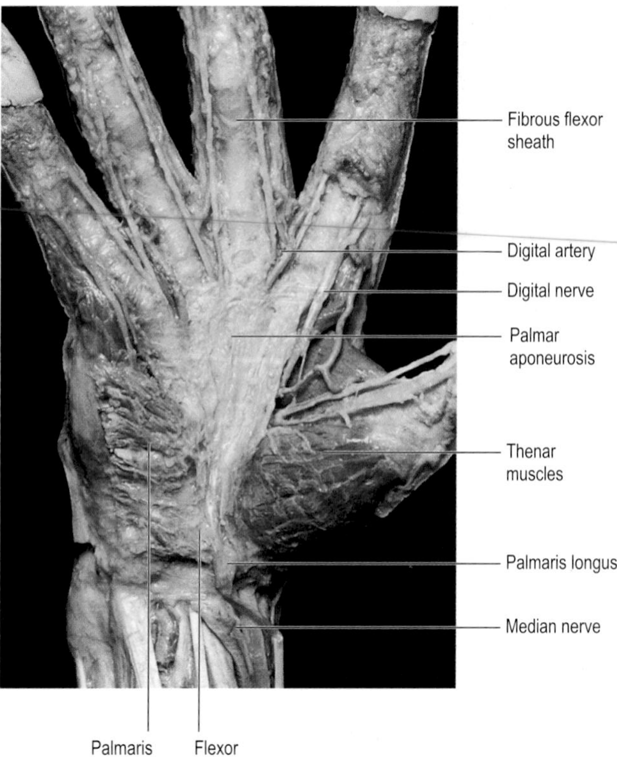


Fig. 2.69 Palmar aponeurosis.

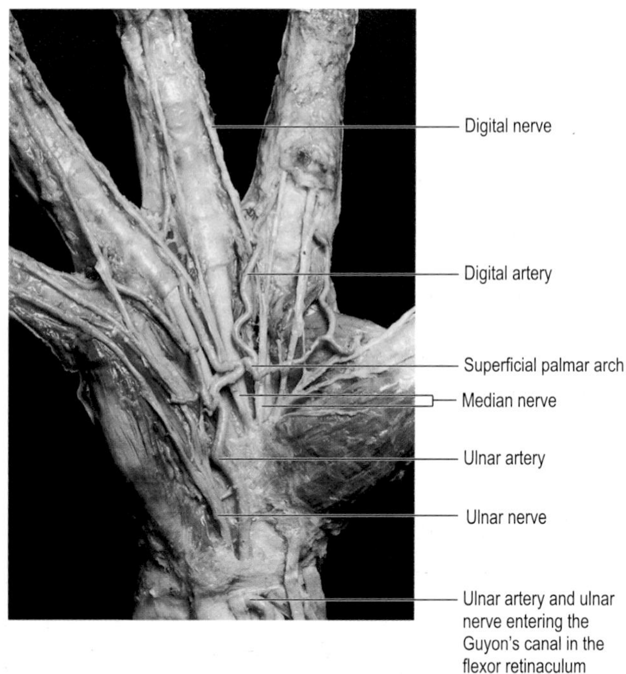


Fig. 2.70 Superficial palmar arch.

superficial branch, which can be palpated as it lies on the hook of the hamate, gives off two digital branches that supply the ulnar one and a half fingers. The deep branch passes deeply between the hypothenar muscles and supplies all the interossei, both heads of the adductor pollicis, the medial two lumbricals and the three hypothenar muscles.

The median nerve (Fig. 2.73) on entering the palm divides into a medial and a lateral branch after giving off the recurrent branch supplying the thenar muscles (Clinical box 2.19). The medial branch divides to supply the ring, middle and the index fingers as well as the second lumbrical

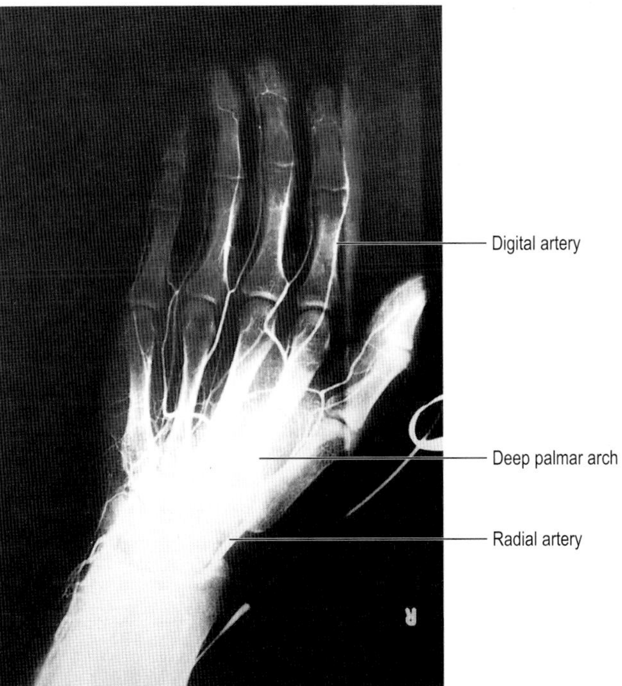


Fig. 2.71 Angiogram of radial artery and the deep palmar arch (the deep palmar arch is partly obscured by the opacity of the metacarpal bones).

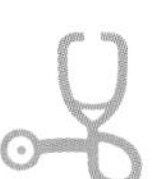

## *Clinical box 2.18*

### Allen's test

The radial artery is usually selected for arterial cannulation (Fig. 2.71). Checking for the integrity of the palmar arches is carried out before cannulation as there is a small risk of thrombosis of the artery. This is done by the Allen's test in which the arterial flow to the hand is stopped by occluding the arteries by firm finger pressure. The hand is then exsanguinated by clenching the fist a few times. The pressure on the radial artery is maintained while that on the ulnar is removed. If the hand flushes rapidly the ulnar inflow is satisfactory. The test is repeated keeping the ulnar artery occluded and releasing the radial artery to test the radial inflow.

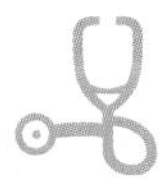

## *Clinical box 2.19*

### Injury to recurrent branch of the median nerve

Distal to the flexor retinaculum the median nerve gives a recurrent branch which curls backwards over the retinaculum to supply the three thenar muscles (Fig. 2.74). The recurrent branch is relatively superficial and can easily be damaged by superficial cuts and incisions in this area. Such an injury will impair the grip by affecting the movements of thumb.

muscle. The lateral branch divides further to supply the radial side of the index finger and the whole of the thumb. The branch to the index finger supplies the first lumbrical.

The palmar digital branches of both ulnar and median at the distal aspect wind around the fingers to supply the skin on the dorsum of the terminal phalanges as well.

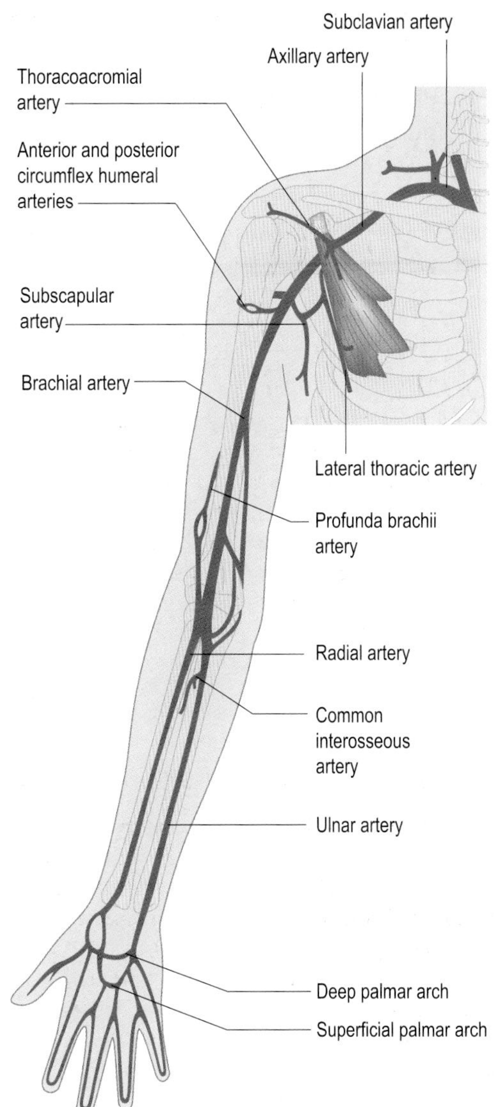


Fig. 2.72 Summary diagram showing the arteries of the upper limb.

### The thenar muscles

There are three muscles in this group – the abductor pollicis brevis, flexor pollicis brevis and the opponens (Fig. 2.74). They take origin from the flexor retinaculum and the adjoining carpal bones. The abductor and the flexor are inserted to the lateral aspect of the first phalanx of the thumb. The opponens lies deep to these two muscles and is inserted to the first metacarpal bone. The three muscles are supplied by the recurrent branch of the median nerve (Clinical box 2.19).

*Test* The abductor pollicis brevis being superficial can easily be tested. Bring the thumb forward at right angles to the plane of the palm against resistance and feel the muscle contracting.

### Movements of the thumb

The following are the movements of the thumb redefined by the International Federation of Societies for Surgery of the Hand (see Fig. 2.75):

- Palmar abduction – In this movement, produced by abductor pollicis brevis, the thumb moves away from the index finger at right angles to the plane of the palm keeping the thumbnail in a plane at right angles to that of the four fingernails.

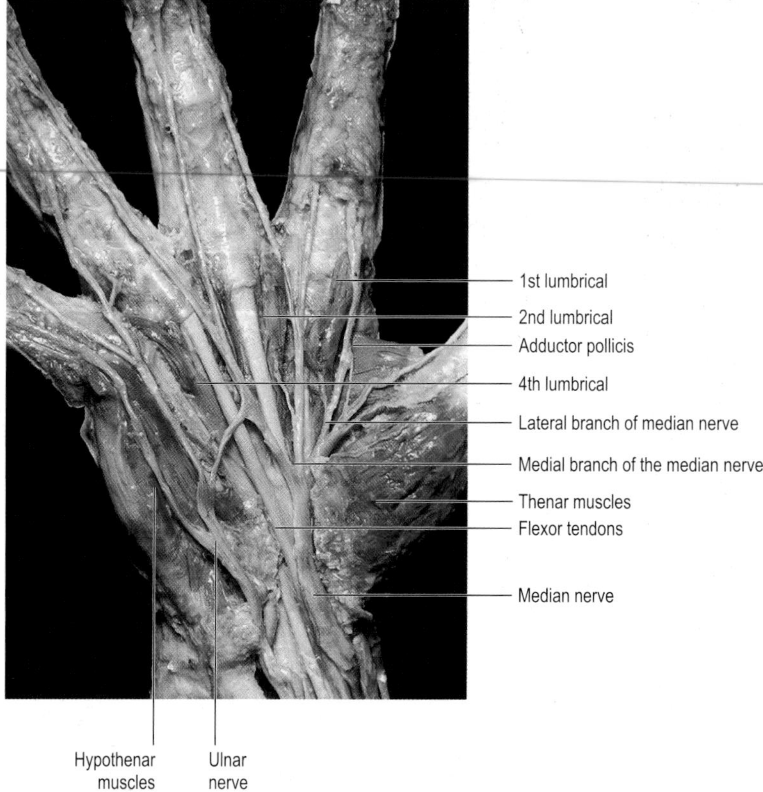


Fig. 2.73 Median and ulnar nerves in the hand (flexor retinaculum is partially removed).

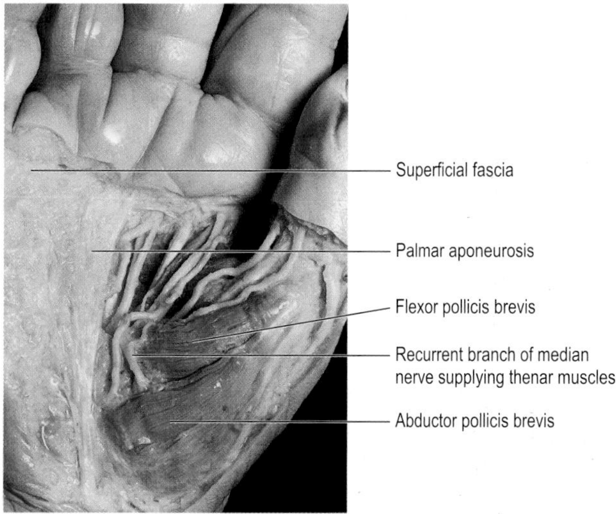


Fig. 2.74 Thenar muscles and the recurrent branch of median nerve.

- Radial abduction – The thumb is moved away from the index finger in the plane of the palm by abductor pollicis longus and extensor pollicis brevis. The opposite movement of adduction is produced by adductor pollicis and can be continued across the palm by flexor pollicis brevis.
- Opposition – In this the pulp of the thumb is made to face the pulp of another finger (as in holding a pin between thumb and index finger) by medially rotating and adducting the first metacarpal bone at its joint with the trapezium. This is done mostly by the opponens pollicis.

### The flexor tendons

The tendons of the flexor digitorum superficialis and profundus lie deep to the superficial palmar arch. The tendons of the profundus lie deep to those of the superficialis. They pass in pairs into the fibrous flexor sheaths of fingers (Fig. 2.76). At the proximal part of each finger the superficialis is tunnelled through by the profundus tendon. A cut on the anterior aspect of the proximal part may thus sever the profundus before cutting the superficialis. The superficialis is inserted to the base of the middle phalanx and the profundus to the terminal phalanx (Fig. 2.77). The tendon of the flexor pollicis longus is inserted to the base of the terminal phalanx of the thumb.

### The lumbrical muscles

There are four lumbrical muscles in the hand, one for each finger. Each muscle takes origin from the flexor digitorum profundus tendon, crosses the root of the finger laterally and is inserted to the dorsal digital expansion at the back of the finger. How the lumbrical muscles of the hand function is not clearly understood. Many anatomists are of the view that the muscles are used to simultaneously flex the metacarpophalangeal and extend the interphalangeal joints. The lateral two lumbricals are usually supplied by the median nerve and the medial two lumbricals by the ulnar nerve.

### The hypothenar muscles

The attachments of the hypothenar muscles – abductor, flexor and opponens digiti minimi – are mirror images of those of the thenar muscles and they act on the little finger. They are supplied by the deep branch of the ulnar nerve.

### Synovial sheath

The flexor tendons are enclosed by synovial sheaths. In the fibrous flexor sheath both tendons are invested by a common synovial sheath. The tendons receive their blood

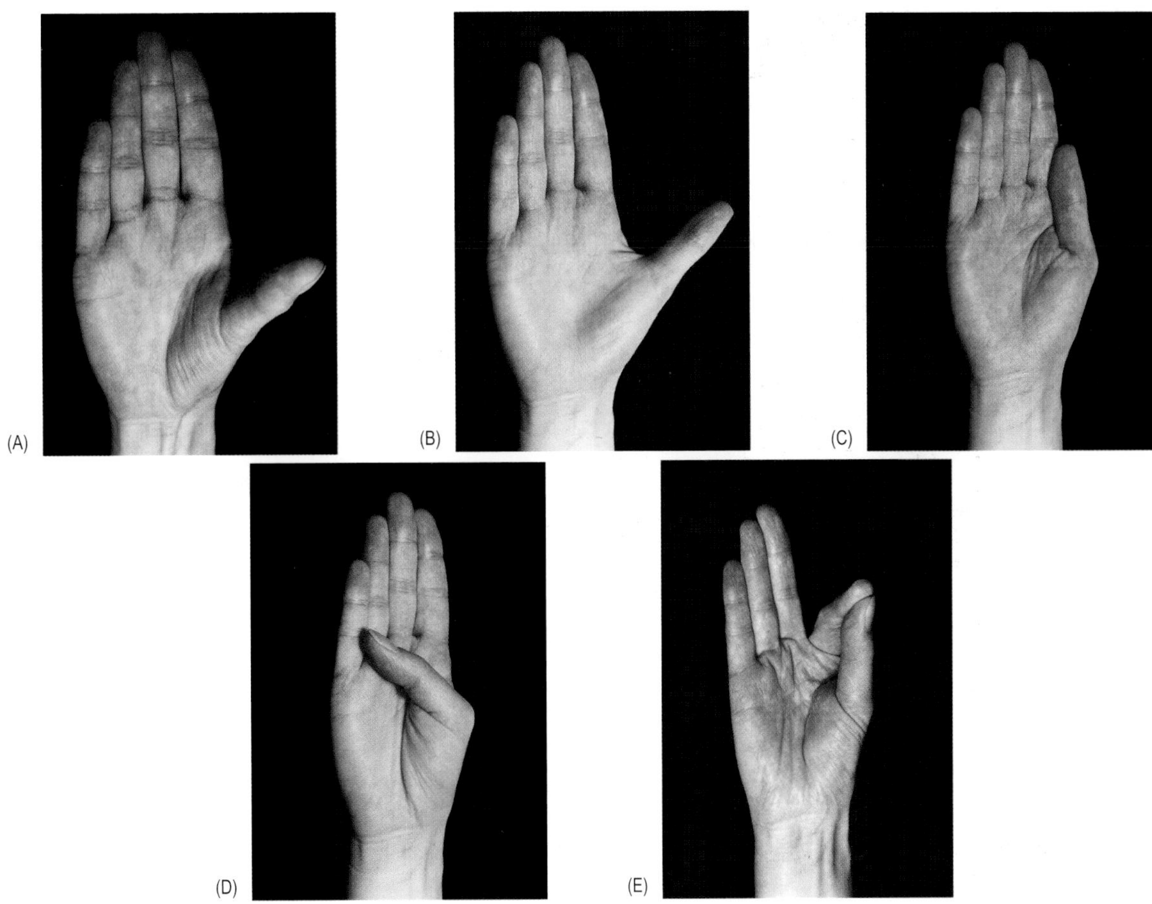


Fig. 2.75 (A) Palmar abduction of thumb. (B) Radial abduction of thumb. (C) Adduction of thumb. (D) Transpalmar adduction of thumb. (E) Opposition of thumb.

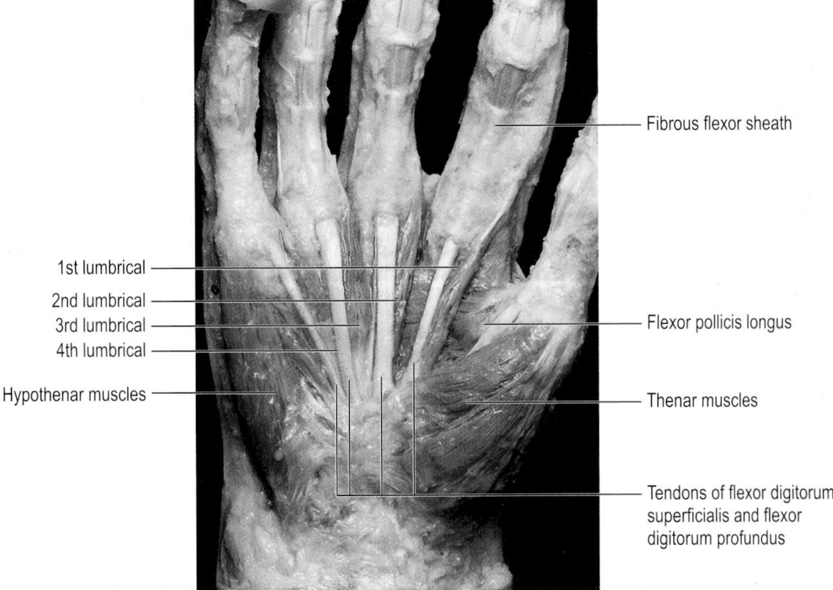


Fig. 2.76 Long flexor tendons, lumbricals and hypothenar muscles.

supply through synovial folds known as vincula, each tendon having two, vincula longa and vincula brevia. The sheath of the little finger is continuous with the ulnar bursa covering the flexor tendons in the palm. The flexor pollicis longus is covered by a single sheath throughout, the radial bursa. The arrangement of the synovial sheaths for these tendons is illustrated in Figure 2.78. ✪ Synovial sheaths can be infected producing tenosynovitis. Infection can spread throughout the sheath. Infection of the sheath of the little finger can thus spread up the distal aspect of the forearm into

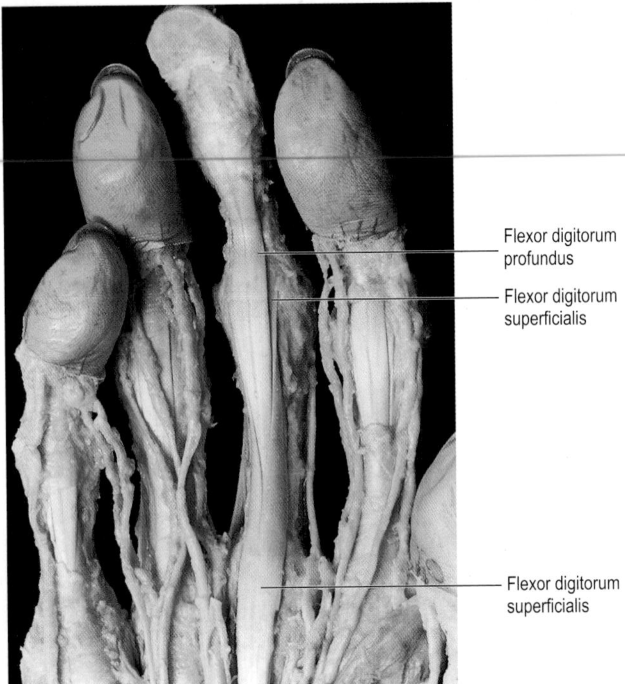


Fig. 2.77 Insertion of flexor digitorum superficialis and flexor digitorum profundus.

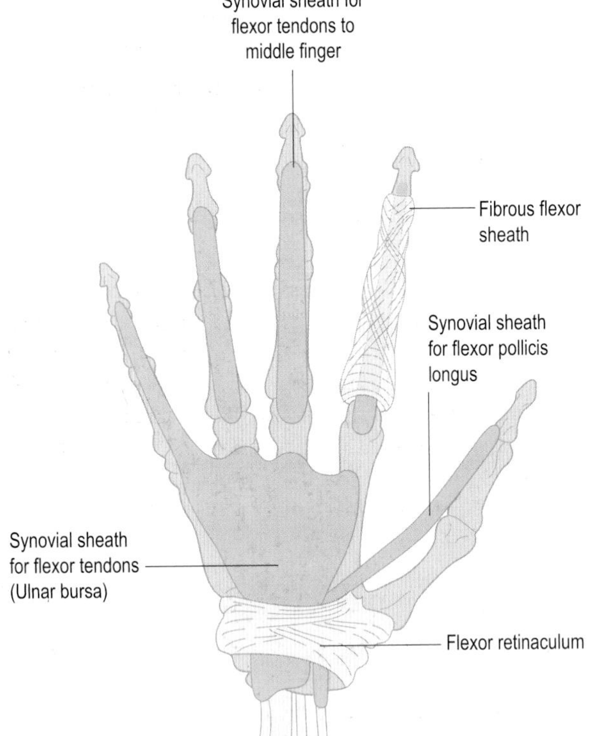


Fig. 2.78 Arrangement of synovial sheaths for the flexor tendons.

the space of Parona (see Clinical box 2.14). See Figure 2.79 and Clinical box 2.20.

### Adductor pollicis

This muscle (Fig. 2.80) located deep in the palm has two heads of origin, the transverse head arising from the shaft of the third metacarpal bone and the oblique head from the bases of the second and third metacarpal bones and the capitate. The two heads converge to its insertion to the

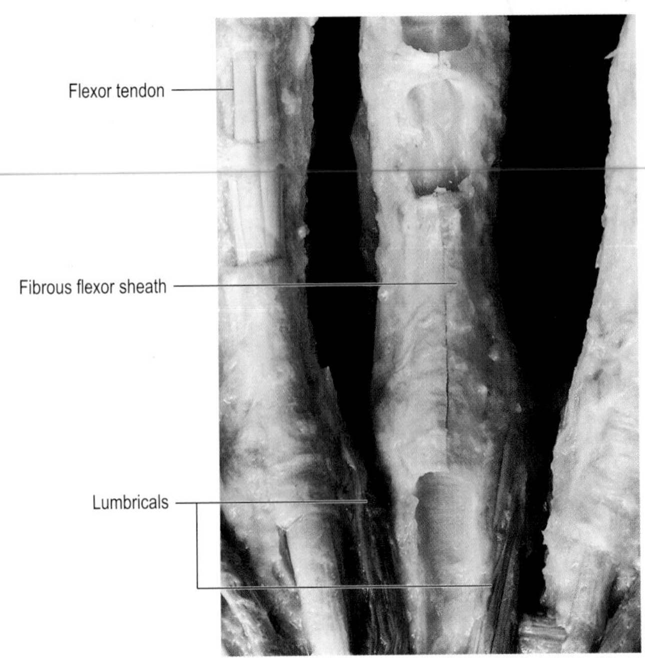


Fig. 2.79 Fibrous flexor sheath.

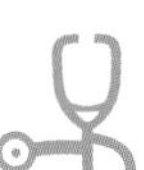

*Clinical box 2.20*

**Trigger finger**

The flexor tendons are held on to the front of the finger by the fibrous flexor sheath lined by synovial membrane (Fig. 2.79). The tendons move inside the sheath during flexion and extension. However narrowing of the space in the sheath can occur by thickening of the sheath or nodular thickening of the tendon. The finger may then click painfully when attempting to bend it, or when the hand is unclenched the affected finger can remain bent and may suddenly straighten with a snap – a 'trigger finger'.

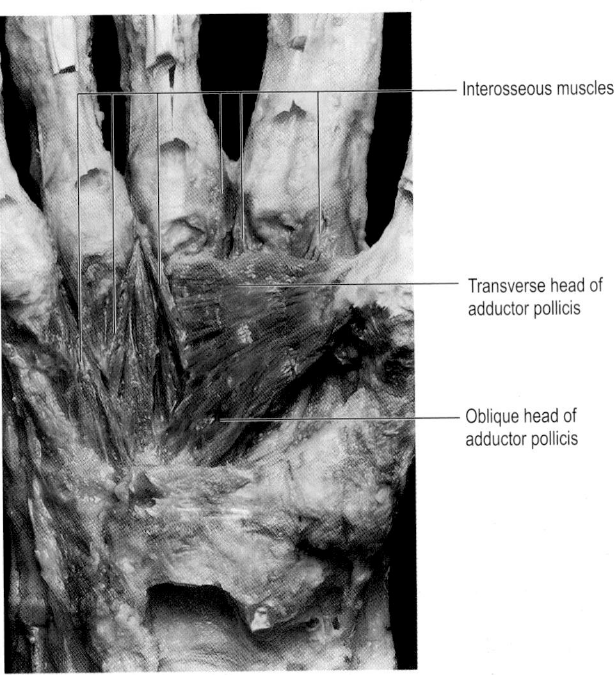


Fig. 2.80 Adductor pollicis.

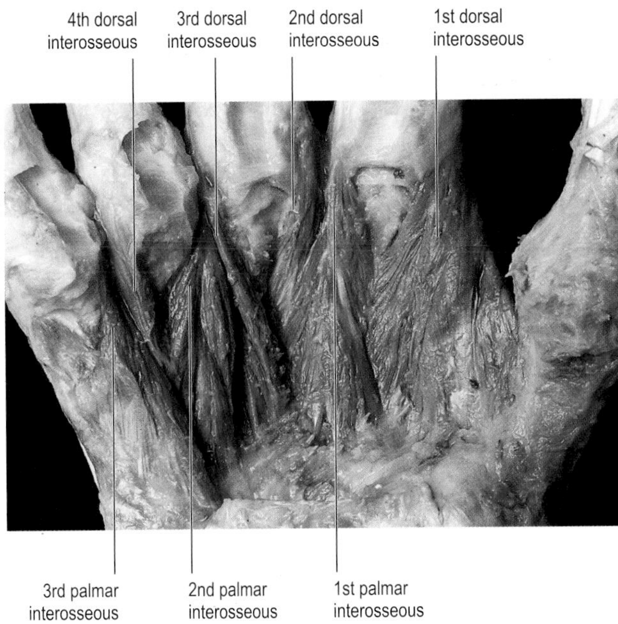


Fig. 2.81 Palmar and dorsal interosseous muscles.

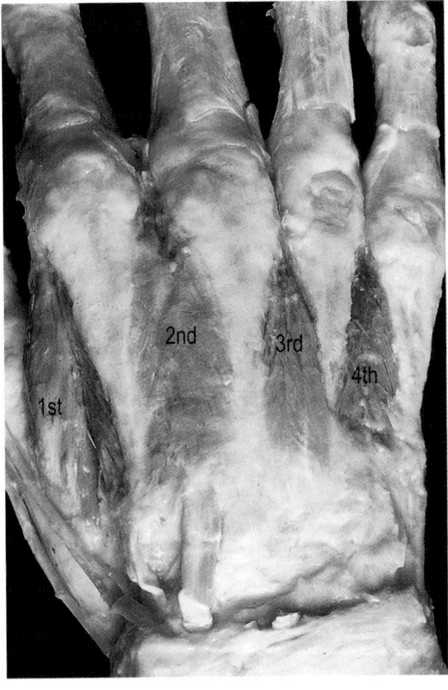


Fig. 2.82 Dorsal interossei seen from the posterior aspect of hand (dorsum of hand).

medial aspect of the first phalanx of the thumb. It is supplied by the deep branch of the ulnar nerve.

### Interosseous muscles

The interosseous muscles (Figs 2.81, 2.82) lie in the interosseus spaces between the metacarpal bones. They are in two groups, palmar and dorsal. The palmar interossei are arranged in such a way that they produce adduction of the fingers by moving them towards the middle finger. The dorsal interossei are abductors of the fingers, i.e. moving the fingers away from the axis of the movement going through the middle of the middle finger. It is easier to work out the arrangement of the interosseous muscles by remembering the words PAD (palmar interossei adducts) and DAB (dorsal interossei abduct). When the palmar and the dorsal interossei act together they, like the lumbricals, can flex the metacarpophalangeal joints and extend the interphalangeal joints. All the interossei are supplied by the deep branch of the ulnar nerve. The interossei and hence the ulnar nerve can be tested by keeping a card between two fingers and asking the patient to hold it firmly. Inability to do so indicates weakness or paralysis of the muscles.

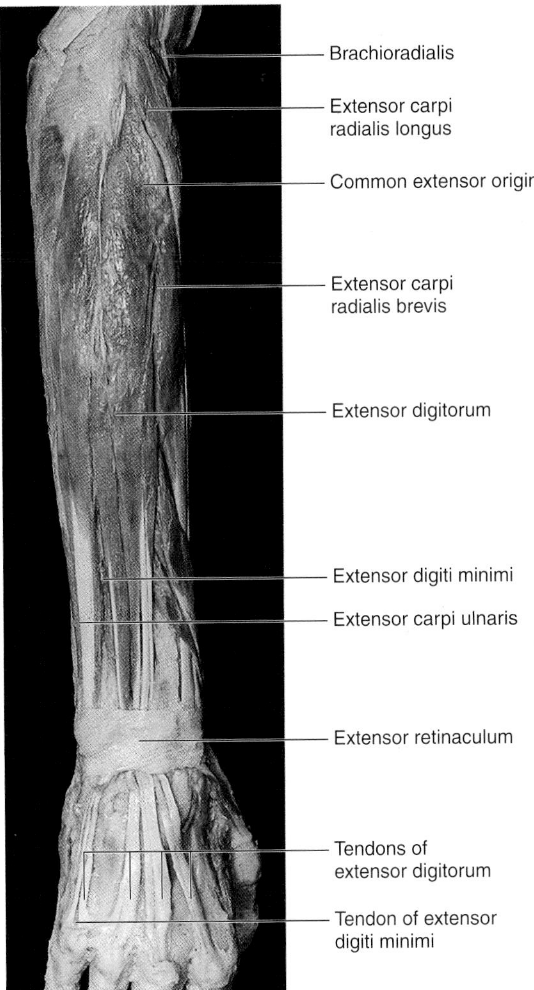


Fig. 2.83 Superficial extensor muscles at the back of forearm.

## Back of the forearm and hand

### The superficial extensor muscles at the back of the forearm

The extensor carpi radialis longus takes origin from the lateral supracondylar ridge just below the origin of the brachioradialis. The extensor carpi radialis brevis, the extensor digitorum, the extensor carpi ulnaris and the extensor digiti minimi (Fig. 2.83) have a common origin from the front of the lateral epicondyle (common extensor origin). The extensors of the carpus are inserted into the metacarpal bones. Four tendons arise from the extensor digitorum which pass deep to the extensor retinaculum to enter the dorsum of the hand where they spread out to reach their insertions on the dorsal aspect of the digits. All these muscles are supplied by the posterior interosseous branch of the radial nerve, except the extensor carpi radialis longus, which like the brachioradialis is supplied by the

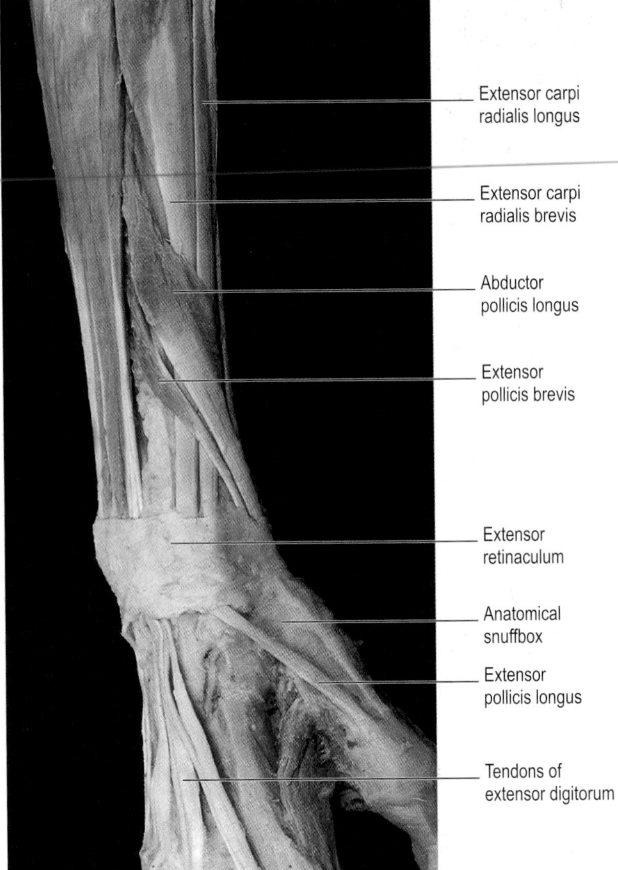


Fig. 2.84 Extensor retinaculum and the extensor tendons on the lateral aspect of wrist and hand.

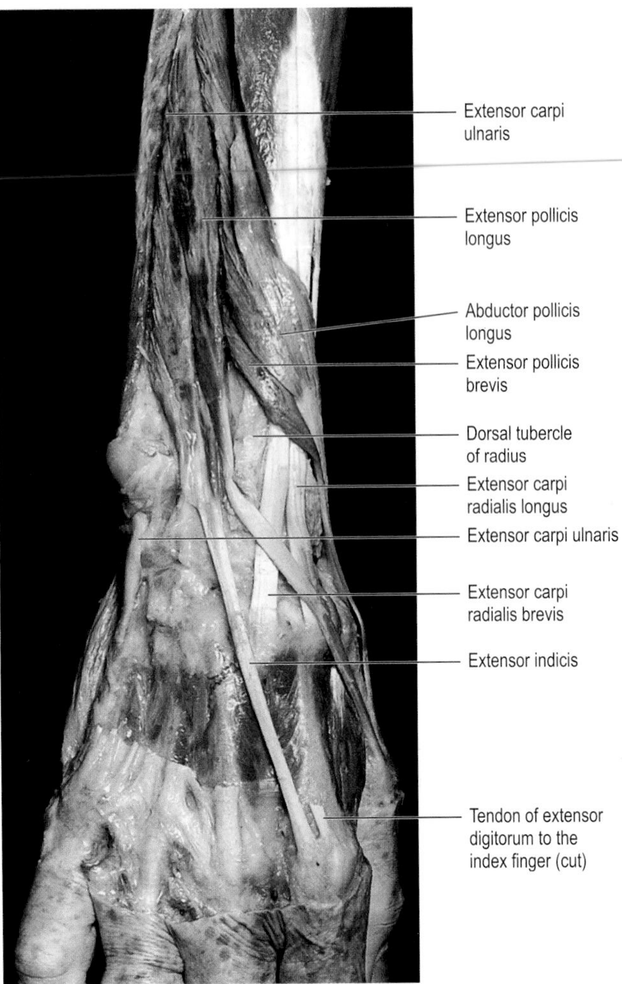


Fig. 2.85 Deep extensors at the back of the forearm (all the superficial extensors except extensor carpi radialis longus and brevis and extensor carpi ulnaris have been removed).

radial nerve just above the elbow (see wrist drop – Clinical box 2.11).

### Extensor retinaculum

The extensor retinaculum (Fig. 2.84) is a thick band of deep fascia attached proximally to the anterolateral border of the radius above the styloid process and distally and medially to the pisiform and triquetral bones. It has no attachment to the ulna. The retinaculum which is comparable to the flexor retinaculum prevents bowstringing of the extensor tendons when the hand is hyperextended. The extensor tendons lie in six separate compartments deep to the retinaculum. Most tendons have their own independent synovial sheaths. The four tendons of the digitorum and the extensor indicis share a common sheath. The abductor pollicis longus and the extensor pollicis brevis can be seen superficially in the distal part of the forearm winding round the radius before passing deep to the retinaculum.

### The deep extensors

This group (Fig. 2.85) contains the long abductor and the extensors of the thumb as well as the extensor indicis. They are attached to both the ulna and radius and the interosseous membrane. ✪ The extensor pollicis longus tendon winding round the dorsal tubercle (Lister's tubercle) of the radius on its way to its insertion to the distal phalanx of thumb can rupture spontaneously or as a consequence of fracture of the lower end of the radius (Colles' fracture). The flexor pollicis longus will then overact, producing a flexion deformity of the distal phalanx of the thumb (hammer thumb). The extensor indicis is an additional extensor for the index finger. Its tendon joins the ulnar side of the extensor digitorum tendon on the index finger. This muscle can be connected on to the tendon of the extensor pollicis longus to repair a hammer thumb.

### Supinator

This muscle (Fig. 2.86) covering the upper part of the back of the radius lies deep to the brachioradialis and the superficial extensors. The muscle is closely related to the radial nerve. The posterior interosseous branch of the radial nerve (deep branch of the radial) passes through the supinator before giving its branches to the extensor muscles in the forearm. The supinator which is inserted into the posterolateral aspect of the upper part of the radius supinates the forearm in the extended position.

### Superficial structures at the dorsum of the hand

The veins in the digits drain into a dorsal venous arch from which the cephalic and basilic veins are formed (Figs 2.88, 2.89). The former crosses the anatomical snuff box and courses upwards along the lateral aspect in the front of the forearm. The basilic vein arising from the medial aspect of the venous arch runs upwards along the posteromedial aspect of the forearm. The superficial branch of the radial

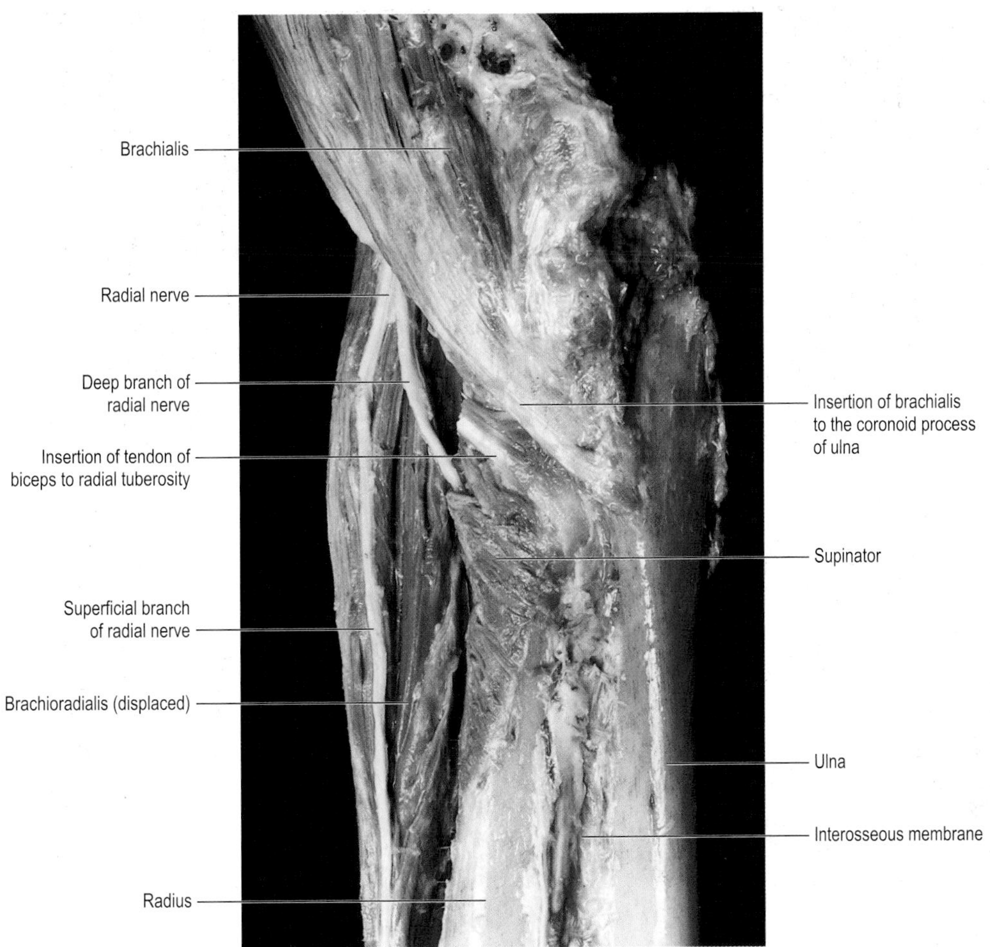


Fig. 2.86 Upper end of radius and ulna with supinator and radial nerve. Right side, oblique view.

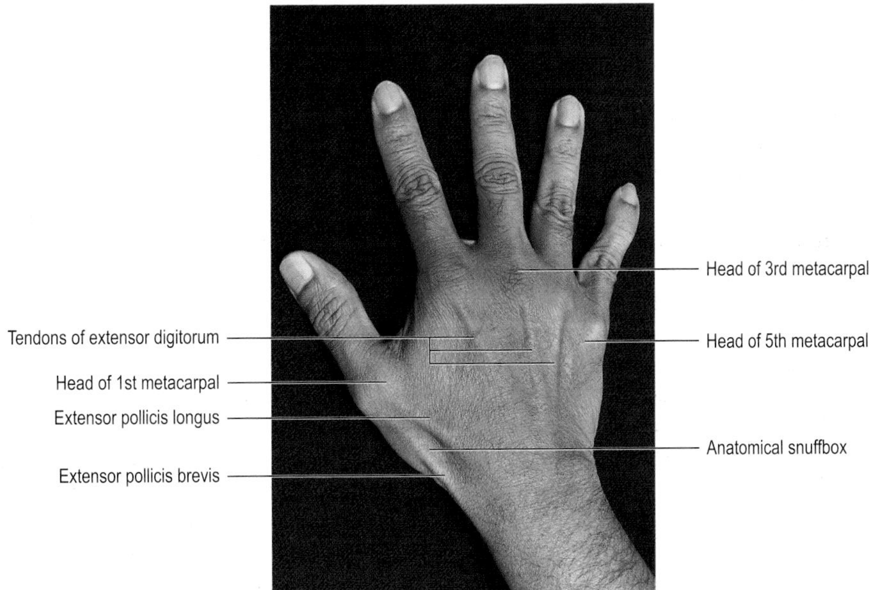


Fig. 2.87 Dorsum of the hand – surface anatomy.

nerve and the dorsal branch of ulnar nerves innervate the skin of the dorsum of the hand and digits. The radial nerve supplies the lateral two and a half or even three and a half fingers (variable) and the corresponding region of the dorsum of the hand. The remaining medial aspect is supplied by the ulnar nerve. The dorsal aspect of the terminal phalanges are supplied by the palmar digital branches (median and ulnar nerves) winding round the borders of the digits to reach the dorsal aspect. The radial artery reaches the anatomical snuff box by winding round the lateral border of the wrist. From there it passes deep to the extensor pollicis longus tendon before piercing the first

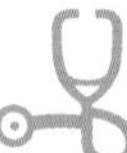

*Clinical box 2.21*

**Dorsum of the hand, anatomical snuff box**

The space proximal to the thumb bounded medially by the extensor pollicis longus and laterally by the tendons of the abductor pollicis longus and the extensor pollicis brevis is the anatomical snuff box (Fig. 2.87). The scaphoid bone forms its floor. The radial artery lies in it and the cephalic vein and the superficial branch of the radial nerve cross it superficially. After a fall on the outstretched hand, tenderness in the anatomical snuff box is suggestive of a fracture of the scaphoid bone. The tendons of the extensor digitorum are also visible as the wrist is extended against resistance. The metacarpal bones are easily palpable on the dorsum of the hand.

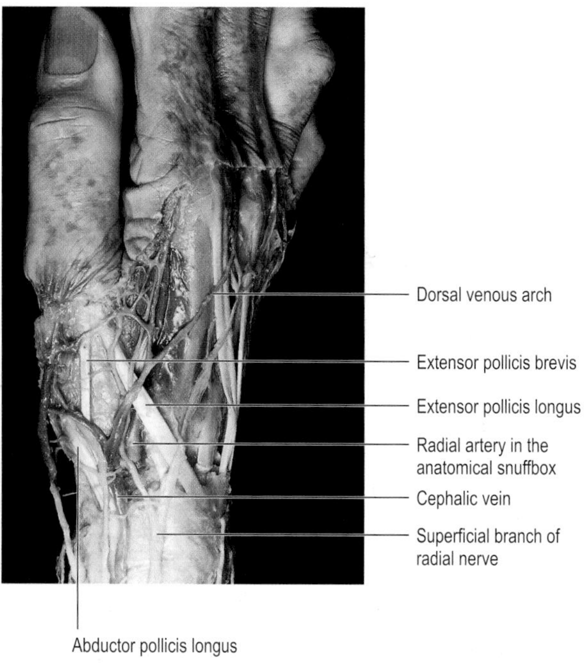


Fig. 2.88 Superficial structures on the dorsum of hand – lateral aspect.

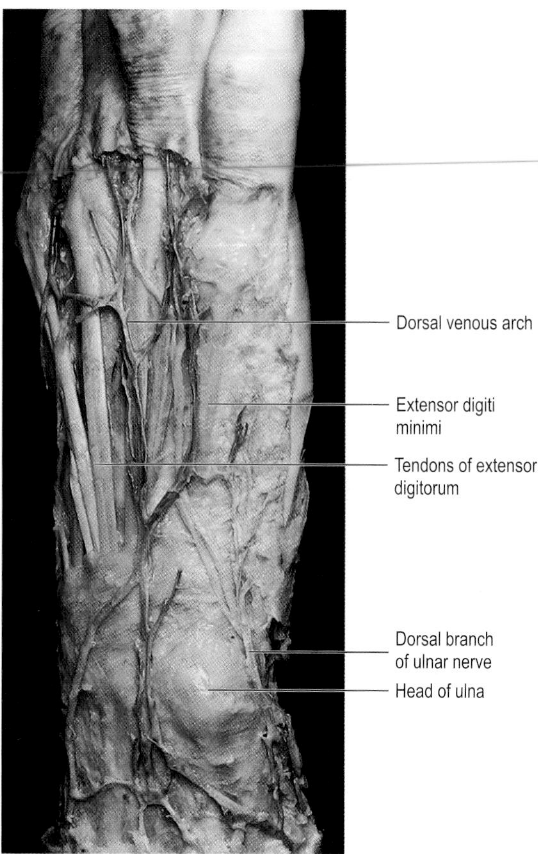


Fig. 2.89 Superficial structures on the dorsum of hand – medial aspect.

dorsal interosseous muscle to reach the palm of the hand to become the deep palmar arch.

### Extensor tendons on the dorsum of the hand

The extensors of the carpus are inserted into the metacarpal bones; the radial (lateral) extensors into the bases of the first and second metacarpal bones and the ulnar extensor into the fifth metacarpal bone. The extensor digitorum forms the extensor expansion at the back of the fingers (see below) and the extensor digiti minimi which divides into two slips reinforces the extensor expansion at the back of the little finger. The extensor indicis is an additional extensor for the index finger. Its tendon joins the ulnar side of the extensor digitorum tendon on the index finger (Fig. 2.90).

The tendons reaching the thumb are inserted as follows:

- abductor pollicis longus to the lateral aspect of the base of the first metacarpal bone
- extensor pollicis brevis to the base of the first phalanx
- extensor pollicis longus to the base of the distal phalanx.

### The extensor expansion (dorsal digital expansion)

At the wrist the extensor digitorum gives rise to four tendons which supply digits 2–5. Each slip forms an expanded hood over the dorsum of the digit (Fig. 2.91). The expansion is attached to the base of the proximal phalanx before dividing into a central and two marginal slips. The central slip is inserted into the base of the middle phalanx. The marginal slips unite together and insert to the base of the distal phalanx. The interossei and the lumbricals are inserted into the proximal part of the extensor expansion.

## The joints of the forearm and hand

### Elbow joint

See Figures 2.92–2.94.

#### Osteology

At the elbow joint the upper surface of the head of radius articulates with the capitulum of the humerus and the trochlea of the humerus with the trochlear notch of the ulna. The capsule of the elbow also encloses the superior radioulnar joint where the head of the radius articulates with the radial notch of the ulna.

#### Relations of the joint

Posteriorly there is the insertion of the triceps to the olecranon (Fig. 2.95). ✪ The ulnar nerve lies on the back of the medial epicondyle on the medial collateral ligament of the joint and may be damaged in a posterior dislocation, by fracture of the medial epicondyle, or by compression of the nerve against it. The brachial artery and the median nerve lie in front of the elbow joint. The radial nerve lies on the

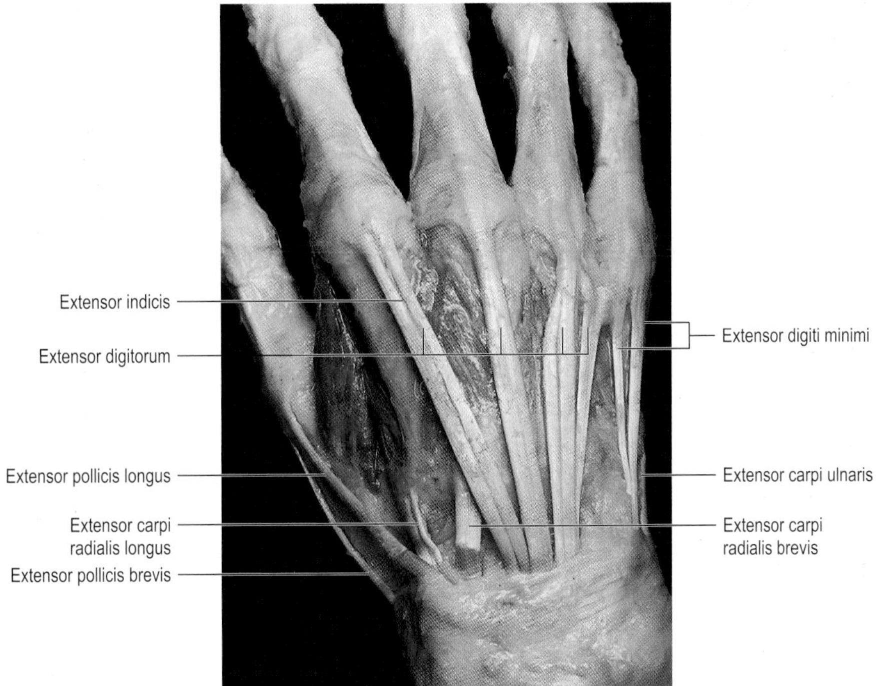


Fig. 2.90 Extensor tendons on the dorsum of hand.

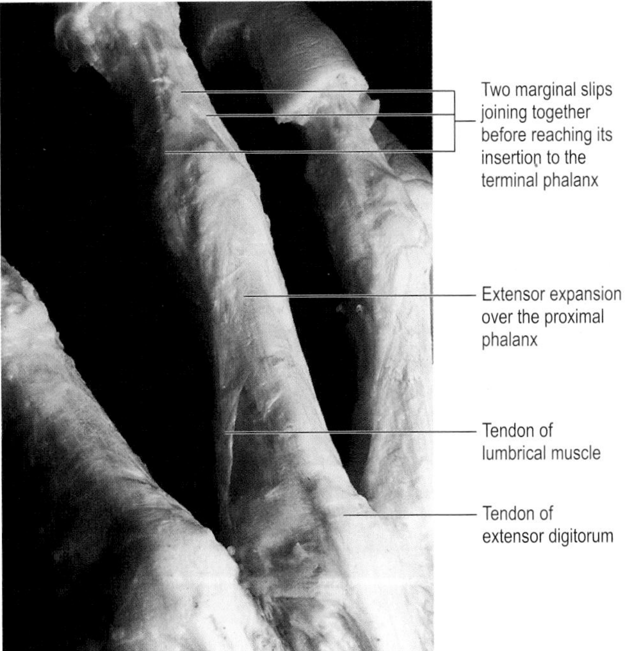


Fig. 2.91 Extensor expansion or dorsal digital expansion.

anterior surface of the lateral epicondyle. Also anteriorly there is the insertion of the tendon of the biceps to the radial tuberosity and that of the brachialis to the coronoid process of the ulna. The common flexor origin from the medial epicondyle and the common extensor origin from the lateral epicondyle are the other anterior relations of the joint.

✪ The surgical approaches to the joint are usually from the medial or the lateral sides. In the medial approach the common flexor origin is detached after displacing the ulnar nerve to expose the capsule. In the lateral approach the common extensor origin is detached. The posterior interosseous nerve is vulnerable if the incision is extended below the level of the head of the radius.

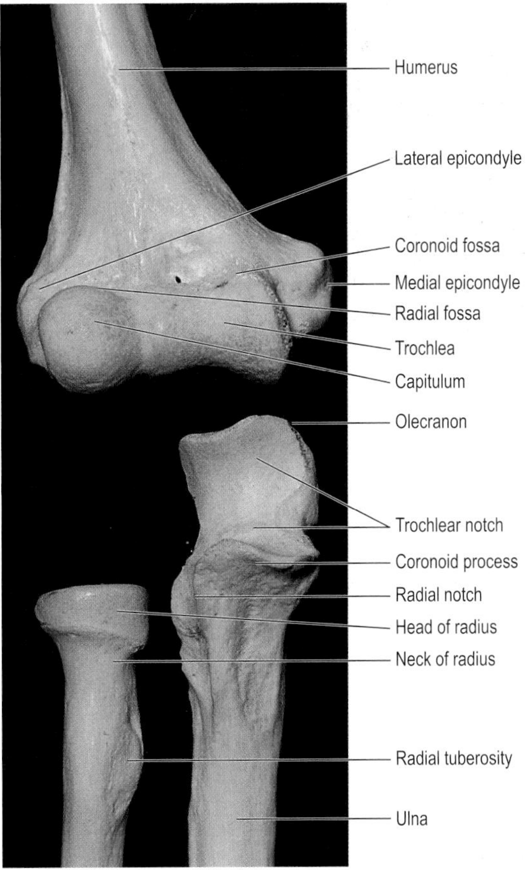


Fig. 2.92 Lower end of humerus and upper ends of radius and ulna – anterior aspect.

## Capsule and the interior of the joint

The elbow joint is a synovial joint. The capsular attachment on the humerus extends from the outer margins of the capitulum and trochlea upwards to enclose the olecranon fossa posteriorly and the coronoid fossa and radial fossa anteriorly (Figs 2.96–2.101). The medial and lateral

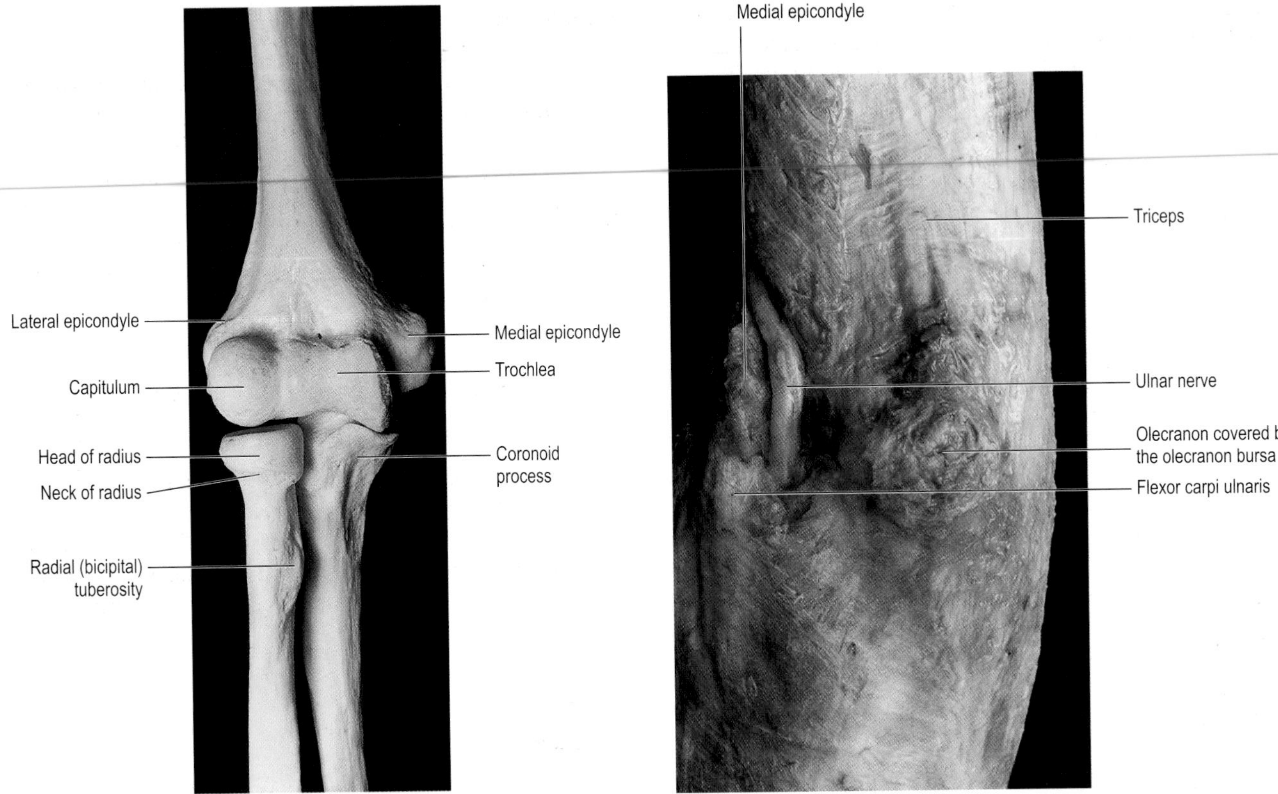


Fig. 2.93 Bones of the elbow in the articulated position – anterior aspect.

Fig. 2.95 Structures related to the posterior aspect of the elbow joint.

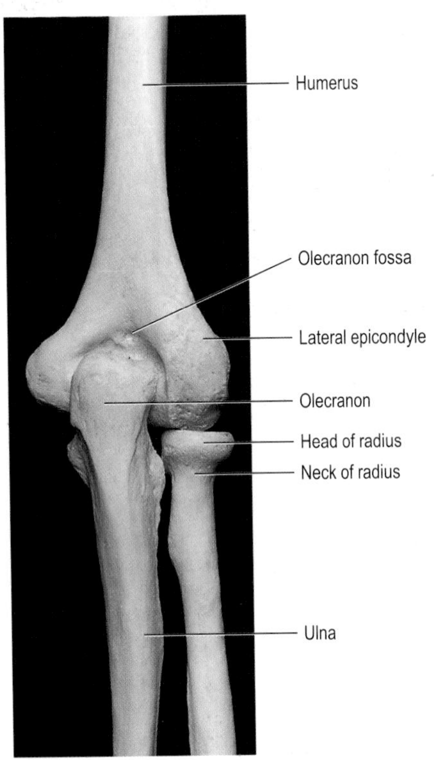


Fig. 2.94 Bones of the elbow joint in the articulated position – posterior aspect.

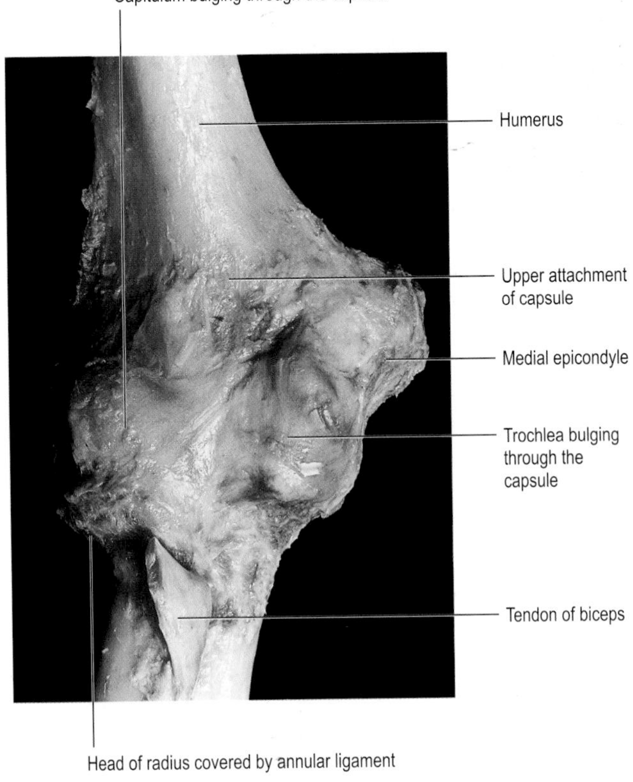


Fig. 2.96 Capsule of the elbow joint – anterior aspect.

epicondyles and the supracondylar ridges are extracapsular. Distally the capsule is attached to the margins of the trochlear notch of the ulna and the annular ligament. It is not directly attached to the radius. The capsule, and the olecranon, coronoid and radial fossae are all lined by synovial membrane.

### Ligaments

The capsule is reinforced by extracapsular ligaments on either side. The triangular medial (ulnar) collateral ligament is attached to the medial epicondyle, coronoid process and the olecranon (Fig. 2.99). The ulnar nerve lies on this ligament. The lateral (radial) collateral ligament extends from the lateral epicondyle to the annular ligament. It is not attached to the radius.

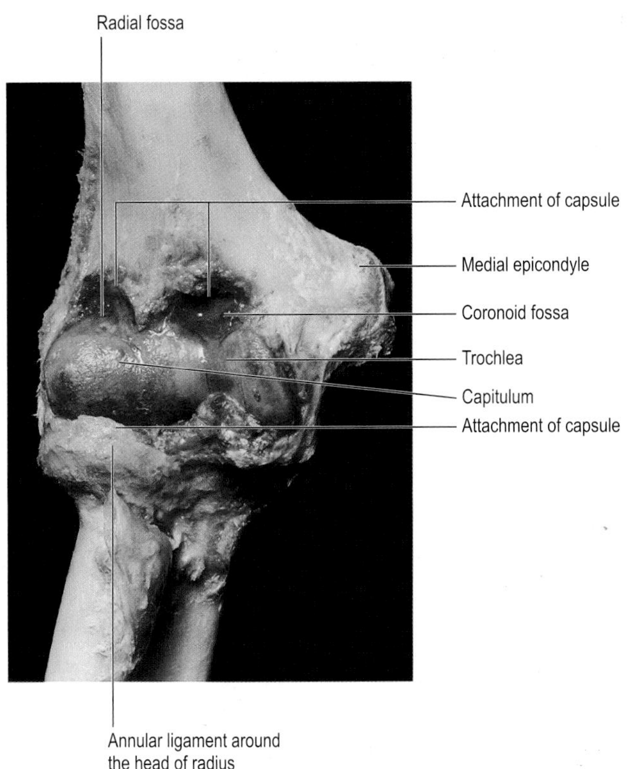


Fig. 2.97 Interior of the elbow joint – anterior aspect.

### Movements

The long axis of the ulna is not in line with that of the humerus but is shifted outwards making the carrying angle of about 170°. An increase of this valgus angle (cubitus valgus) due to fractures or epiphyseal injuries will stretch the ulnar nerve. The normal carrying angle of the elbow joint causes the axis of movements to be in an oblique plane. Flexion is about 140° and is done primarily by the brachialis and the biceps muscles and extension by the triceps muscle. See Clinical box 2.22.

## The radioulnar joints: pronation and supination

The radius and ulna articulate with each other at the superior and inferior radioulnar joints. In the superior radioulnar joint, which shares the capsule of the elbow joint, the head of the radius articulates with the radial notch of the ulna. The two bones are held together by the annular

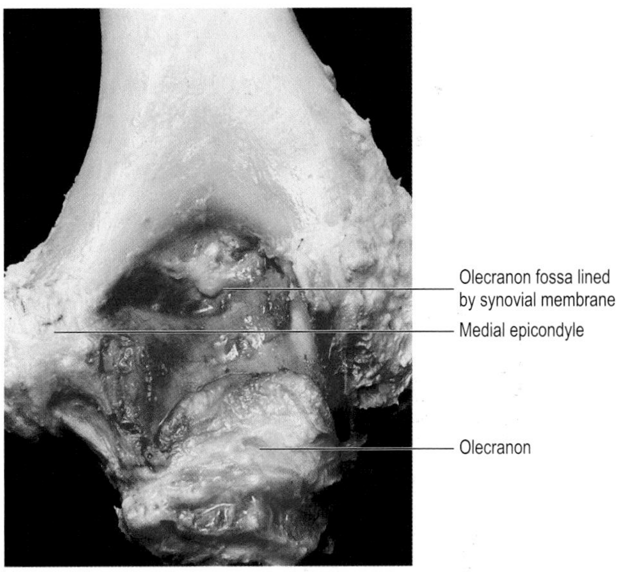


Fig. 2.98 Interior of the elbow joint – posterior aspect (elbow in semiflexed position).

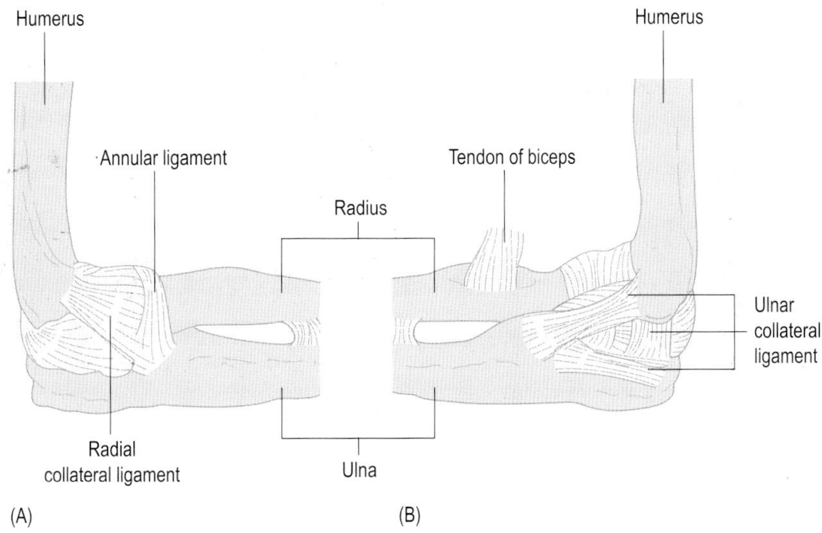


Fig. 2.99 Right elbow joint: (A) lateral view; (B) medial view.

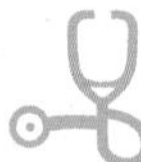

## Clinical box 2.22

### Tennis elbow, Golfer's elbow and Student's elbow

Overuse of muscles and tendons can lead on to pain and inflammation around the elbow joint. In tennis elbow, also known as lateral epicondylitis, the muscles involved are the extensors of the wrist which has a common origin from the lateral epicondyle. Though the actual cause of the condition is not clearly known, it is thought to be due to microscopic tears of the tendinous attachment of the muscles to the epicondyle. Pain is on the lateral aspect of the elbow and is worse when the wrist is extended and a grip is made.

Golfer's elbow or medial epicondylitis is a counterpart of tennis elbow where the pain is on the medial aspect of the elbow and forearm especially when gripping objects. Though called golfer's elbow it can occur in carpenters and others who move their wrist repeatedly gripping tools.

Student's elbow is caused by inflammation of the olecranon bursa and hence is also known as the olecranon bursitis. The bursa overlies the olecranon at the back of the elbow.

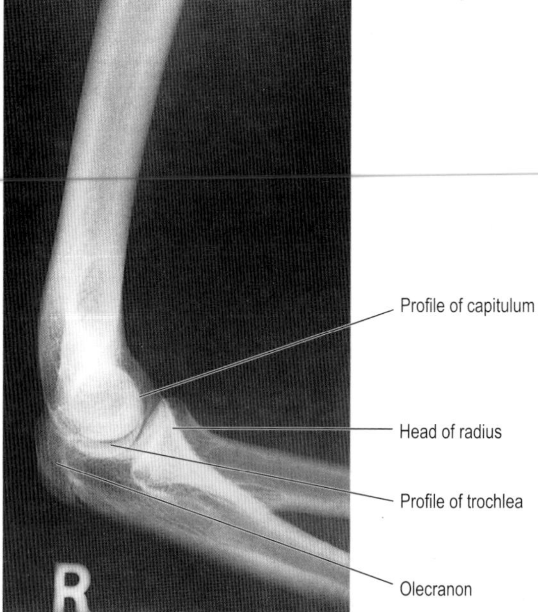


Fig. 2.101 Lateral radiograph of the elbow joint – semi-flexed position.

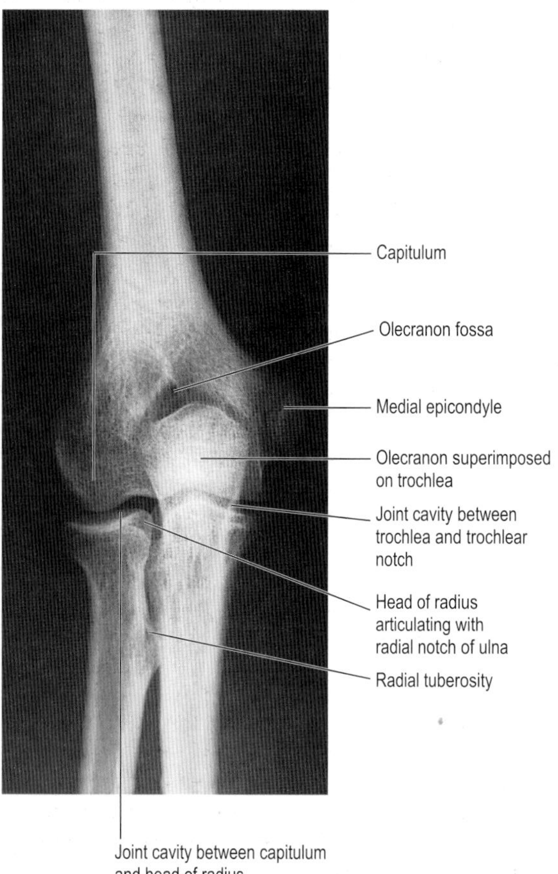


Fig. 2.100 Anteroposterior radiograph of elbow joint.

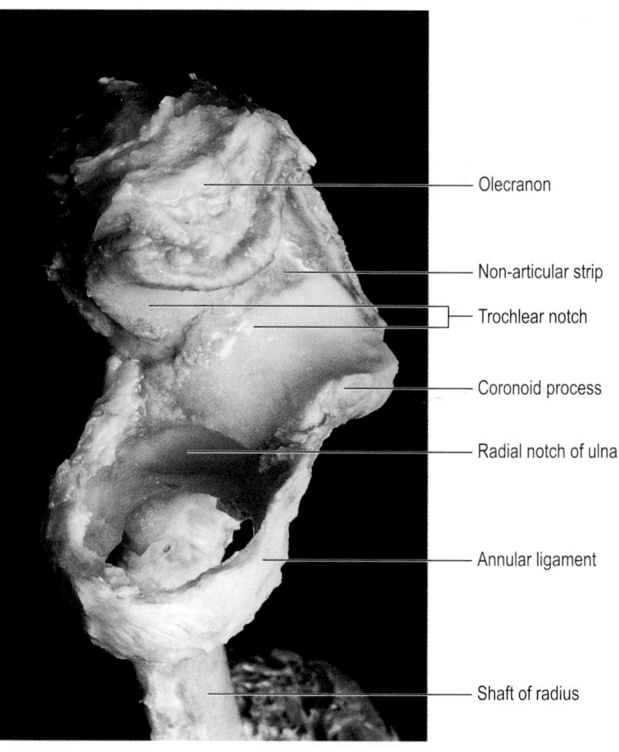


Fig. 2.102 Annular ligament after removal of the upper end of radius. Viewed from above.

ligament (Fig. 2.102). The ligament is attached to the anterior and posterior margins of the radial notch of the ulna but is not attached to the radius. It circles round the head and neck of the radius. The upper end of the radius is totally free of ligamentous attachments enabling the radius to rotate freely inside the annular ligament. The inferior radioulnar joint between the head of the ulna is outside the capsule of the wrist joint. Here a triangular fibrocartilagenous disc extends from the ulnar notch of the radius to the fossa at the base of the ulnar styloid. The radius and ulna are also connected by the interosseous membrane (Fig. 2.103).

At the superior and inferior radioulnar joints the radius rotates inwards to produce pronation (Fig. 2.104). Pronation makes the palm of the hand face backwards in the anatomical position or downwards if the arm is flexed (Fig. 2.105). This movement is produced by the pronator teres

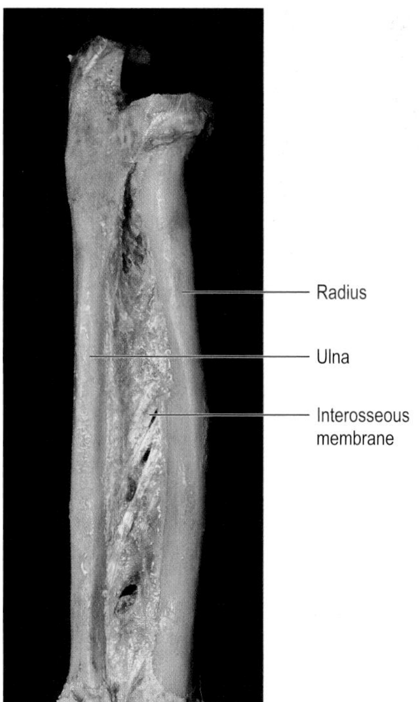


Fig. 2.103 Interosseous membrane – posterior aspect (right side).

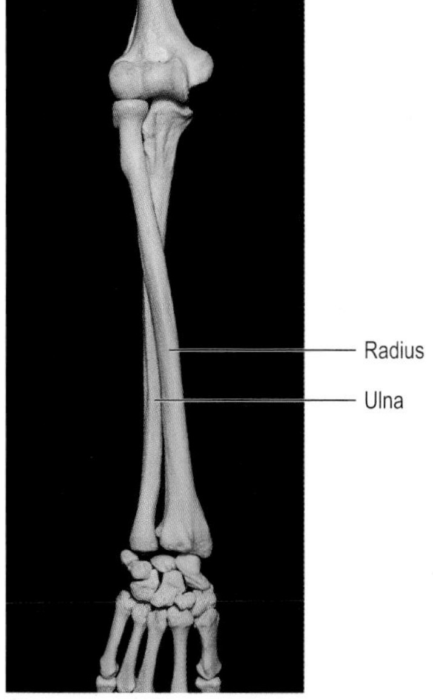


Fig. 2.104 Radius and ulna in pronation. Note that the radius crosses over the ulna carrying the hand with it.

and the pronator quadratus. The opposite movement is supination in which the radius rotates outwards. In the flexed position of the elbow, the bicep acts as a powerful supinator. Supination is weak when the elbow is extended and is done by the supinator muscle. The axis of pronation and supination is across a line passing through the head of the radius to the styloid process of the ulna. However the ulna is not entirely stationary during these movements. Its distal end moves slightly posterolaterally during pronation and anteromedially in supination. About 140° of rotation of the forearm can take place during pronation and supination. It can however be further increased by rotation of the humerus and the scapula. See Clinical box 2.23.

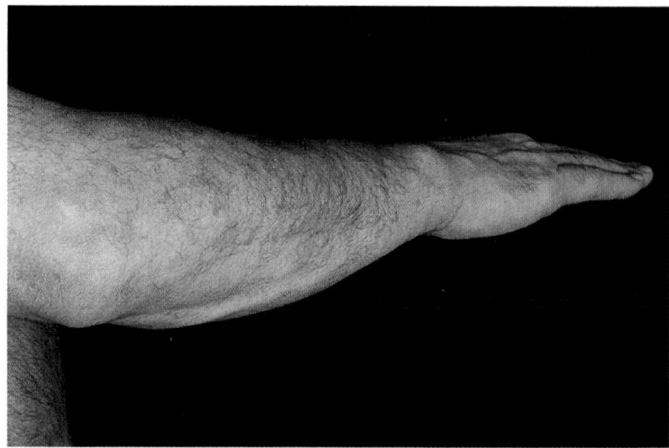

Fig. 2.105 Pronation of forearm.

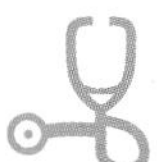

### *Clinical box 2.23*

**Injuries of forearm bones and joints**

A fall on the outstretched hand can cause a fracture at the lower half shaft of the radius and dislocate the inferior radioulnar joint. This is known as the Galeazzi fracture-dislocation. It is analogous to the Monteggia fracture-dislocation where the fracture is at the upper half of the shaft of the ulna along with dislocation of the superior radioulnar joint. More commonly seen is a Colles' fracture almost always caused by a fall on the outstretched hand producing a dinner-fork deformity. The radius is fractured transversely a few centimetres above its lower end. The lower fragment may be displaced backwards and laterally and is tilted backwards, making the lower articular surface face backwards instead of slightly forwards as it normally does.

In a young child a sudden pull on the forearm may result in the head of the radius being pulled partly outside the annular ligament. This injury is termed a 'pulled elbow'. In children the head of the radius is not fully formed and the annular ligament is circular. The annular ligament is of conical shape in the adult, facilitating a better grip on the radius.

## The wrist joint

A number of synovial joints are present at the wrist region. The radiocarpal joint, also known as the wrist joint, is a biaxial joint. The midcarpal joint, between the two rows of carpal bones, and the intercarpal joint between the carpal bones (Fig. 2.106) are synovial joints with irregular joint cavities. These joint cavities communicate with each other and with those of the carpometacarpal joints and intermetacarpal joints (between the bases of the metacarpals).

At the wrist joint (radiocarpal joint) the scaphoid, lunate and triquetral bones articulate proximally with the distal end of the radius and the triangular fibrocartilagenous disc connecting the distal end of radius and ulna (Figs 2.108, 2.109). The radius articulates with the scaphoid and the lunate. The head of ulna which does not take part in the

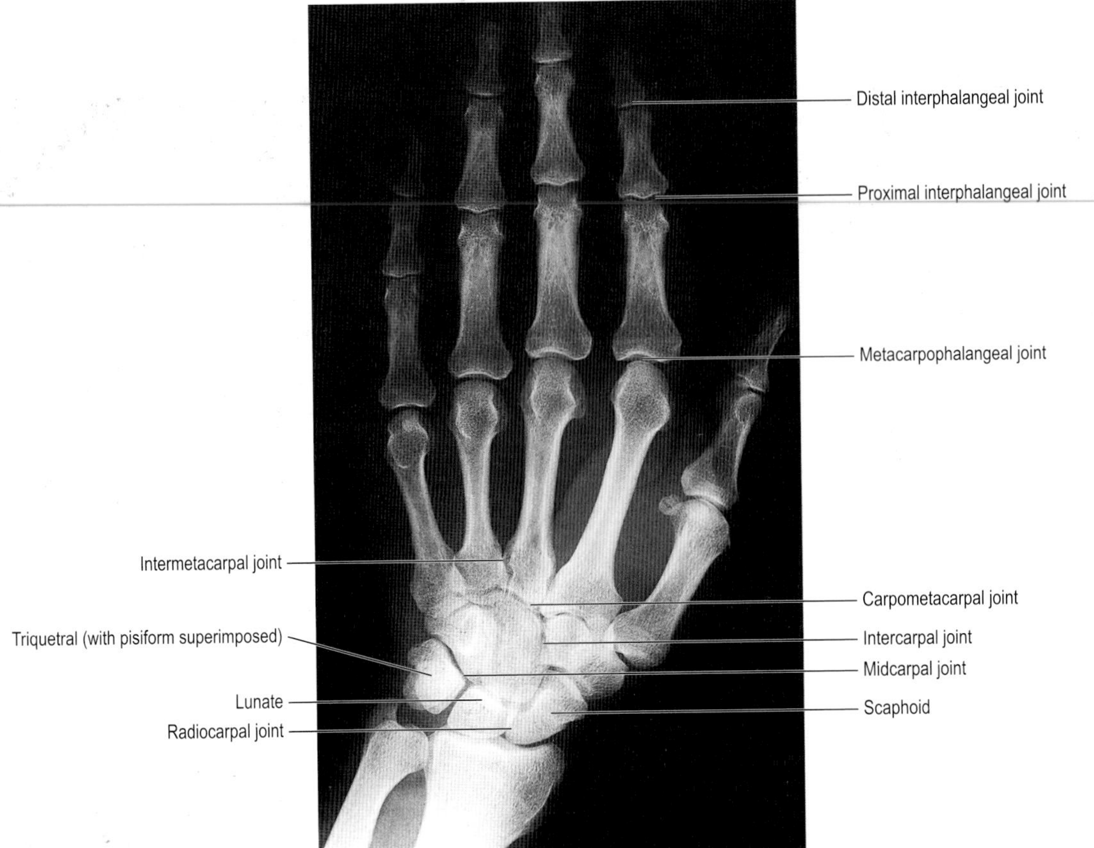


Fig. 2.106 Radiograph of joints of wrist and hand.

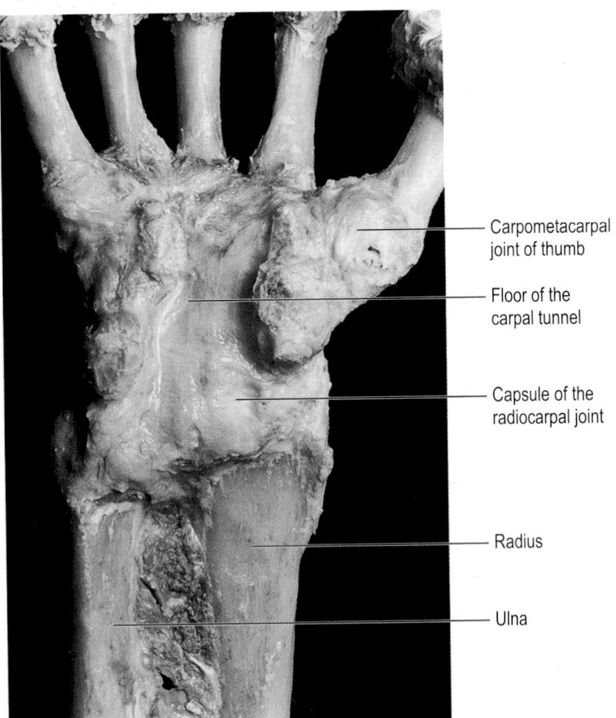


Fig. 2.107 Capsule of radiocarpal joint and the floor of carpal tunnel formed by capsule of midcarpal and intercarpal joints.

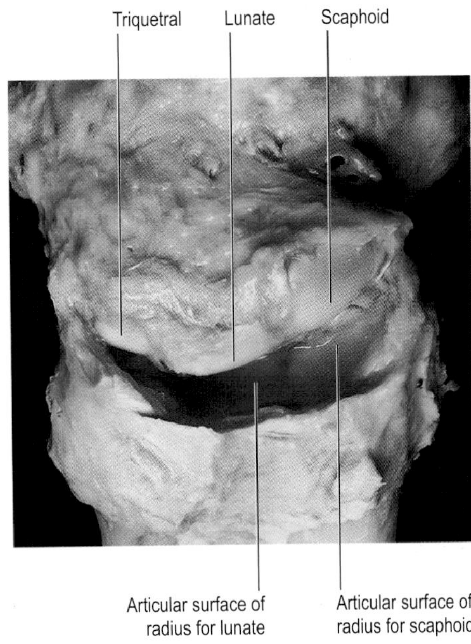


Fig. 2.108 Interior of wrist joint – anterior view.

formation of the joint is separated from the triquetral by the fibrocartilagenous disc which also separates the wrist joint from the inferior radioulnar joint. A capsule (Fig. 2.107) which is reinforced by palmar, dorsal and radial and ulnar collateral ligaments surrounds the joint.

## Movements

Movements of the wrist joint are accompanied by similar movements at the midcarpal joint which is between the carpal bones. The range of movements and the muscles producing them are given below:

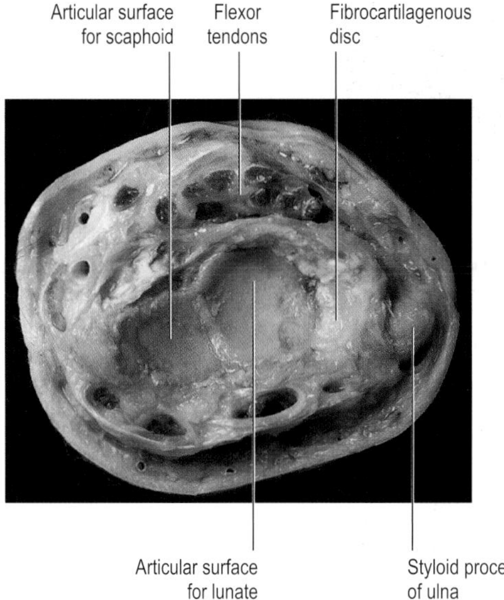


Fig. 2.109 Transverse section at the level of wrist joint showing the distal articular surface (for scaphoid and lunate) of the radius and the fibrocartilagenous disc connecting radius and ulna onto which the triquetral articulates.

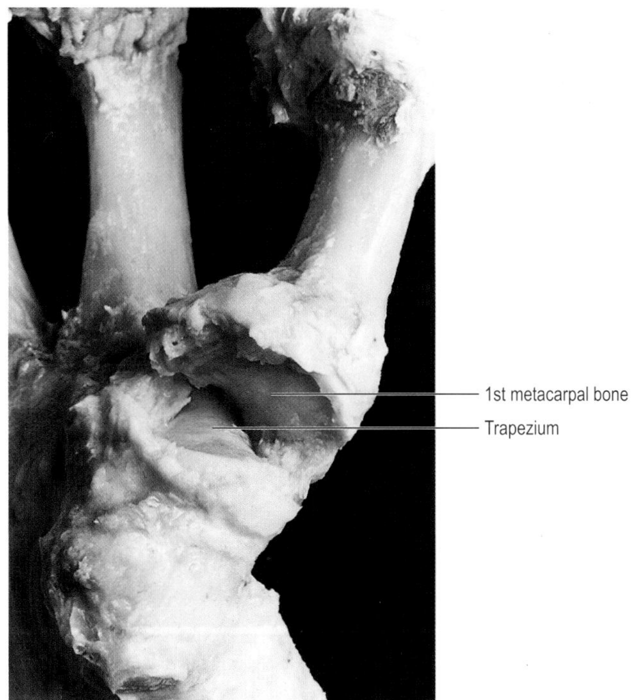


Fig. 2.110 Interior of carpometacarpal joint of thumb.

| Movement | Muscles |
|---|---|
| Flexion — about 80° mostly at the midcarpal joint | Flexor carpi radialis and flexor carpi ulnaris aided by the long flexors of the digits and thumb and the abductor pollicis longus |
| Extension about 60° mostly at the wrist joint | Extensor carpi radialis longus and brevis and extensor carpi ulnaris assisted by extensors of the fingers and thumb |
| Abduction — limited to 15° due to radial styloid process projecting down | Flexor carpi radialis and extensor carpi radialis longus and brevis assisted by abductor pollicis longus |
| Adduction — about 45° | Flexor carpi ulnaris and extensor carpi ulnaris |

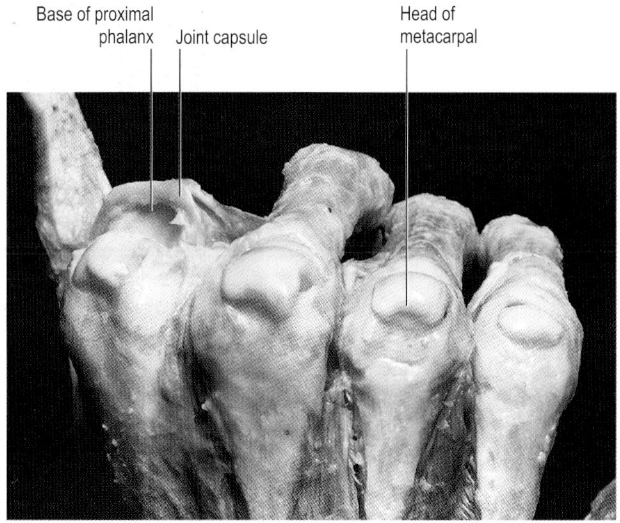


Fig. 2.111 Metacarpophalangeal joints.

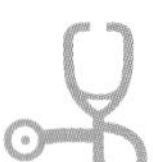

*Clinical box 2.24*

**Bennett's fracture**

This is a fracture of the base of the first metacarpal bone involving the carpometacarpal joint of the thumb. This is usually sustained as a result of a blow to the point of the thumb as can occur in boxing.

Surgical approach to the joint is usually through the dorsal surface between the tendons of the extensor pollicis longus and the extensor digitorum and the indicis as this area has no major vessels or nerves. Also see Clinical box 2.11.

### Carpometacarpal joint of the thumb

The joint is between the trapezium and the first metacarpal bone and has a separate joint cavity (Fig. 2.110). This is where most of the movements of the thumb take place. The articular surfaces are reciprocally saddle-shaped to facilitate versatility of thumb movements including opposition. See Clinical box 2.24.

### The metacarpophalangeal joints

These are synovial joints allowing flexion and extension as well as abduction and adduction (Fig. 2.111). They lie along the distal skin crease of the palm where the prominence of the metacarpal heads can be easily felt. The joints are thus proximal to the interdigital webs. The palmar ligaments of these joints are strong fibrocartilagenous pads which are connected to each other by the deep transverse metacarpal ligament. These joints lie on the arc of a circle. Because of this when the fingers are extended they diverge from each other, whereas when they are flexed they crowd together in the palm. The collateral ligaments of the joints are taut in flexion and this limits abduction and adduction of the fixed joints.

The interphalangeal joints are hinge joints allowing only flexion and extension without any abduction and adduction. Their collateral ligaments are taut in all positions of the joints.

# Chapter 3
# Thorax



## The thoracic cage and the intercostal space

The bony thoracic cage is formed by the 12 thoracic vertebrae at the back, the sternum in front and 12 pairs of ribs in between (Fig. 3.1). The upper seven pairs of ribs articulate anteriorly direct with the sternum through their respective costal cartilages. The costal cartilage of ribs 8, 9 and 10 articulates with that of the rib above. These ribs with the xiphisternum form the lower costal margin. The lowermost point of the thoracic cage is the 10th costal cartilage.

The space between two adjacent ribs is known as the intercostal space. Thus there are 11 intercostal spaces on each side.

The junction between the manubrium and the body of the sternum is the sternal angle. The second costal cartilage articulates at the sternal angle (Figs 3.1, 3.2). This is an important landmark and corresponds to the level of the lower border of the 4th thoracic vertebra. The seventh costal cartilage anteriorly articulates at the junction between the body of the sternum and the xiphisternum. The 8th, 9th and 10th ribs each articulate with the rib above. The 11th and 12th ribs are the floating ribs as they have no connection to bone or cartilage in front. See Clinical box 3.1.

### Surface anatomy

The sternal angle is palpable on the surface as a transverse ridge (Fig. 3.1). This landmark is used to palpate the second costal cartilage and the second rib. It is possible to identify the other ribs as well as intercostal spaces by counting down from the second rib.

The first rib is not palpable as it is under the clavicle. Ribs 11 and 12 are rudimentary, confined to the back covered by muscles and hence are not palpable.

### The intercostal space

The intercostal space (Fig. 3.3) contains the external intercostal, the internal intercostal and the innermost intercostal muscles arranged in three layers. The neurovascular bundle, consisting of the intercostal nerve and vessels, lies in between the internal and the innermost intercostals.

The external intercostal muscle fibres are directed downwards and forwards. In the anterior part the muscle fibres are replaced by a membrane. The internal intercostal fibres lie in the opposite direction to those of the external. The neurovascular bundle lies between the internal and the innermost intercostal muscles. ✪ If it is necessary to insert a chest drain or a needle into the intercostal space it is always placed in the lower part of the space to avoid damage to the neurovascular bundle (which lies along the lower border of the rib along the upper part of the space). The neurovascular bundle consists of, from above downwards, intercostal vein, artery and nerve. See Clinical box 3.2.

The intercostal nerves are the anterior rami of the first 11 thoracic nerves. These supply the intercostal muscles, the skin of the chest wall as well as the parietal pleura. The lower intercostal nerves, 7th downwards, supply the

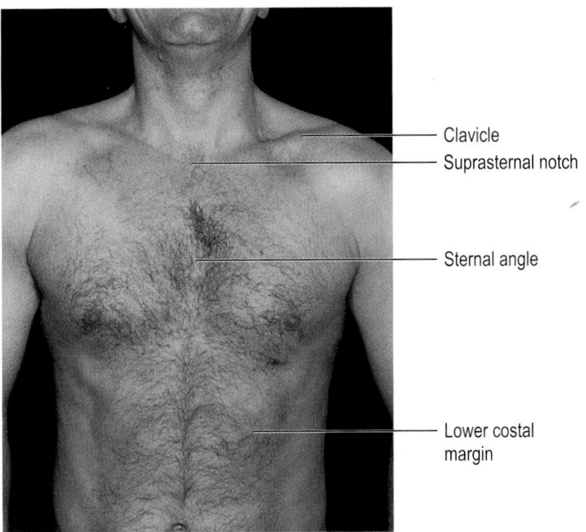


Fig. 3.1 Surface anatomy of the chest wall.

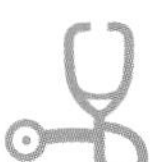

*Clinical box 3.1*

**Rib fractures and 'stove-in-chest'**

Rib fractures can be fracture of a single rib or can be multiple fractures and are caused by direct blow on the rib or by a crush injury. In a severe crush injury several ribs can fracture in front as well as behind producing a loose segment of chest wall disconnected from the rest. This is known as a 'stove-in-chest'. The loose segment may show paradoxical movements during respiration i.e. moves inwards during inspiration and blows out during expiration. Stove-in-chest is a serious condition needing urgent intubation and positive pressure ventilation using a respirator as well as a chest drain.

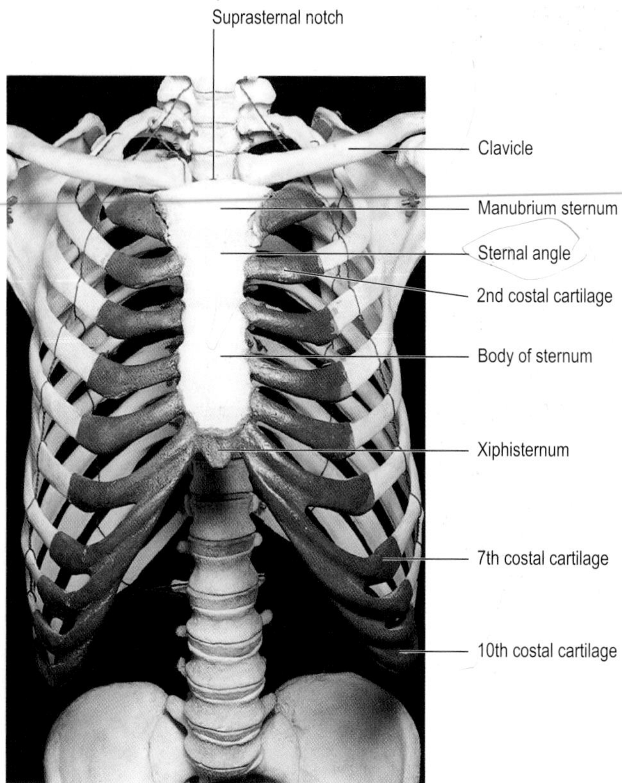


Fig. 3.2 Bony thoracic cage.

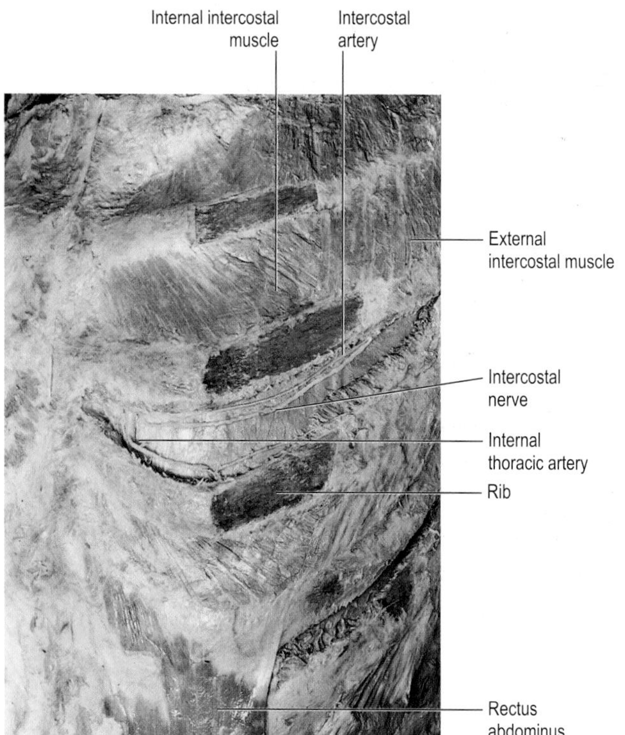


Fig. 3.3 Intercostal spaces (left side).

anterior abdominal wall as well. ✪ Segments of skin supplied by the intercostal nerves are common sites of vesicles in Herpes zoster, a viral infection affecting the spinal nerve ganglia spreading through the intercostal nerves.

The internal thoracic artery, a major artery on the anterior aspect of the chest wall, is a branch of the subclavian artery and it descends vertically downwards lying about 1cm

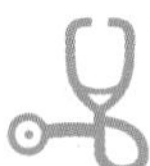

### *Clinical box 3.2*

**Thoracocentesis, insertion of a chest drain**

Insertion of a chest tube into the pleural cavity is required to remove large amounts of serous fluid, blood, pus or air. The site of insertion of the tube is usually at the 5th intercostal space just anterior to the midaxillary line on the affected side. This site will avoid the tube going through the pectoral muscles which lie more anteriorly and will avoid possible damage of liver (right side) and spleen (left side) which are overlapped by the pleural cavity more inferiorly (see Clinical box 3.3). Nerve to serratus anterior lies at the level of insertion of the tube and may be damaged occasionally, causing winging of the scapula (see Clinical box 2.1).

A needle thoracocentesis done in a critically ill patient with tension pneumothorax may be life saving. An over the needle catheter is inserted into the pleural cavity on the side of the tension pneumothorax through the second intercostal space in the midclavicular line. Insertion medial to the midclavicular line has a potential danger of damaging the great vessels in the mediastinum.

The needle or chest drain is always inserted superior to the rib (lower part of the intercostal space) to avoid damaging the neurovascular bundle. Damage of the intercostal nerve will cause neuritis and pain (neuralgia) and puncture of the vessels may result in bleeding into the pleural cavity (haemothorax).

The parietal pleura, the periosteum and other structures in the area of needle insertion and chest drain have rich innervation and hence a good local anaesthesia is required for procedures mentioned above.

lateral to the sternum. In the sixth intercostal space it divides into its two terminal branches, the musculophrenic and superior epigastric arteries, the latter entering the anterior abdominal wall by passing through the diaphragm

The anterior intercostal arteries are branches of the internal thoracic artery or those of its musculophrenic branch. Most of the posterior intercostal arteries are derived from the descending thoracic aorta. ✪ Anastomoses between the anterior and posterior intercostal arteries are important collateral channels for circulation in cases of obstruction to the blood flow in the aorta anywhere beyond the origin of the left subclavian artery.

## The thoracic cavity, lungs and pleura

The thoracic cavity contains on either side the right and left lungs surrounded by the pleural cavities and the mediastinum in between.

### The lungs and pleural cavities

See Figures 3.4–3.11. The right lung is subdivided into superior, middle and inferior lobes by an oblique fissure and a horizontal fissure (Figs 3.4 and 3.5). The left lung usually has only two lobes, a superior and an inferior with an oblique fissure in between. Each lung has an apex which extends about 3cm above the clavicle into the neck, a costal surface, a mediastinal surface and a base or diaphragmatic

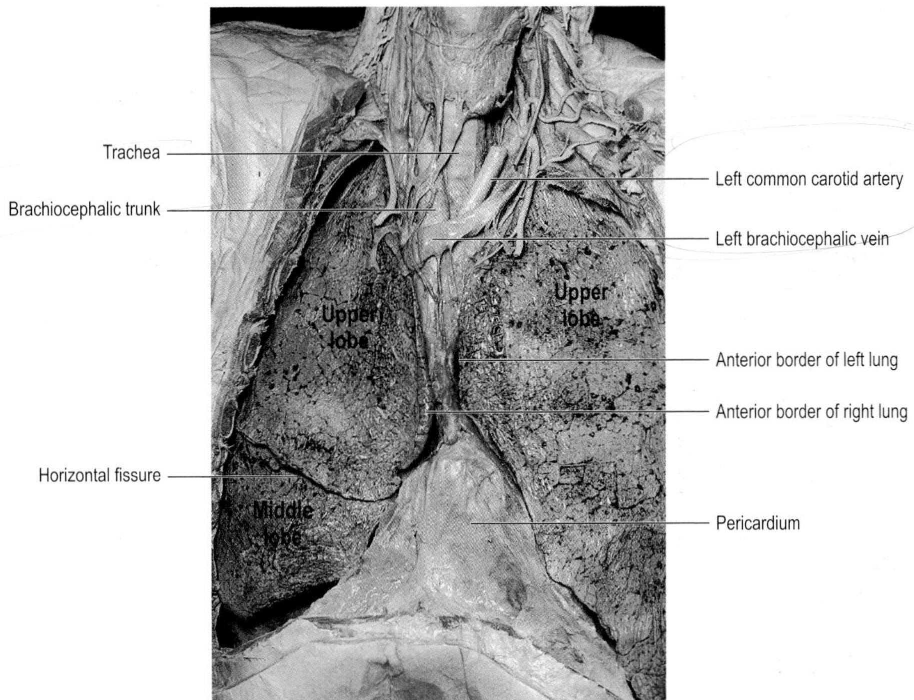


Fig. 3.4 The lungs in situ – anterior aspect.

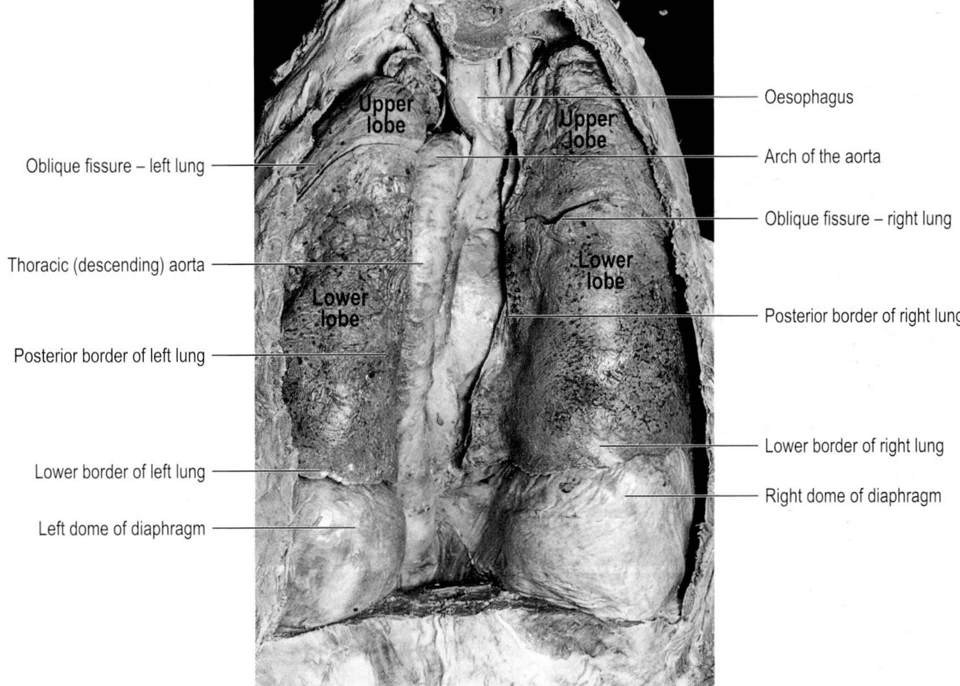


Fig. 3.5 The lungs in situ – posterior aspect.

surface (Figs 3.6 and 3.7). The anterior border of the lung separates the costal and the mediastinal surfaces whereas the lower border is between the costal and the diaphragmatic surface (Fig. 3.6).

The root of the lung connects the lung to the mediastinum and consists of, anterior to posterior, two pulmonary veins, the pulmonary artery and the bronchus. The pulmonary veins are at a lower level compared with the pulmonary artery (Figs 3.7 and 3.8). The area where these structures enter the lung is the hilum of the lung. These structures are enclosed in a sleeve of pleura which loosely hangs down in its lower part as the pulmonary ligament. The right main bronchus gives off the superior lobar bronchus outside the lung. All the branches of the left bronchus are given off inside the lung. The root of the lung also contains the bronchial arteries supplying the bronchi and bronchioles, the pulmonary plexus of autonomic nerves innervating the lung as well as the lymph nodes draining the lung. The phrenic nerve lies in front of the root of the lung and the vagus nerve behind.

✪ The right bronchus is shorter, wider and more vertical than the left. The angle between the two bronchi is about

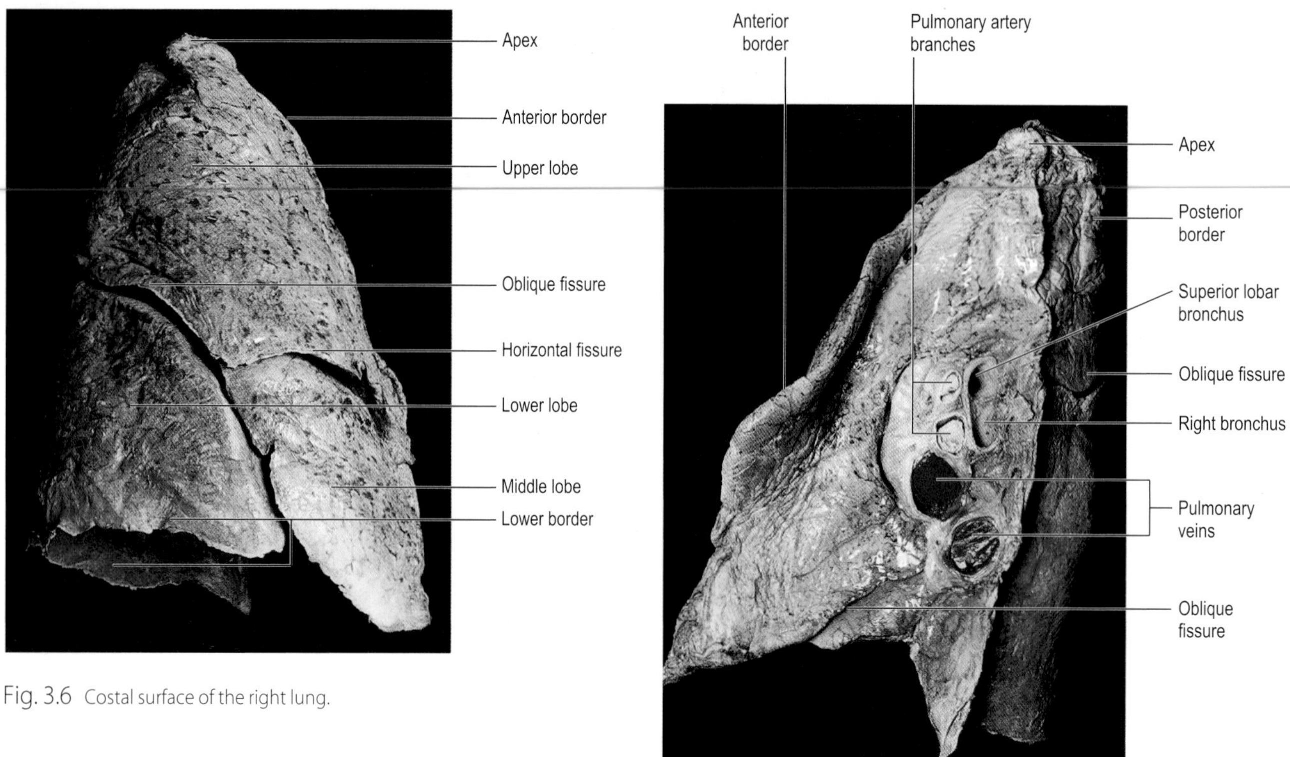


Fig. 3.6 Costal surface of the right lung.

Fig. 3.7 Mediastinal surface of the right lung.

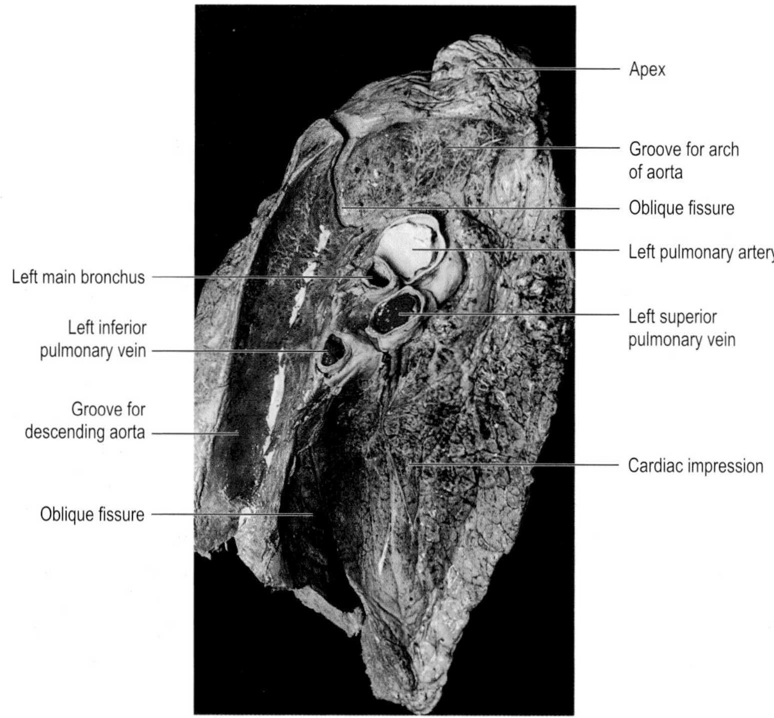


Fig. 3.8 Mediastinal surface of the left lung.

70° in the adult; 25° to the right and 45° to the left from the midline. Therefore foreign bodies getting into the trachea tend to go to the right bronchus rather than into the left. At birth the bifurcation angle is about 110° with both bronchi angulating equally from the midline (55° each way).

The lung is surrounded by the pleural cavity, the potential space between the two layers of pleura. The outer parietal layer of pleura lines the thoracic cavity and the inner visceral or pulmonary layer closely fits on to the surface of the lung. The two layers become continuous with each other at the root of the lung. The parietal pleura lining the diaphragm is known as the diaphragmatic pleura and that lining the mediastinum as the mediastinal pleura. See Clinical box 3.3.

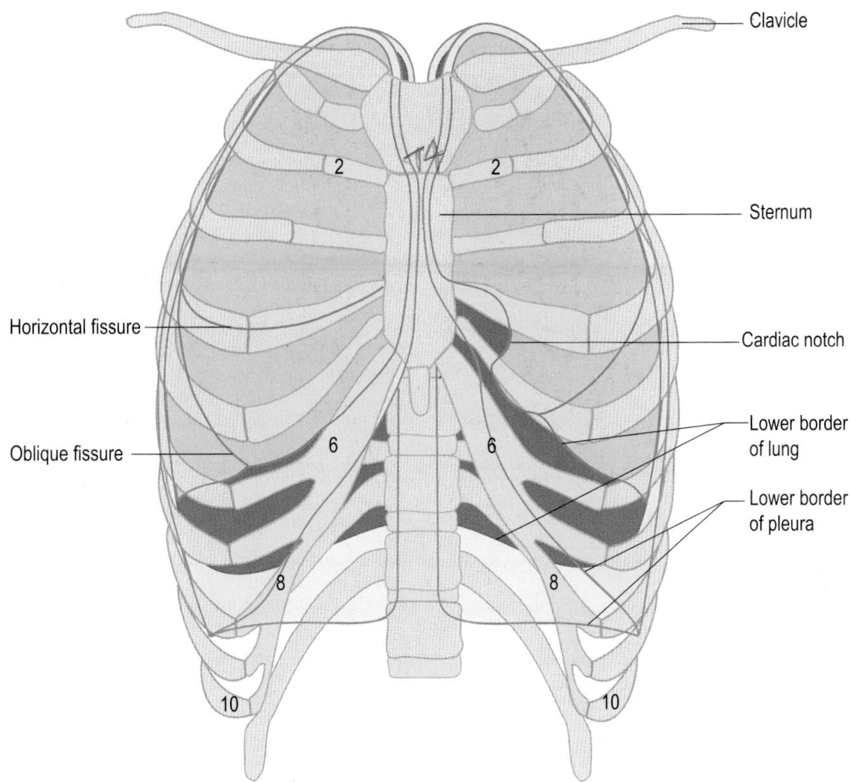


Fig. 3.9 Surface relationship of the lungs and pleural cavities. The numbers indicate those of the ribs and costal cartilages.

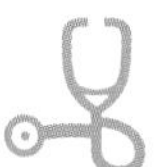

## *Clinical box 3.3*

### Surface anatomy of the lung and pleura

Knowledge of the extent of the lung and pleura is clinically important (Fig. 3.9). Their lower parts overlap abdominal organs such as the liver, kidney and spleen. On the apical pleura lie the subclavian vessels and the brachial plexus. The stellate ganglion of the sympathetic trunk lies behind the apex of the lung and pleura on the neck of the first rib. Pancoast's tumour affecting the apex of the lung may involve these structures when it spreads locally. Cannulation of the subclavian vein may inadvertently produce a pneumothorax (air in the pleural cavity) resulting in collapse of the lung. (See Root of the neck p. 186) Procedures such as exposure of the kidney, kidney and liver biopsies may also produce pneumothorax. This is due to the fact that the diaphragm is dome shaped and hence the lower parts of the lung and pleura overlap the upper abdominal organs (separated, of course, by the diaphragm).

When the lung fields are markedly hyperinflated, as in emphysema, the liver is pushed down by the diaphragm and may be palpable.

The apex of the lung and the surrounding pleural cavity extends about 3cm above the medial part of the clavicle. The apical pleura is covered by a fascia, the suprapleural membrane (Sibson's fascia), attached to the inner border of the first rib. This fascia prevents the lung and pleura expanding too much into the neck during deep inspiration.

From the apex, the anterior border of the pleural cavity descends behind the sternoclavicular joint to reach the midline at the level of the sternal angle. (Here the two pleural cavities are close to each other.) The anterior limit of the right pleural cavity descends vertically downwards in the midline from the sternal angle to the level of the sixth costal cartilage. From there the lower border extends laterally, crossing the eighth rib in the midclavicular line, the 10th rib in the midaxillary line and then ascends to the middle of the 12th rib at the back. The posterior border then ascends almost vertically upwards in the paravertebral region. A midline sternotomy (splitting of the sternum) is done to open up the chest cavity for cardiac surgery. During this procedure the right lung and pleura will be seen extending up to the midline, and occasionally even beyond, just behind the sternum.

From the sternal angle the anterior border of the left pleural cavity deviates laterally to the lateral border of the sternum. The extent of the lower and the posterior margins are similar to those on the right.

The surface marking of the lung is the same as that of the pleura except for the lower margin and the cardiac notch (Fig. 3.9). The lower margin of the lung is about two ribs higher than the lower margin of the pleura. Because of the bulge of the heart and pericardium, the anterior border of the left lung deviates laterally from the sternal angle to the apex of the heart (usually in the fifth intercostal space a little inside the midclavicular line) producing the cardiac notch. The oblique fissure of the lung lies along the sixth rib on both sides and the horizontal fissure of the right lung extends anteriorly from the midaxillary line along the fourth rib.

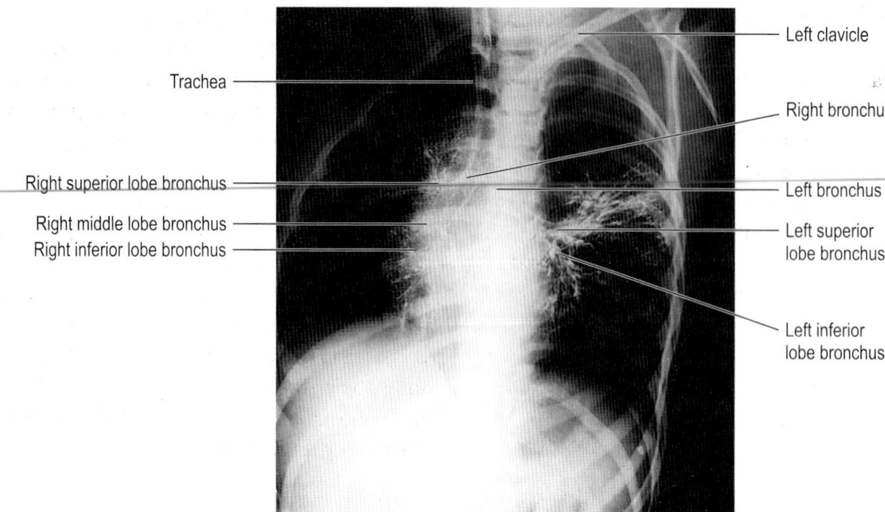


Fig. 3.10 Bronchogram – left anterior oblique view.

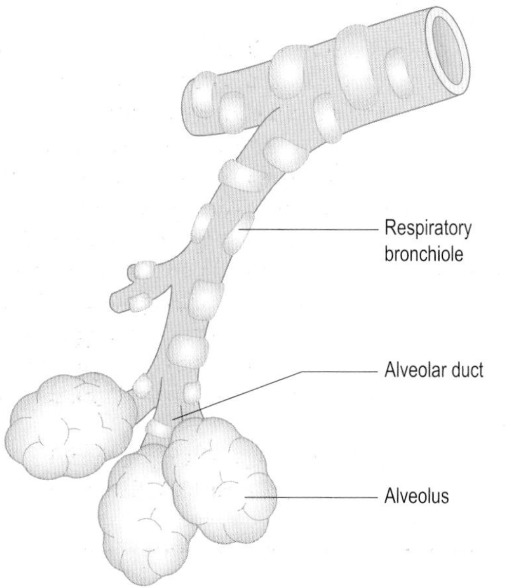


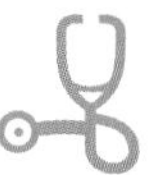

Fig. 3.11 The bronchioles and alveoli.

## *Clinical box 3.4*

### Bronchopulmonary segments

A bronchopulmonary segment is defined as the area of lung ventilated by a tertiary (branch immediately following the lobar branch) division of the bronchial tree. Each segment has its own bronchus and a pulmonary artery branch. Pulmonary veins are intersegmental. There are 10 such segments for the right lung and nine for the left. Conditions such as lung abscess may be localised to these segments and patients can be positioned accordingly to facilitate postural drainage. Secretions collected in anterior segments drain better if the patient lies on the back, and posterior ones in the prone position.

Lumen of the trachea, main bronchi and the commencement of the segmental bronchi can be visualised during bronchoscopy.

### The trachea, bronchi and bronchioles

The trachea, which is slightly to the right of the midline, divides at the carina into right and left main bronchi. ✪ The right main bronchus is more vertical than the left and, hence, inhaled material is more likely to pass into it. The right main bronchus divides into three lobar bronchi (upper, middle and lower), whereas the left only into two (upper and lower) (Fig. 3.10). Each lobar bronchus divides into segmental and subsegmental bronchi. There are about 25 generations of bronchi and bronchioles between trachea and the alveoli; the first 10 are bronchi and the rest bronchioles (Fig. 3.11). The bronchi have walls consisting of cartilage and smooth muscle, epithelial lining with cilia and goblet cells, submucosal mucous glands and endocrine cells containing 5-hydroxytryptamine. The bronchioles are tubes less than 2mm in diameter and are also known as small airways. They have no cartilage or submucosal glands. Their epithelium has a single layer of ciliated cells but only few goblet cells and Clara cells secreting a surfactant-like substance. See Clinical box 3.4.

### The alveolar ducts and alveoli

Each respiratory bronchiole supplies approximately 200 alveoli via alveolar ducts. There are about 300 million alveoli in each lung and their walls have type I and type II pneumocytes. Type II pneumocytes are the source of surfactant. The type I pneumocytes and the endothelial cells of adjoining capillaries constitute the blood–air barrier, the thickness of which is about 0.2–2µm.

## The heart

### Borders and surfaces of the heart

The heart has an anterior or sternocostal surface, formed mostly by the right ventricle, an inferior or diaphragmatic surface, formed mostly by the left ventricle, a base or posterior surface, formed by the left atrium, and an apex, formed entirely by the left ventricle. The borders of the heart (Fig. 3.12) are the right border, formed by the right atrium, the inferior border, formed by the right ventricle, the left or obtuse border, formed mostly by the left ventricle with the left auricle at its superior end (Fig. 3.13).

The apex beat is defined as the lower-most and lateral-most cardiac pulsation in the precordium, normally felt inside the midclavicular line in the fifth left intercostal space (approximately 6cm to the left of the midline) (Fig. 3.13). However it is felt in the anterior axillary line when lying on the left side. The right border of the heart extends from the third to the sixth right costal cartilage approximately 3cm to the right of the midline, the inferior border from the lower end of the right border to the apex, and the left border from the apex to the second left intercostal space approximately 3cm from the midline. See Clinical box 3.5.

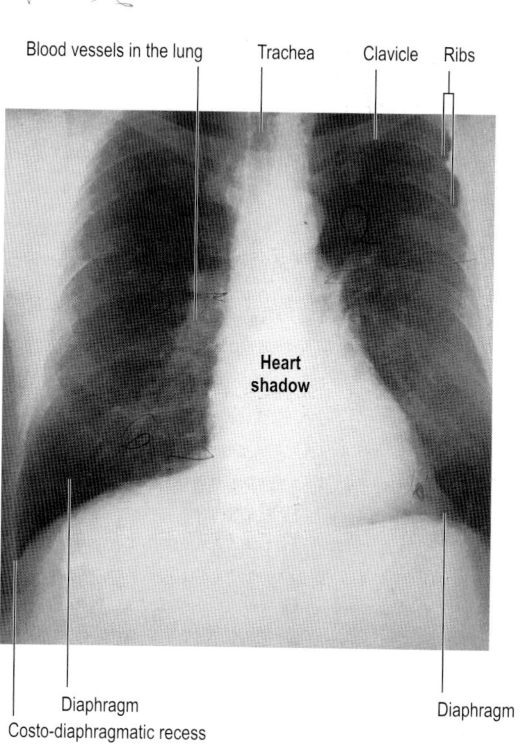


Fig. 3.12 Posteroanterior radiograph of the chest.

## Blood supply of the heart

The heart muscle is supplied by the right and left coronary arteries and is drained by the cardiac veins (Figs 3.14–3.19). The coronary arterial supply is of great clinical importance. Its occlusion is the chief cause of death in the western world.

The right coronary artery arises from the anterior aortic sinus. It passes between the pulmonary trunk and the right atrium to lie in the atrioventricular groove (Fig. 3.14). It winds round the inferior border to reach the diaphragmatic surface where it anastomoses with the terminal part of the left coronary artery. It gives off an artery to the sinoatrial node, the right (acute) marginal artery and the posterior interventricular artery, which is also known as the posterior descending artery (Fig. 3.15).

### Clinical box 3.5
**Apex beat**

Apex beat is the lower and lateral-most cardiac pulsation in the precordium, its normal site being just medial to the midclavicular line in the fourth or fifth left intercostal space. It may be normally felt in the anterior axillary line when lying on the left side. There are abnormal forms of apex beats in various clinical conditions.

A heaving apex beat which is forceful and sustained may be present in hypertension and aortic stenosis (pressure overload) whereas a thrusting one which is forceful but not sustained is a sign of mitral or aortic regurgitation (volume overload). A tapping apex beat is a sudden but brief pulsation and occurs in mitral stenosis.

Apex beat may be missing (i.e. not palpable) in obesity, pleural effusion, pericardial effusion and emphysema.

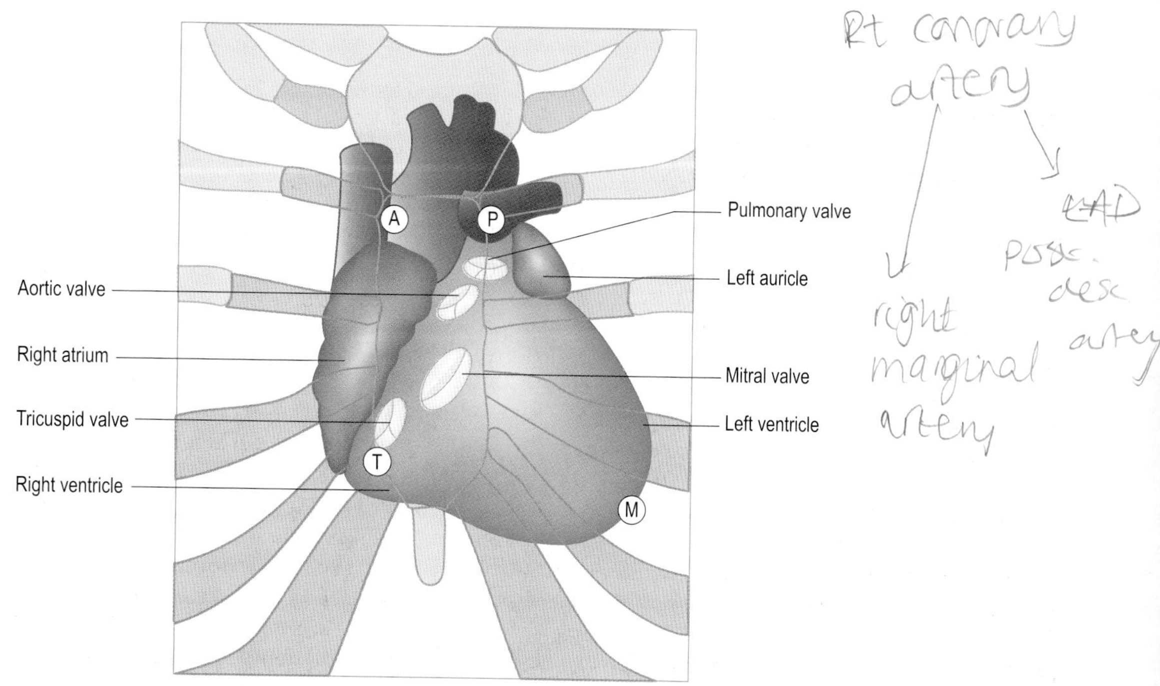


Fig. 3.13 Surface projections of the heart. A, P, T and M indicate auscultation areas for the aortic, pulmonary, tricuspid and mitral valves.

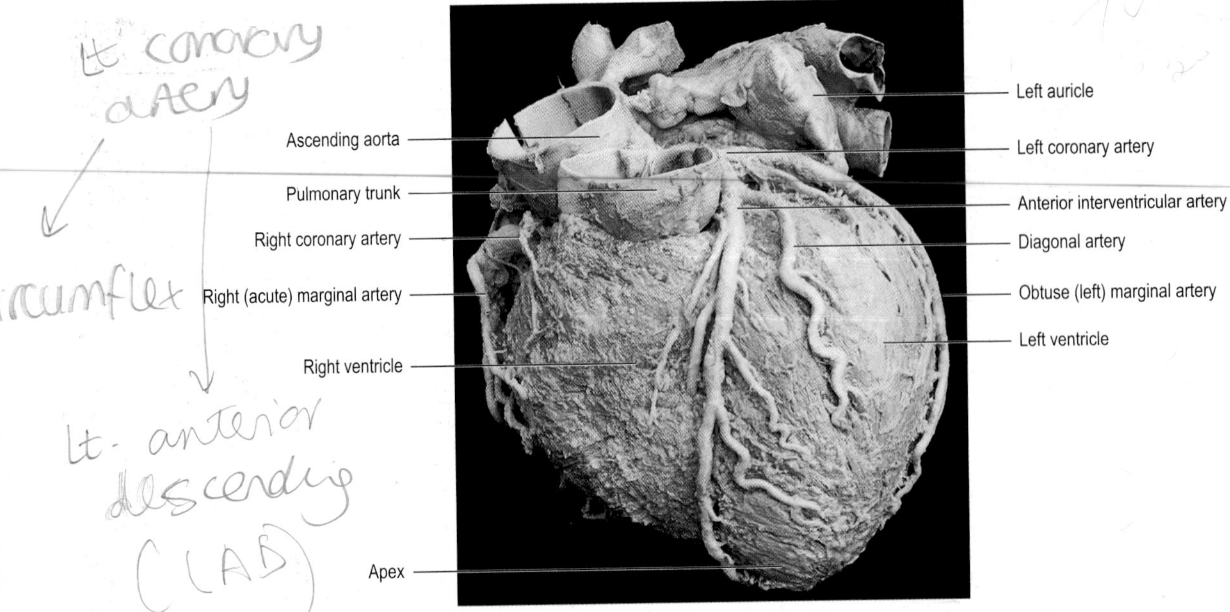


Fig. 3.14 Coronary arteries – anterior aspect of the heart.

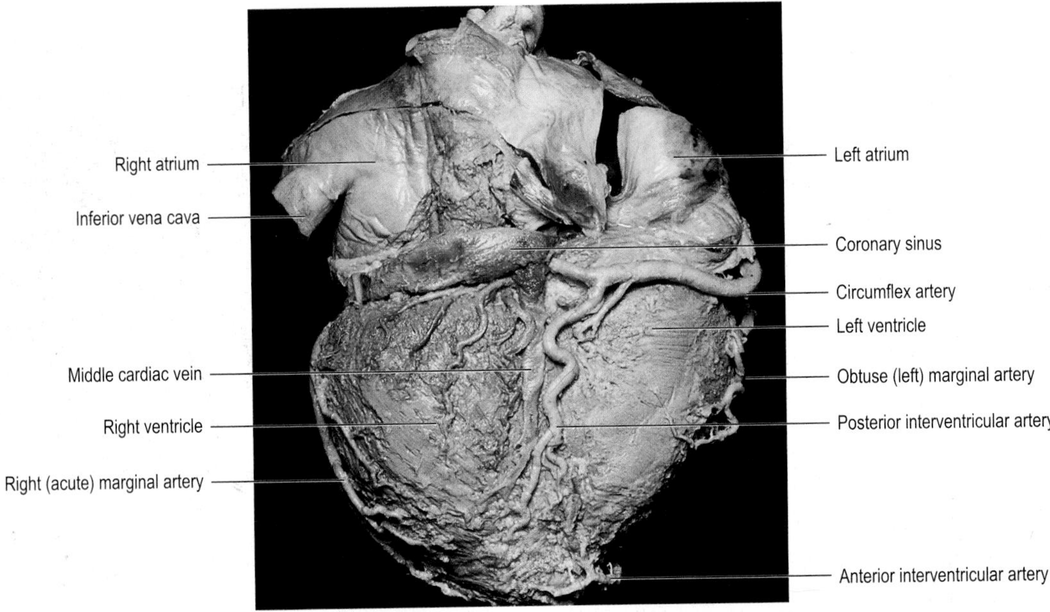


Fig. 3.15 Coronary arteries – posteroinferior aspect of the heart.

The left coronary artery arises from the left posterior aortic sinus. It passes behind the pulmonary trunk and the left auricle to reach the atrioventricular groove where it divides into the circumflex and the anterior interventricular (anterior descending) arteries, both of equal size (Figs 3.14, 3.15). The circumflex artery winds round the left margin where it gives off the left (obtuse) marginal artery and reaches the diaphragmatic surface to anastomose with the right coronary artery. The anterior descending artery (LAD), also known as the 'widow maker' because many men die of blockage of this artery, descends in the interventricular septum and gives off ventricular branches, septal branches as well as the diagonal artery. It then winds round the apex reaching the diaphragmatic surface to anastomose with the posterior descending artery. The main stem of the left coronary artery varies in length between 4mm and 10mm. In 10% of the population in whom the left coronary is larger and longer than usual – 'left dominance' – the posterior descending artery arises from it instead of from the right coronary. Another 10% have 'co-dominant' coronary circulation where both left and right coronaries contribute equally to the posterior interventricular artery. In a third of the population the left main stem divides into three branches instead of two, the third being a branch lying between the circumflex and the anterior descending on the lateral aspect of the left ventricle.

The blood supply of the conducting system is of clinical importance. In about 60% of the population the sinoatrial node is supplied by the right coronary and in the rest by the circumflex branch of the left coronary. However occasionally (3%) it can have a dual supply. The atrioventricular node is supplied by the right coronary in 90% and the circumflex in 10%.

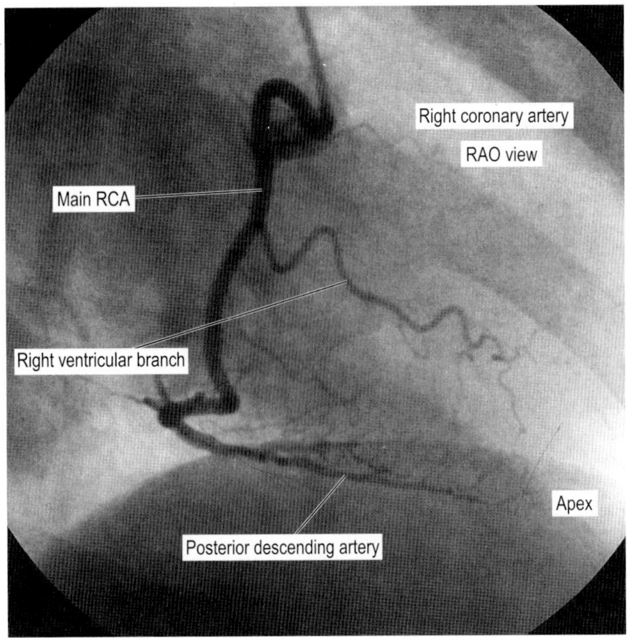


Fig. 3.16 Right coronary arteriogram – right anterior oblique view.

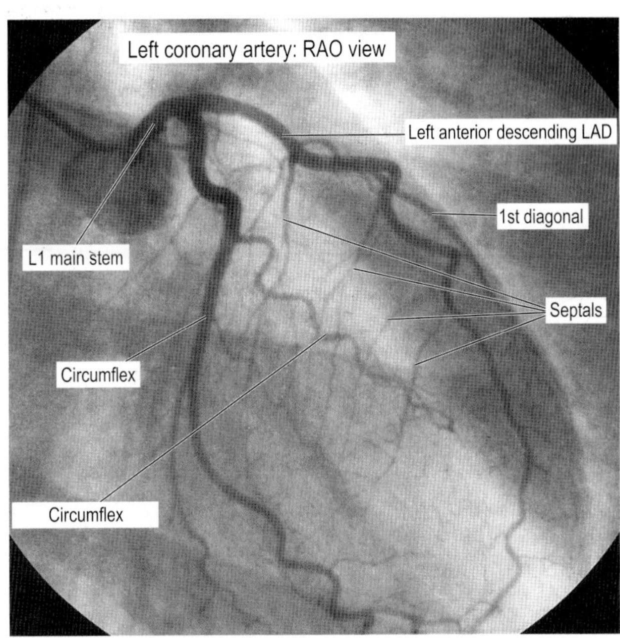


Fig. 3.18 Left coronary arteriogram – right anterior oblique view.

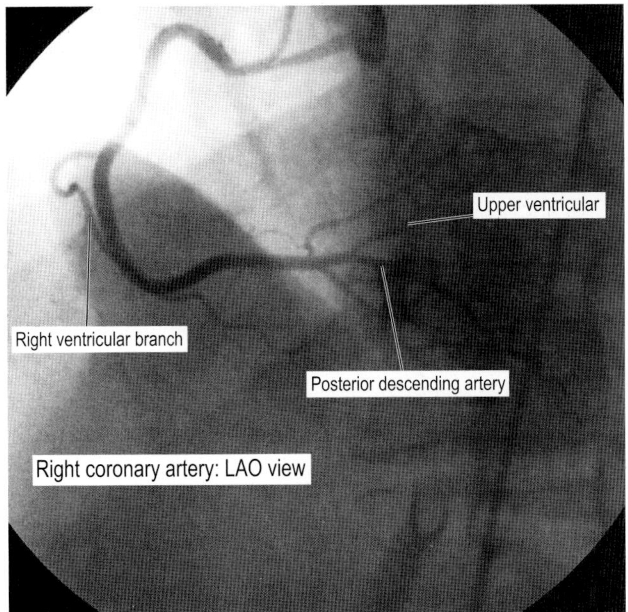


Fig. 3.17 Right coronary arteriogram – left anterior oblique view.

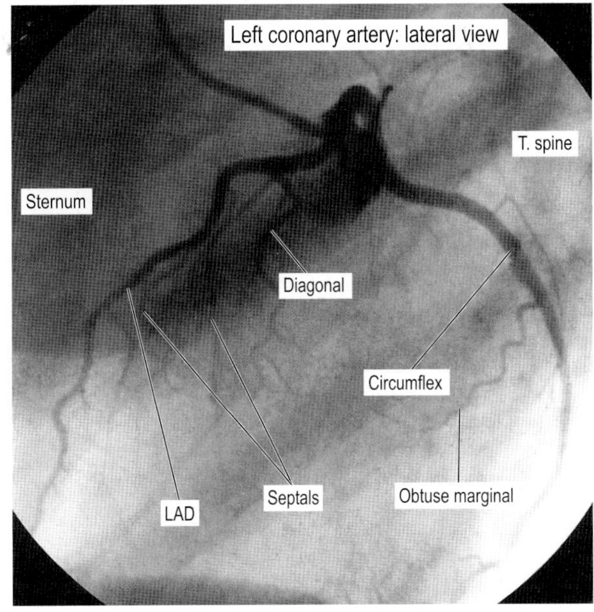


Fig. 3.19 Left coronary arteriogram – lateral view.

Cardiac veins accompany the arteries. Most of them are tributaries of the coronary sinus, a sizable vein lying in the posterior part of the atrioventricular groove and opening into the right atrium. The great cardiac vein accompanies the anterior interventricular artery; the middle cardiac vein accompanies the posterior interventricular artery and the small cardiac vein accompanies the marginal artery. Anterior cardiac veins seen on the anterior wall of the right ventricle drain directly into the right atrium. Additionally there are very small veins on the various walls – venae cordis minimae, draining directly into the cardiac cavity. See Clinical box 3.6.

## The pericardium

The heart lies within the pericardial cavity, in the middle mediastinum. The pericardial cavity is similar in structure and function to the pleural cavity. The pericardium provides a friction-free surface for the heart to accommodate its sliding movements.

Components of the pericardium are the fibrous pericardium and the serous pericardium, the former being a collagenous outer layer fused with the central tendon of the diaphragm. The serous pericardium consists of a parietal layer which lines the inner surface of the fibrous pericardium and a visceral layer which lines the outer surface of the heart and the commencement of the great vessels. The pericardial cavity is the space between the parietal and the visceral layers.

Two regions of the pericardial cavity have special names. The transverse sinus of the pericardial cavity lies between the ascending aorta and the pulmonary trunk in front and the venae cavae and the atria behind. The pericardial space

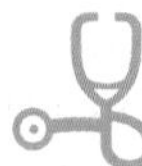

## Clinical box 3.6

### Coronary artery disease

Occlusion of a coronary artery or its branch causes myocardial infarction which is cell death of the cardiac musculature due to inadequate blood supply. A partial occlusion may manifest as angina which typically is felt as a deep pain in the sternal area radiating to the left arm and left side of the neck.

The changes caused by occlusion are based on the distribution of the coronary artery branches. Right coronary artery occlusion leads to inferior myocardial infarction, often associated with dysrhythmia (abnormal heart beats) due to ischaemia of SA node and/or AV node, parts of the conducting system. Occlusion of the left coronary artery or its branches leads to anterior and/or lateral myocardial infarction, often with substantial ventricular damage and very poor prognosis.

Coronary arteries and their branches can be visualised by selectively catheterising each coronary artery and injecting a radio-opaque dye (usually iodine-containing).

Several procedures are now available to treat coronary artery disease. In an angioplasty a catheter with a small inflatable balloon attached to its tip is passed into the coronary artery (via the femoral, external and common iliac and aorta). The balloon is inflated to widen the artery by flattening the atheromatous plaque. In the coronary artery bypass graft operation a small segment of the great saphenous vein is connected to the ascending aorta or to the coronary artery proximal to the obstruction and the distal end of the segment is then attached to the coronary artery distal to the narrowing bypassing the obstruction. The radial artery and the internal thoracic artery are also commonly used for bypass surgery.

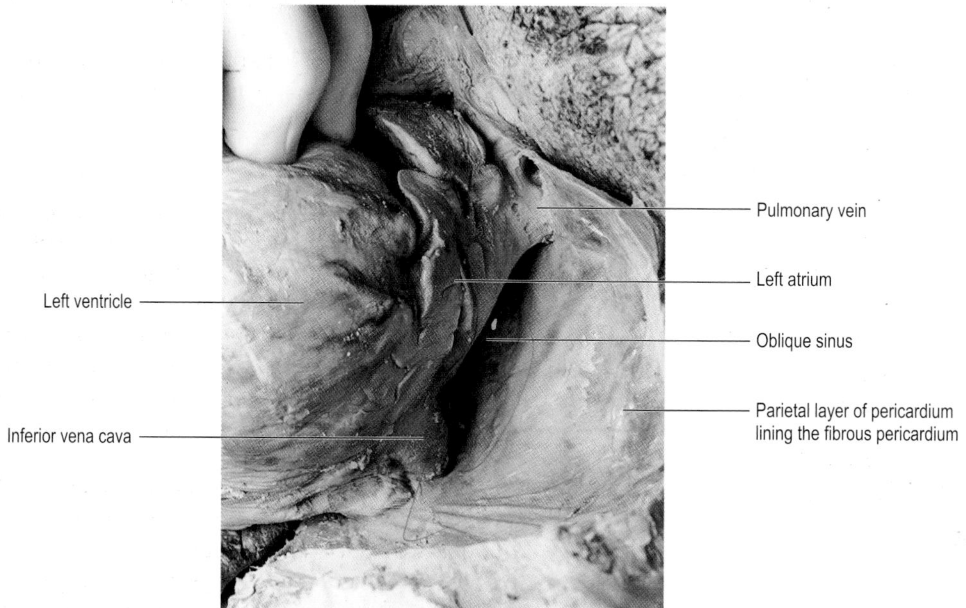


Fig. 3.20 Pericardial cavity opened up and the heart lifted up to show the oblique sinus.

behind the left atrium is the oblique sinus (Fig. 3.20). The oblique sinus separates the left atrium from the oesophagus.

Anteriorly the pericardium is related to the sternum, third to sixth costal cartilages, lungs and the pleura. Posterior relations are oesophagus, descending aorta and T5–T8 vertebrae. Laterally on either side lie the root of the lung, mediastinal pleura and the phrenic nerve. Innervation of the fibrous and the parietal layer of serous pericardium is by the phrenic nerves. Pericardial pain originates in the parietal layer and is transmitted by the phrenic nerves. The pericardial cavity is closest to the surface at the level of the xiphoid process of sternum and the sixth costal cartilages. See Clinical box 3.7.

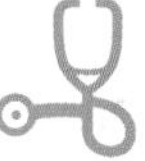

## Clinical box 3.7

### Pericardiocentesis

Diseases of the pericardium can cause accumulation of fluid or blood in the pericardial cavity. Blood can also accumulate in the pericardial cavity as a result of trauma. To remove fluid or blood from the pericardial cavity a needle is inserted into the angle between the xiphoid process and the left seventh costal cartilage and is directed upwards at an angle of 45° towards the left shoulder. The needle passes through the central tendon of the diaphragm before entering the pericardial cavity.

## Interior of the chambers of the heart

### The right atrium

The right atrium (Fig. 3.21) has a smooth and a rough part which are separated by a vertical ridge, the crista terminalis, extending between the superior and inferior venae cavae which bring systemic venous blood into the smooth part of the atrium. The coronary sinus opens anterior to the opening of the inferior vena cava. Developmentally the smooth part of the atrium is derived from the sinus venosus of the primitive cardiac tube and the rough part which has muscular ridges known as musculae pectinatae from the primitive atrium. The fossa ovalis (Fig. 3.21), an oval depression on the interatrial wall, is the remnant of the foramen ovale in the fetus. Before birth the foramen ovale allowed blood to flow from the right atrium to the left atrium bypassing the lungs. At birth when the lungs begin to function the foramen ovale closes to produce the fossa ovalis.

## The right ventricle

The right ventricular wall is thicker than that of the atrium. The tricuspid orifice is guarded by the tricuspid valve which has an anterior, posterior and a septal cusp. The interior of the ventricle has muscular ridges known as trabeculae carneae as well as the anterior, posterior and septal (small) papillary muscles and the chordae tendineae (Fig. 3.22). The chordae tendineae connect the papillary muscles to the tricuspid valve cusps. ✪ These prevent the valve cusps being everted into the atrium during ventricular systole. Failure of this mechanism due to breakage of the papillary muscle or chordae tendineae causes tricuspid incompetence and regurgitation of blood back into the atrium during ventricular systole. When this happens blood from the atrium can pool back into the liver and the neck veins causing enlarged neck veins and palpable liver as the superior and inferior venae cavae do not have valves.

The septomarginal trabecula (moderator band) is a muscular ridge extending from the interventricular septum to the base of the anterior papillary muscle of the heart. The moderator band is a part of the conducting system of the heart which regulates the cardiac cycle.

The infundibulum leads on to the orifice of the pulmonary trunk. The pulmonary orifice has the pulmonary valve with three semilunar cusps. Each cusp has a thickening in the centre of its free edge.

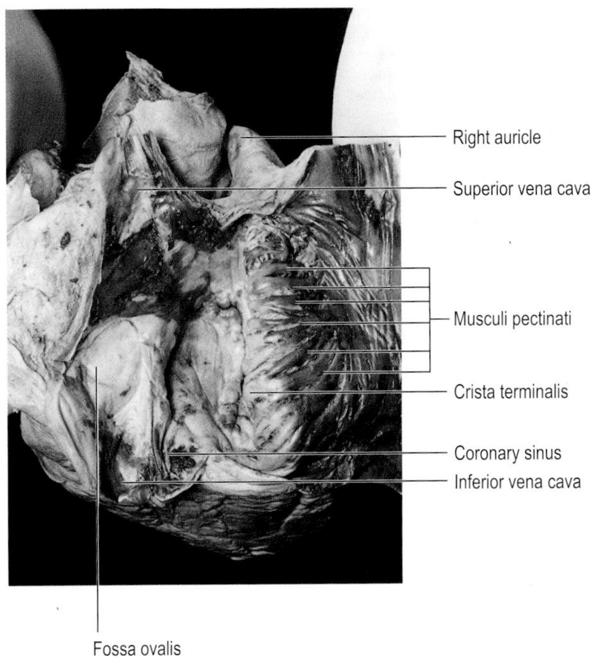


Fig. 3.21 Interior of the right atrium.

## The left atrium

The left atrium which develops by a combination of absorption of the pulmonary veins as well as from the primitive atrium has the openings of the four pulmonary veins. The mitral orifice separates the left atrium from the left ventricle.

## The left ventricle

The walls of the left ventricle are about three times thicker than those of the right ventricle because of the increased resistance of the systemic circulation compared with that of the pulmonary circulation. The mitral orifice is guarded by the mitral valve with an anterior and a posterior cusp. The large anterior cusp lies between the aortic and mitral orifices. The trabeculae carneae, papillary muscles and chordae tendineae are similar to those in the right ventricle. The aortic orifice has the aortic valve (Fig. 3.23) with the three semilunar aortic cusps, one anterior and two posterior in the anatomical position of the heart. These are thicker than those of the pulmonary valves to cope with the increased pressure. Alongside each cusp there is a dilation, the aortic sinus. The coronary arteries originate from the

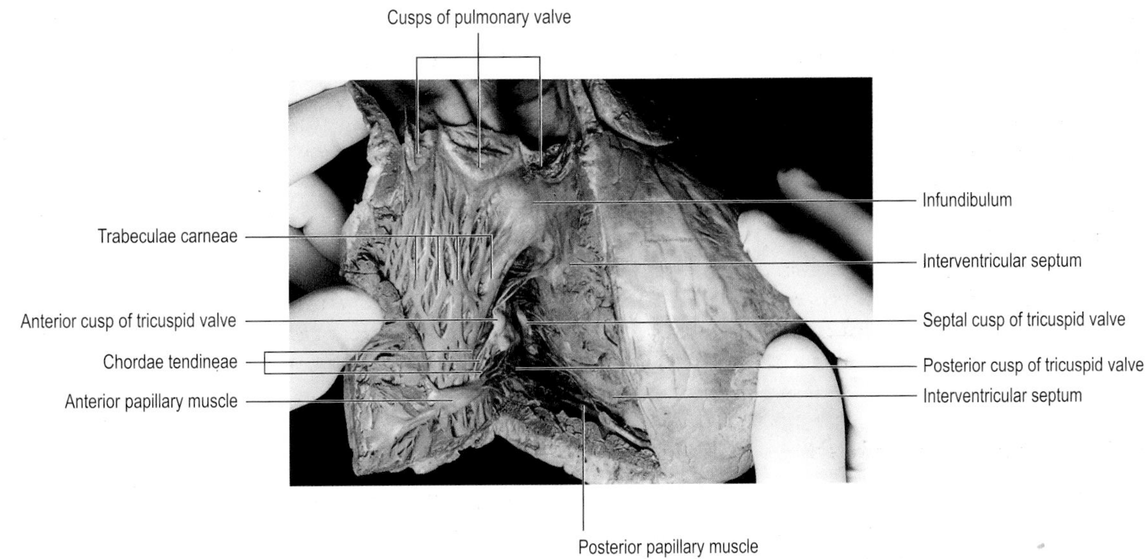


Fig. 3.22 Interior of the right ventricle.

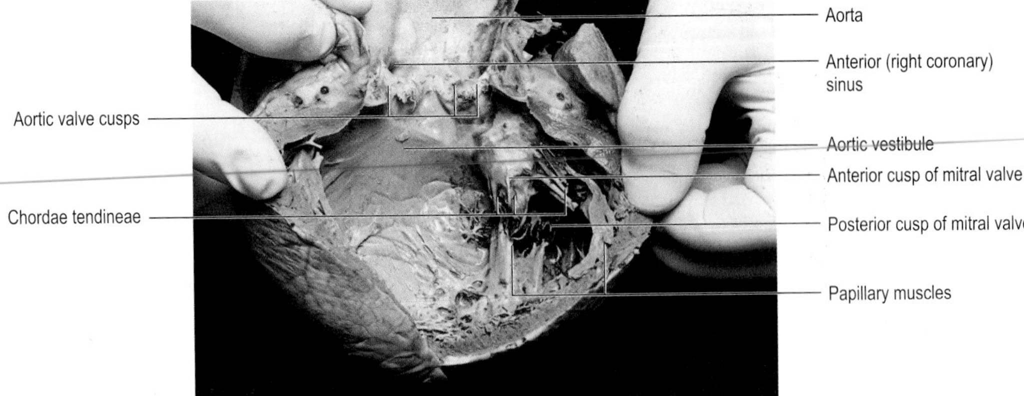


Fig. 3.23 Interior of the left ventricle.

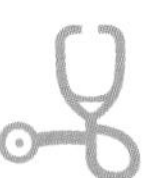

## Clinical box 3.8

### Valves, heart sounds and murmurs

The valves between the atria and the ventricles, i.e. the tricuspid and the mitral valves, prevent regurgitation of blood from the ventricles back into the atria during ventricular contraction (systole). Similarly the pulmonary and aortic valves prevent regurgitation during diastole (relaxation of ventricle) from these vessels back into the ventricles. Closure of the tricuspid and mitral valves occurs at the beginning of systole and causes the first heart sound and closure of the aortic and pulmonary valves, which happens at the beginning of diastole, the second sound. Thus the interval between the first and the second heart sounds is the period of ventricular systole and that between the second and the next first sound is the diastole. A hissing sound heard during systole is a systolic murmur and that during diastole is a diastolic murmur. Murmurs are caused by blood flow through narrow orifice or leaking valves. Pulmonary or aortic valve stenosis (narrowing) cause systolic murmur. It can also be heard in mitral or tricuspid incompetence (regurgitation). A diastolic murmur, on the other hand, is a characteristic of mitral or tricuspid stenosis. It is also a sign of aortic or pulmonary valve incompetence.

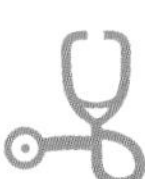

## Clinical box 3.9

### Areas of auscultation

The two heart sounds and the abnormal murmurs are caused by turbulence and vibrations inside the ventricles, the aorta or the pulmonary trunk. This is best heard where the particular chamber or vessel is closer to the surface. Thus the mitral valve closure produces vibrations in the left ventricle and the sound is best heard where the left ventricle is closer to the surface, i.e. where the apex beat is felt. Mitral valve therefore is auscultated at the apex, tricuspid at the lower end of sternum pulmonary valve at the second intercostal space on the left side just outside the lateral border of sternum, and the aortic valve in the second intercostal space close to the lateral border of the sternum on the right side (Fig. 3.13).

sinuses, the right from the anterior (also known as the right coronary sinus) and the left from the left posterior aortic sinus (also known as the left coronary sinus). The interventricular septum which has the muscular and the membranous parts bulges into the right ventricle and separates the left ventricle from the right. See Clinical boxes 3.8 and 3.9.

### The conducting system of the heart

Specialised cardiac muscle cells initiate and regulate the heart-beat. The sinoatrial node (SA node) or 'pacemaker of the heart' initiating the heart-beat is situated in the right atrium at the upper end of the crista terminalis (Fig. 3.24). From there the cardiac impulse spreads through the atrial musculature to reach the AV node (atrioventricular node) which is situated in the interatrial septum near the opening of the coronary sinus. After a brief pause there the impulse passes into the atrioventricular bundle of His (AV bundle). The AV bundle which starts from the AV node passes

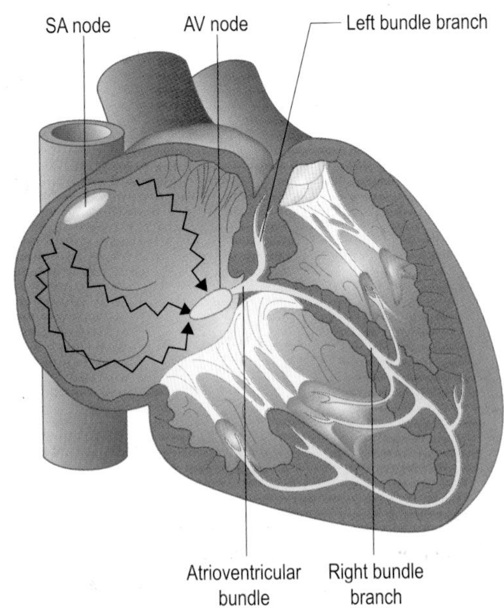


Fig. 3.24 The conducting system of the heart.

through the fibrous ring at the atrioventricular junction to reach the membranous part of the interventricular septum where it divides into a right and left bundle branch. The atrioventricular bundle is the only pathway through which impulses can reach the ventricles from the atrium. The left

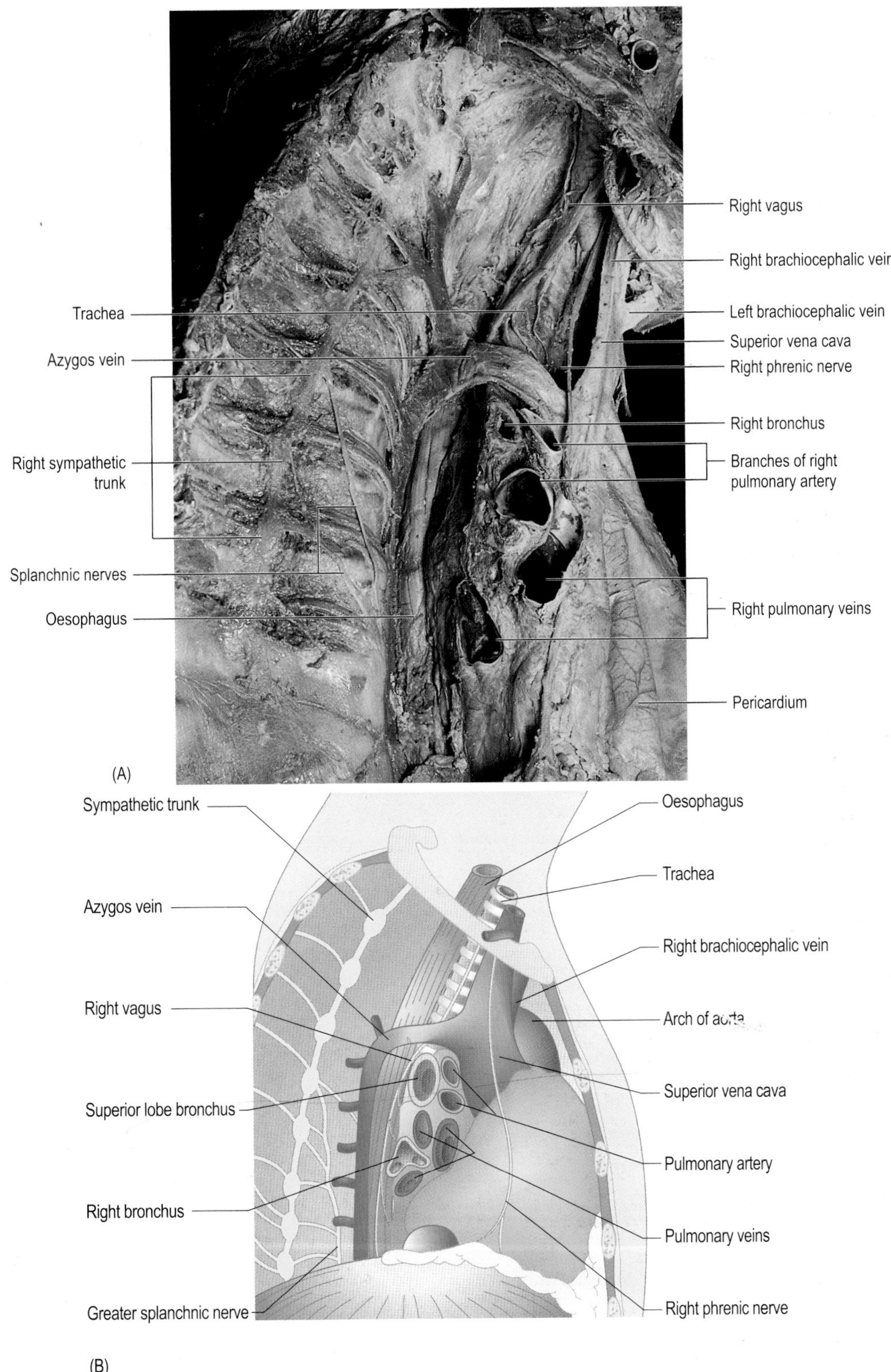


Fig. 3.25 a & b Right side of the mediastinum after removal of the right lung and pleura. Viewed from the right side.

and right bundles descend towards the apex and break up into Purkinje fibres which activate the musculature of the ventricle in such a way that the papillary muscles contract first followed by the simultaneous contraction of both the ventricles from apex towards the base.

## The mediastinum

The mediastinum is the region between the two pleural cavities. It contains the heart, great vessels, trachea, oesophagus and many other structures. The mediastinum is divided into four parts for descriptive purposes. The superior mediastinum lies above the horizontal plane joining the sternal angle to the lower border of T4 vertebra. The middle mediastinum contains the heart and pericardium; the anterior mediastinum is in front of this and the posterior mediastinum behind.

## The brachiocephalic vein and the superior vena cava

The brachiocephalic vein, one on each side, is formed by the union of the subclavian and the internal jugular veins. The right and left brachiocephalic veins join together to form the superior vena cava which drains into the right atrium (Fig. 3.25).

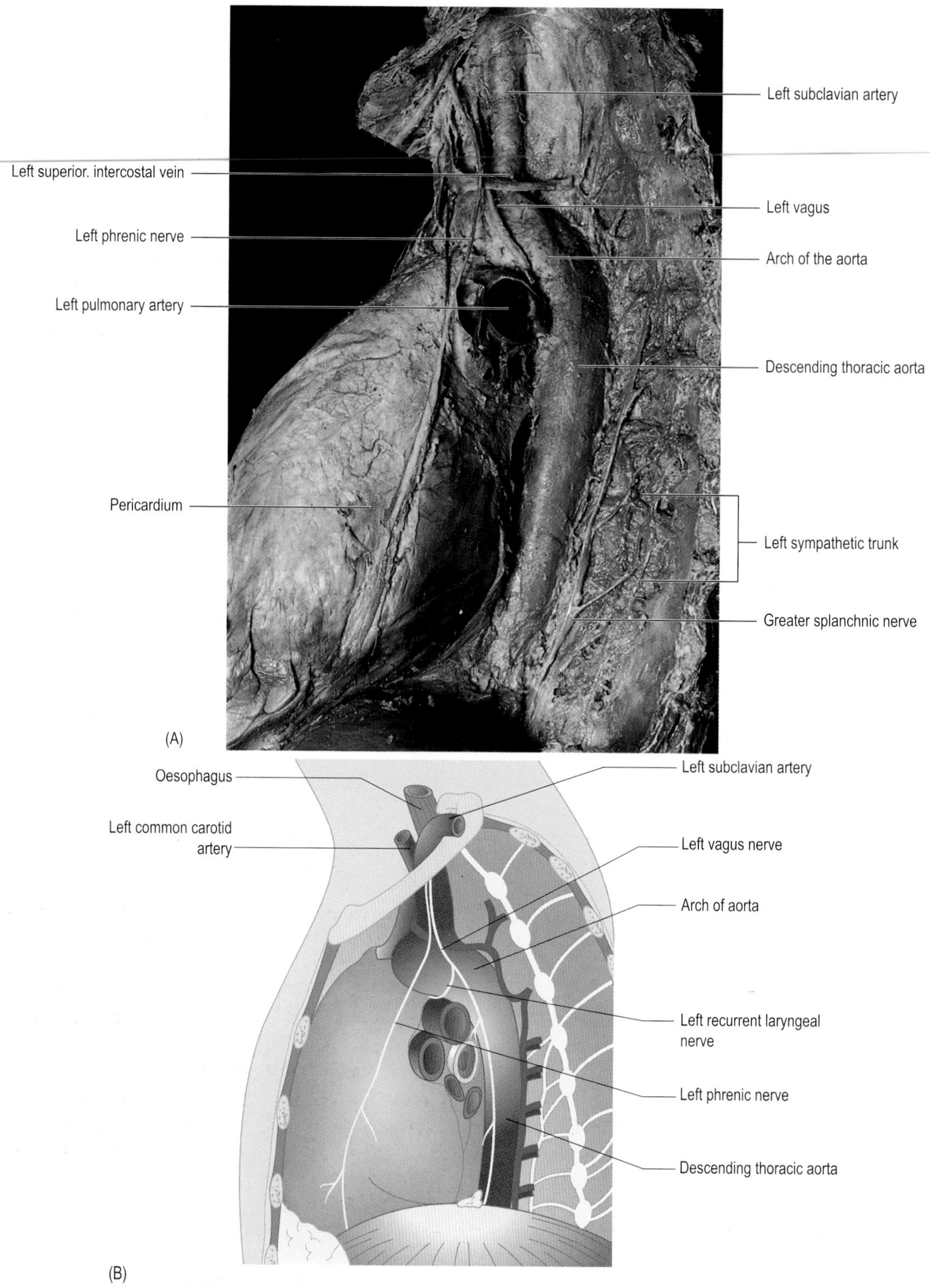


Fig. 3.26 A & B Left side of the mediastinum.

The azygos vein which receives segmental veins from the thoracic and posterior abdominal walls (intercostal and lumbar veins) joins the superior vena cava.

## The phrenic nerves

The right and left phrenic nerves are formed in the cervical plexus (C3, 4, 5). Besides supplying the diaphragm they give sensory innervation to pleura, pericardium and peritoneum (all starting with 'p'!). The thoracic part of the right phrenic nerve (Fig. 3.25) reaches the diaphragm lying on the surface of the right brachiocephalic vein, the superior vena cava, the right side of the heart and pericardium (where it lies in front of the root of the lung) and the inferior vena cava. In other words it lies on the big veins and the right atrium.

The left phrenic nerve crosses the arch of the aorta (Figs 3.26, 3.27). It descends in front of the root of the lung then lies on the pericardium as it descends to reach the diaphragm

## The right and left vagus nerves

The right vagus nerve lies on the trachea (Fig. 3.25) and crosses behind the root of the lung and breaks up into

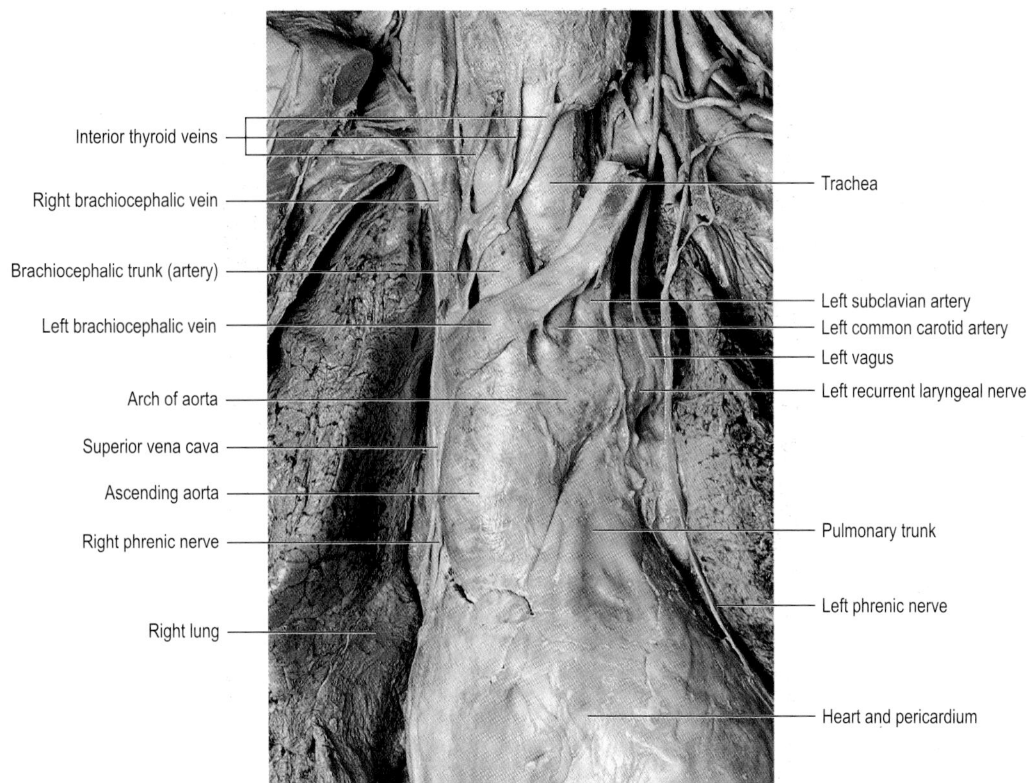


Fig. 3.27 Structures in the superior mediastinum seen after removal of the thoracic cage and the parietal pleura. The lungs have been retracted to expose the structures.

branches on the oesophagus forming the oesophageal plexus. It leaves the thorax by passing along with the oesophagus through the diaphragm as the posterior gastric nerve.

The left vagus, like the left phrenic nerve, crosses the arch of the aorta (Figs 3.26, 3.27). It crosses behind the root of the left lung (the phrenic nerve descends in front). The left vagus gives off an important branch, the left recurrent laryngeal nerve, as it crosses the arch of the aorta. The left recurrent laryngeal nerve winds round the ligamentum arteriosum, a fibrous connection between the left pulmonary artery and the arch of the aorta. The ligamentum arteriosum is the remnant of the ductus arteriosum which shunts blood from the pulmonary trunk to the aorta in the fetus. The recurrent laryngeal nerve ascends to the neck lying in the groove between the trachea and the oesophagus and supplies the muscles and mucous membrane of the larynx.

Carcinoma of the oesophagus, mediastinal lymph node enlargement and aortic arch aneurysm may compress the left recurrent laryngeal nerve to cause change in voice.

Below the root of the lung the left vagus, like the right, breaks up into branches contributing to the oesophageal plexus and leaves the thorax by passing along with the oesophagus through the diaphragm as the anterior gastric nerve.

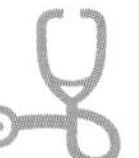

*Clinical box 3.10*

**Arch of the aorta**

The arch of the aorta hooks over the left bronchus and lies on the left side of the trachea and oesophagus with the left recurrent laryngeal nerve lying between the two. An aneurysm of the arch of the aorta can occlude the left bronchus and collapse the left lung. It can produce a change in voice due to compression of the left recurrent laryngeal nerve. Pathology of the aorta, trachea, bronchus and the oesophagus tend to involve one another due to their close relationship. Pulsation of the arch of the aorta is visible during bronchoscopy and oesophagoscopy.

## Arch of the aorta

The ascending aorta commencing from the left ventricle continues upwards and to the left over the root of the left lung as the arch of the aorta (Figs 3.26–3.28). It then descends down to become the descending thoracic aorta. The arch of the aorta commences at the level of the sternal angle and ends at the lower border of T4. It is entirely confined to the superior mediastinum. It has three branches: the brachiocephalic trunk which divides into the right common carotid and the right subclavian arteries, the left common carotid artery and the left subclavian artery (Fig. 3.28). The left vagus and the left phrenic nerves cross the arch of the aorta. The small vein lying across the arch of the aorta is the left superior intercostal vein. This drains the second and third left intercostal spaces and in turn drains into the left brachiocephalic vein (Fig. 3.26). See Clinical box 3.10.

## The trachea

The trachea (Figs 3.27, 3.29, 3.30) extends from the lower border of the cricoid cartilage in the neck to the tracheal bifurcation at the level of the lower border of the T4 vertebra. In the living, in the erect posture, the tracheal bifurcation is at a lower level. The trachea is about 15cm long, the first 5cm

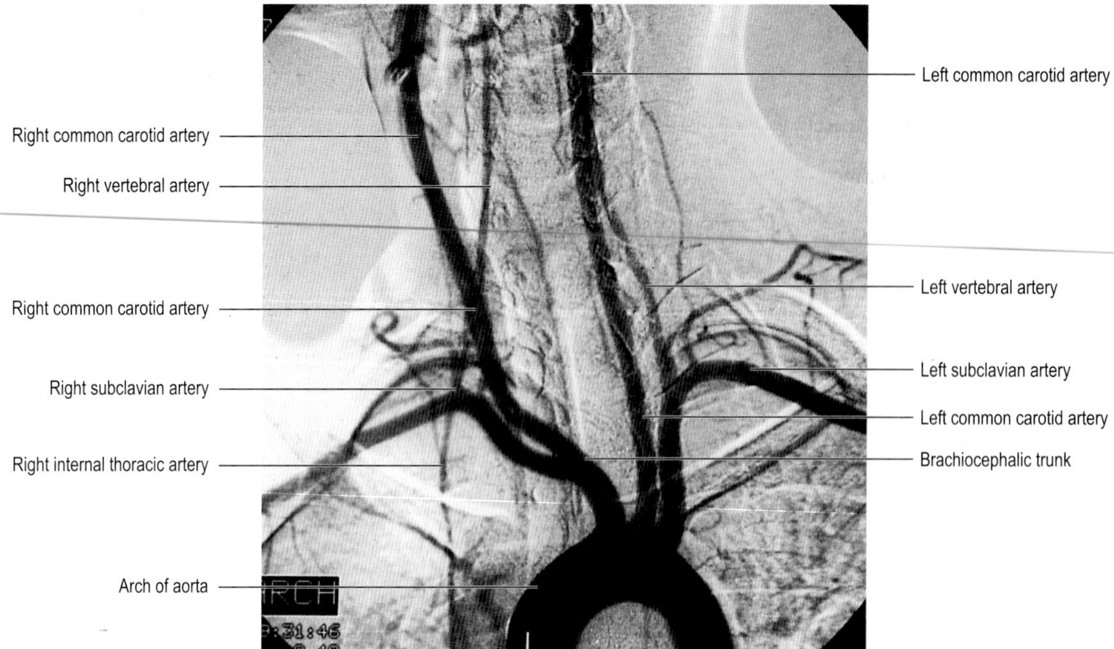


Fig. 3.28 Arch aortogram.

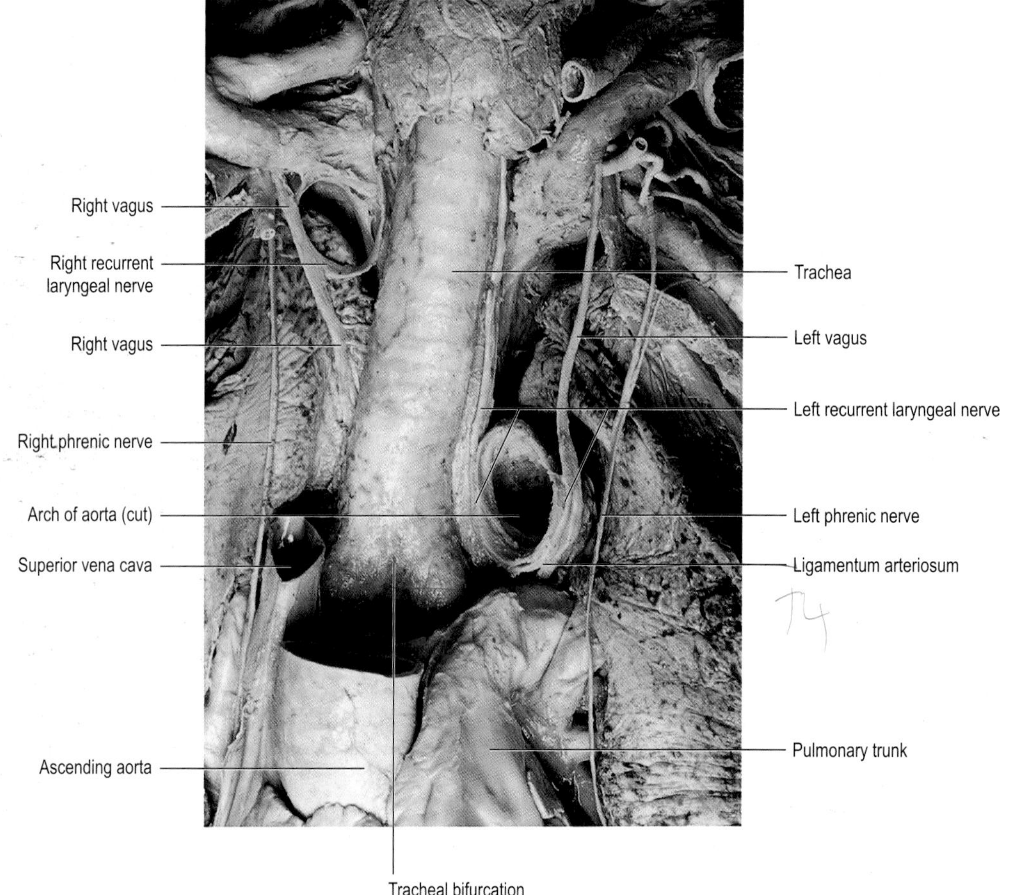


Fig. 3.29 Superior mediastinum – deeper aspect. Part of the arch of the aorta and its branches, the superior vena cava and the brachiocephalic veins have been removed.

being in the neck. The cervical part of the trachea lies in the midline and is easily palpable.

The diameter of the lumen of the trachea is correlated to the size of the subject and has approximately the same diameter as his/her index finger. It is made up of 15–20 'C'-shaped cartilaginous rings which prevent it from collapsing. The gap in the cartilage is at the back and is bridged by the trachealis muscle which allows the trachea to constrict and dilate. It is elastic enabling it to stretch during swallowing and its diameter changes during coughing and sneezing.

The thoracic part of the trachea is in the superior mediastinum. Anteriorly it is related to the left brachiocephalic vein, the commencement of the

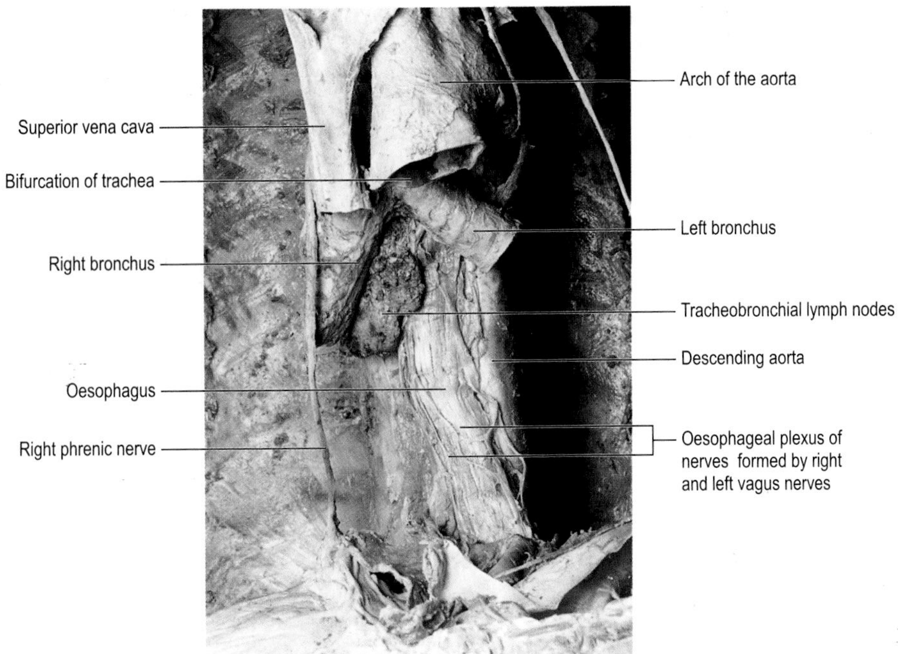


Fig. 3.30 The superior and posterior mediastinum seen after removal of the heart, pericardium, lungs and pleura.

brachiocephalic artery and the left common carotid artery. The posterior relations are the oesophagus and the left recurrent laryngeal nerve. To the left of it lies the arch of the aorta and on its right side the azygos vein. The lung and pleura are also related to it on either side, the left lung and pleura being pushed away slightly by the arch of the aorta.

The angle of bifurcation of the trachea in the adult is such that the right main bronchus is more vertical than the left. The right bronchus is shorter, wider and more vertical than the left. The angle between the two bronchi is about 70° in the adult; 25° to the right and 45° to the left from the midline. ✪ Therefore foreign bodies getting into the trachea tend to go to the right bronchus than into the left. At the time of birth the bifurcation angle is bigger, about 110° with both bronchi angulating equally from the midline (55° each way), with no difference in the angulation of the right and left main bronchi.

✪ The cartilage at the tracheal bifurcation is the keel-shaped carina which projects into the lumen as a vertical ridge. Flattening of this ridge is a sign of alteration of the bifurcation angle, often due to enlargement of the tracheobronchial group of lymph nodes located near the bifurcation.

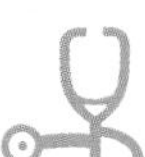

*Clinical box 3.11*

**Coarctation of aorta**

In this condition the aorta is narrowed, usually, just distal to the origin of the left subclavian artery. Blood flow to the lower part of the body is reduced. Branches of the aorta above the narrowing enlarge and this facilitates collateral channels via the internal thoracic, superior epigastric and musculophrenic arteries. Blood will flow bypassing the narrowing via the anterior intercostal branches of the internal thoracic and musculophrenic into the posterior intercostal arteries and the distal part of the aorta. Enlarged intercostal arteries may cause radiologically visible notching of the lower border of the ribs.

### The descending (thoracic) aorta

The descending aorta, also known as the thoracic aorta (Figs 3.26, 3.30), commences where the arch of the aorta ends at the lower border of T4 vertebra. It lies on the left side of the vertebral column in the upper part of the posterior mediastinum. As it descends it curves to the right and at its lower part it lies in front of the vertebral column. It leaves the posterior mediastinum in the midline at the level of T12 vertebra by passing between the crura of the diaphragm. The two hemiazygos veins lie behind it. The oesophagus crosses anterior to it from right to left. The descending aorta gives off nine pairs of posterior intercostal arteries, a pair of subcostal arteries, two bronchial arteries for the left lung and small branches to the oesophagus.

✪ Radicular arteries arise from the posterior intercostal arteries to supply the spinal cord. One such artery (usually from the 10th or 11th intercostal space) is large and is known as the great radicular artery or artery of Adamkiewicz. Blood flow through radicular arteries may be interfered with during aortic surgery producing ischaemia of the spinal cord and resulting in paraplegia. See Clinical boxes 3.11 and 3.12.

### The oesophagus

The oesophagus starts as a continuation of the pharynx at the level of C6 vertebra and ends by entering the stomach at the cardiac orifice. The thoracic part of the oesophagus lies in the superior and posterior mediastinum and enters the abdomen by piercing the diaphragm at the level of T10 vertebra. In the superior mediastinum it lies behind the trachea with the arch of the aorta lying on its left side. The left recurrent laryngeal nerve lies in the groove between the trachea and the oesophagus. The left main bronchus crosses in front of the oesophagus and the part below that is related to the left atrium. The arch of the aorta, the left main bronchus and the left atrium produce indentations on the oesophagus which can be seen clearly on a radiograph taken after barium swallow (Fig. 3.31).

✪ The close relationship of the oesophagus and the left atrium is made use of in determining left atrial enlargement in mitral stenosis. Barium swallow may show displacement of the oesophagus by the enlarged atrium. The lumen of the oesophagus is narrower at its commencement, where the left bronchus crosses it and where it passes through the diaphragm to enter the stomach. These are sites where foreign bodies swallowed are usually impacted and where strictures develop after swallowing caustic fluids. They are also common sites for carcinoma of the oesophagus.

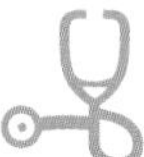

*Clinical box 3.12*

**Dissecting aneurysm**

In dissecting aneurysm the part of the wall of the aorta (tunica media) splits into two layers creating a false lumen in the wall. Entry of blood into this cavity can occlude branches of the aorta at that site. The thoracic aorta is the most common artery affected in this process. The most prominent symptom of this condition is a very sudden onset of excruciating pain which may radiate to the back and shoulder. If the condition occurs proximal to the origin of the left subclavian artery it can occlude the coronary arteries and the head and neck vessels.

✪ In the posterior mediastinum the oesophagus is closely related to the descending aorta (see above). Pathology of one can affect the other. Carcinoma of the oesophagus may spread into the aorta to cause severe bleeding. An aneurysm

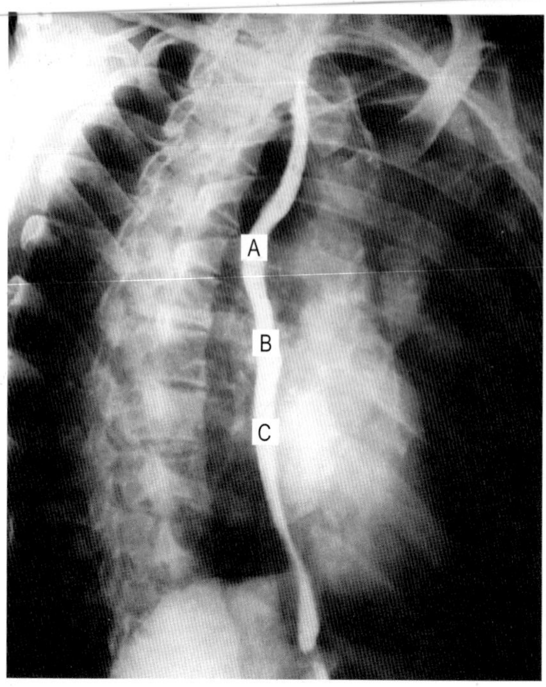


Fig. 3.31 Oblique radiograph of the thorax during a 'barium swallow' outlining the oesophagus. The three indentations produced by the arch of the aorta (A), left bronchus (B) and the left atrium (C) are seen well.

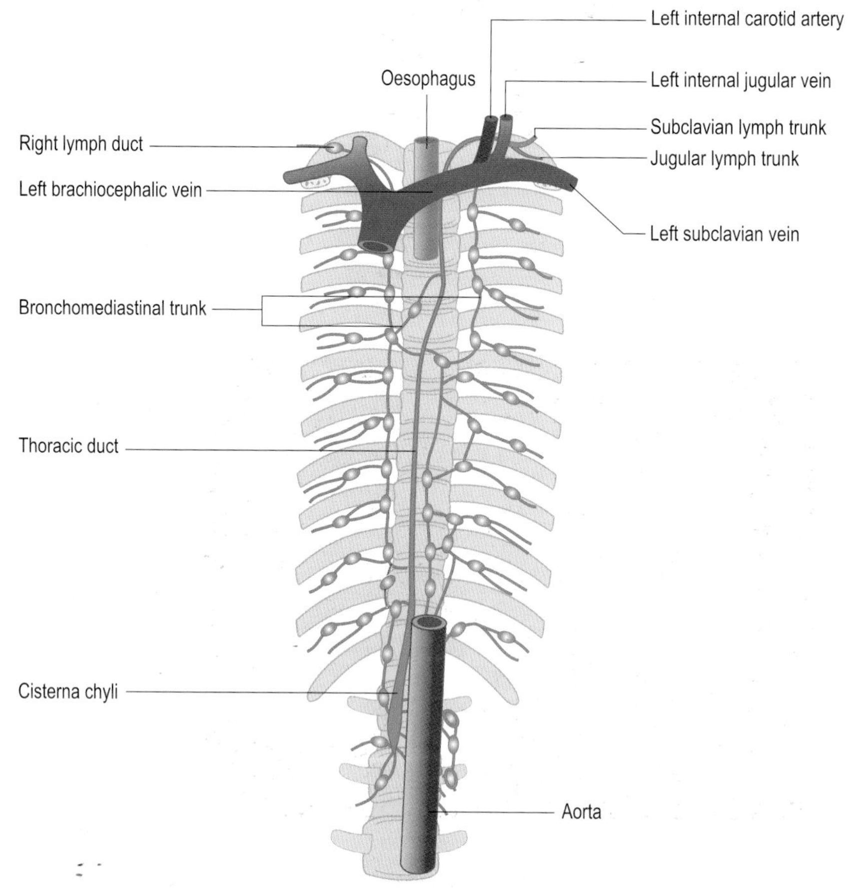


Fig. 3.32 Cisterna chyli, thoracic duct and right lymph duct.

of the aorta may compress the oesophagus to cause difficulty in swallowing (dysphagia).

### Thoracic duct

The thoracic duct, a large lymph duct, starts as the continuation of the cysterna chyli in the abdomen, passes through the thorax and enters the neck lying on the left border of the oesophagus (Fig. 3.32). In the neck it arches to the left, lying in the plane between the carotid sheath and vertebral arteries, to enter the junction between the subclavian and internal jugular veins. It carries lymph from the whole body except that from the right side of thorax, right upper limb, right side of head and neck and the lower lobe of right lung.

### The azygos vein

The azygos vein enters the thorax through the aortic opening of the diaphragm and passes upwards lying on the vertebral bodies and arching over the root of the right lung to drain into the superior vena cava. The azygos vein receives the lower eight posterior intercostal veins of the right side and the right superior intercostal vein (Fig. 3.33).

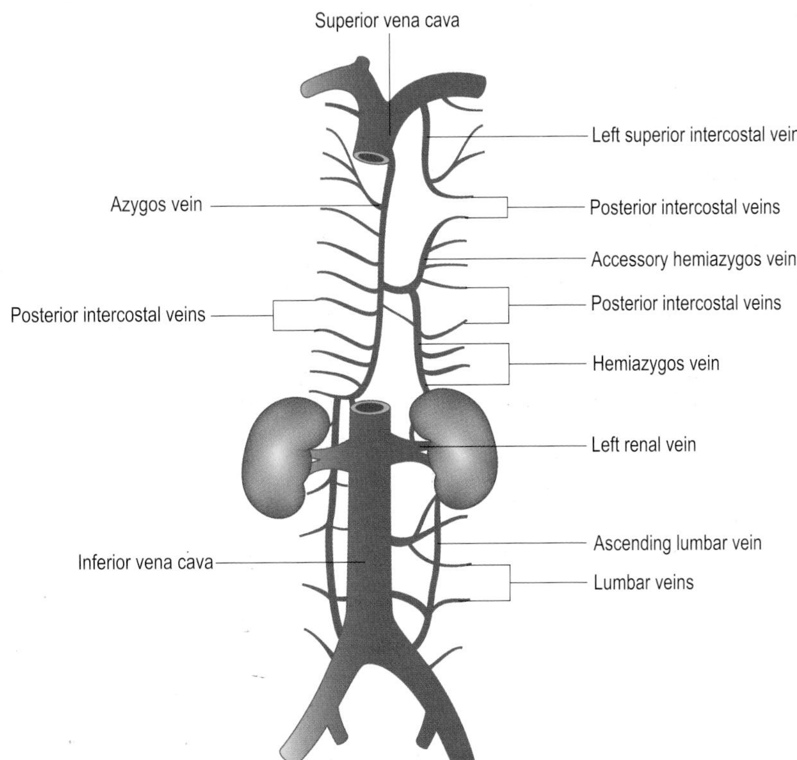


Fig. 3.33 Veins of the posterior chest and abdominal wall.

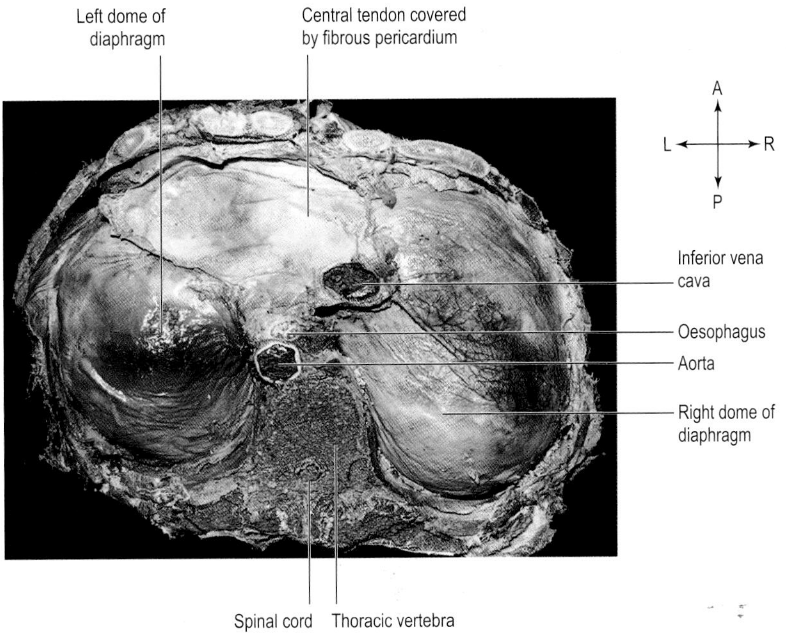


Fig. 3.34 Diaphragm viewed from above.

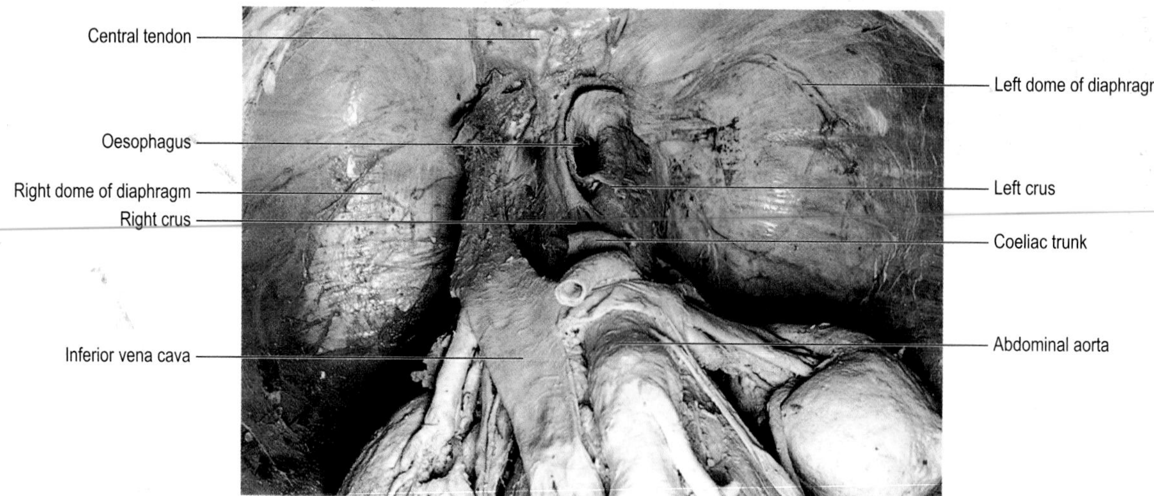


Fig. 3.35 Diaphragm viewed from below. Liver, stomach, spleen and the small and large intestines have all been removed.

The hemiazygos veins which receive the intercostal veins of the left side drain into the azygos vein.

## The sympathetic trunk

The sympathetic trunks (see Figs 3.25, 3.26) lie on each side of the vertebral column, extending from the base of the skull to the coccyx where the two chains fuse together. Each trunk contains a number of sympathetic ganglia, the thoracic region having about 11 ganglia which lie on the neck of the ribs. The ganglia are closely related to the intercostal nerves from which they receive preganglionic fibres as white rami communicantes. The postganglionic fibres from the ganglia go back to the intercostal nerves as grey rami communicantes. The thoracic ganglia give off the greater, lesser and least splanchnic nerves to supply the abdominal viscera. The splanchnic nerves are preganglionic fibres which will synapse in collateral ganglia displaced from the sympathetic trunk (e.g. coeliac ganglion) in the abdomen.

## Diaphragm

The diaphragm (Figs 3.34, 3.35) separates the thoracic and abdominal cavities. It transmits the inferior vena cava, the oesophagus, the sympathetic trunk and the splanchnic nerves. The aorta passes behind the diaphragm between its two crura. The peripheral part of the diaphragm is muscular whereas its central part, the central tendon, is fibrous. Its upper surface fuses with the fibrous pericardium. The muscular part is attached to the upper lumbar vertebrae and the intervertebral discs through the right and left crura. Fibres of the diaphragm also take origin from the medial and lateral arcuate ligaments which are thickenings of the fascia overlying the psoas major and the quadratus lumborum muscles on the posterior abdominal wall. Besides these vertebral attachments the diaphragm is attached to the inner aspects of the lower six ribs and costal cartilages, as well as to the xiphoid process of the sternum. The aortic opening lies at the level of T12 and transmits the abdominal aorta, thoracic duct and the azygos vein. The oesophagus passes through the left crus with the fibres of the right crus looping around it at the level of T10. The oesophageal orifice also transmits the vagus nerves and the left gastric vessels. The inferior vena caval opening which lies more anteriorly in the central tendon of the diaphragm at the level of T8 also transmits the right phrenic nerve. The sympathetic trunk enters the abdomen by passing under the medial arcuate ligament and the splanchnic nerves by piercing the crura.

✪ The nerve supply of the diaphragm, both sensory and motor, is by the phrenic nerve and hence pain due to diaphragmatic irritation is felt in the shoulder region as a referred pain. There is additional supply of sensory nerves to the peripheral aspect by the intercostal nerves. On contraction the diaphragm descends down to increase the vertical diameter of the thoracic cavity. It thus acts as the major muscle of inspiration. The abdominal pressure is increased by contraction of the diaphragm and hence it contributes importantly to functions such as defecation, micturition and parturition.

✪ Injury to the phrenic nerve will paralyse the corresponding half of the diaphragm resulting in paradoxical movement during respiration. Instead of descending during inspiration the paralysed side gets pushed upwards by the abdominal viscera. This can be detected radiographically.

# Chapter 4
# Abdomen



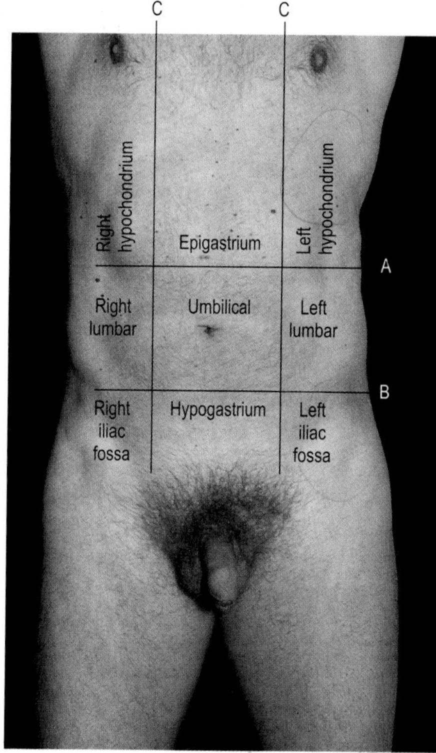


Fig. 4.1 Regions of the abdomen. A: Transpyloric plane, B: Transtubercular plane, C: Midclavicular line.

## Surface anatomy, regions of the abdomen

The various regions of the abdomen referred to in the description of surface anatomy and in the localisation of pathology are shown in Fig. 4.1. The lower costal margin extends from the xiphoid process of the sternum to the 10th costal cartilage (Fig. 4.2). The transpyloric plane passing across the lower border of L1 vertebra lies halfway between the suprasternal notch and the pubic symphysis. This plane passes through the pylorus, the neck of the pancreas, the duodenojejunal flexure, the fundus of the gallbladder and the hila of the kidneys. It can also be drawn by connecting the tips of the ninth costal cartilages. The subcostal plane passing through the lower margin of the 10th costal cartilage cuts across the L3 vertebra.

✪ For descriptive purposes the abdomen is divided into nine regions (Fig. 4.1) by two horizontal and two vertical planes. The transpyloric and transtubercular (connecting the tubercles of the iliac crest) are the horizontal planes, the two midclavicular lines the vertical. The nine regions are the epigastrium, the right and left hypochondrium, the umbilical region, the right and left lumbar region, the hypogastrium (or the suprapubic region) and the right and left iliac fossa. References to these regions are made in relation to location of viscera, localisation of pain and location of an abdominal mass.

### Dermatomes of the anterior abdominal wall

Skin of the abdominal wall is innervated segmentally by the spinal nerves T7 just below the xiphoid process of the sternum, L1 in the suprapubic region and the segments in between in the region between the two. T10 segment is at the level of the umbilicus. ✪ As in the thoracic wall, segments of skin supplied by the intercostal nerves are common sites of vesicles in Herpes zoster (shingles), a viral infection affecting the spinal nerve ganglia spreading through the intercostal nerves.

### Fasciae of the anterior abdominal wall

Unlike most of the rest of the body the anterior abdominal wall has no deep fascia. The superficial fascia has two layers,

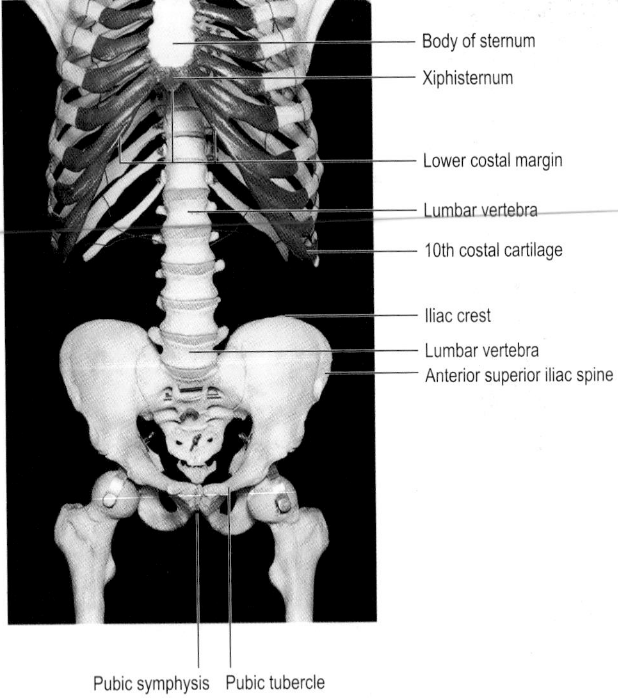


Fig. 4.2 Bony thoracic cage and pelvis.

a fatty layer (Camper's fascia) underneath which is a membranous (fibrous) layer (Scarpa's fascia). The fatty layer is continuous with the superficial fascia of the rest of the trunk and lower limbs whereas the membranous layer extends into the perineum as the Colles' fascia prolonging onto the scrotum, penis and labia majora. It also extends into the upper part of the thigh where it fuses with the deep fascia of the thigh.

## Muscles of the anterior abdominal wall

The anterior abdominal wall has three flat muscles, i.e. external oblique, internal oblique and transversus, which are fleshy laterally and aponeurotic in front. The aponeuroses ensheath the rectus abdominis muscle and fuse in the midline to form the linea alba. The linea alba extends from the pubic symphysis to the xiphoid process of the sternum.

### External oblique

This arises from the lower eight ribs and is inserted into the iliac crest, pubic tubercle and pubic crest (Figs 4.3, 4.4, also see Fig. 4.84). Between the anterior superior iliac spine and the pubic tubercle its lower curved free border forms the inguinal ligament. The anterior part of the aponeurosis contributes to the anterior wall of the rectus sheath.

### Internal oblique

This arises from the lumbar fascia, the iliac crest and the lateral two-thirds of the inguinal ligament (Fig. 4.4). The majority of its fibres run upwards and medially at right angles to the fibres of the external oblique. The fibres arising from the inguinal ligament arch over the spermatic cord to fuse with the aponeurosis of the transversus to form the conjoint tendon which extends behind the cord to be attached to the pubic crest.

### Transversus abdominis

This arises from the inner surface of the lower six ribs, the lumbar fascia, the iliac crest and the lateral third of the inguinal ligament (Fig. 4.5). The major part of the muscle is inserted to the linea alba via an aponeurosis which contributes to the posterior wall of the rectus sheath. The fibres from the inguinal ligament fuse with similar fibres from the internal oblique to form the conjoint tendon.

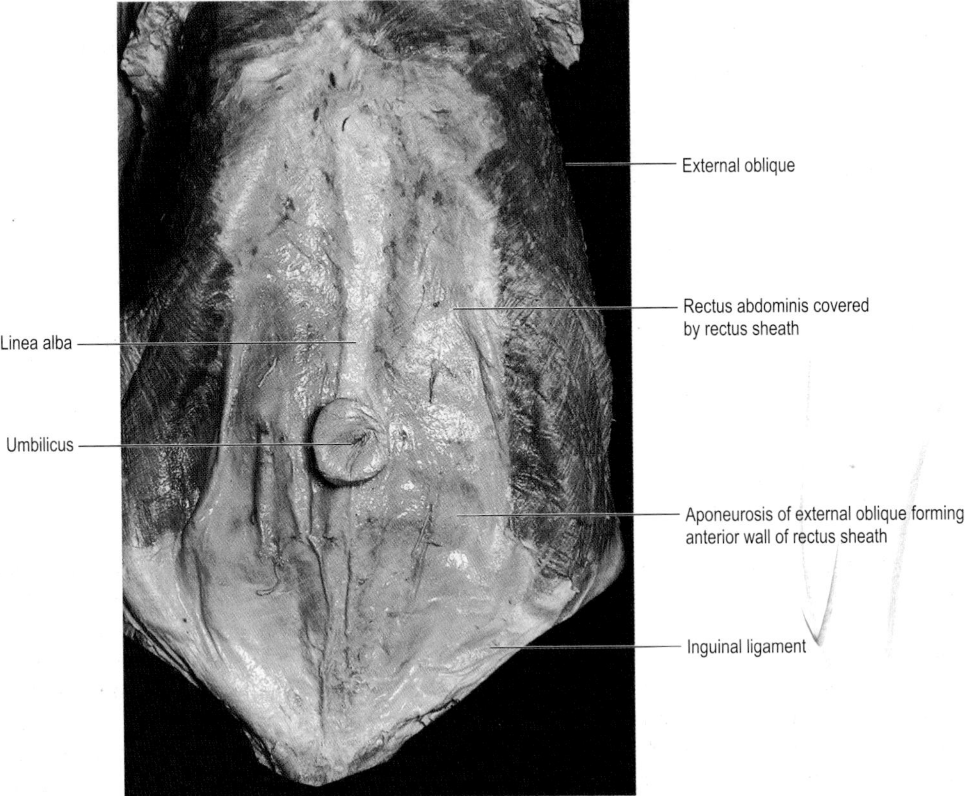


Fig. 4.3 External oblique, rectus sheath and linea alba.

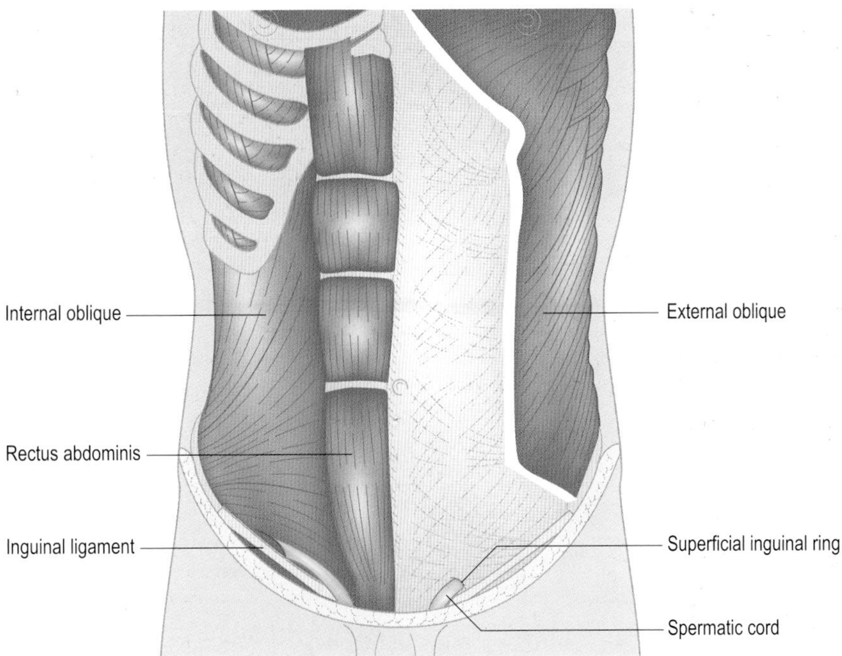


Fig. 4.4 Muscles of the anterior abdominal wall – anterior view. The external oblique has been removed on the right hand side.

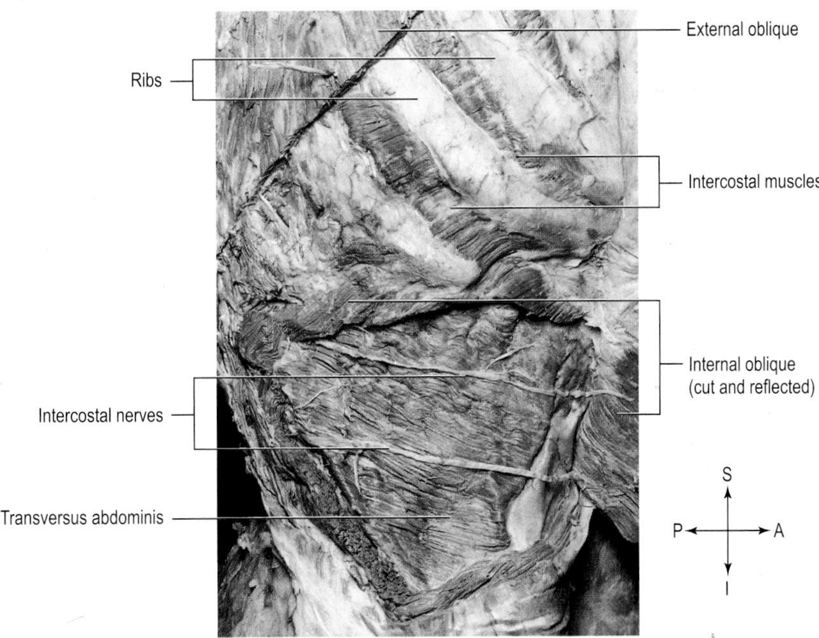


Fig. 4.5 The neurovascular plane of the anterior abdominal wall. The nerves of the anterior abdominal wall (7th–11th intercostal nerves and the subcostal nerve) accompanied by blood vessels lie between the internal oblique and transversus abdominis.

## Transversalis fascia

This is a layer of fascia deep to the transversus abdominis separating it from the parietal peritoneum and extraperitoneal fat. It extends above as the fascia lining the under-surface of the diaphragm and posteriorly as the fascia covering the psoas major muscles.

## Rectus abdominis

This muscle lying on either side of the midline arises from the pubic symphysis and pubic crest to be inserted to the fifth, sixth and seventh costal cartilages (Figs 4.3, 4.4). The anterior surface of the muscle has three tendinous intersections, one at the level of the xiphoid, one at the umbilicus and the third halfway between these two levels. The intersections are adherent to the anterior wall of the rectus sheath but not to the posterior.

## Nerve supply

The abdominal muscles, like the skin over the anterior abdominal wall, are segmentally innervated by spinal nerves T7 to L1. The distribution can be remembered by knowing that T7 supplies the region near the xiphoid, T10 the region of the umbilicus and L1 the suprapubic region. The nerves and the accompanying intercostal vessels (Fig. 4.5) lie between the internal oblique and transversus (neurovascular plane). This is similar to the neurovascular plane of the thoracic wall where it is between the second and third layers of muscles.

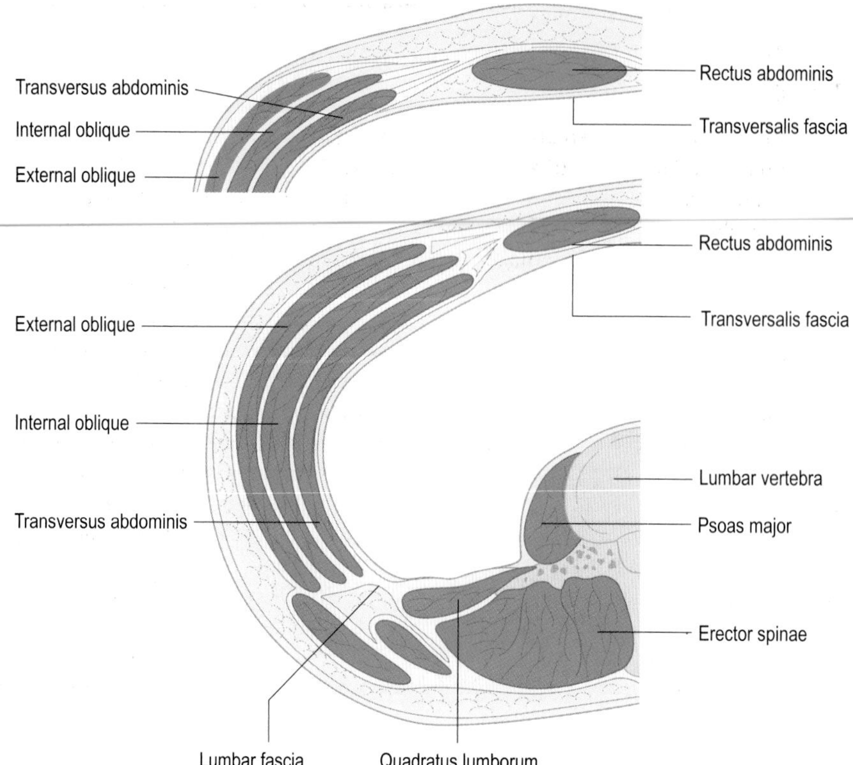


Fig. 4.6 Transverse section of the abdominal wall, showing the arrangement of muscles, lumbar fascia and rectus sheath. The upper figure shows the rectus abdominis and the formation of the rectus sheath below the arcuate line.

### The rectus sheath

The arrangement of the rectus sheath (Fig. 4.6) which strengthens the rectus and gives additional support to this region of the abdomen is as follows:

- Above the costal margin where the muscle is attached to the costal cartilages the sheath's anterior wall is by external oblique aponeurosis only.
- From the costal margin to a point midway between the pubic crest and umbilicus the internal oblique aponeurosis splits to enclose the rectus. The anterior aspect of the sheath thus formed is reinforced by the external oblique aponeurosis and the posterior aspect by the transversus.
- Below the point halfway between the umbilicus and the pubic crest the aponeurosis of the external oblique, internal oblique and transversus pass in front of the rectus. Thus the sheath is deficient posteriorly in this region. The posterior wall of the rectus sheath thus has a free border halfway between the umbilicus and the pubic crest. This is known as the arcuate line of Douglas. The inferior epigastric artery enters the rectus sheath at this point to anastomose with the superior epigastric artery.

The rectus sheath contains, besides the rectus abdominis, the terminal parts of the T7–L1 nerves and accompanying vessels as well as the superior and inferior epigastric vessels. See Clinical box 4.1.

## The inguinal canal

The inguinal canal (Figs 4.7–4.9) is a slit-like space in between the muscles of the anterior abdominal wall, above the medial half of the inguinal ligament. It contains the spermatic cord and the ilioinguinal nerve in the male and the round ligament of the uterus and the ilioinguinal nerve in the female. It is about 6cm long and extends from the deep inguinal ring to the superficial inguinal ring (external ring). The deep inguinal ring is a defect in the transversalis fascia about 1 cm above the midpoint of the inguinal ligament. The superficial inguinal ring, which is above and medial to the pubic tubercle, is a defect in the external oblique aponeurosis.

### Walls of the inguinal canal

The anterior wall (i.e. structures in front of the spermatic cord) is formed by the external oblique aponeurosis reinforced laterally by fibres of the internal oblique. The posterior wall (structures behind the spermatic cord) throughout is formed by the transversalis fascia and is reinforced medially by the conjoint tendon.

### Roof and floor of the inguinal canal

The roof of the canal (structures above the cord) is formed by the arched fibres of the transversus and the internal oblique. The floor, on which the spermatic cord lies, is formed by the inguinal ligament. The lacunar ligament (pectineal part of the inguinal ligament or Gimbernat's ligament), which is the continuation of the attachment of the inguinal ligament to the pubic ramus, is an additional structure on the floor in the medial part of the canal. See Clinical box 4.2.

## Testis, epididymis and the spermatic cord

See Figures 4.10–4.13. The testis which lies within the scrotum has the following coverings:

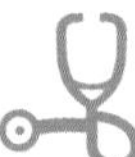

## Clinical box 4.1

### Abdominal incisions

Most incisions for surgical access to the abdomen are through the anterior abdominal wall. The choice of a particular incision will depend on the operation performed. A good incision should allow maximum access, leaving an unobtrusive scar with minimal damage to the muscles and nerves. A weak scar can cause an incisional hernia

In a **midline incision** the linea alba is cut. Rapid access is possible by this route as the linea alba, being fibrous tissue, has fewer blood vessels to ligate. A midline incision below the umbilicus is slightly more difficult than the one above as the linea alba narrows considerably in the lower part of the abdomen.

A **paramedian** incision is placed about 2–4cm lateral to the midline. The anterior layer of the rectus sheath is encountered deep to the skin and subcutaneous tissue. This is adherent to the muscles on three locations where the tendinous intersections of the rectus are adherent to the anterior layer of the sheath and has to be carefully released. The rectus is pushed laterally to avoid traction on the nerves and vessels entering it from the lateral aspect. The posterior layer of the sheath and peritoneum together form a tough membrane and this is incised together after making sure that no part of the bowel is adherent to it. Only the transversalis fascia, peritoneum and fat are present below the arcuate line of Douglas as all three aponeuroses lie in front of the rectus. The inferior epigastric artery, which lies in the sheath deep to the rectus, may need ligation in a low paramedian incision.

A right **subcostal (Kocher)** incision is used for biliary surgery. It extends from the midline parallel to and 3cm below the costal margin. The anterior layer of the rectus sheath and the rectus abdominis are divided. The superior epigastric artery or its branches seen deep to the rectus are ligated and divided. The 7th intercostal nerve lies above the incision, but the 8th and 9th nerves may be encountered. Cutting more than two intercostal nerves should be avoided as it may weaken the rectus.

**Lanz incision** is commonly used to approach the appendix. This is a transverse incision about 2cm above the anterior superior iliac spine extending up to the lateral border of the rectus. External oblique, internal oblique and transversus muscles are split in the direction of their fibres. Care should be taken not to damage the ilioinguinal and iliohypogastric nerves which supply the internal oblique and transversus fibres forming the conjoint tendon. Weakening of the conjoint tendon can cause a direct inguinal hernia.

The Lanz incision replaces the oblique incision at the McBurney's point (McBurney's incision) as it is more in line of the skin crease and hence leaves a cosmetically better scar.

**Pfannenstiel's incision** is a transverse incision in the suprapubic region commonly used for pelvic surgery. The anterior layer of rectus is incised transversely following a transverse incision of the skin just above the symphysis pubis. The rectus muscles are separated or incised transversely. Deep to the rectus the transversalis fascia and the peritoneum are incised, taking care not to injure the urinary bladder.

For **laparoscopic surgery**, carbon dioxide is introduced into the peritoneal cavity through a needle to increase its space. A trocar/port is placed into the now insufflated peritoneal cavity and a laparoscope which has a small camera attachment is introduced into the abdomen which allows visualisation inside the abdominal cavity on video screens. Additional trocar ports are then placed to introduce laparoscopic instruments, such as graspers, dissectors and scissors.

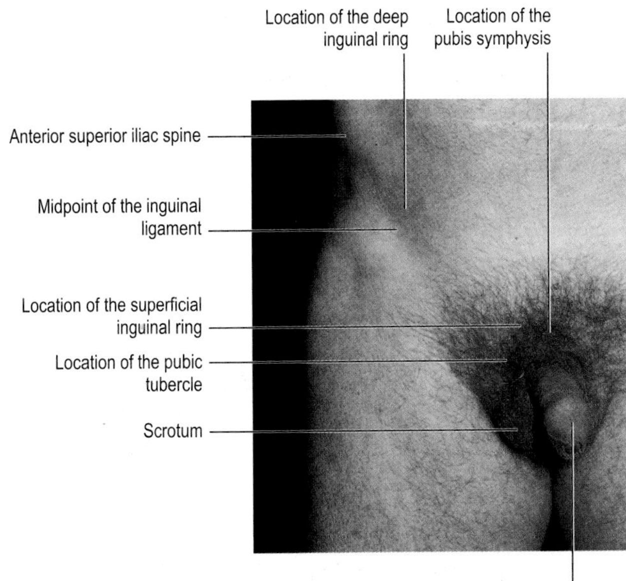


Fig. 4.7 Surface anatomy of the groin.

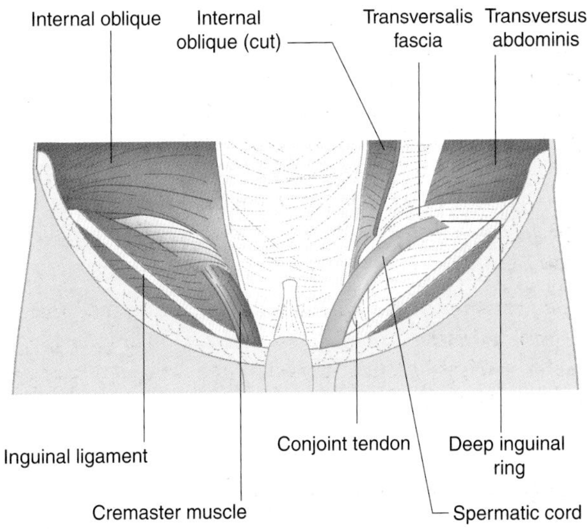


Fig. 4.8 Inguinal region in the male. On the right-hand side of the external oblique has been removed; on the left-hand side the external oblique and internal oblique have been partially removed.

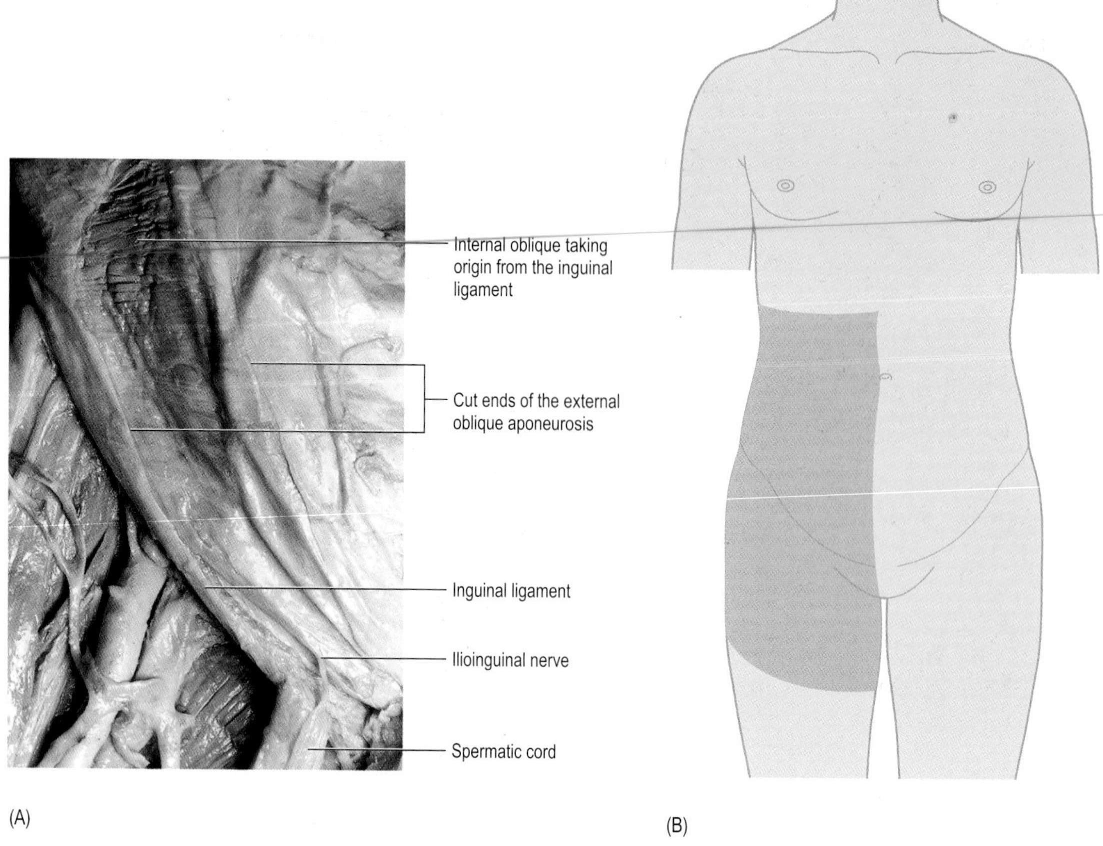


Fig. 4.9 (A) External oblique aponeurosis cut to show the internal oblique fibres arching over the spermatic cord. Also seen is the ilioinguinal nerve between the external oblique aponeurosis and the internal oblique. (B) Region dissected.

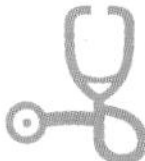

## *Clinical box 4.2*

### Inguinal hernias

Part of the intestine or peritoneal fold can herniate through the inguinal canal as an inguinal hernia. The peritoneal sac in which the hernia is contained is known as the hernial sac. These hernias are more common in the male as the canal is bigger. Inguinal hernias protrude through the external (superficial) ring above and medial to the pubic tubercle. This may have to be distinguished from a femoral hernia which comes through the femoral ring which is below and lateral to the pubic tubercle.

An indirect inguinal hernia comes through the deep inguinal ring and hence traverses the whole extent of the canal. It is often caused by a persistent processus vaginalis and hence may be congenital. It is contained inside the coverings of the spermatic cord. If large enough it emerges through the external ring and descends into the scrotum. The inferior epigastric artery which lies medial to the deep ring is a guide to determine the type of hernia. The neck of the sac (the point of entry on the abdominal wall), being at the deep inguinal ring, is lateral to the inferior epigastric artery.

A direct inguinal hernia on the other hand invaginates the posterior wall of the canal. It does not descend into the scrotum as the conjoint tendon which it invaginates will not stretch that far. The neck of the hernia, at operation, will be seen medial to the inferior epigastric artery.

- scrotal skin
- dartos muscle (muscle developed in the superficial fascia)
- external spermatic fascia
- cremaster muscle and fascia
- internal spermatic fascia
- tunica vaginalis.

The testis measures about 4cm from its upper pole to the lower pole, 3cm from anterior border to posterior border and about 2.5cm from its medial to lateral surface. The left testis is at a lower level than the right. The testis has a fibrous capsule, the tunica albuginea, which in turn is surrounded by a double-layered serous membrane, the tunica vaginalis. The internal structure consists of a large number of lobules separated by septae, each lobule containing between one and three seminiferous tubules within which the sperms are produced.

The epididymis lies on the posterolateral aspect of the testis. The groove between the testis and epididymis is the sinus epididymis. The epididymis has an upper part or head and a lower part which continues as the ductus deferens. The epididymis is also covered by tunica vaginalis except along its posterior border. The seminiferous tubules drain into an irregular series of ducts known as the rete testis from which efferent tubules enter the head of the epididymis. Sperms produced in the seminiferous tubules of the testis are stored in the epididymis and the ductus before ejaculation. The ductus deferens which joins the duct

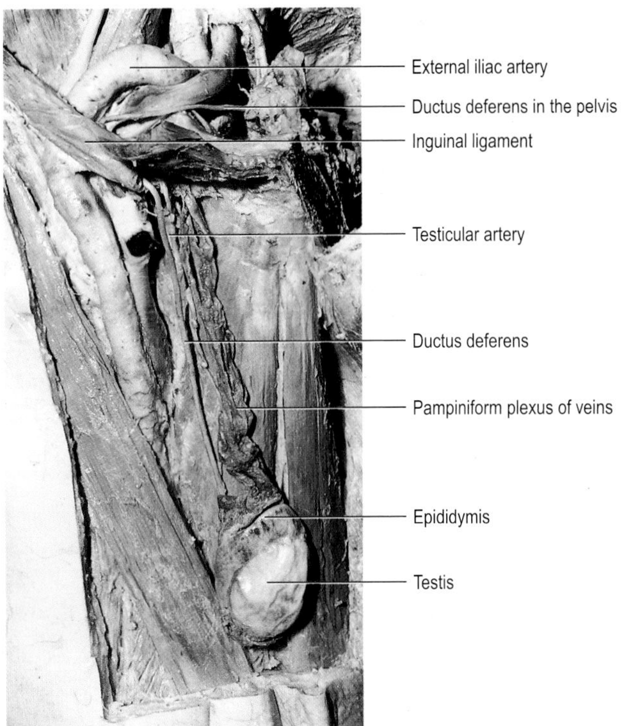


Fig. 4.10 Contents of the scrotum and spermatic cord dissected and displaced on to the front of the thigh.

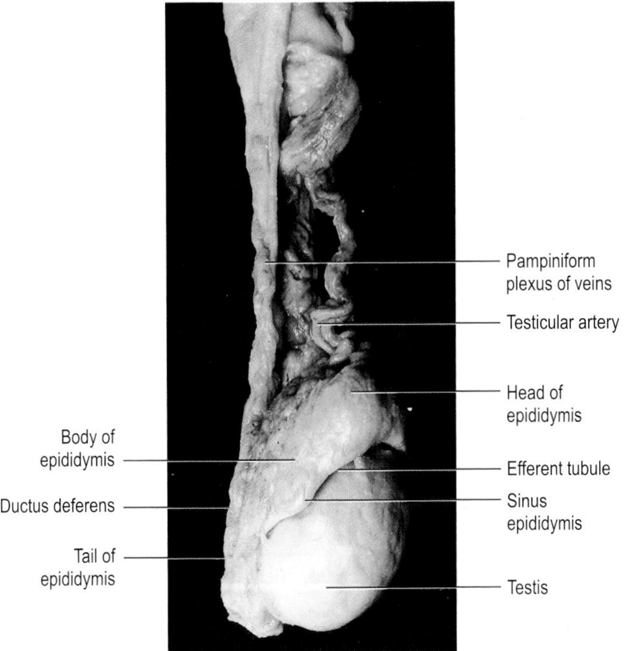


Fig. 4.11 Testis, epididymis and the contents of the spermatic cord after removal of their coverings.

of the seminal vesicle to form the ejaculatory duct in turn enters the prostatic part of the urethra and transports sperm to the urethra.

✪ The testis and the epididymis at their upper ends may have embryological remnants known as appendix testis and appendix epididymis respectively. These small pedunculated bodies may undergo torsion.

✪ The testis lies outside the body cavity in the scrotum where it is maintained at a temperature 2–3°C lower than the body temperature. Failure to descend into the scrotum causes failure of spermatogenesis.

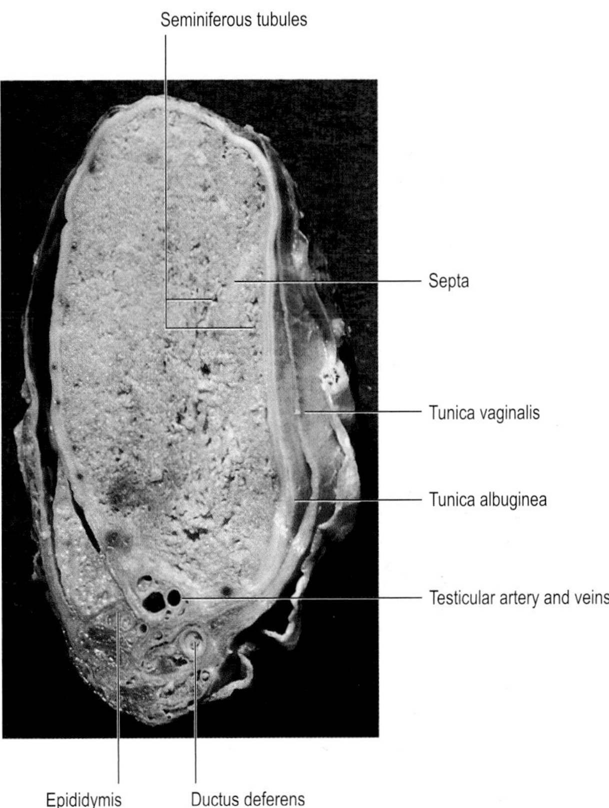


Fig. 4.12 Transverse section of left testis and epididymis.

### Blood supply

The testis and epididymis are suspended by the spermatic cord containing their arterial supply, venous and lymphatic drainage and nerve supply. The testis develops in the L2/L3 vertebral region and drags its vascular, lymphatic and nerve supply from this region to the scrotum. ✪ Testicular and renal pain may mimic each other. Testicular pain hence can radiate to the loin and renal pain often is referred to the scrotum.

The arterial supply is via the testicular artery which is a branch of the abdominal aorta given off just below the level of origin of the renal arteries. The venous drainage is via the pampiniform plexus of veins which become a single testicular vein before terminating in the inferior vena cava on the right side and the left renal vein on the left side. ✪ The lymphatics of the testis and epididymis accompany the blood vessels and drain into the para-aortic lymph nodes. Upper abdomen must therefore be palpated when searching for secondary lymphatic spread from a carcinoma of the testis. See Clinical boxes 4.3 and 4.4.

### The spermatic cord

The spermatic cord (Figs 4.10, 4.11, 4.13) contains the ductus deferens (vas deferens), the testicular artery and the pampiniform plexus of veins. Other structures in the cord are the cremasteric artery, the artery to the vas, nerve to the cremaster, sympathetic nerves and the lymphatics of the testis and epididymis. Because of its passage through the inguinal canal the spermatic cord acquires three coverings, i.e. the external spermatic fascia from the external oblique aponeurosis at the superficial inguinal ring, the cremasteric muscle and fascia from the internal oblique, and the internal spermatic fascia from the transversalis fascia at the deep inguinal ring.

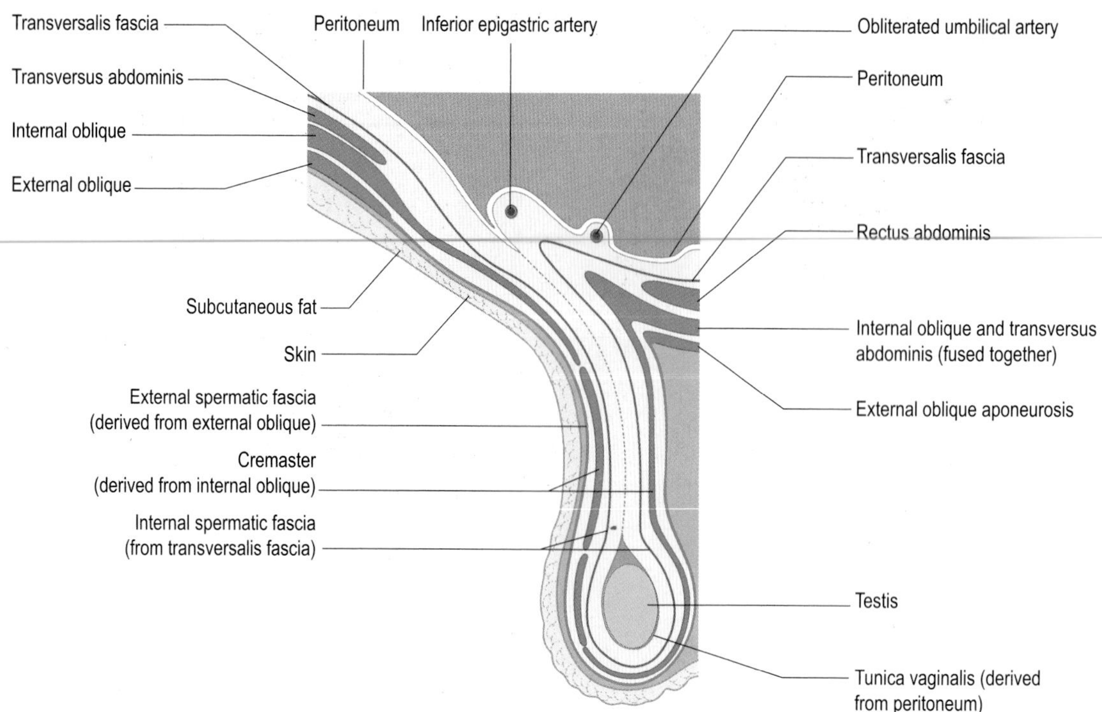


Fig. 4.13 Schematic diagram of the inguinal canal, and the coverings of testis and spermatic cord.

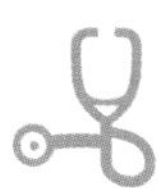

### *Clinical box 4.3*

**Descent of the testis**

The testis develops on the posterior abdominal wall at the level of L2/L3 vertebrae from the genital ridge, a mesodermal outgrowth medial to the mesonephros from which the renal tissues are developed. As the testis enlarges, it migrates downwards. At the 3rd month of intrauterine life it reaches the iliac fossa and enters the inguinal canal in the 7th month. At the 8th month it is at the superficial inguinal ring and finally reaches the scrotum by the 9th month. A mesodermal strand known as the gubernaculum accompanied by a peritoneal sac, the processus vaginalis, precedes the testicular descent. The testis, after descent invaginates the lower part of the processus vaginalis from behind. Part of the processus (peritoneum) around the testis forms the tunica vaginalis and rest of the processus obliterates.

An undescended testis or cryptorchid testis is a condition where the testicular descent is arrested anywhere in its normal path. Testis may remain in the abdomen or in the inguinal canal. Androgenic activity of undescended testis is normal whereas spermatogenesis is defective or absent. Undescended testes are more prone to malignancies.

An ectopic testis is seen when the testicular migration takes an abnormal route into the suprapubic region, perineum or thigh. Ectopic testis, unlike the undescended, has a long spermatic cord and can easily be replaced in the scrotum surgically without causing any tension.

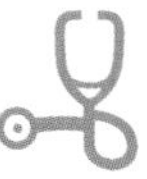

### *Clinical box 4.4*

**Hydrocoele**

Hydrocoele, which manifests as a swelling of the scrotum, is caused by distension of the tunica vaginalis by collection of fluid between it and the testis. This may be idiopathic (due to no apparent cause) or as secondary to testicular diseases. It can also occur where the processus vaginalis is not fully obliterated. In a congenital hydrocoele the fluid collection will extend into the peritoneal cavity due to the presence of an unobliterated processus vaginalis. In the infantile type the processus is obliterated in the proximal half and hence the fluid only extends up to the external ring. In hydrocoele of the cord the processus is obliterated proximally and distally and hence fluid collection is confined to the cord but not around the testis.

✪ Varicocoele is a condition caused by dilated tortuous pampiniform plexus of veins. The condition, which may be felt as a 'bag of worms' while palpating the scrotum, is more commonly present on the left side. As the left testicular veins drain into the left renal veins it may be a sign of a malignant tumour in the left kidney. See Clinical box 4.5.

## The peritoneal cavity

The peritoneal cavity of the abdomen is a potential space between the parietal and the visceral layers of peritoneum. The parietal peritoneum lines the inner surface of the abdominal and pelvic wall. The visceral peritoneum is the continuation of the parietal peritoneum and it invests many of the abdominal organs. In some organs such as duodenum, ascending and descending colon and kidneys only the anterior surfaces of the organs are covered by the peritoneum, making them retroperitoneal organs. Peritoneal membranes connecting the parietal peritoneum to the visceral peritoneum have different names in different regions. The mesentery connects the small intestine,

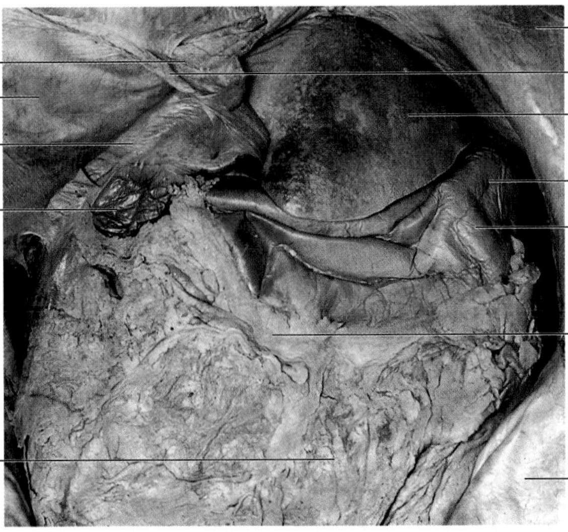

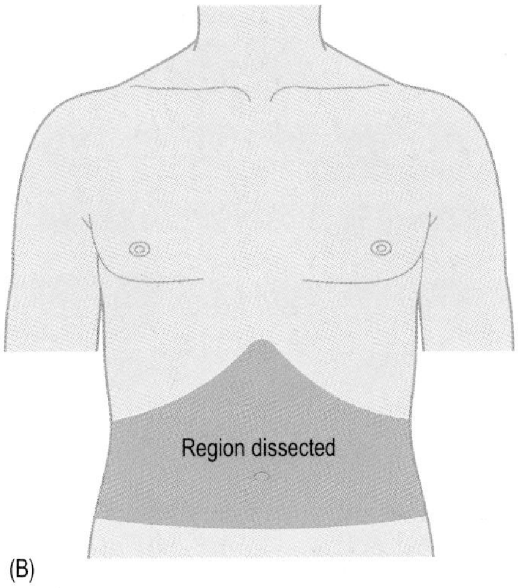

Fig. 4.14 Abdomen opened up to show the upper part of the peritoneal cavity and related organs.

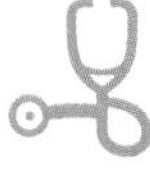

## *Clinical box 4.5*

**Vasectomy**

Male sterilisation is done by bilateral vasectomy. The vas deferens (ductus deferens) can easily be felt through the skin at the root of the scrotum as it has a very firm feel compared with all the other structures forming the spermatic cord. Incision is made on the skin over the vas (often under local anaesthesia) and the surrounding cremaster muscle fibres are separated to expose the ductus deferens. It is then ligated and cut and the wound is finally closed.

mesocolon the large intestine, omentum is attached to the stomach, and the peritoneal ligaments connect the liver.

✪ In the male the peritoneal cavity is a closed sac, but in the female the ends of the uterine tubes open into the peritoneal cavity resulting in a communication with the exterior via the cavity of the tube, the uterus and the vagina. This is a potential source of infection of the peritoneal cavity from the exterior.

The peritoneal cavity is subdivided into a greater sac and a smaller lesser sac or the omental bursa. The greater sac is connected to the lesser sac through the epiploic foramen or the foramen of Winslow. The greater sac is subdivided into a supracolic and an infracolic compartment by the transverse colon and the transverse mesocolon.

The falciform ligament, a double-layered fold of peritoneum, extends from the umbilicus onto the liver holding a cord-like ligamentum teres (which is the obliterated umbilical vein) in its free edge (Fig. 4.14). The right layer of the falciform ligament covers the right lobe of the liver and gets reflected onto the diaphragm as the coronary ligament. The left layer of the falciform ligament after enclosing the left lobe is reflected onto the diaphragm as the left triangular ligament.

After enclosing the liver the peritoneum extends from the liver to the lesser curvature of the stomach and to the first part of the duodenum as the lesser omentum. The two-layered lesser omentum has a right free border (Figs 4.15, 4.16, 4.19) which contains the common bile duct, the hepatic artery and the portal vein.

Along the lesser curvature the lesser omentum splits to enclose the stomach. Along the greater curvature of the stomach it reforms again as the greater omentum. The greater omentum hangs down like an apron from the greater curvature. Two layers from the greater curvature pass down as the anterior two layers of the greater omentum and fold on themselves to go upwards and backwards as its two posterior layers. The posterior layers split to enclose the transverse colon and continue on to the anterior aspect of the pancreas as the transverse mesocolon

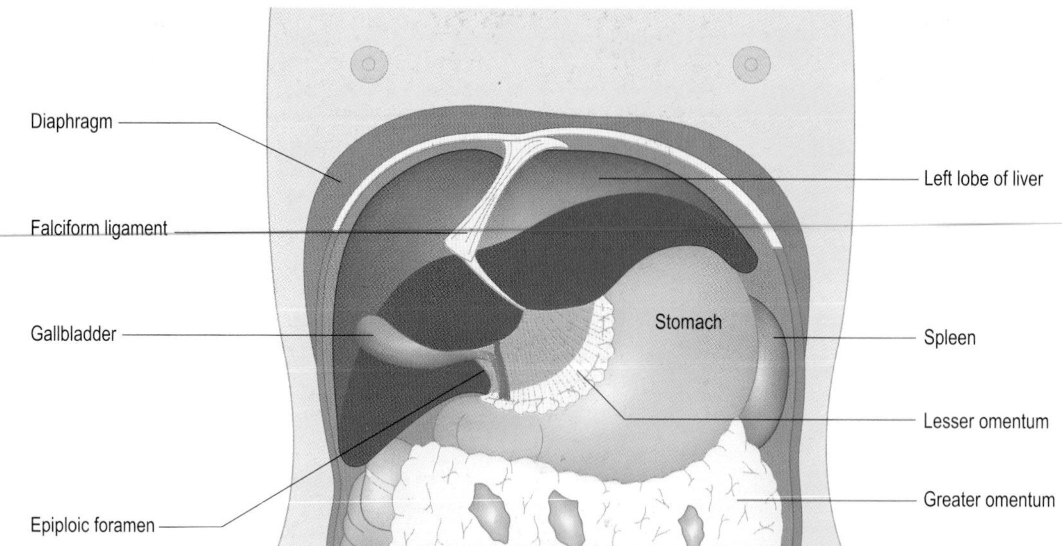


Fig. 4.15 Liver, stomach, lesser omentum – anterior view.

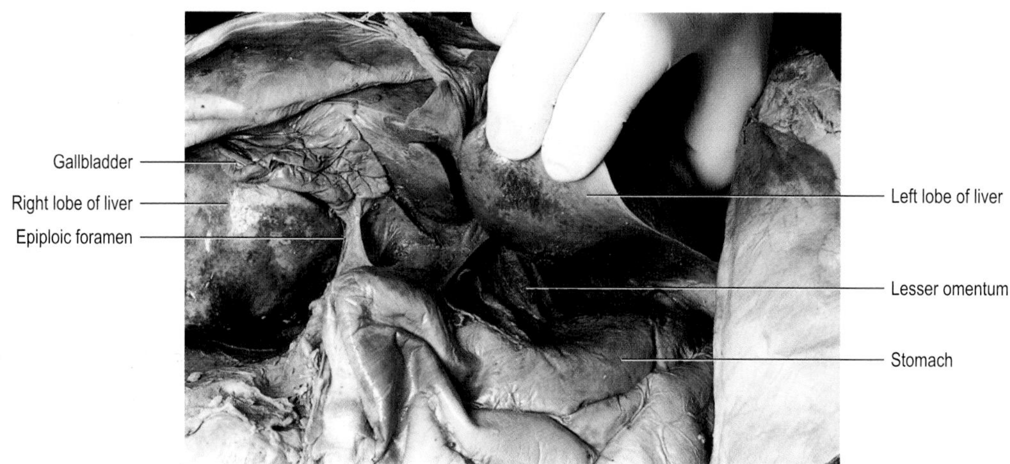


Fig. 4.16 Liver, stomach and lesser omentum.

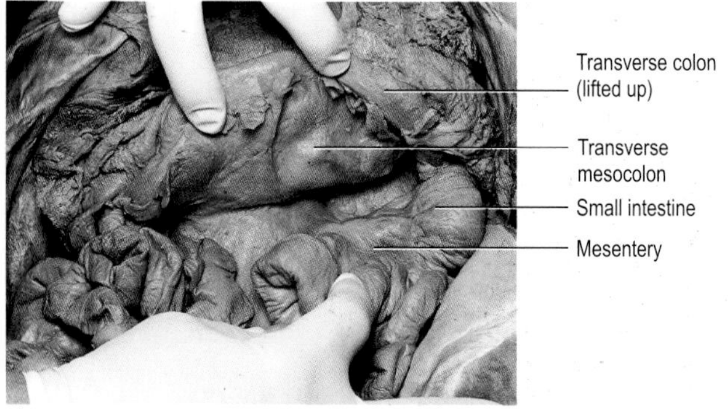


Fig. 4.17 Transverse colon, transverse mesocolon, small intestine and the mesentery.

(Fig. 4.17). From this attachment the upper layer continues as the parietal peritoneum of the posterior abdominal wall and that lining the diaphragm to be reflected back onto the liver. The lower layer from the attachment of the transverse mesocolon similarly continues downwards as the parietal peritoneum of the lower part of the posterior abdominal wall and then onto the pelvic viscera, ultimately becoming the parietal peritoneum of the anterior abdominal wall (Fig. 4.18). The parietal peritoneum of the posterior abdominal wall, however, is interrupted in two places. It is reflected to enclose the jejunum and ileum forming the mesentery of the small intestine and also further down it is interrupted where it is reflected to enclose the sigmoid colon forming the sigmoid mesocolon, the peritoneal membrane connecting the sigmoid colon to the abdominal and pelvic wall. The line of attachment of the mesentery to the posterior abdominal wall is known as the root of the mesentery.

From the greater curvature of the stomach the greater omentum extends to the left as the gastrosplenic ligament which splits to invest the spleen and continues onto the left kidney as the lienorenal ligament (Fig. 4.19).

In the pelvis the peritoneum covers the front and sides of the upper third of the rectum and only the front of its middle third. In the male, from the rectum it is reflected on to the upper surface of the urinary bladder and from there to the anterior abdominal wall. The peritoneal space between the rectum and the bladder is the rectovesical pouch.

In the female the reflection from the rectum is onto the posterior wall of the upper third of the vagina and then over

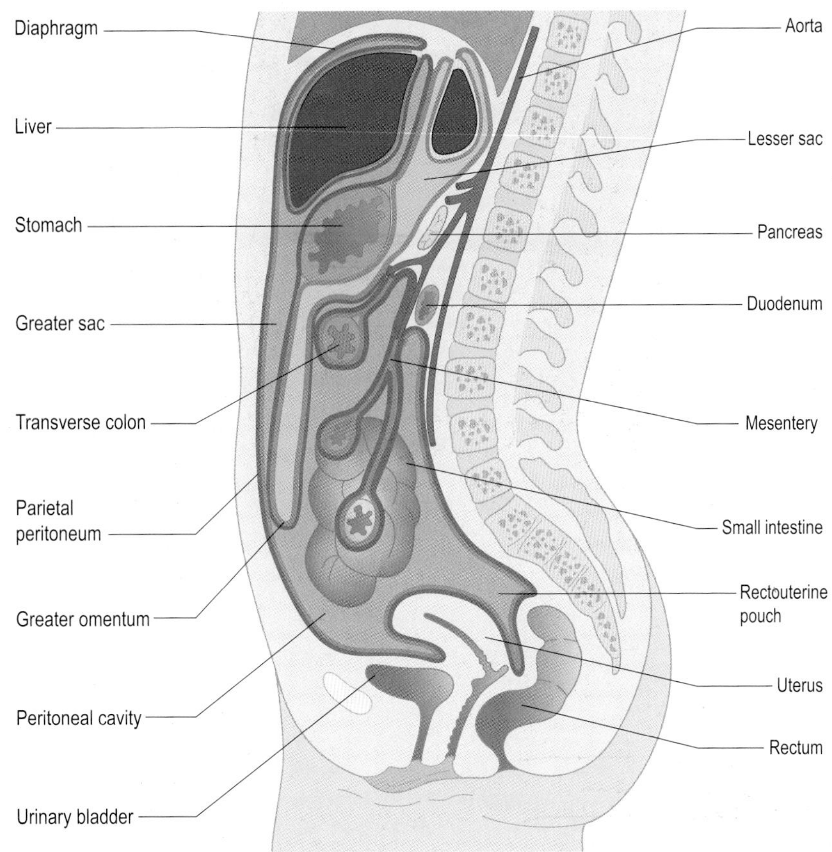


Fig. 4.18 Peritoneum and peritoneal cavity – midline sagittal section.

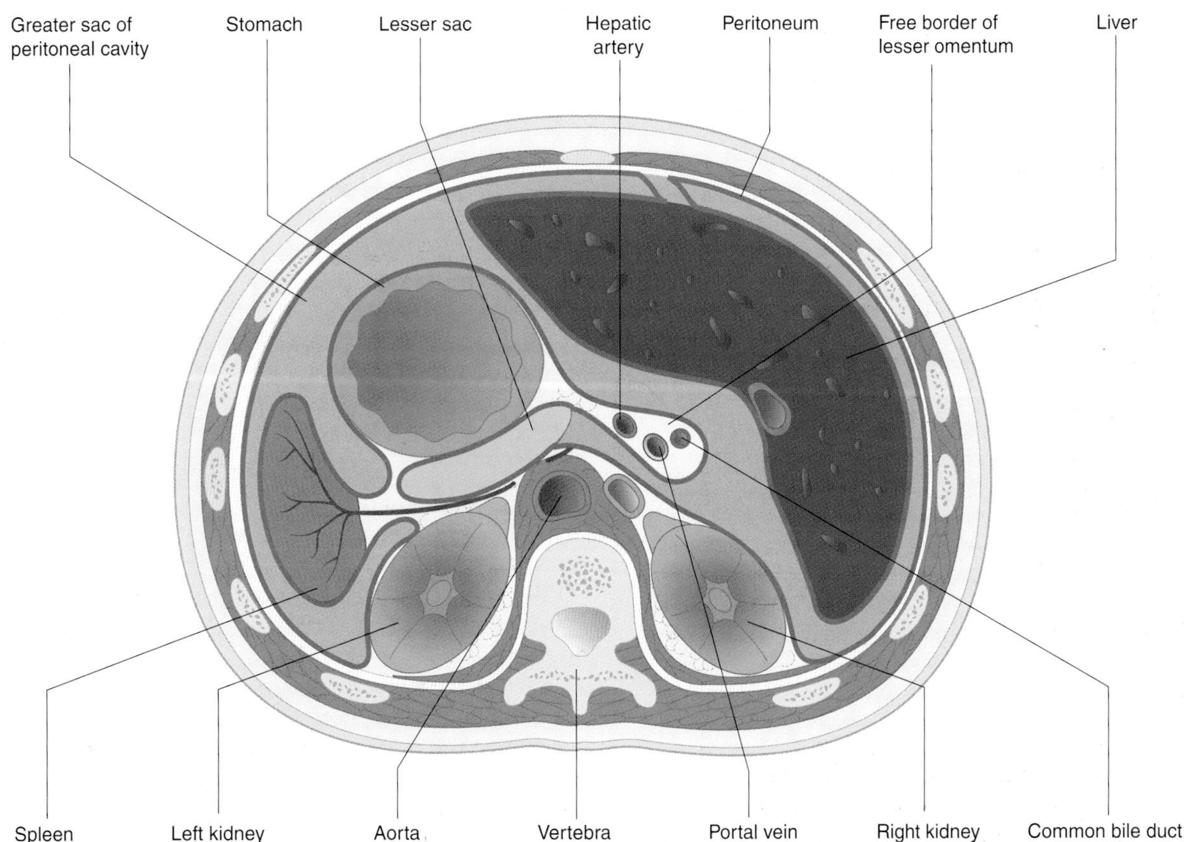


Fig. 4.19 Peritoneum and peritoneal cavity – transverse section at the level of vertebra T12.

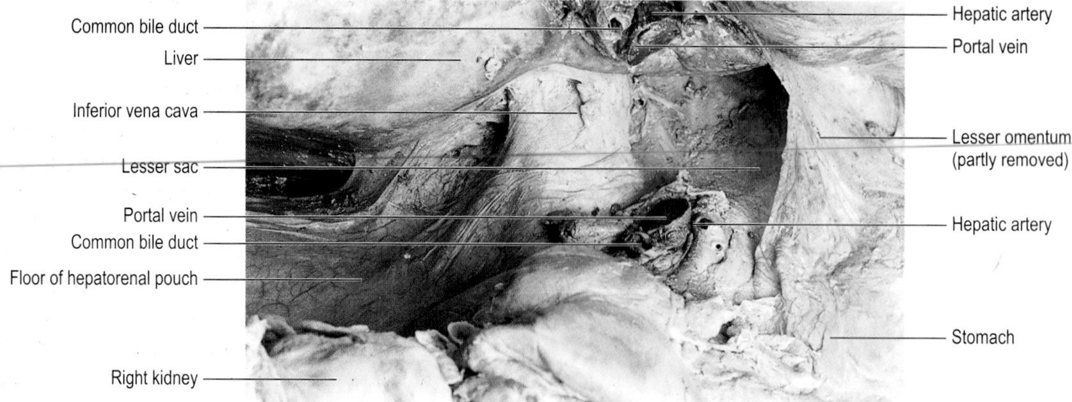


Fig. 4.20 Lesser sac seen after partial removal of the lesser omentum. Transverse colon and the right side of the lesser omentum were removed to obtain this dissection.

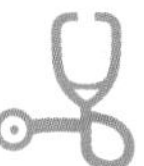

## *Clinical box 4.6*

### Development of the gut

The gastrointestinal tract is developed from an endodermal tube which is known as the primitive gut which is held on to the body wall by the dorsal and ventral mesentery. It has three parts, the foregut, midgut and the hindgut (Fig. 4.21). These are supplied by the three gut arteries viz. the coeliac trunk, the superior mesenteric artery and the inferior mesenteric artery. The parts derived from the foregut, supplied by the coeliac trunk, extend up to the region of the duodenum where the bile duct enters. The midgut extends from the region of the duodenum where the bile duct enters to the junction between the middle and distal third of the transverse colon and is supplied by the superior mesenteric artery. The hindgut, supplied by the inferior mesenteric artery, extends beyond the midgut up to the dentate line of the anal canal.

During development the foregut (from which the stomach and the proximal half of the duodenum develops) rotates so that its left wall becomes its anterior surface and the right wall becomes posterior.

The midgut forms a loop with cranial and caudal limbs whose apex is connected to the yolk sac by the vitellointestinal duct. The caecum develops in the caudal limb. The yolk sac disappears and the vitellointestinal duct becomes a fibrous strand. If it remains patent it becomes the Meckel's diverticulum (see Clinical box 4.7).

The location of the apex of the midgut loop hence is the location of the Meckel's diverticulum i.e. about 2 feet (60cm) proximal to the ileocaecal valve. Therefore the duodenum beyond the entry of the bile duct, the jejunum and most of the ileum are derived from the cranial limb of the midgut loop whereas its caudal limb gives rise to the distal 2 feet (60cm) of the ileum, the caecum and the large intestine up to the junction between the right two-thirds and the left third of the transverse colon. The midgut loop herniates into the umbilical cord in the 5th week of intrauterine life where it remains until the 10th week. When it returns to the abdominal cavity the cranial (proximal) limb (small intestinal components) returns first and then the caudal (distal) limb. The loop also rotates anticlockwise around the axis of the superior mesenteric artery (Fig. 4.21). This order of return and the rotation make the large gut components lie anterior to those of the small gut. Occasionally reverse rotation occurs making the duodenum lie in front of the transverse colon and the superior mesenteric artery.

Rapid proliferation of the mucosa of the gut wall obliterates its lumen in the early stage. Re-canalisation normally takes place. Failure to do so results in atresia or stenosis of part of the bowel. This may be caused by damage to the blood supply resulting in ischaemic changes.

the posterior upper and anterior surfaces of the uterus to the bladder. Between the uterus and the rectum is the rectouterine pouch and between the uterus and the bladder is the uterovesical pouch.

The lesser sac is a part of the peritoneal cavity that lies behind the lesser omentum and the stomach and it also extends into the greater omentum. (The rest of the peritoneal cavity is known as the greater sac.) The lesser sac extends to the left up to the spleen where the sac is bounded by the gastrosplenic and lienorenal ligaments. To the right aspect of the lesser sac is the epiploic foramen through which it communicates with the greater sac of peritoneum.

✪ The epiploic foramen has the following important boundaries:

- Anteriorly – the free border of the lesser omentum containing the bile duct, hepatic artery and the portal vein (Figs 4.19, 4.20). The hepatic artery can be compressed here between the finger and thumb to stop haemorrhage from a torn cystic artery during cholecystectomy. This is known as Pringle's manoeuvre.
- Posteriorly – the inferior vena cava.
- Inferiorly – the first part of the duodenum.
- Superiorly – the caudate process of the liver.

See Clinical box 4.6.

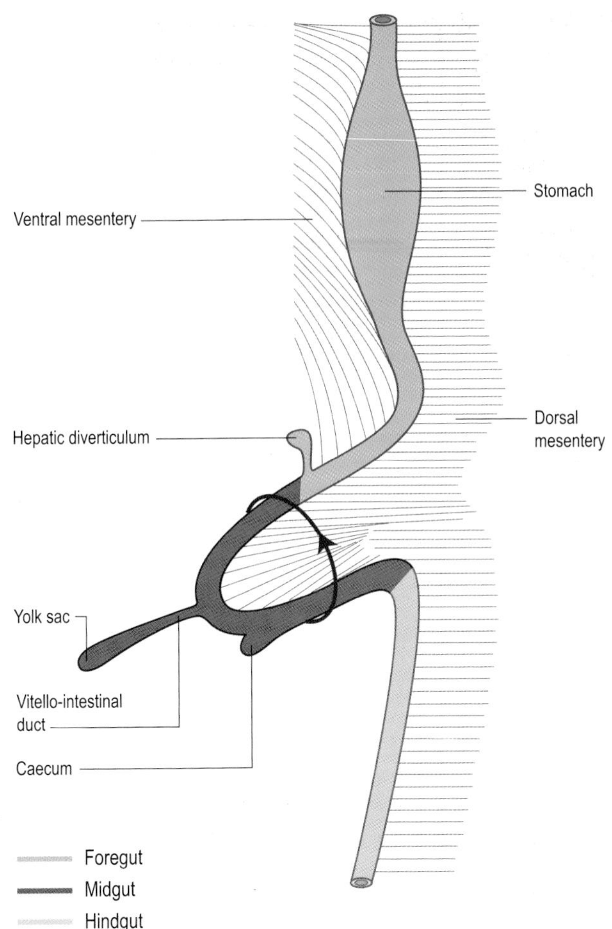


Fig. 4.21 Development of the gut. Arrow shows the direction of rotation of the midgut loop.

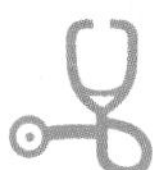

### *Clinical box 4.7*

**Meckel's Diverticulum**

Meckel's (ileal) diverticulum is a remnant of the vitellointestinal duct (connection between the midgut and the yolk sac) of the developing gut. It is present only in 2% of individuals. This may be seen about 2 feet (60cm) proximal to the ileocaecal junction in the antemesenteric border of the ileum. The Meckel's diverticulum may often have pancreatic or gastric mucosa as a lining, resulting in ulceration and bleeding. The vitellointestinal duct may rarely persist as a fistula connecting the intestine to the umbilicus. It can also present as a 'raspberry tumour' at the umbilicus (persistent red mucosa of the duct).

## Oesophagus and stomach

### Abdominal part of the oesophagus

The oesophagus extends from the pharynx in the neck via the thorax to the cardiac end of the stomach (Figs 4.22, 4.23). Its abdominal part, which is about 2.5cm long, lies behind the left lobe of the liver and the left triangular ligament. The oesophagus enters the abdominal cavity by passing through the right crus of the diaphragm at the level of the 10th thoracic vertebra.

✪ The lower oesophageal sphincter and the external 'sphincter' formed by crural fibres of the diaphragm are the two major anatomical sphincter mechanisms to prevent gastro-oesophageal reflux. The lower oesophageal sphincter is formed by specialised circular muscle fibres in the region passing through the diaphragm, the abdominal part being kept closed by tonic contraction of muscle. The sphincter, which relaxes only during swallowing and during vomiting, is controlled by intramural plexuses of enteric nervous system. The neural release of nitric oxide may aid relaxation. The tone of the diaphragm, the phreno-oesophageal membrane, which connects the oesophagus to the surrounding right crus of diaphragm, and the intra-abdominal pressure also exert a sphincteric effect.

### Stomach

The parts of the stomach are shown in Figure 4.22. The stomach has two borders – the greater and lesser curvatures, two surfaces, the anterior and posterior surfaces, and two orifices, the cardia and pylorus. It is approximately 'J'-shaped but its shape and its size are very variable. It can lie transversely as the 'steer-horn' type. Between the cardia and

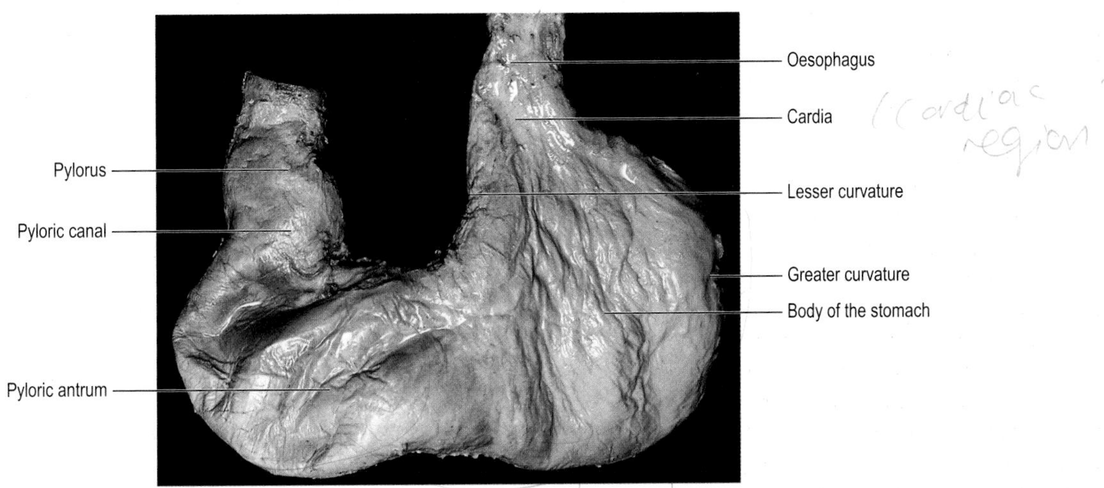


Fig. 4.22 Parts of the stomach (contracted horizontal type of stomach – 'steer-horn' type).

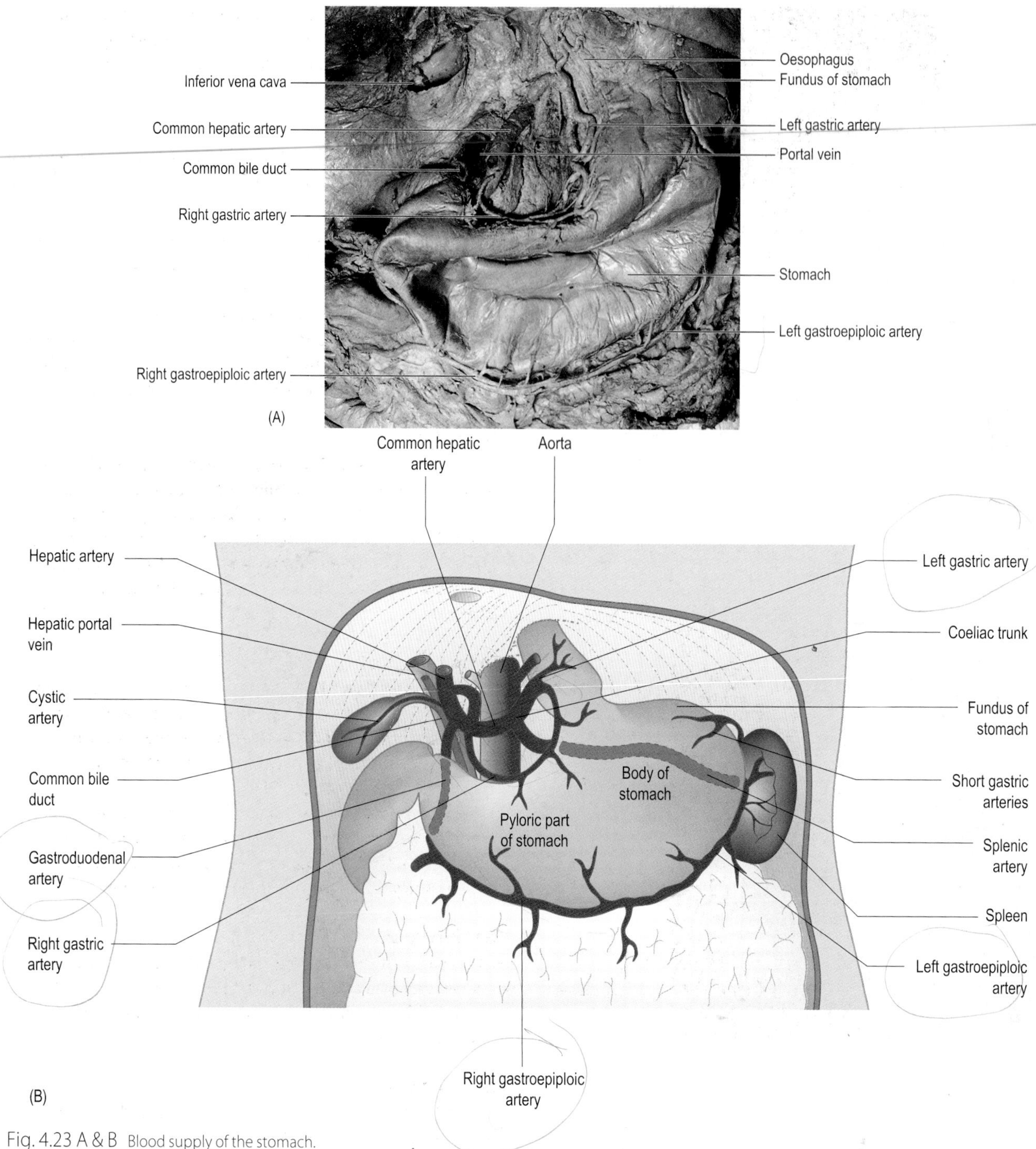


Fig. 4.23 A & B Blood supply of the stomach.

the pylorus lies the body and the pyloric part of the stomach, the latter having an expanded pyloric antrum which is proximal to the narrow pyloric canal. At the junction between the pyloric canal and the first part of the duodenum is the pyloric sphincter. ✪ This is a well-marked sphincter and is palpable at operation. Its position corresponds to a vertical vein on the surface – the pre-pyloric vein of Mayo. The part of the stomach projecting upwards from the cardia is the fundus (Figs 4.23–4.25).

Anteriorly the stomach is related to the anterior abdominal wall and the left lobe of the liver. Posteriorly it is related to the diaphragm, aorta, pancreas, left kidney, and suprarenal gland and the spleen with the lesser sac of peritoneum intervening between these and its posterior surface (see Figs 4.18, 4.19).

## Blood supply of the stomach

Rich arterial anastomoses are present along the greater and lesser curvatures. The left and right gastric arteries (Fig. 4.23) anastomose along the lesser curvature, the right and left gastroepiploic arteries and the short gastric arteries along the greater curvature of the stomach. ✪ The gastroduodenal artery, a branch of the common hepatic artery, lies behind the first part of the duodenum and can bleed when a peptic ulcer on the posterior wall erodes into it.

## Lymphatic drainage

✪ The lymphatics accompany the blood vessels. Lymphatics accompanying the splenic artery branches drain to the nodes along the upper border of the pancreas, nodes at the hilum of the spleen and then into the coeliac group of

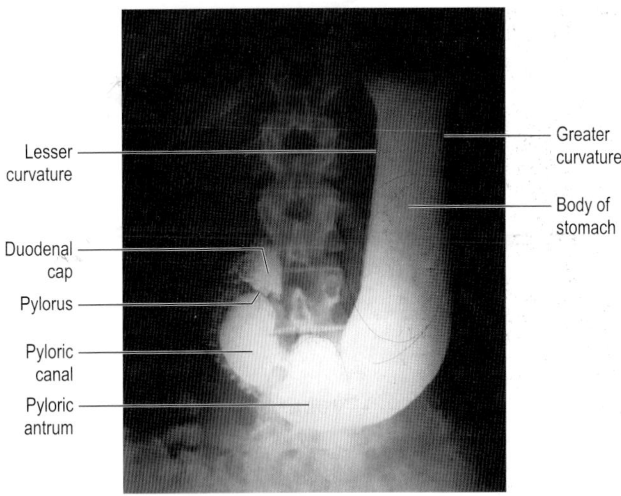


Fig. 4.24 Radiograph of the stomach after barium meal where barium sulphate is used as a contrast medium. The fundus is filled with gas (air) as the patient is in the erect position. Pylorus is seen as a gap in the barium proximal to the duodenal cap which is the first part of the duodenum.

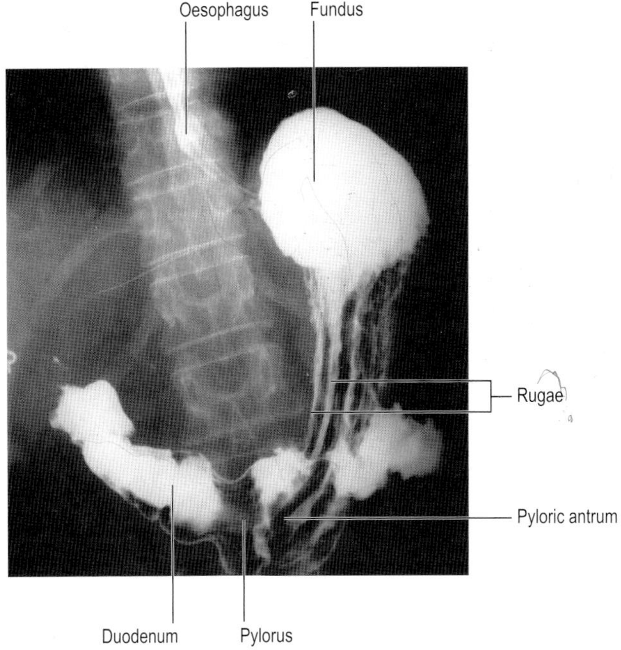


Fig. 4.25 Radiograph of the stomach after barium meal. The patient is in the recumbent position. The fundus is well outlined. Rugae, the longitudinal folds of mucosa are also well seen.

lymph nodes. Similarly branches of the hepatic artery are also accompanied by lymphatic vessels which too eventually reach the coeliac nodes. When the stomach is affected by carcinoma secondaries can also spread in a retrograde manner and affect the lymph nodes at the porta hepatis. These may block the bile duct to cause obstructive jaundice.

### Nerve supply

The stomach is supplied by the two vagus nerves as the anterior and posterior gastric nerves. These nerves are related to the oesophagus. The anterior gastric nerves (from the left vagus) lie on the anterior surface of the oesophagus and the posterior gastric nerves (right vagus) behind. ✪ The vagus constitutes the motor and secretory nerve supply of the stomach. Vagotomy (division of vagus) reduces acid secretion from the stomach.

## The duodenum

The small intestine, the major site of digestion and absorption, extends from the pylorus of the stomach to the ileocaecal junction. It is 2–7m long. The first 25cm is the duodenum (Figs 4.26–4.28), the next two-fifths is the jejunum and the distal three-fifths is the ileum.

The duodenum is C-shaped and it curves around the head of the pancreas. It is divided into four parts. Except for the first 2–3cm the entire duodenum is retroperitoneal.

### The first part

The first part is about 5cm long. Posteriorly it is related to the gastroduodenal artery, bile duct and the portal vein (Figs 4.23, 4.27). ✪ A duodenal ulcer on the posterior wall can erode into the artery causing haematemesis (vomiting of blood) and melaena (altered blood in stool). Anteriorly this part of the duodenum is related to the liver and gallbladder.

### The second part

✪ The bile duct (Fig. 4.27) and the pancreatic duct enter the major duodenal papilla on the posteromedial wall about 10cm from the pylorus. This point also is the junction between the foregut and midgut components of the developing gastrointestinal tract

The accessory pancreatic duct of Santorini opens a little above. The second part of the duodenum is related posteriorly to the hilum of the right kidney and the ureter and anteriorly it is crossed by the transverse colon.

### The third part

As this part runs horizontally to the left it crosses the inferior vena cava and the aorta. It is crossed anteriorly by the root of the mesentery and the superior mesenteric vessels (Fig. 4.26).

### The fourth part

This part ascends vertically and turns abruptly to end as the duodenojejunal flexure. ✪ A peritoneal fold, the ligament of Treves from the right crus of diaphragm, is an identification point for the duodenojejunal flexure at operation.

### Blood supply

The duodenum is supplied by the superior and the inferior pancreaticoduodenal arteries. The former is a branch of the gastroduodenal artery and the latter that of the superior mesenteric. Along the curved border of the duodenum these arteries anastomose and supply the duodenum and the head of the pancreas.

## Jejunum and ileum

Unlike the duodenum, the jejunum and ileum (Figs 4.29, 4.30) are very mobile because of the mesentery (Fig. 4.18) by which they are anchored to the posterior abdominal wall. The root of the mesentery, which is about 15cm long, extends from

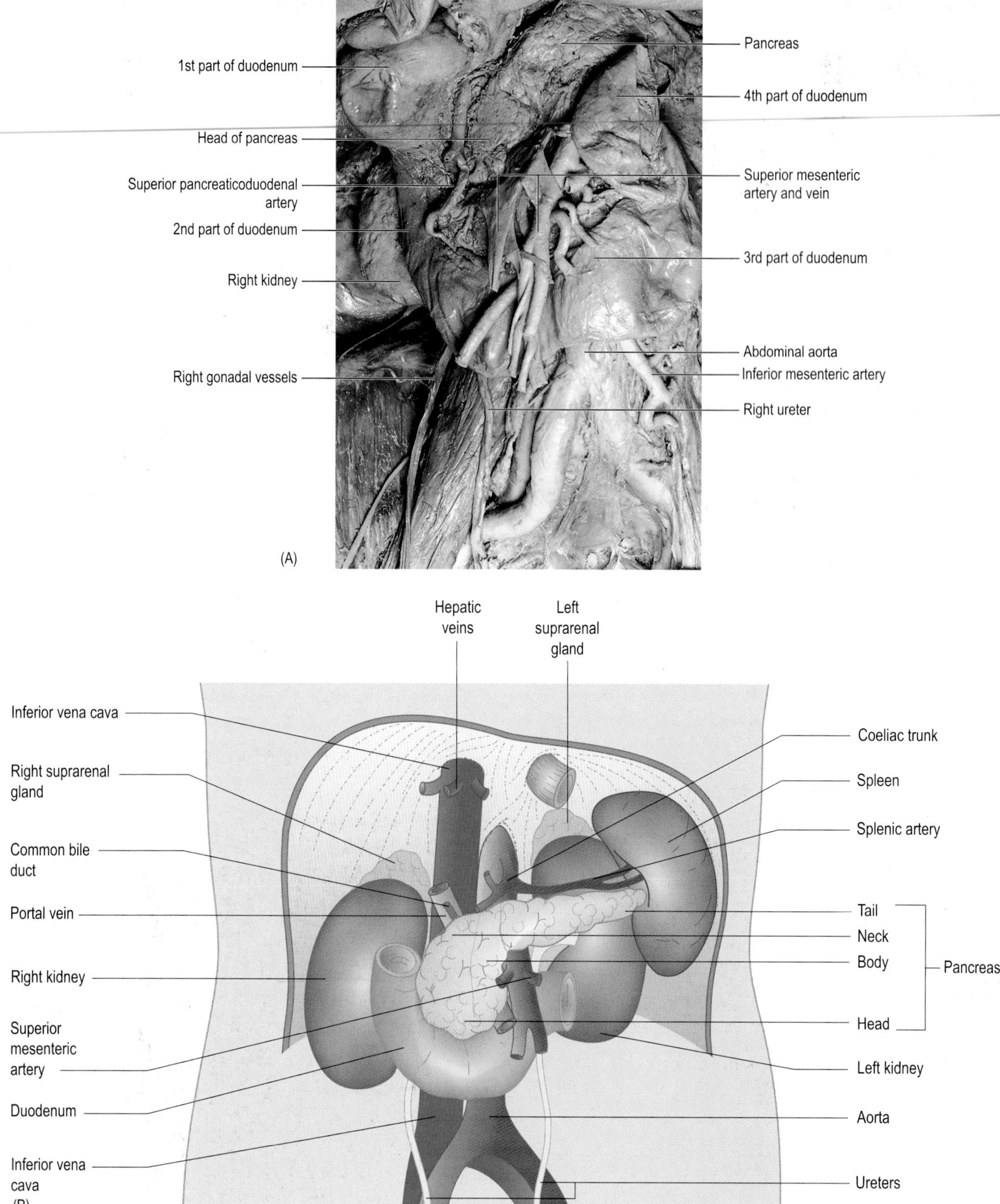


Fig. 4.26 (A) Dissection of the posterior abdominal wall showing duodenum and the related structures. (B) Pancreas, duodenum and the related structures.

the duodenojejunal flexure obliquely downwards and to the right to the ileocaecal junction. It crosses the third part of the duodenum, the aorta, the inferior vena cava, the right ureter and the right gonadal arteries. The superior mesenteric artery, a branch of the abdominal aorta, enters the mesentery as it crosses the third part of the duodenum. The mesentery also contains the superior mesenteric vein, lymphatics and lymph nodes as well as autonomic nerves.

Transition between the jejunum and ileum is gradual. There is no landmark between the two. It is important for the surgeon to distinguish a loop of the jejunum from that of the ileum but there are few anatomical factors to assist. ✪ The jejunal and ileal branches from the superior mesenteric artery form arcades from which terminal vessels – vasae rectae – supply the gut wall. The jejunum has only one or two arcades, making the vasae rectae longer than that of the ileum (Fig. 4.29). The number of arcades are more in the ileal mesentery which have relatively short vasae rectae. The jejunum has a thicker wall due to circular folds or valvulae conniventes or plicae circulares which increase the surface area of the mucosa. These are more numerous in the jejunum than in the ileum (Fig. 4.30).

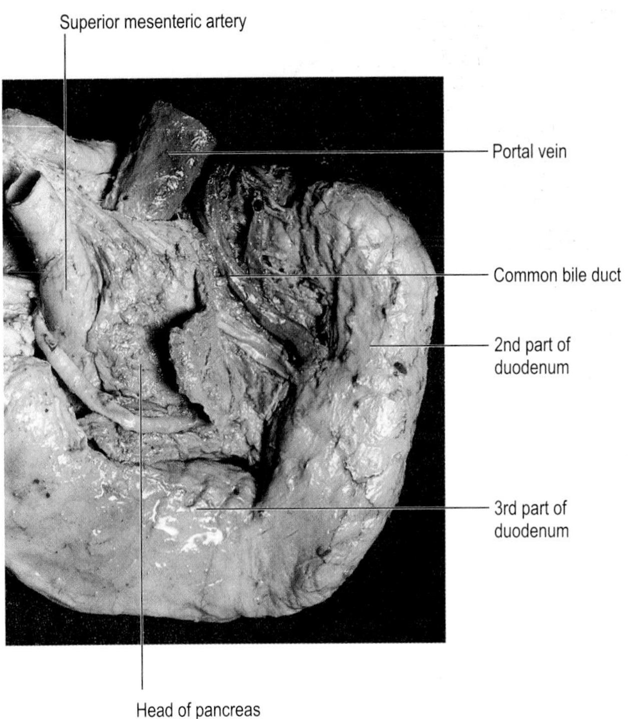


Fig. 4.27 Posterior aspect of the duodenum and the head of pancreas.

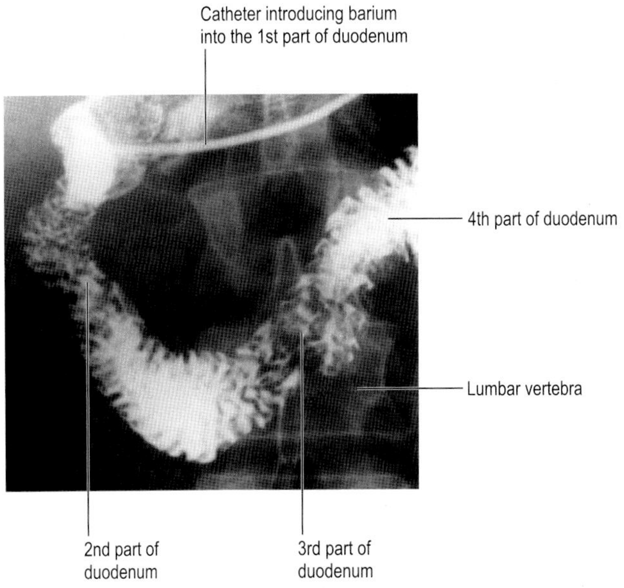


Fig. 4.28 Radiograph of the duodenum outlined by barium sulphate. Barium is broken up by circular folds in the duodenum.

The veins corresponding to the arterial branches drain into the superior mesenteric vein and then into the hepatic portal vein.

✪ Loops of small intestine may get twisted around abnormal peritoneal bands or adhesions, producing a volvulus. A volvulus can result in intestinal obstruction and strangulation of its blood supply. Malrotation of the gut during development may result in a very short root of the mesentery and this may also produce a volvulus. See Clinical box 4.7.

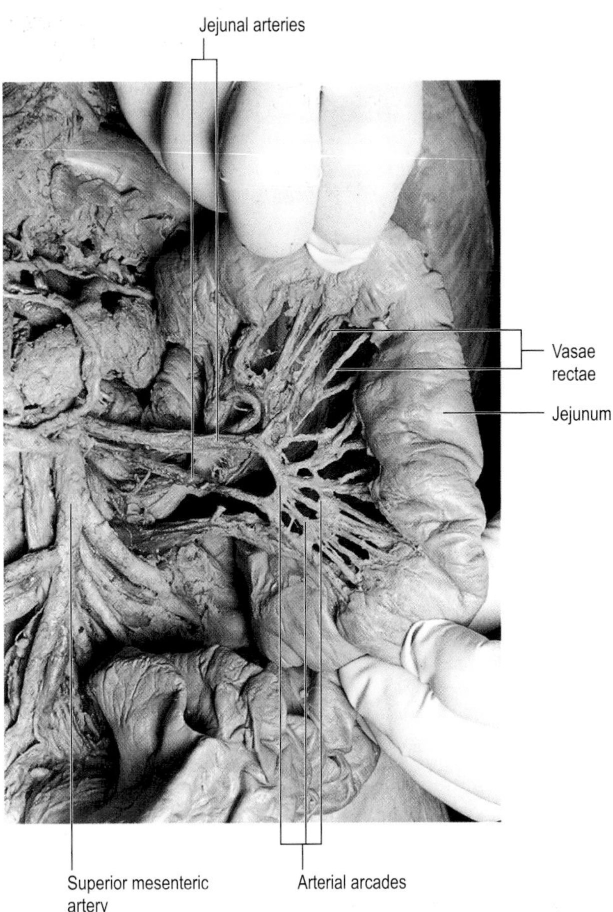


Fig. 4.29 Jejunal arteries, arterial arcades and vasae rectae.

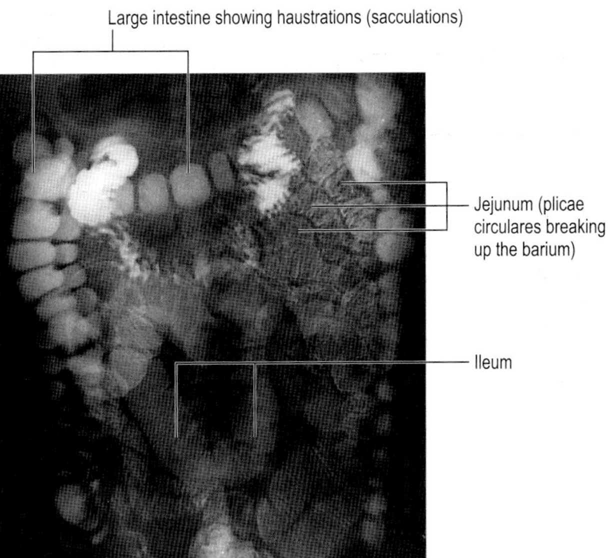


Fig. 4.30 Radiograph of the abdomen after barium meal showing jejunum, ileum and parts of the large intestine.

## Large intestine

The large intestine (Figs 4.31–4.43) consists of the caecum, ascending colon, transverse colon, descending colon and the sigmoid colon. The transverse and sigmoid colon have their own mesentery (the transverse and sigmoid mesocolon) and hence are mobile. The ascending and the

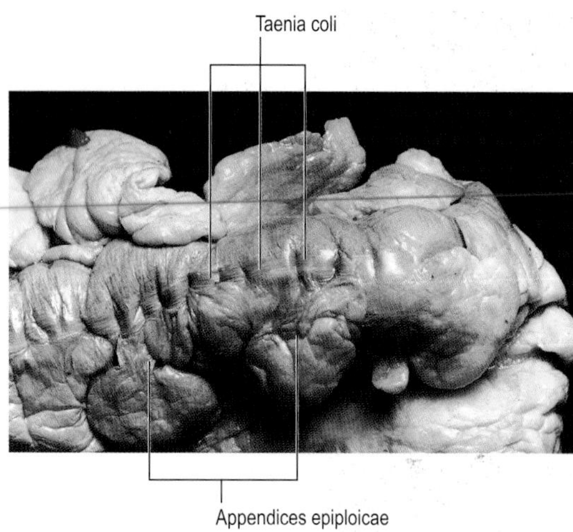


Fig. 4.31 Large intestine – taenia coli and appendices epiploicae.

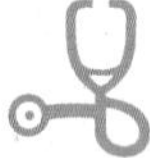

### Clinical box 4.8
**Appendicitis**

Inflammation of the appendix is known as appendicitis. The abdominal pain of appendicitis is somewhat unique. Inflammation follows obstruction of its lumen which causes swelling and stretching of the visceral peritoneum. This causes a vague pain in the region of the umbilicus in the early stage. It is a referred pain transmitted through sympathetic afferents to T10 segment of the spinal cord which falsely refers it to the umbilical region. At a later stage the parietal peritoneum is inflamed when the pain gets localised in the right iliac fossa at the McBurney's point.

The appendicular artery is functionally an end artery, thrombosis of which in appendicitis causes gangrene of the appendix leading to perforation.

The lumen of the appendix is relatively wide in infants but it is almost obliterated in old age. As appendicitis starts with obstruction of the lumen it is rare in infants and the elderly.

Appendicectomy is often done through a Lanz incision (see Clinical box 4.1). The caecum is mobilised and the appendix, if not visible, identified by tracing the taenia coli. The appendicular mesentery containing the vessels and the root of the appendix are then tied and removed. The stump is finally invaginated into the caecum.

descending colon are retroperitoneal structures. The caecum often has peritoneum reflected on to its posterior wall forming a retrocaecal recess and hence may be mobile.

✪ The presence of taenia coli, haustrations and appendices epiploicae distinguish the large intestine from the small intestine. Taenia coli are longitudinal bands of muscle. There are three of them and they converge together at the root of the appendix (root of the appendix can be identified at operation by tracing the taenia coli). Sacculations caused by the pull of the taenia coli are known as haustrations. Appendices epiploicae are fat lobules covered by peritoneum. They are more abundant in the sigmoid colon.

### The caecum

The caecum (Figs 4.33, 4.37–4.39) which is the dilated blind-ending commencement of the large intestine is located in the right iliac fossa. The ileocaecal valve (Fig. 4.39) at the termination of the ileum is located on the left side at the junction between the caecum and the ascending colon. Although the lips of the valve may to a certain extent prevent colonic content getting into the ileum, the sphincteric action of the valve is thought to be poor. Tumours in the caecum

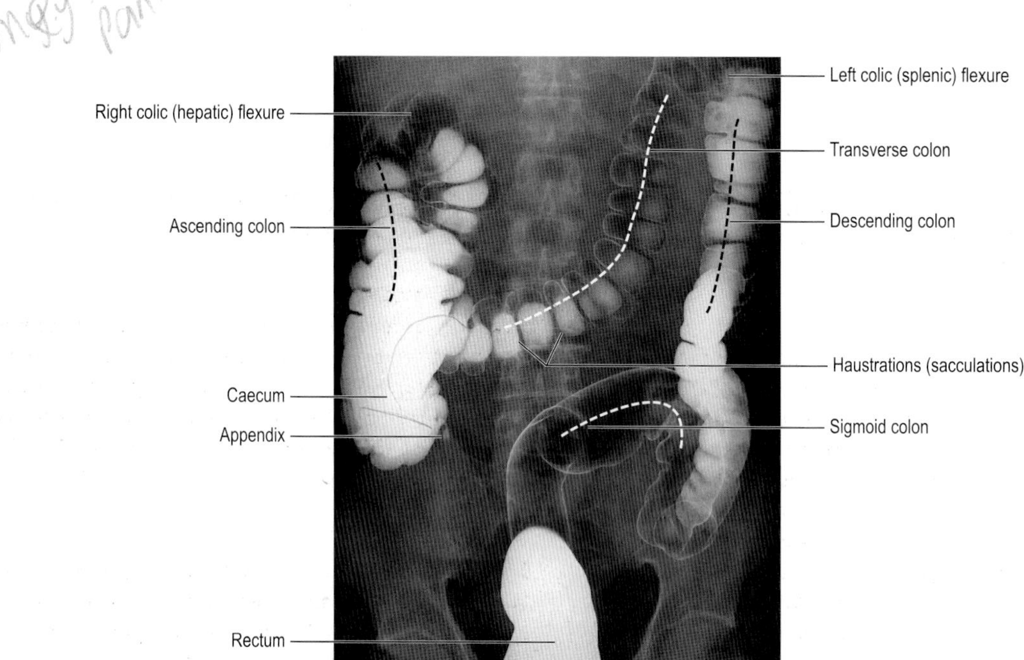


Fig. 4.32 Radiograph of the large intestine and rectum after barium enema.

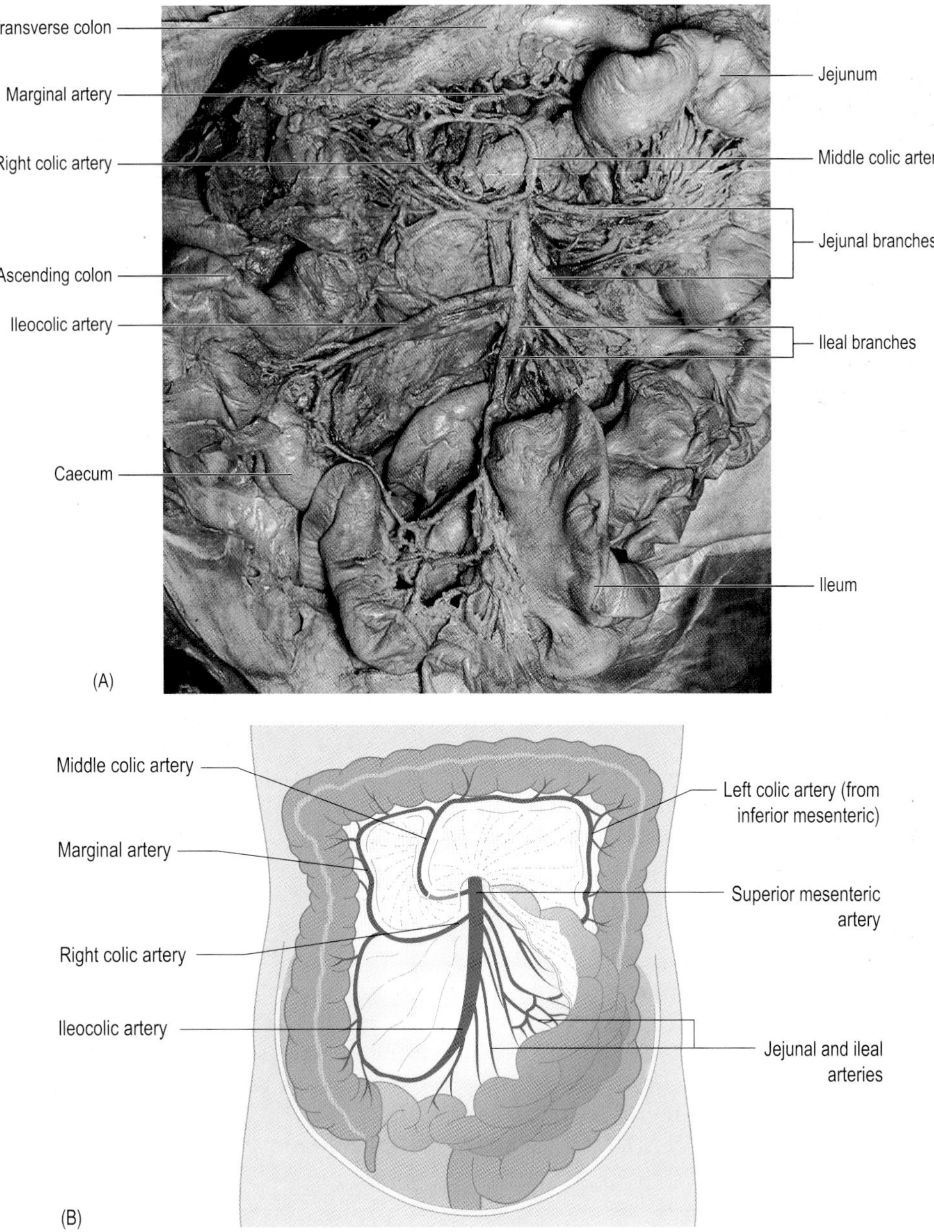


Fig. 4.33 A & B The distribution of the superior mesenteric artery.

may grow to a large size without causing obstruction until they involve the ileocaecal junction. Appendices epiploicae are not present on the caecum.

## The appendix

✪ The appendix (Figs 4.37, 4.38) is attached to the posteromedial aspect of the caecum. Its size and position are variable. In about 75% of cases it is retrocaecal, whereas in about 20% it hangs into the pelvis. The other possible locations are paracaecal, preileal (in front of ileum) and postileal. The three taenia coli merge at the root of the appendix. However the appendix itself is devoid of taenia and appendices epiploicae. It has a mesentery which contains the appendicular artery, which is a branch of the ileocolic artery or that of one of its caecal branches.

The surface marking of the appendix is the McBurney's point, which is the junction between the lower third and the upper two-thirds of the line connecting the anterior superior iliac spine to the umbilicus. See Clinical box 4.8.

## Ascending colon

From the caecum the ascending colon extends superiorly towards the liver where it turns to the left to become the hepatic flexure. ✪ Posteriorly its upper part is related to the duodenum, the right kidney and the ureter which all can be injured when this part of the colon is mobilised during a right hemicolectomy.

## Transverse colon

The transverse colon extends from the right colic flexure to the left colic flexure and it lies across the abdomen. The right and left hepatic flexures are fixed points between which the transverse colon hangs downwards to a variable level. It is mobile as it has the transverse mesocolon which is attached to the anterior surface of the pancreas where it

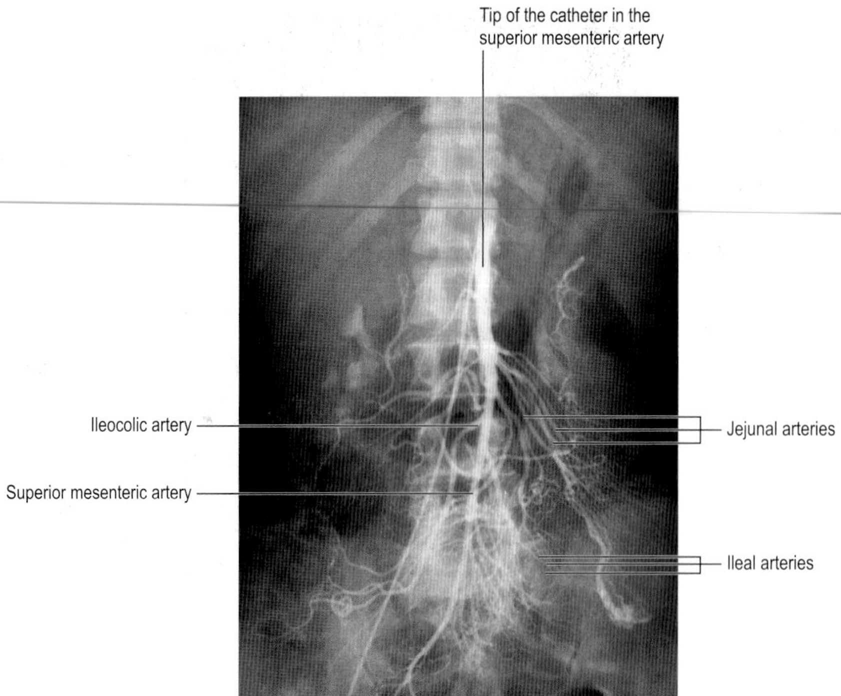


Fig. 4.34 Superior mesenteric arteriogram.

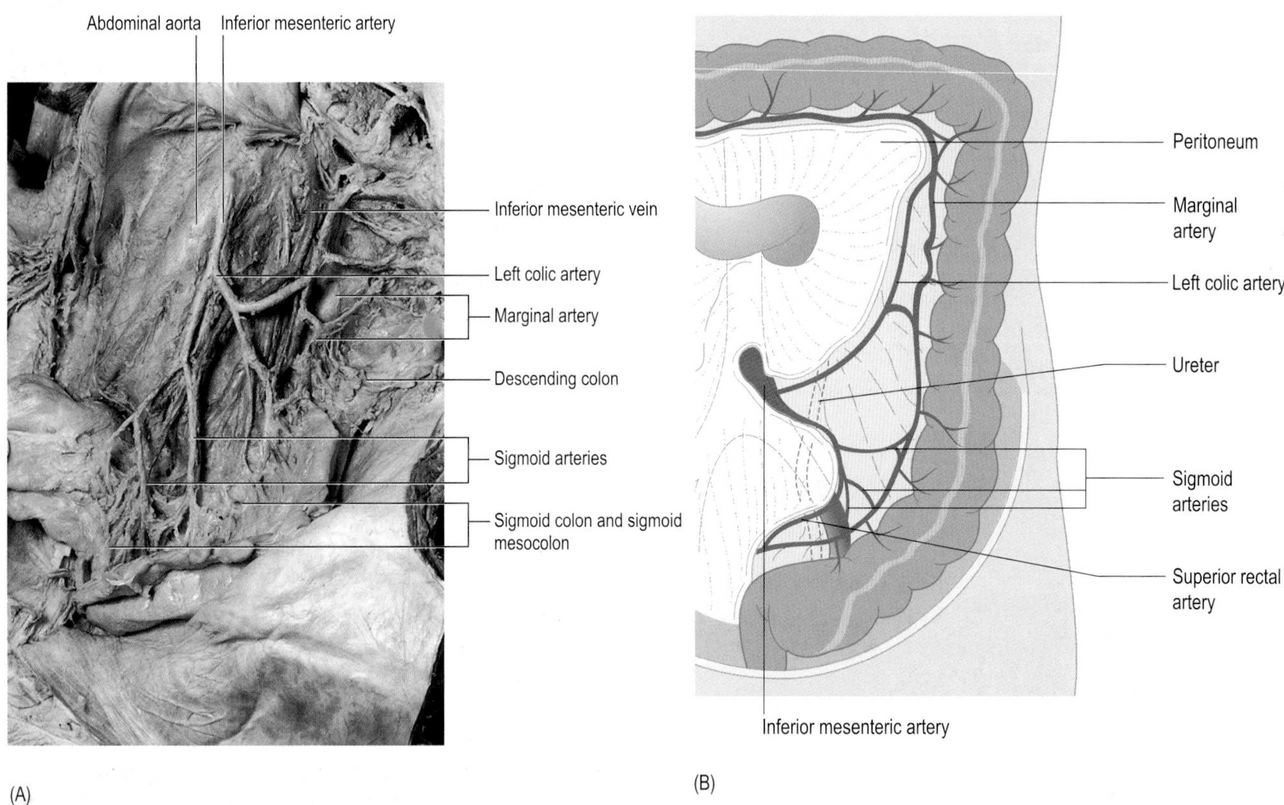


Fig. 4.35 A & B The distribution of the inferior mesenteric artery.

becomes continuous with the parietal peritoneum (see Figs 4.17, 4.18). The transverse mesocolon which contains the middle colic vessels divides the greater sac into supracolic and infracolic compartments.

### Splenic flexure and the descending colon

The splenic flexure lies at a higher level compared with the hepatic flexure (Fig. 4.32). It is held on to the diaphragm by a peritoneal fold, the phrenicocolic ligament on which the spleen sits. It turns downwards as the descending colon, which, like the ascending colon, is retroperitoneal. The descending colon lies on the posterior abdominal wall muscles and is closely related to the left ureter. ✪ Close relationship of the splenic flexure to the spleen and the tail of the pancreas are taken care of while performing a left hemicolectomy.

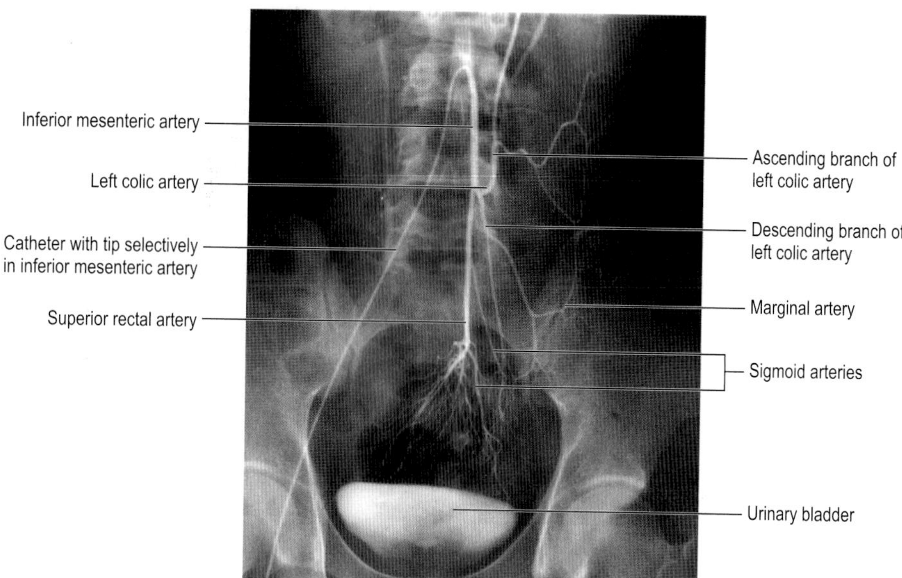


Fig. 4.36 The inferior mesenteric artery angiogram.

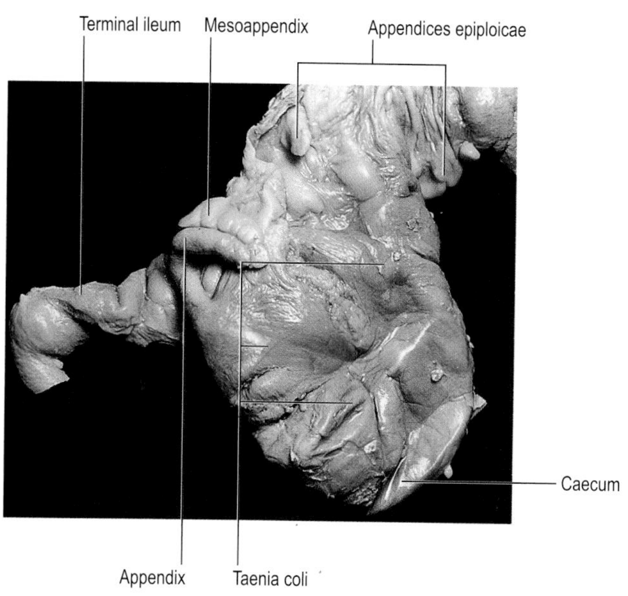


Fig. 4.37 Posterior aspect of the caecum with a retrocaecal appendix.

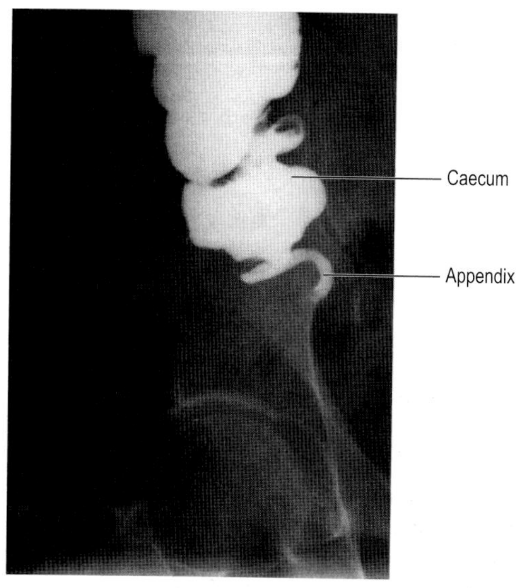


Fig. 4.38 Radiograph of caecum and appendix following barium enema.

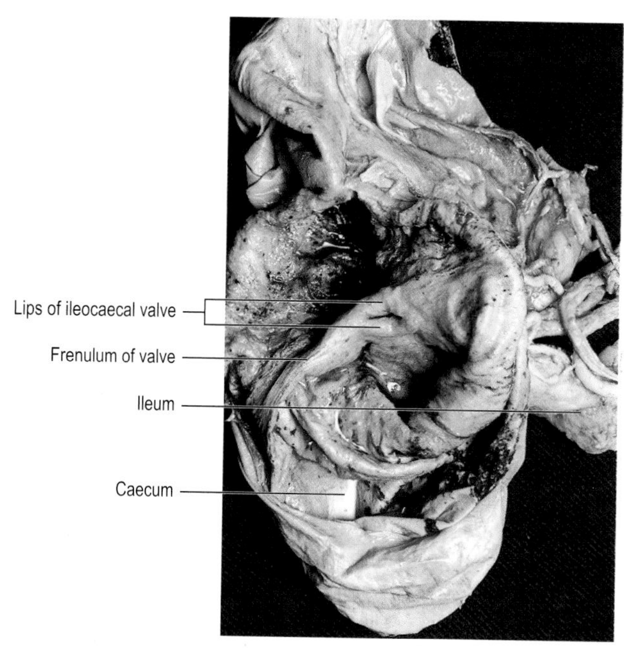


Fig. 4.39 Interior of the caecum showing the ileocaecal valve.

## Sigmoid colon

The sigmoid colon (Fig. 4.32; see also Fig. 4.81) extends from the pelvic brim to the rectosigmoid junction. It has a mesentery which makes it hang down into the pelvic cavity where it is closely related to the urinary bladder in the male and the uterus and vagina in the female. The sigmoid mesocolon has an inverted 'V'-shaped attachment to the pelvic wall. The apex of the attachment is at the bifurcation of the common iliac artery where it is closely related to the left ureter and the inferior mesenteric vessels lying medial to the ureter. ✪ Diverticulitis of the sigmoid colon can give rise to vesicocolic or vaginocolic fistulae. The appendices epiploicae are most numerous in the sigmoid colon.

## Blood supply and lymphatic drainage of the large intestine

The large intestine is supplied by the superior and inferior mesenteric arteries (Figs 4.33–4.36). The branches of the

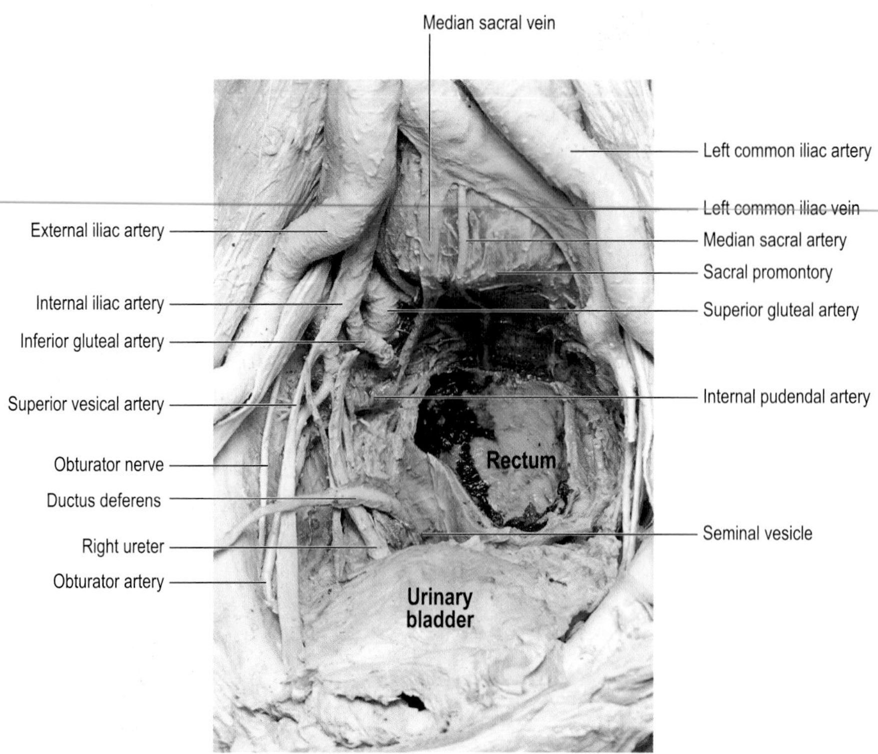


Fig. 4.40 Dissection of the male pelvis after removal of the sigmoid colon. The rectum, urinary bladder and the related structures are viewed from above.

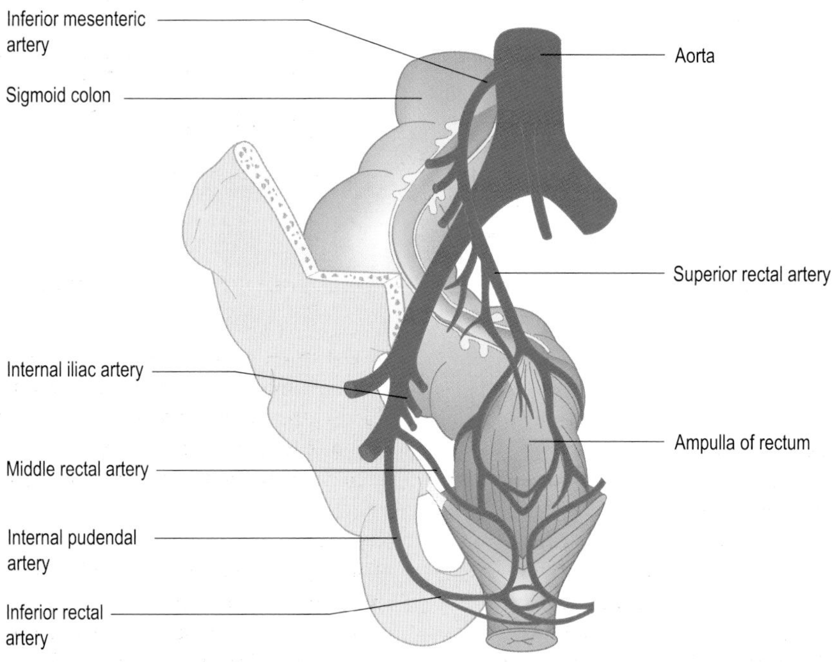


Fig. 4.41 Arterial supply of the rectum and anal canal – posterior view.

superior mesenteric artery are the ileocolic, right colic and the middle colic arteries (Figs 4.33–4.34). The ileocolic also gives off the anterior and posterior caecal arteries and the appendicular artery. The ascending colon is supplied by the right colic artery and the right branch of the middle colic artery. The middle colic artery (from the superior mesenteric) through its right and left branches supplies the right two-thirds of the transverse colon. The inferior mesenteric artery gives off the left colic arteries which supply the left third of the transverse colon and the descending colon. It also gives off the sigmoidal arteries to supply the sigmoid colon (Figs 4.35–4.36). The inferior mesenteric artery continues into the pelvis as the superior rectal artery. ✪ The colic arteries form a series of anastomoses giving rise to the marginal artery of Drummond which extends from the ileocolic to the colorectal junction. A good blood supply to the colon is maintained through the marginal artery even if one or two colic arteries are ligated. The weakest part of the anastomosis is near the splenic flexure where the superior and inferior mesenteric branches meet. Deficiency of blood supply can lead to ischaemic colitis.

Lymphatic drainage of the large intestine follows the course of the arteries. The primary nodes lie along the wall of the gut from where efferents go to the nodes along the branches of the superior and inferior mesenteric vessels

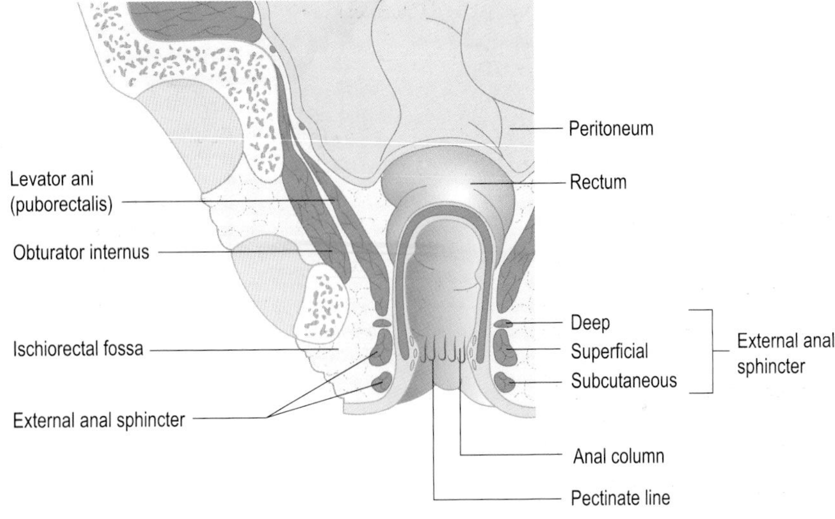


Fig. 4.42 Section through the pelvis showing the sphincters of the anal canal.

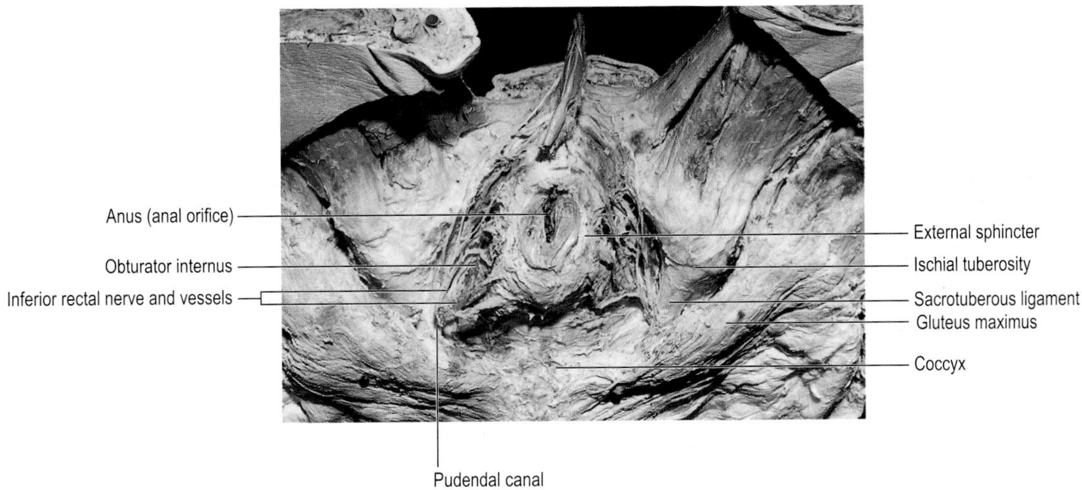


Fig. 4.43 The anal canal and the two ischiorectal fossae. The anococcygeal body is removed to show the continuity of one fossa to the other.

and finally into the nodes around the superior mesenteric artery.

✪ The colic arteries are ligated during hemicolectomies often as a treatment of carcinoma of the colon. In a right hemicolectomy the ileocolic, right colic and the right branch of the middle colic are ligated to remove the terminal part of the ileum, the caecum, the ascending colon and the hepatic flexure. In a left hemicolectomy the left colic vessels are ligated. Ligation is done very close to their origin from the parent arteries to ensure the removal of the associated lymph nodes en-bloc. The right and left colic vessels cross the ureters as they go towards the colon, a point taken care of by the surgeon during ligation of these vessels.

## Rectum and anal canal

The rectum (Figs 4.40–4.43) starts at the level of the third piece of sacrum and ends in front of the coccyx. The lower part of the rectum is expanded to form the ampulla of the rectum. Unlike the sigmoid colon the rectum has no mesentery, appendices epiploicae or taenia coli. Peritoneum covers the anterior and lateral aspect of the upper third but only the anterior aspect of the middle third.

The lower third of the rectum lying below the pelvic peritoneum is completely extraperitoneal. The rectum follows the curvature of the sacrum and also has three lateral flexures. Its upper part is convex to the left, middle part convex to the right and lower part again convex to the left.

### Relations

The upper part of the rectum is related in front to the rectovesical pouch containing coils of ileum and sigmoid colon. In the male the lower part is related anteriorly to the seminal vesicles, ductus and bladder and the ends of the ureters and the rectouterine pouch, whereas in the female the vagina and the posterior fornix and the uterine cervix form the immediate relations. A layer of fascia (Denonvillier's) separates these anterior structures from the rectum. ✪ In surgical mobilisation of rectum during abdominoperineal resection the plane of dissection should be on the rectal side of the fascia to avoid injury to anterior structures

Posteriorly the rectum is related to the sacrum, coccyx, the sacral nerves, the median sacral artery and the sacral veins. A fascia, known as the Waldeyer's fascia, separates the rectum from these structures and contains the plexus of veins draining the rectum.

✪ During surgery dissection should be done on the rectal side of Waldeyer's fascia to avoid bleeding from sacral veins.

Rectal cancer spreading posteriorly causes sciatic pain. On the lateral aspect of the rectum there is a lateral ligament formed by condensation of fascia around middle rectal vessels. Also related are the ureter, sympathetic chain and the superior and inferior hypogastric plexuses. During rectal surgery damage to ureters should be avoided and both the superior and inferior hypogastric plexuses, which are autonomic nerve plexuses in the pelvis, should be kept intact to avoid sexual dysfunction.

The rectum has no mesentery. However the surgeon often refers to the pelvic fascia surrounding the rectum as the mesorectum. As it contains lymph nodes it is removed with the rectum in the treatment of rectal carcinoma.

### Anal canal

The space below the pelvic diaphragm is defined as the perineum. The rectum passes through the pelvic diaphragm to become the anal canal in the perineum. The anal canal, which is about 4cm long, passes downwards and backwards from the anorectal junction to the anus, the external opening. It is surrounded by the internal sphincter which is the continuation of the circular muscle fibres of the rest of the gut (smooth muscle) and an external sphincter which is a striated muscle. The lining mucosa show vertical columns, anal columns or columns of Morgagni (Fig. 4.42). Their lower ends are connected by folds forming the anal valves or valves of Ball. Behind the valves are small anal sinuses into which the anal glands open. The line along which the anal valves are arranged is the dentate or pectinate line. It represents the junction between endoderm and ectoderm. The anal canal above the dentate line is lined by columnar epithelium and the part below, derived from the ectoderm, is lined by stratified squamous epithelium. ✪ A carcinoma of the upper anal canal therefore is an adenocarcinoma and that of the lower anal canal is a squamous cell carcinoma. Also due to the developmental differences the part above the dentate line is supplied by autonomic nerves and is insensitive to ordinary pain stimuli, whereas the lower part is supplied by somatic nerves making it painful to ulceration, to injections and instrumentations.

### Blood supply of the rectum and anal canal

The arterial supply of the rectum and anal canal is illustrated in Figure 4.41. The superior rectal artery supplies the whole of the rectum and the upper part of the anal canal up to the dentate line, and the inferior rectal artery supplies the lower part of the anal canal and the rectum and its supply may extend up to the peritoneal reflection of the rectum. The small middle rectal artery may supply only the muscle coats of the rectum. The arteries are accompanied by veins. The tributaries of the superior rectal vein drain into the portal vein whereas the middle and inferior rectal veins drain into the internal iliac vein. Hence the anorectal region is a site of portosystemic anastomosis.

✪ A rectal examination (by a finger passed per anal canal and rectum) allows palpation of the prostate in the male but rarely the seminal vesicles. In the female the cervix, the perineal body and rarely the ovaries are felt. The anorectal ring, coccyx and sacrum and ischial spines can be felt in both sexes.

### Ischiorectal fossa

The ischiorectal fossa (Figs 4.42, 4.43) is a fat-containing space which allows expansion of the anal canal. ✪ The ischiorectal fossa can get infected, forming an ischiorectal abscess which may need surgical intervention. It is a wedge-shaped space bounded laterally by the obturator internus muscle and medially by the levator ani and the anal canal. The anal canal here is surrounded by its external sphincter. The obturator internus takes origin from the inner aspect of the obturator membrane covering the obturator foramen. The ischiorectal fossa is crossed by the inferior rectal nerves and vessels from lateral to medial side. These are branches of the internal pudendal nerves and vessels which lie on the lateral wall of the fossa in the pudendal canal (Alcock's canal) in the fascia covering the obturator internus.

The two ischiorectal fossae are separated in the midline behind the anal canal by a fibromuscular partition, the anococcygeal body, which has an opening in its upper portion through which the two ischiorectal fossae communicate with each other. Infection from one fossa can readily pass on to the other side through this communication. See Clinical boxes 4.9 and 4.10.

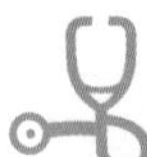

*Clinical box 4.9*

**Haemorrhoids**

Haemorrhoids are classified as internal and external. Internal haemorrhoids (piles) are dilated tortuous veins which are tributaries of the superior rectal veins. A pile mass typically is covered by the rectal mucosa and contains the corresponding branch of the artery besides the tortuous veins. It can prolapse and hence may get strangulated. An external haemorrhoid is nothing but ruptured subcutaneous vein. It is painful.

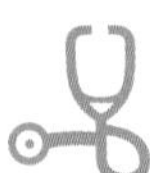

*Clinical box 4.10*

**Perianal abscesses**

Abscesses around the anal canal can be submucous (under the mucosa), subcutaneous (under the skin) or in the ischiorectal fossa (ischiorectal abscess). During examination of a perianal abscess it is important to verify whether it opens into the anal canal (fistula in ano). These are painful conditions which need incision and drainage. If there is a fistula its tract has to be laid open. In doing so one should avoid damaging the anorectal ring (p. 116) which is the major sphincter of the rectum and anal canal.

## Liver

The liver occupies a major part of the upper abdominal cavity. It is supplied by the hepatic artery and the hepatic portal vein and is drained by the hepatic veins which join the inferior vena cava. Bile produced by the liver drains into the second part of the duodenum via the biliary duct system.

✪ Normal liver is not palpable except in small children and in patients with emphysema where the diaphragm is at a lower level. On palpation the sharp inferior border is felt as the liver moves down on deep inspiration. The movement is due to the attachment of the liver to the diaphragm via the hepatic veins and the inferior vena cava.

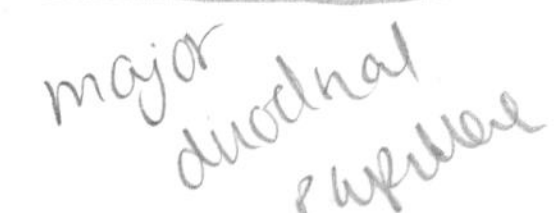

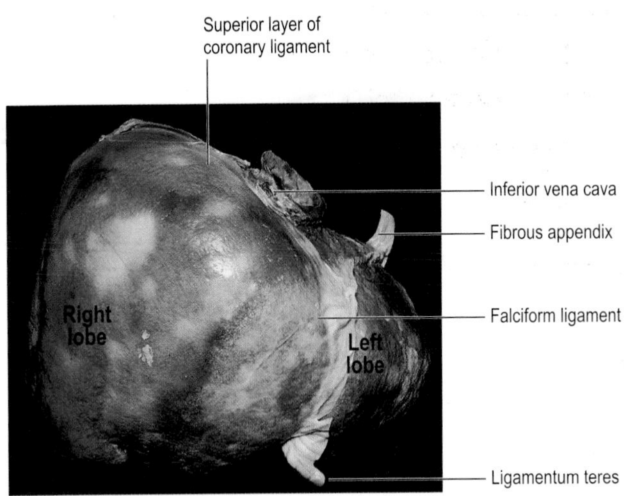


Fig. 4.44 Anterior and right surfaces of the liver.

The liver has diaphragmatic and visceral surfaces, the former subdivided into posterior superior, right and anterior surfaces which are not demarcated by sharp borders. The sharp inferior border of the liver separates the anterior and right surfaces from the visceral surface. Most main vessels and ducts enter or leave the liver at the porta hepatis on the visceral surface. The hepatic veins however leave the liver to enter the inferior vena cava on the posterior surface.

## Peritoneal relations

The liver (Figs 4.44–4.49) is completely covered by peritoneum except in the bare area which is bounded by the two layers of the coronary ligament and the inferior vena cava. The liver is divided into right and left lobes by the falciform ligament (Figs 4.44, 4.48). The right layer of the falciform ligament covers the right lobe of the liver and gets reflected onto the diaphragm as the coronary ligament. The gap between the upper and lower layers of the coronary ligament is the bare area. The right end of the coronary ligament is known as the right triangular ligament. The peritoneum covering the right lobe of the liver also continues downwards onto the stomach as the posterior layer of the lesser omentum. The left layer of the falciform ligament after enclosing the left lobe is reflected onto the diaphragm as the left triangular ligament. It extends downwards as the anterior layer of the lesser omentum.

## Lobes of the liver

The liver is divided into right and left lobes by the falciform ligament (Figs 4.44, 4.48). The larger right lobe has two well-defined small lobes, the caudate lobe and a quadrate lobe on its posterior and inferior aspect respectively. The former is bounded by the inferior vena cava and a fissure which holds the ligamentum venosum (remnant of the ductus venosus which was a vein during fetal life shunting blood from the portal vein to the inferior vena cava) and the latter by the gallbladder and the groove for the ligamentum teres (remnant of the left umbilical vein).

## Visceral and posterior surfaces of the liver

✪ The porta hepatis on the visceral surface of the liver (Figs 4.45–4.48) is where major vessels and ducts enter or leave the liver. From posterior to anterior the porta hepatis has the portal vein, the right and left hepatic arteries and the right and left hepatic ducts (i.e. vein, artery and duct – VAD from back to front). (Fig. 4.46) The ducts, being in front, are more accessible to surgery. It also contains lymph nodes and nerves.

The gallbladder lies in a shallow fossa on the visceral surface. The visceral surface of the left lobe is related to the stomach and duodenum. The left lobe of the liver lies in front of the oesophagus which can be exposed by cutting the left triangular ligament and mobilising the left lobe. The right kidney and right colic flexure (hepatic flexure) (Fig. 4.45) are related to the right lobe, the kidney being posterior to the colon. The right adrenal gland is related to the bare area on the posterior surface of the right lobe. The bare area is bounded by the two layers of the coronary ligaments and the inferior vena cava. See Clinical boxes 4.11, 4.12 and 4.13.

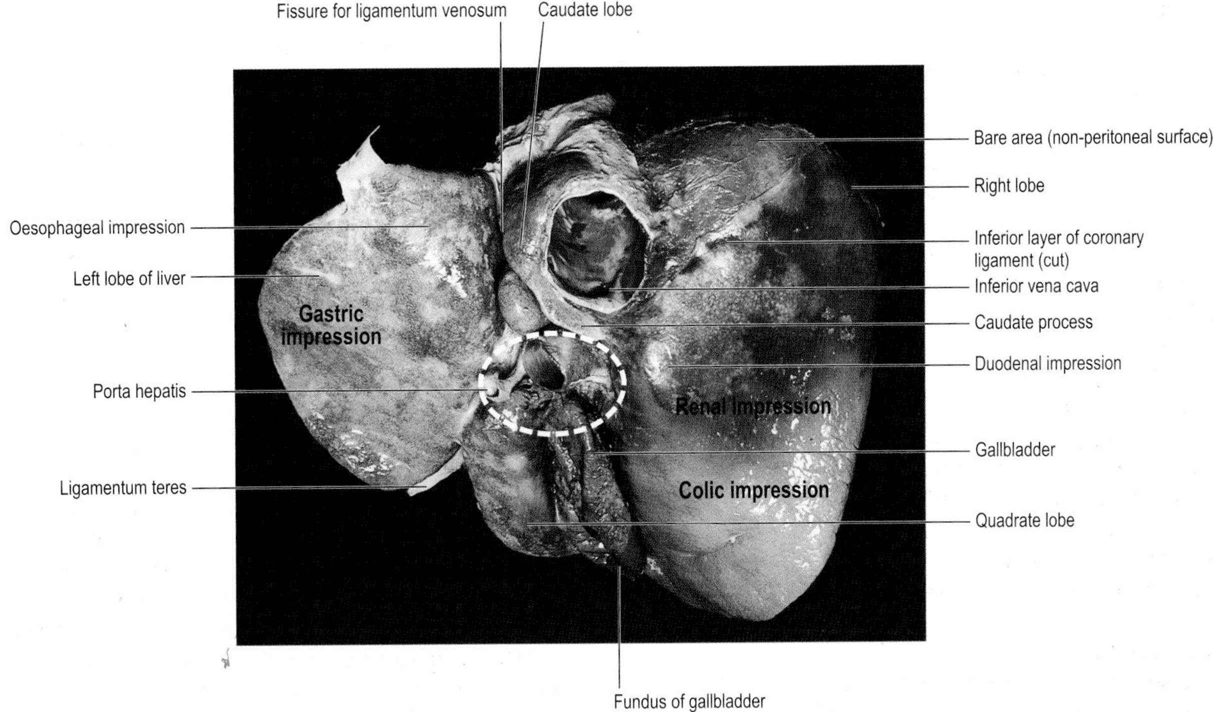


Fig. 4.45 Visceral (inferior) surface of the liver.

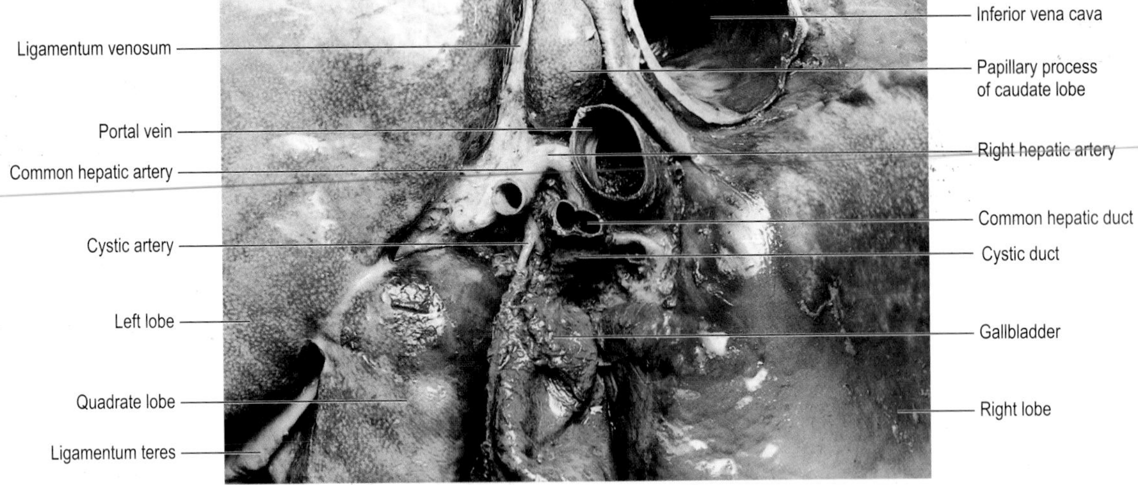


Fig. 4.46 Inferior surface of the liver. Structures at the porta hepatis.

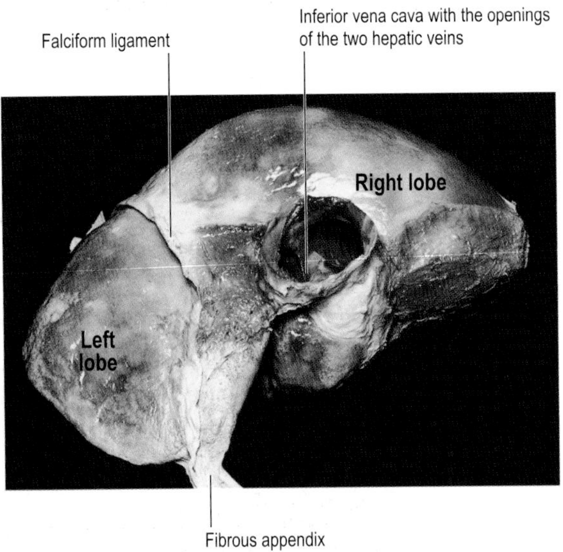


Fig. 4.47 Superior surface of the liver.

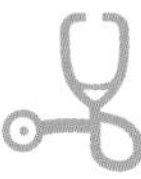

## *Clinical box 4.12*

### Functional (vascular) lobes and segments of the liver

Besides the demarcation of the liver into right and left anatomical lobes by the falciform ligament it can also be divided into functional (vascular) lobes and segments. The divisions into vascular lobes and segments are made use of in hepatic resections. The demarcation between the functional left and right lobes is a plane connecting the gallbladder fossa to the inferior vena cava, making the quadrate lobe as parts of the functional left lobe. The left functional lobe thus is larger than the anatomical left lobe. The right branch of the common hepatic artery and the right branch of the portal vein supply the right functional lobe whereas the left functional lobe is supplied by the left branch of the vessels. Similarly the right and left hepatic ducts drain the corresponding functional lobes. Each functional lobe thus has its own arterial and portal venous blood supply and drainage system. The patterns of blood supply and biliary drainage of the caudate lobe make it belong to both the functional lobes. Each functional lobe is further divided into segments based on the intrahepatic branching pattern of the vessels and ducts. Each functional lobe has four such segments.

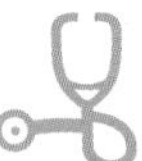

## *Clinical box 4.11*

### Subphrenic and subhepatic spaces

These spaces between the liver and the diaphragm are clinically important as they are sites of subphrenic abscess formation. The right and left subphrenic spaces lie on either side of the falciform ligament between the anterior surface of the liver and the diaphragm. The right subhepatic space or the hepatorenal pouch (of Rutherford Morrison) (Figs 4.20, 4.49) is one of the most dependent parts of the peritoneal cavity in the recumbent position (the other being the rectovesical or rectouterine pouch). The space is between the peritoneum covering the liver in front and the right kidney behind. Intestinal content can easily gravitate into it as sequelae of perforated appendix, duodenal ulcer or perforated diverticulitis and become infected, giving rise to subphrenic abscess. The left subhepatic space is the lesser sac.

## Anatomy of the biliary tract

For descriptive purposes the gallbladder (Figs 4.50–4.52) is divided into fundus, body and neck, the latter continuing as the cystic duct. The fundus, which projects out from the inferior border of the liver, is located at the level of the ninth costal cartilage in the midclavicular line on the right side. The right and left hepatic ducts, which collect the bile from the liver, join to form the common hepatic duct, which in turn is joined by the cystic duct to form the common bile duct. The common bile duct lies in the free border of the lesser omentum along with the hepatic artery and the portal vein. ✪ Lower down it passes behind the duodenum and the head of the pancreas, and hence a tumour of the head of the pancreas can block the common bile duct to produce obstructive jaundice.

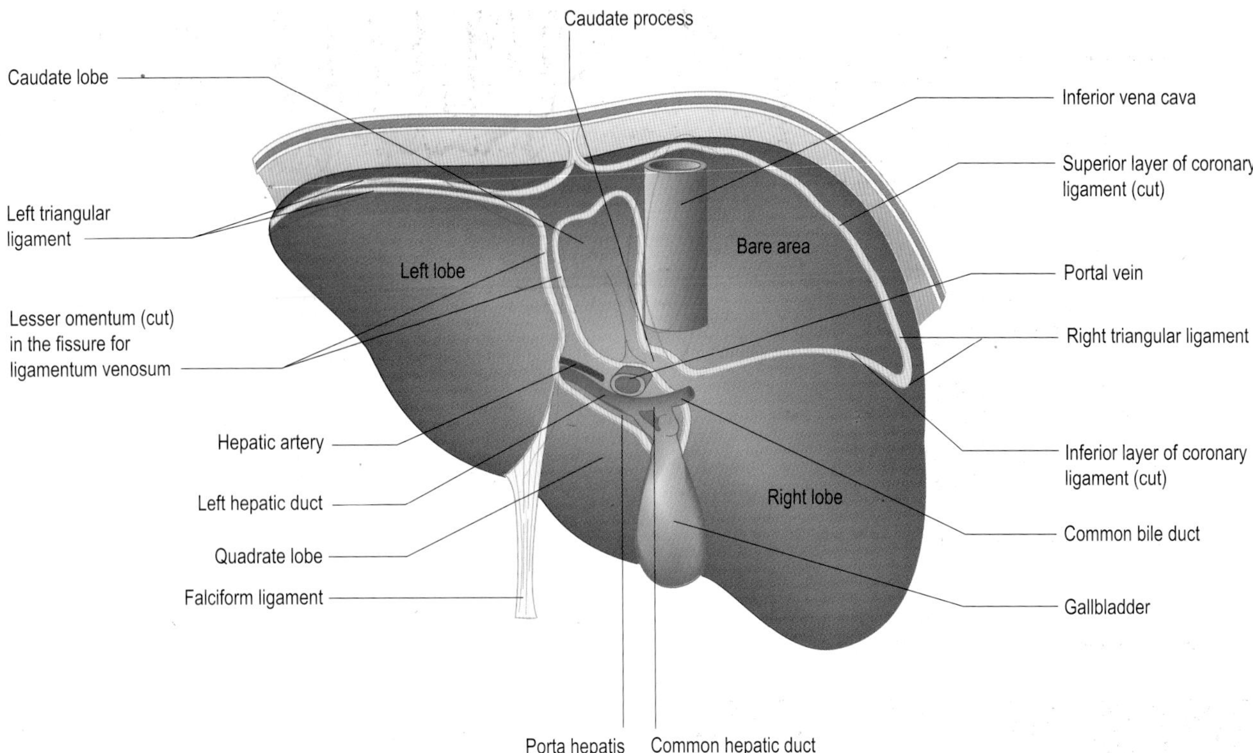


Fig. 4.48 Liver – posterior view.

## Clinical box 4.13

### Blood supply of the liver

About 25% of the total blood supply of the liver reaches it via the hepatic artery and the remaining 75% through the low pressure portal vein. Blood leaves the liver through the hepatic veins which join the inferior vena cava. There are usually three hepatic veins, draining roughly the left, middle and the right thirds of the liver. The left hepatic vein lies in the plane passing through the falciform ligament, i.e. the plane between the anatomical left and right lobe, whereas the middle hepatic vein lies in the plane separating the right and left functional lobes which is the plane connecting the gallbladder fossa to the inferior vena cava. Presence of these veins in these positions can complicate hepatic resection. Besides the three major hepatic veins there are a number of small veins draining the right lobe which enter the inferior vena cava directly. These may be the only veins draining the liver when the main veins are thrombosed, as in Budd–Chiari syndrome.

✪ Before its termination the common bile duct is joined by the pancreatic duct to form the ampulla of Vater. The ampulla and the ends of the two ducts are surrounded by sphincteric muscles, the whole constituting the sphincter of Oddi. The hepatopancreatic ampulla terminates at the papilla of Vater on the posteromedial wall of the second part of the duodenum about 10cm distal to the pylorus where it can be cannulated to perform an ERCP (Fig. 4.52).

The gallbladder is supplied by the cystic artery, usually a branch of the right hepatic artery and by small arteries from its liver bed. ✪ Gangrene of the gallbladder is rare even if the cystic artery is thrombosed in cholecystitis as the blood supply from the liver bed is significant. The cystic artery lies in the Calot's triangle bounded by the cystic duct, common

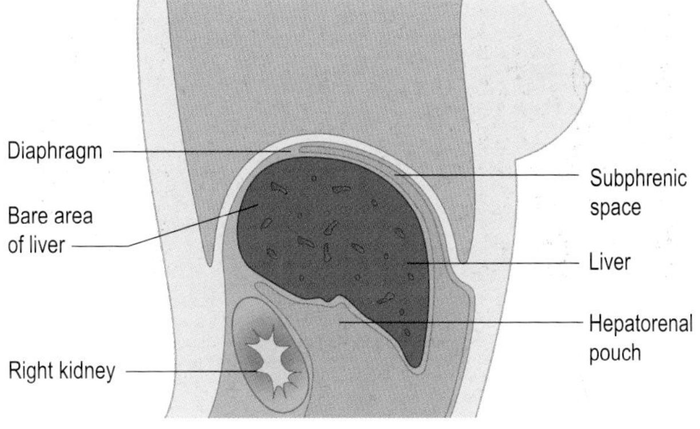


Fig. 4.49 The subdiaphragmatic spaces.

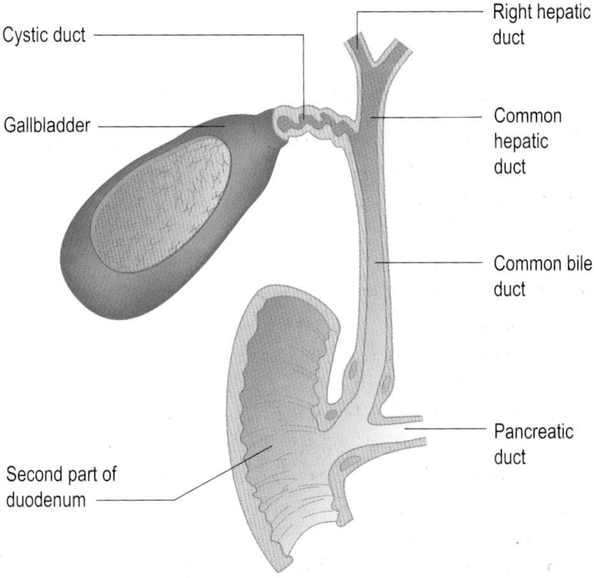


Fig. 4.50 Biliary system.

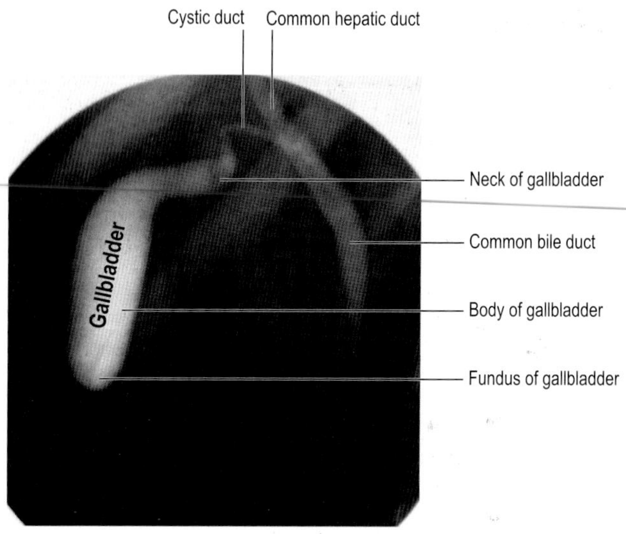


Fig. 4.51 Cholecystogram.

hepatic duct and the liver where it is identified and ligated during cholecystectomy (removal of gallbladder). Variations in the origin of the artery are common and are important to the surgeon. The presence of a cystic vein accompanying the artery is uncommon. The venous return is by small veins in the gallbladder bed entering the substance of the liver and then into the hepatic veins.

✪ The common bile duct is supplied by branches from the cystic artery and the gastroduodenal artery. There is a good anastomosis between these two sets of arteries which is helpful if the cut ends of the bile duct has to be anastomosed when torn.

✪ Variation to the pattern of the biliary duct system is common. The cystic duct may join the right hepatic duct or the common bile duct. Failure to appreciate these variations may result in errors in gallbladder surgery.

## Pancreas

The pancreas, lying transversely across the posterior abdominal wall, has four parts: head, neck, body and tail (Figs 4.26, 4.53). ✪ Most of it is retroperitoneal. The tail of the pancreas, which is in the lienorenal ligament, reaches the hilum of the spleen. It is vulnerable when this ligament is ligated in splenectomy. The head of the pancreas is moulded to the 'C'-shaped concavity of the duodenum. Its posterior surface is related to the inferior vena cava, and the right and left renal veins, and is indented or even tunnelled by the common bile duct (Figs 4.27, 4.54). ✪ As the bile duct is intimately related to the head of the pancreas, carcinoma of the head of pancreas blocks the bile duct to produce obstructive jaundice. This may be an early manifestation of the disease. The lower part of the head hooks behind the superior mesenteric vessels as the uncinate process of the pancreas.

The hepatic portal vein is formed behind the neck of the pancreas which lies in the transpyloric plane. The body of the pancreas crosses the abdominal aorta and the left kidney (Fig. 4.26). The head of the pancreas is supplied by branches from the arterial arcade formed by the superior and inferior pancreaticoduodenal arteries. The body and tail of the pancreas is supplied by the splenic artery and is drained by the splenic vein. The splenic artery runs along its upper border whereas the splenic vein, which is slightly at a lower level, is related to its posterior surface.

The main pancreatic duct extends from the tail of the pancreas to where it terminates at the hepatopancreatic ampulla in the second part of the duodenum (Figs 4.53, 4.55). Interlobular ducts join the main duct almost vertically, giving it a 'herring bone' appearance. ✪ The main pancreatic duct (of Wirsung) in about 80% of the population joins the bile duct and together they form the hepatopancreatic ampulla of Vater which opens at the major duodenal papilla in the second part of the duodenum approximately 10cm distal to the pylorus. The accessory pancreatic duct opens at the minor duodenal papilla about 2cm proximal to the major papilla. The accessory duct drains the uncinate process and lower part of the head. There are communications between the two ducts. See Clinical box 4.14.

## Spleen

The spleen (Fig. 4.56) has diaphragmatic and visceral surfaces. The diaphragm separates the spleen from ribs 9–11 as well as the left lung and pleura. ✪ A stab wound in the lower part of

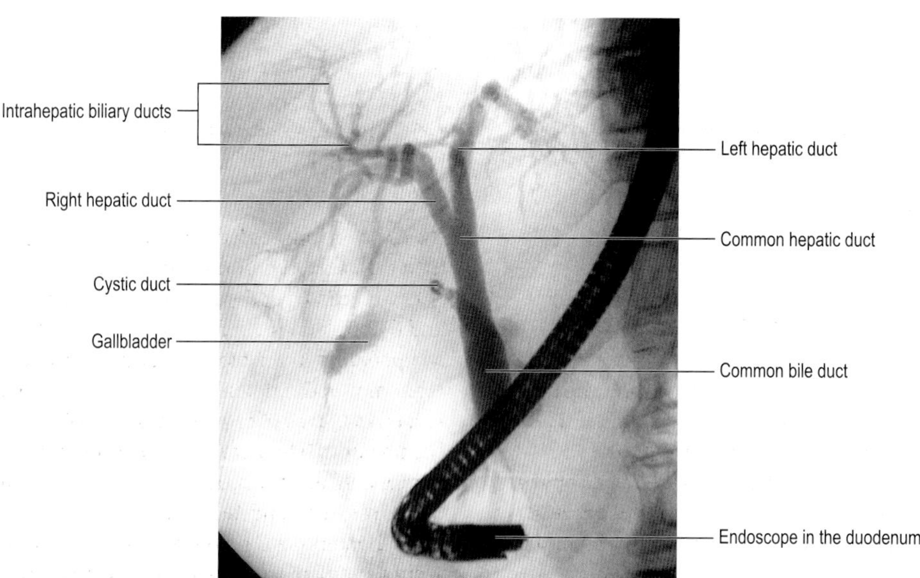


Fig. 4.52 Radiograph of the biliary tract visualised by ERCP (endoscopic retrograde cholangiopancreatogram).

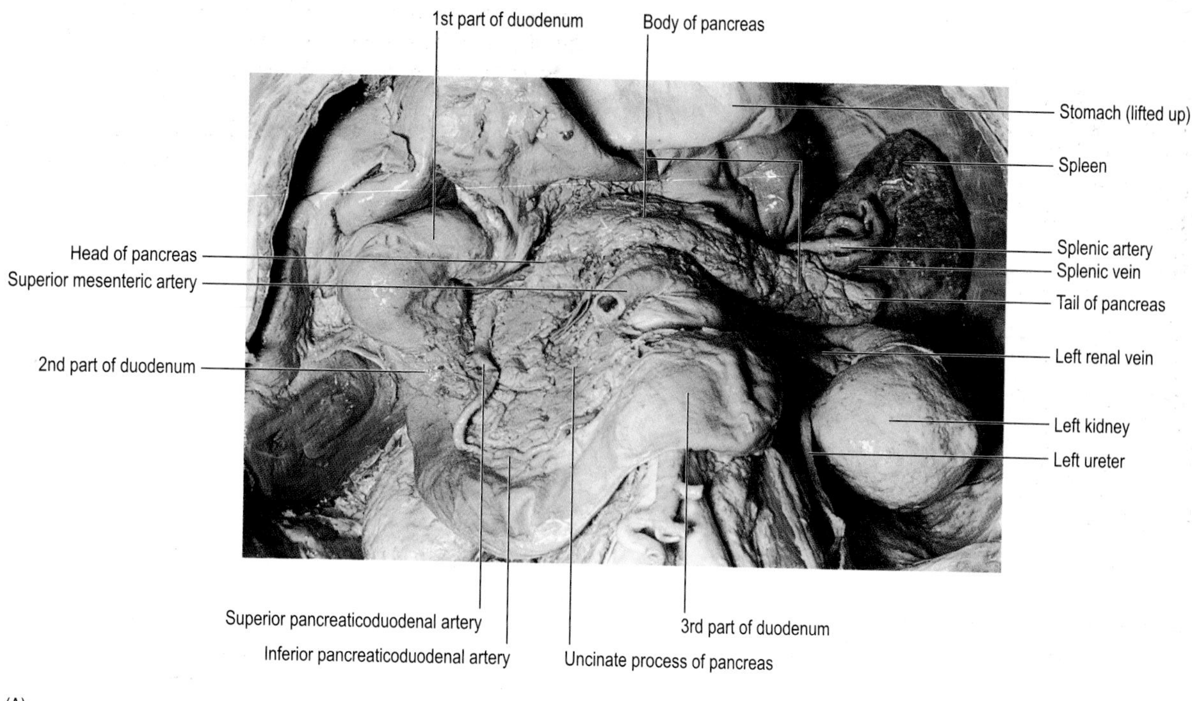


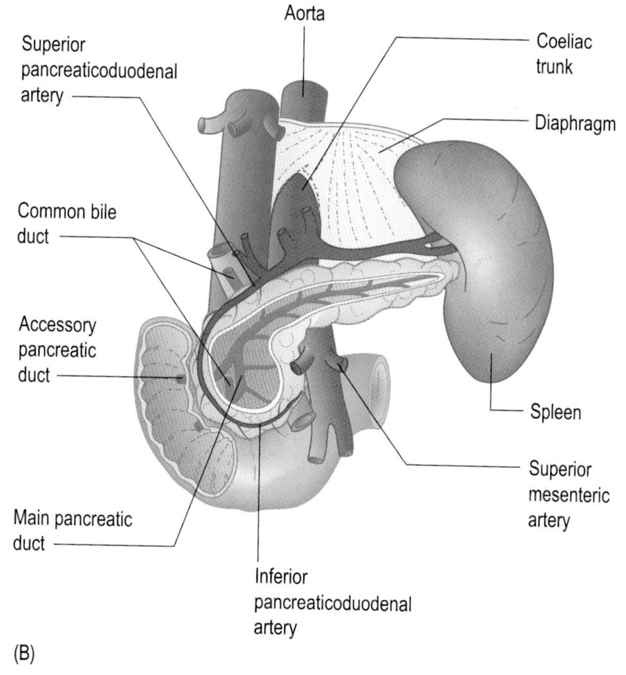


Fig. 4.53 (A) Dissection of the posterior abdominal wall showing pancreas and the related structures – anterior aspect. (B) The common bile duct, pancreatic ducts and the arterial arcades along the inner border of duodenum.

### *Clinical box 4.14*

#### **Pseudopancreatic cyst**

This condition is a collection of pancreatic juice and debris in the lesser sac of peritoneum following the rupture of the pancreatic duct in acute pancreatitis. The lesser sac lies in front of the pancreas, behind the stomach and extends upwards behind the liver and downwards into the layers of the greater omentum. Only a layer of parietal peritoneum intervenes between lesser sac and the pancreas and other retroperitoneal structures.

the chest wall on the left side may enter the pleural cavity before entering the spleen through the diaphragm. The visceral surface is related to the stomach, the splenic flexure of the colon and the left kidney. An injury on the left side of the abdomen in its upper part may affect any of these structures. The spleen is often ruptured by blunt trauma. The hilum of the spleen is related to the tail of the pancreas, the splenic vessels and the lymph nodes. The spleen is almost completely invested by peritoneum and is connected to the stomach and the left kidney by gastrosplenic and lienorenal ligaments respectively.

✪ The spleen is developed by the fusion of small accumulation of lymphoid tissue in the dorsal mesentery. Hence it has a notch. An accessory spleen may be present, often in the hilum of the spleen. It can also be present wherever there

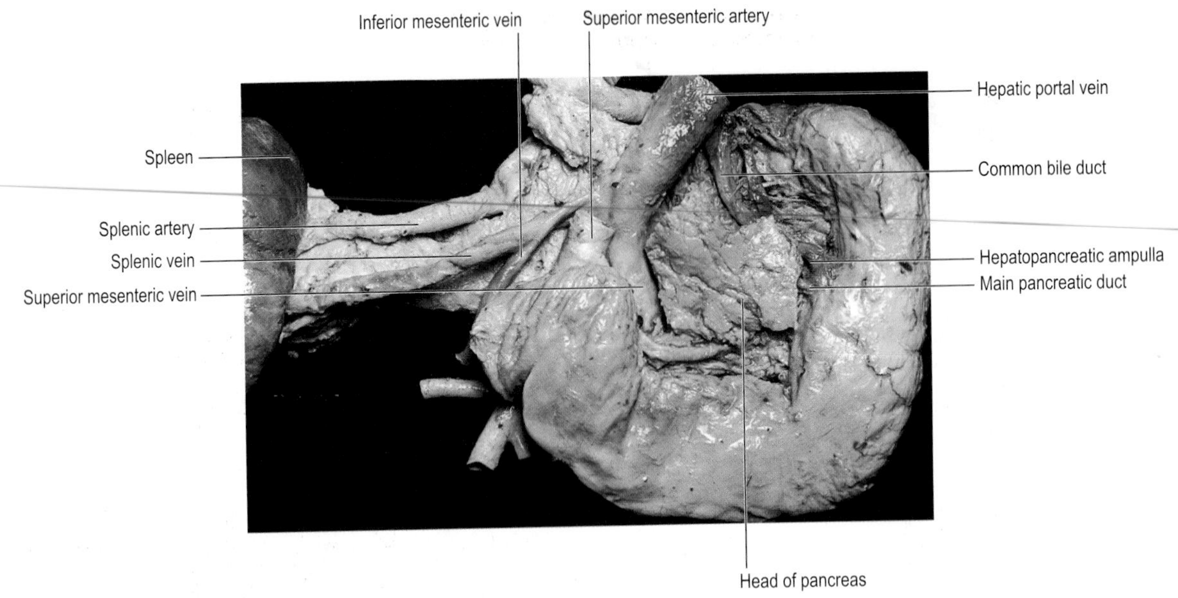


Fig. 4.54 Posterior aspect of the pancreas with the related structures. Formation of partal vein.

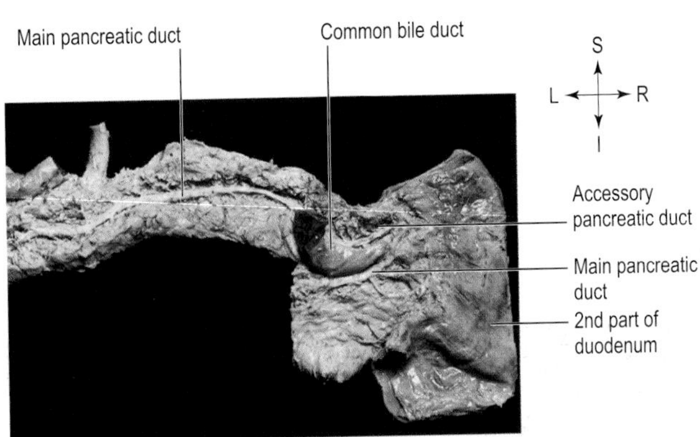


Fig. 4.55 The pancreatic ducts seen from the posterior aspect.

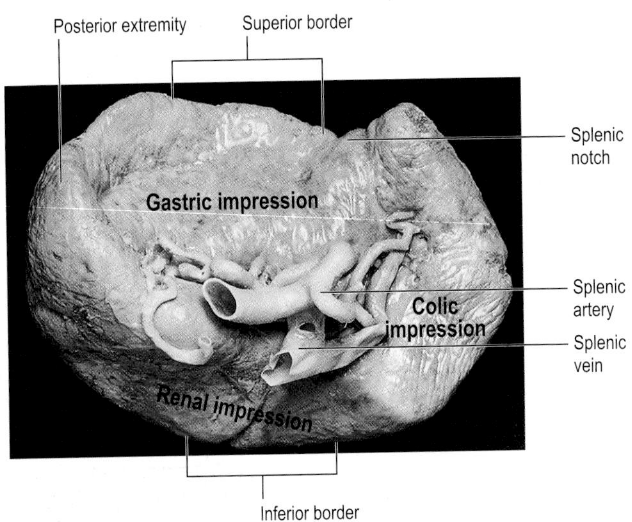


Fig. 4.56 The visceral surface of the spleen.

is mesentery, in the omentum, small bowel mesentery or even associated with testis and ovary. See Clinical box 4.15.

## The coeliac trunk

The coeliac trunk (Figs 4.23b, 4.57, 4.58) is the first major branch of the abdominal aorta and arises immediately below the aortic opening in the diaphragm. Its branches supply the lower part of the oesophagus, the stomach and the first half of the duodenum, as well as the liver, pancreas and the spleen.

The coeliac trunk divides into three branches: the common hepatic artery, the splenic artery and the left gastric artery. The common hepatic artery ascends to the porta hepatis in the free border of the lesser omentum lying to the left of the common bile duct in front of the portal vein (see Fig. 4.23). It gives off the right gastric artery and the gastroduodenal artery. The coeliac trunk is the artery of the foregut and hence the supply by its branches extends up to the region of the entrance of the bile duct in the duodenum, which is the junction between the foregut and midgut.

## The coeliac plexus

The coeliac plexus (Fig. 4.59) is the largest sympathetic plexus and surrounds the coeliac trunk. The plexus receives the greater and lesser splanchnic nerves (p. 70) and also a branch from the

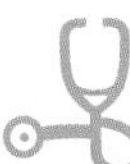

### *Clinical box 4.15*

**Palpation of spleen**

Normal spleen is not palpable. It has to enlarge two to three times its normal size before it is palpable. The spleen may be enlarged in many conditions. It is sometimes difficult to distinguish it from an enlarged left kidney. It is palpated under the left costal margin. The direction of the splenic enlargement from the subcostal region is downwards and towards the right iliac fossa. It is felt as a firm swelling with rounded borders. A notch may often (not always) be felt in the lower medial border of the spleen. The upper border of the enlarged spleen cannot be felt (it is not possible to reach above the swelling). The swelling descends on inspiration because of its intimate relation to the diaphragm. It is dull on percussion as it is not overlapped by coils of the gut.

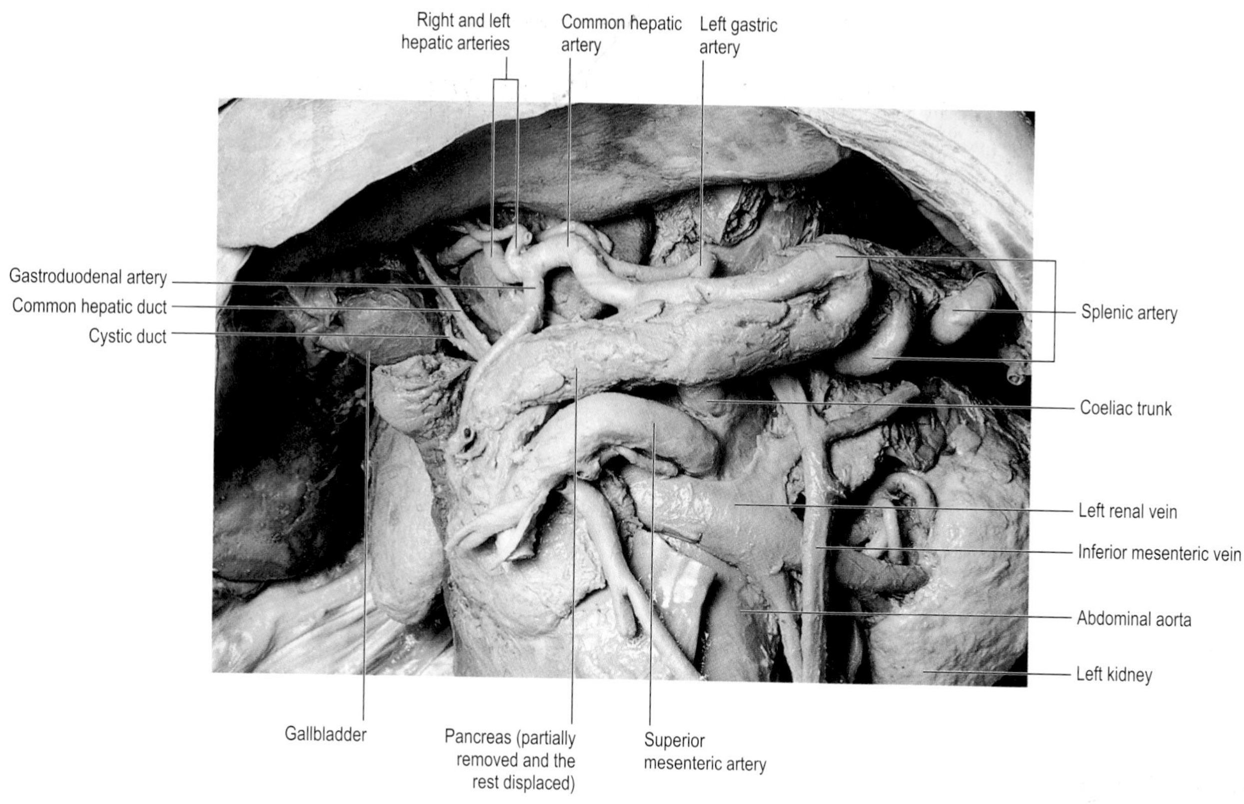


Fig. 4.57 Dissection of the posterior abdominal wall showing the branches of the coeliac trunk and the related structures. Stomach, small intestine, large intestine and the associated peritoneal membranes have been removed.

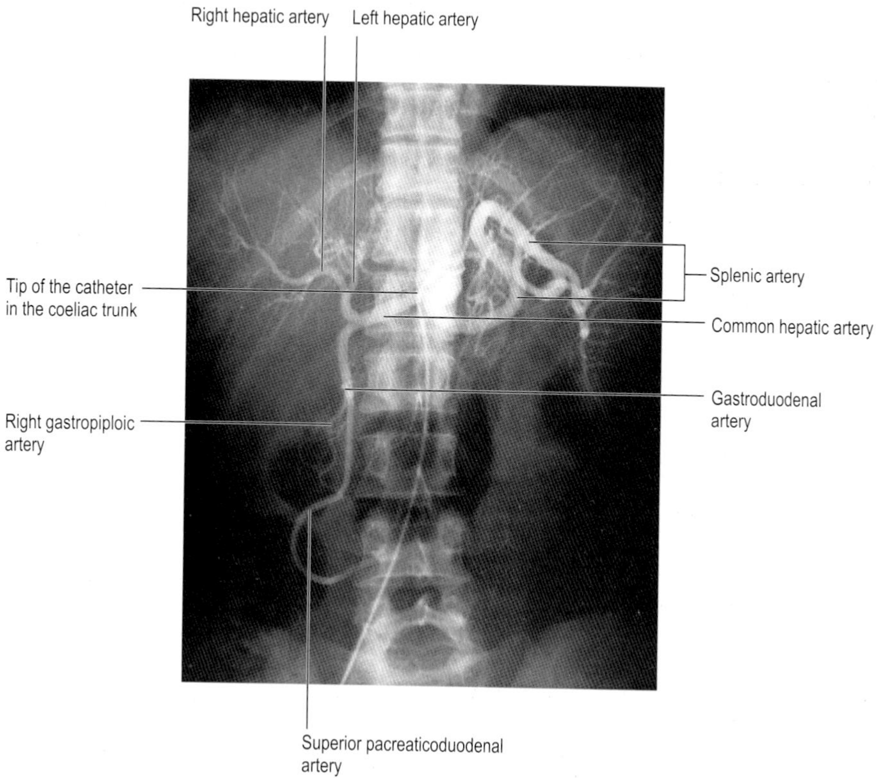


Fig. 4.58 Coeliac trunk arteriogram.

right vagus. The two coeliac ganglia, in which the preganglionic fibres of the splanchnic nerves synapse, lie on the crura of the diaphragm. Each ganglion is about 2cm in diameter. A large contribution of preganglionic fibres from the plexus supply the adrenal medulla. The rest of the plexus descends over the abdominal aorta and is distributed to the abdominal viscera as plexuses accompanying the branches of the aorta.

✪ Pain from the abdominal viscera is transmitted through the afferent sympathetic fibres in the coeliac plexus. Blocking the coeliac plexus with an anaesthetic drug is therapeutically used to relieve intractable abdominal pain produced by conditions such as chronic pancreatitis and carcinoma of the pancreas.

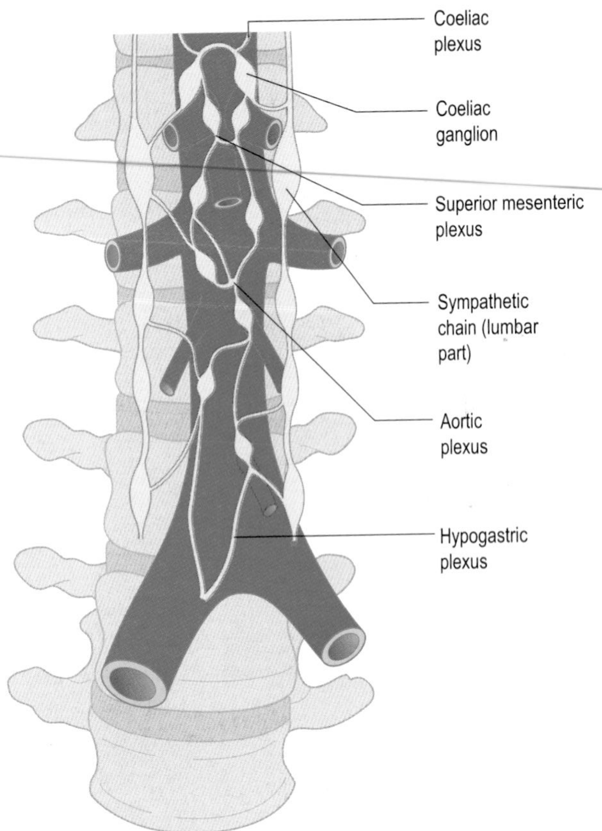


Fig. 4.59 Prevertebral autonomic sympathetic plexuses.

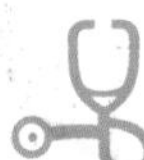

### *Clinical box 4.16*

**Portal hypertension**

Blood flow through the portal vein can be blocked by a number of causes resulting in an increase in portal venous pressure. The conditions include cirrhosis of the liver, thrombosis or congenital obliteration of the portal vein or congenital stenosis of the hepatic veins. When the portal venous pressure rises above 10–12mmHg (normal 5–8mmHg), as in cirrhosis of the liver, the sites of portosystemic anastomoses dilate. It also causes splenomegaly. There are certain sites of portosystemic anastomoses outside the liver where the portal vein tributaries anastomose with those of the systemic veins. The main sites of anastomoses are those under the mucosa of the lower end of oesophagus, rectum, retroperitoneal regions such as the bare area of the liver and posterior aspect of the ascending and descending colon and the umbilical area via the paraumbilical vein. The most important are the oesophageal veins, as rupture of the oesophageal varices can produce life-threatening haematemesis.

## The hepatic portal vein

The hepatic portal vein (Figs 4.60, 4.61) is formed by the union of the superior mesenteric and the splenic veins behind the neck of the pancreas. The inferior mesenteric vein may join the splenic vein or the superior mesenteric vein. The portal vein thus drains blood from most of the gastrointestinal tract. Blood then traverses the liver in the hepatic sinusoids and empties into the central veins through which it reaches the inferior vena cava. In its course towards the porta hepatis the portal vein lies behind the first part of the duodenum and the free border of the lesser omentum. See Clinical box 4.16.

## The adrenal (suprarenal) glands

The adrenal (suprarenal) glands (Figs 4.26b, 4.62) lie on the upper poles of the kidneys overlapping on to the anterior surface. The right gland lies behind the bare area of the liver and its lower part is behind the hepatorenal pouch. The

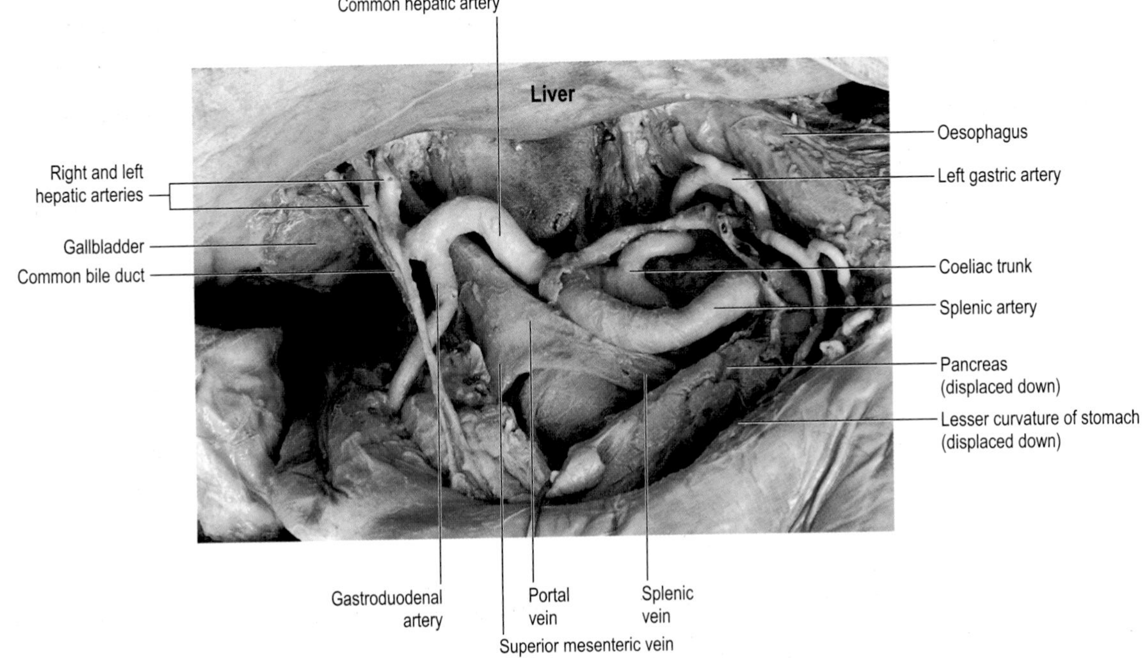


Fig. 4.60 Formation of the portal vein and the branches of the coeliac trunk seen after the removal of the lesser omentum. Stomach and pancreas have been displaced downwards.

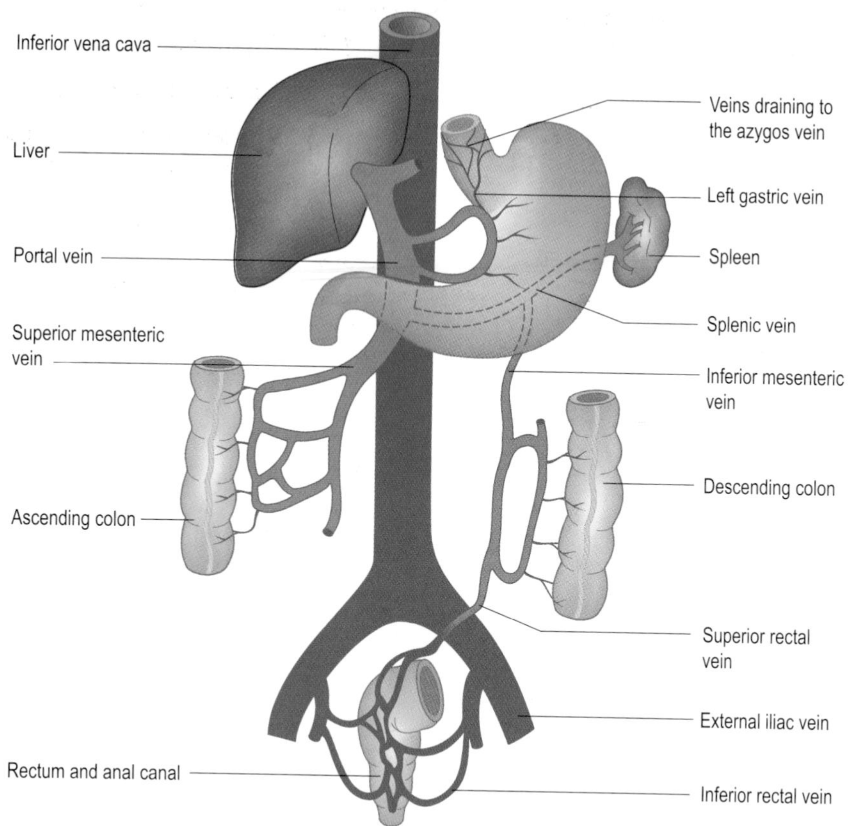


Fig. 4.61 Formation of the portal vein and the portosystemic anastomoses.

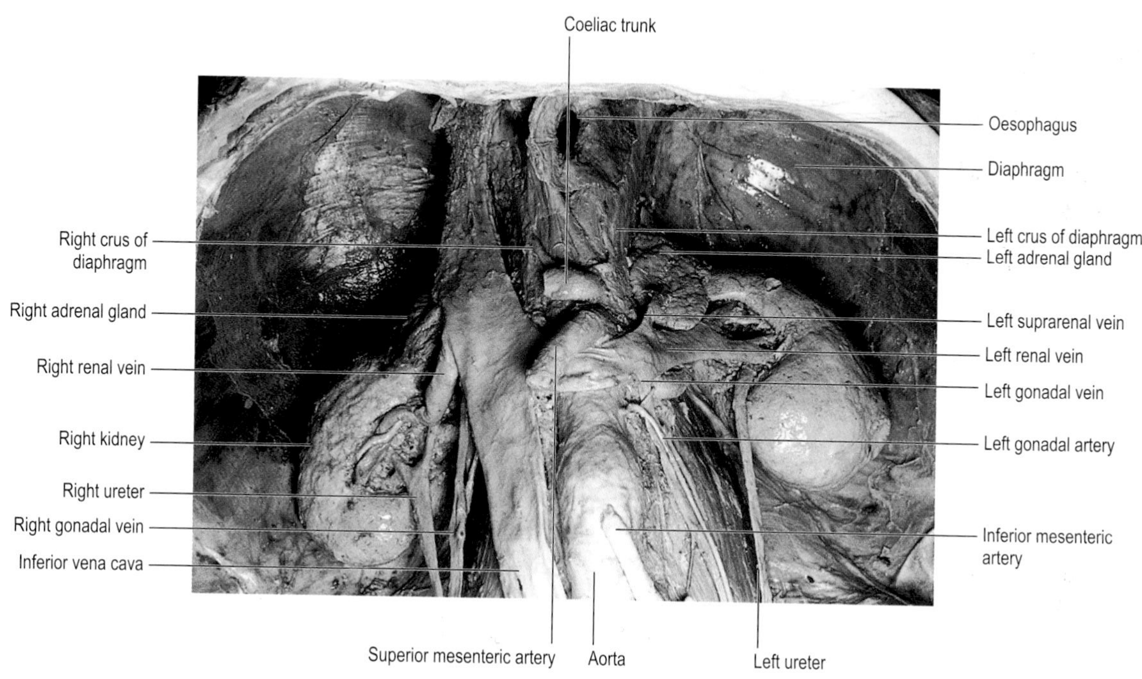


Fig. 4.62 Structures in the upper part of the posterior abdominal wall. Stomach, intestines, liver, pancreas and spleen have all been removed.

inferior vena cava overlaps it medially. Posteriorly lies the diaphragm. The left adrenal gland lies on the left crus of diaphragm. Its upper part is anteriorly related to the stomach separated by the lesser sac. Its lower part lies behind the pancreas and the splenic artery.

Each gland is supplied by three arteries and drained by one vein. The arterial supply is derived by branches from the aorta, renal artery and the inferior phrenic artery. The right adrenal vein is a short vein and it joins the inferior vena cava whereas the left adrenal vein drains into the left renal vein.

✪ The position of the right gland behind the liver, its proximity to the inferior vena cava and the short adrenal vein makes adrenalectomy of the right side more difficult than on the left.

## The abdominal aorta

The thoracic aorta enters the abdomen by passing between the two crura of the diaphragm behind the median arcuate ligament to become the abdominal aorta (Figs 4.63–4.65). It

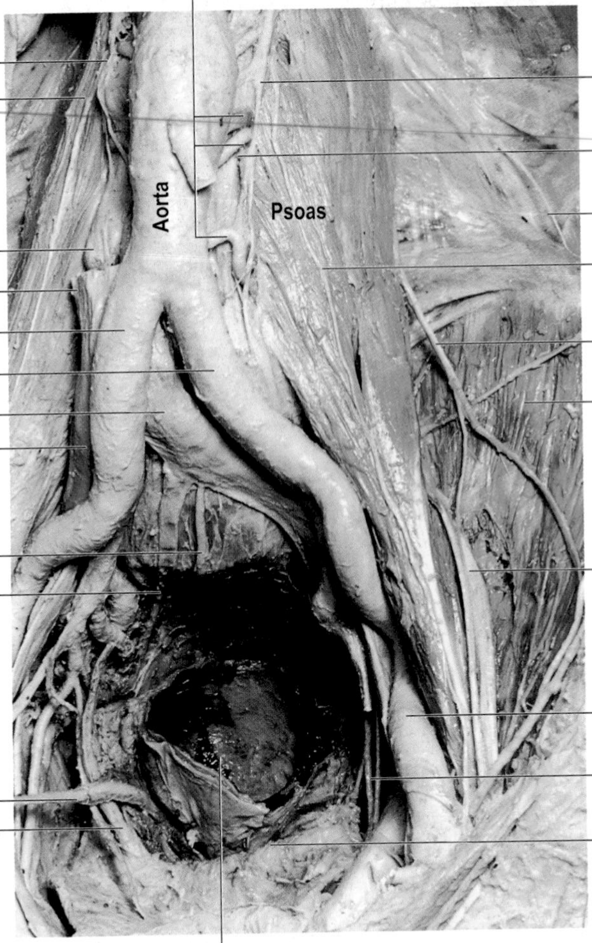

Lumbar arteries and vein
Right lumbar sympathetic trunk
Aorta
Psoas
Inferior vena cava
Right and left common iliac arteries
Right and left common iliac veins
Presacral veins
Ductus deferens
Right ureter
Rectum
Left lumbar sympathetic trunk
Iliohypogastric nerve
Genitofemoral nerve
Lateral cutaneous nerve of thigh
Iliacus
Femoral nerve
External iliac artery
Obturator nerve and artery
Urinary bladder

Fig. 4.63 Lower part of the posterior abdominal wall and pelvis.

Upper pole of the right kidney
Catheter in the abdominal aorta
4th lumbar vertebra
R
Left kidney
Right and left renal arteries
Lumbar arteries
Bifurcation of the aorta
Left external iliac artery
Right and left common iliac arteries
Left internal iliac artery

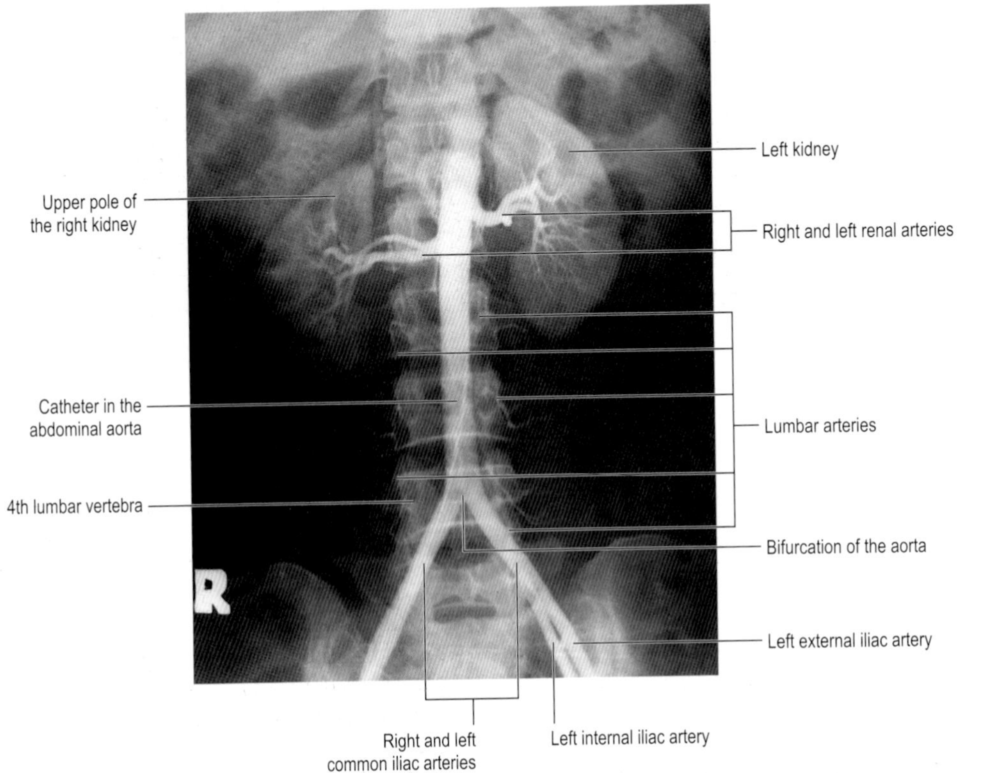

Fig. 4.64 Arteriogram of the abdominal aorta.

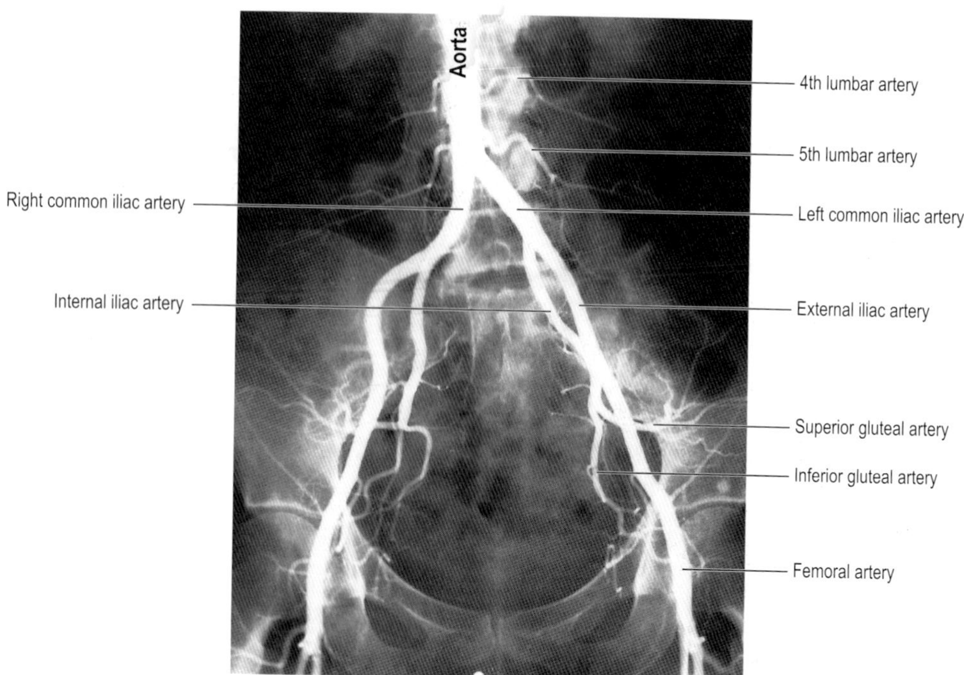


Fig. 4.65 Arteriogram of the lower part of abdominal aorta and the iliac arteries.

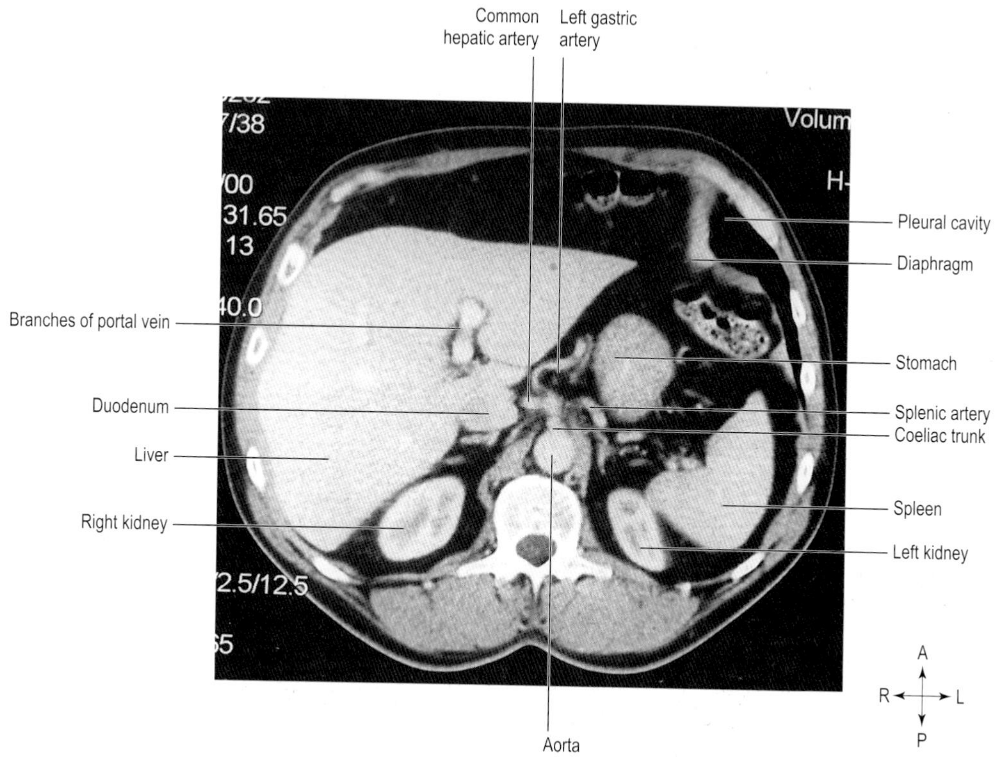


Fig. 4.66 CT scan at the level of the coeliac trunk after injection of intravascular contrast medium.

lies on the bodies of the lumbar vertebrae and inclines slightly to the left as it descends. The abdominal aorta bifurcates into two common iliac arteries in front of the body of the fourth lumbar vertebra (Figs 4.63–4.65).

✪ The surface marking of the aorta extends from a point just above the transpyloric plane in the midline to a point just to the left of the midline in a plane connecting the highest points of the iliac crest.

Branches can be grouped into three categories. The unpaired visceral branches are the three gut arteries – coeliac trunk, superior mesenteric artery and the inferior mesenteric artery. The paired visceral branches are the suprarenal, renal and gonadal arteries. The branches to the abdominal wall are the paired inferior phrenic and the lumbar arteries as well as the unpaired median sacral artery. The lumbar arteries (usually four in number) branching off from the sides of the aorta accompany the lumbar veins. The median sacral artery arising from the bifurcation of the aorta enters the pelvis, anastomoses with the sacral arteries and supplies the pelvic wall.

### Relations

Relations of the abdominal aorta can be seen in Figures 4.26, 4.53, 4.57, 4.66–4.70. The pancreas and the

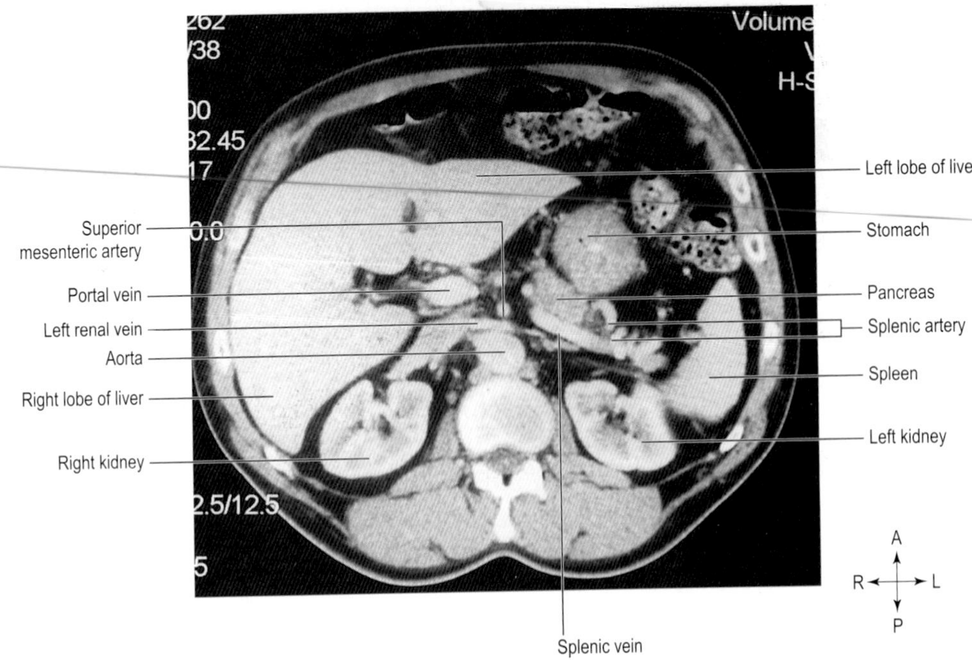


Fig. 4.67 CT scan at the level of the splenic artery after injection of intravascular contrast medium.

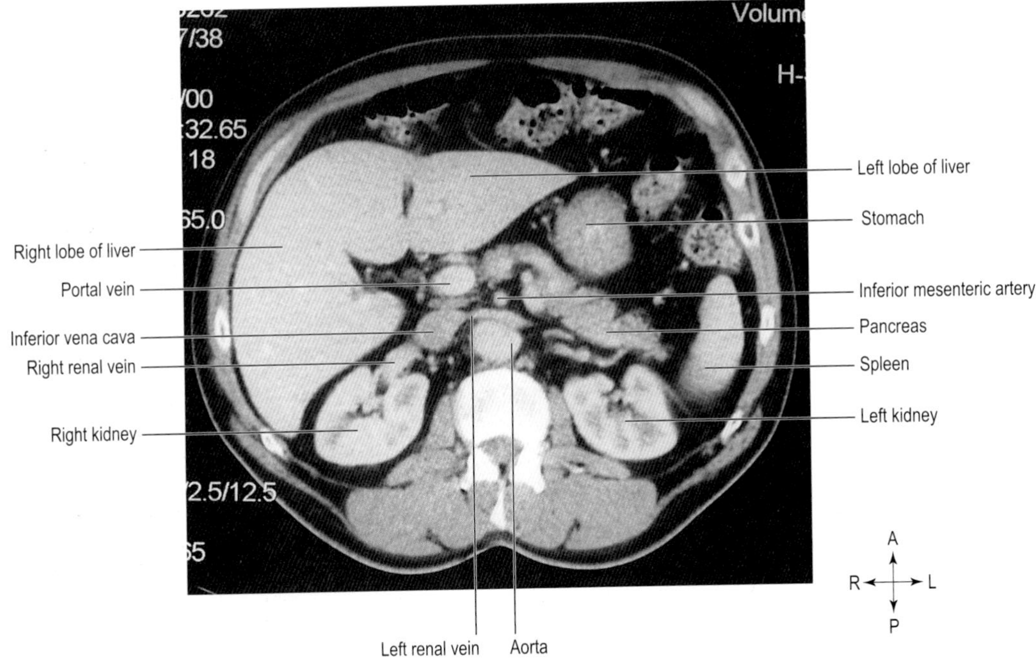


Fig. 4.68 CT scan at the level of the renal veins after injection of intravascular contrast medium.

splenic vein cross the aorta in between the origin of the coeliac trunk and the superior mesenteric arteries. Between the origins of the superior and inferior mesenteric arteries the aorta is crossed by the third part of the duodenum and the left renal vein. ✪ An aortic aneurysm in this area can bleed into the duodenum. Removal of an aneurysm may require ligation of the left renal vein. The third and fourth left lumbar veins cross behind the aorta.

✪ A tumour of the pancreas or mass of para-aortic lymph nodes transmitting aortic pulsation can be mistaken for an aneurysm of the aorta.

## The inferior vena cava

The inferior vena cava (Figs 4.63, 4.68–4.71; see also Fig. 4.26), lying close to the abdominal aorta on its right side, is longer than the aorta. It commences in front of the fifth lumbar vertebra by the union of two common iliac veins. It lies on the lumbar vertebrae and the right crus of the diaphragm and enters the thorax by piercing the central tendon of the diaphragm at the level of T8 vertebra. It crosses the right gonadal, the right renal and the right inferior phrenic arteries and overlaps the right lumbar sympathetic trunk. In the infracolic compartment the inferior vena cava, lying

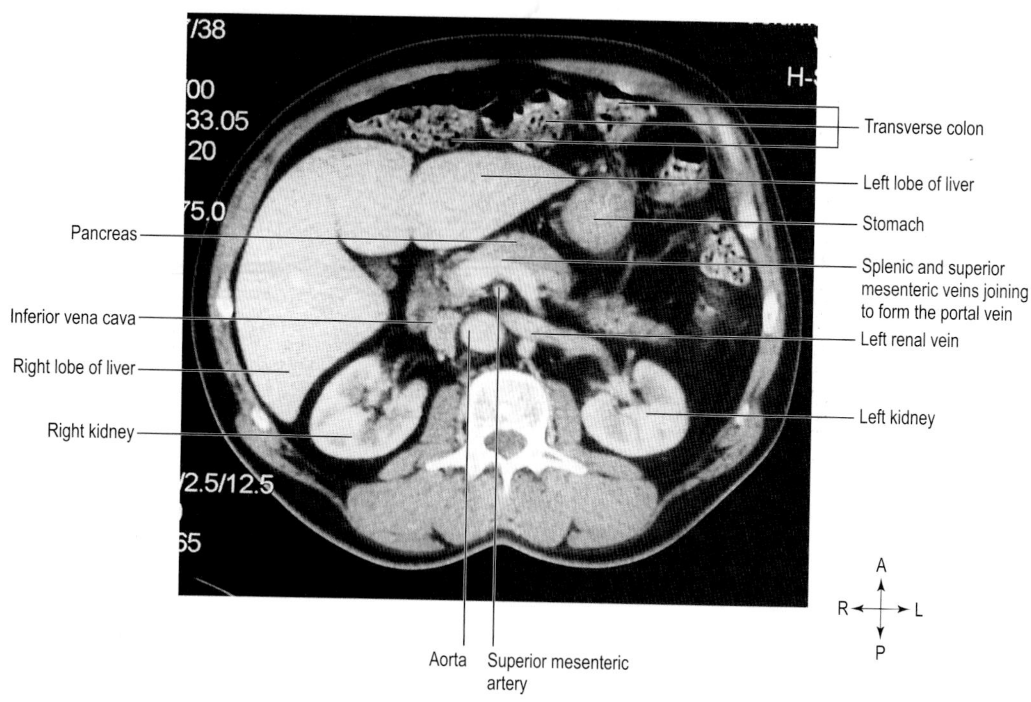


Fig. 4.69 CT scan at the level of the formation of the portal vein after injection of intravascular contrast medium.

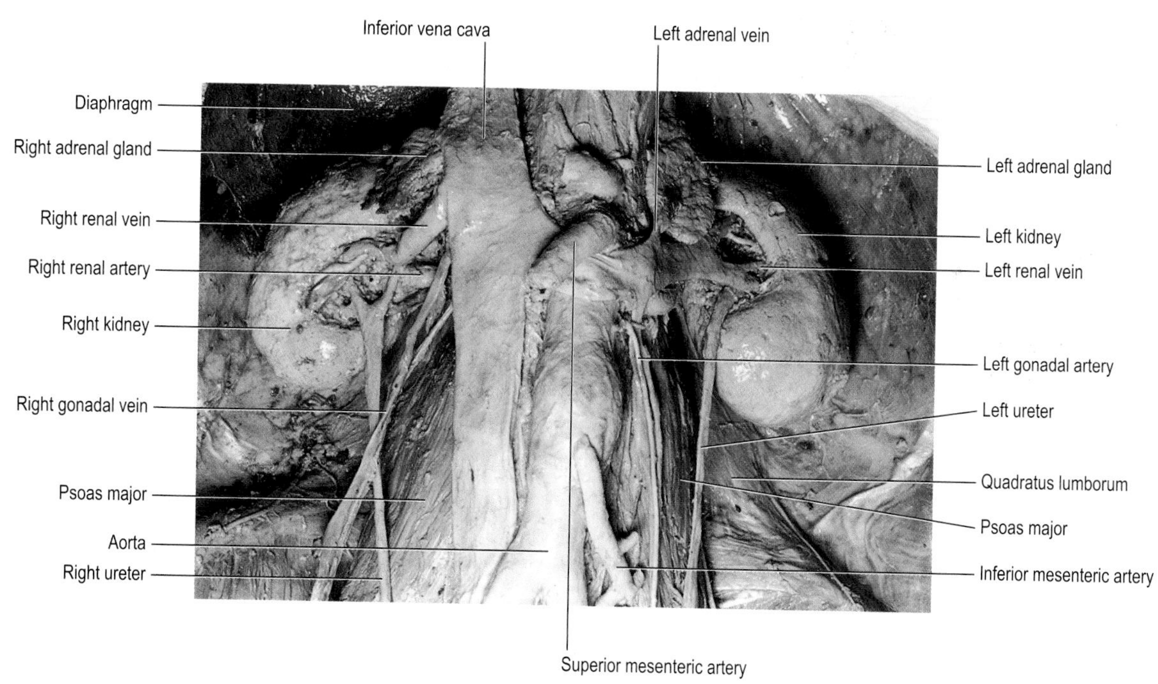


Fig. 4.70 The kidneys and the related structures.

behind the parietal peritoneum, is crossed by the root of the mesentery, the right gonadal artery and the third part of the duodenum. In the supracolic compartment the peritoneum covering the inferior vena cava forms the posterior wall of the epiploic foramen and above that level it lies behind the bare area of the liver. ✪ The vein–artery relationship alters as the inferior vena cava ascends. At its commencement the inferior vena cava lies behind the common iliac artery (Fig. 4.63), whereas in the upper part it lies in a plane anterior to that of the aorta. The surface marking is by a vertical line 2.5cm to the right of the midline extending from the intertubercular plane to the right sixth costal cartilage.

## Tributaries

Besides the two common iliac veins, the lumbar veins, the right gonadal veins, the renal veins, the right suprarenal vein, the right inferior phrenic vein and the three hepatic veins and several accessory hepatic veins drain into the vena cava. The left gonadal veins, the left adrenal vein and the left inferior phrenic vein are tributaries of the left renal vein.
✪ As the left renal vein crosses in front of the aorta it may have to be ligated and divided during surgery for aortic aneurysm. If this is done to the right of where its tributaries enter, the left kidney may survive by opening of anastomotic channels to drain the kidney. The inferior vena cava and its

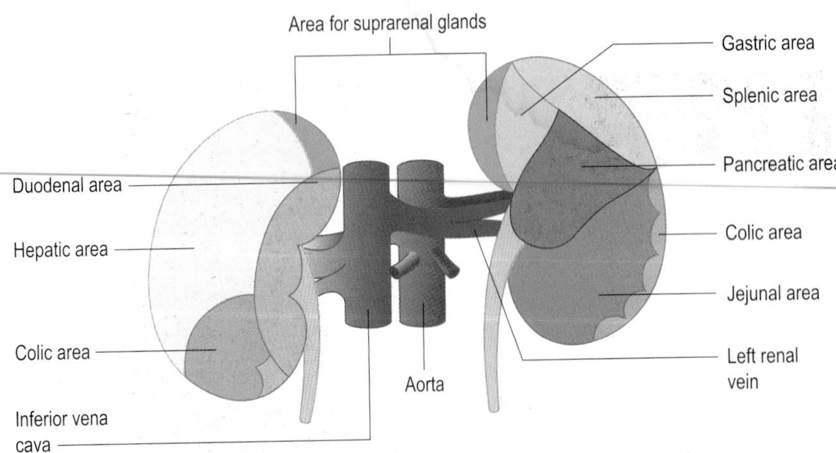


Fig. 4.71 Anterior relations of the kidneys.

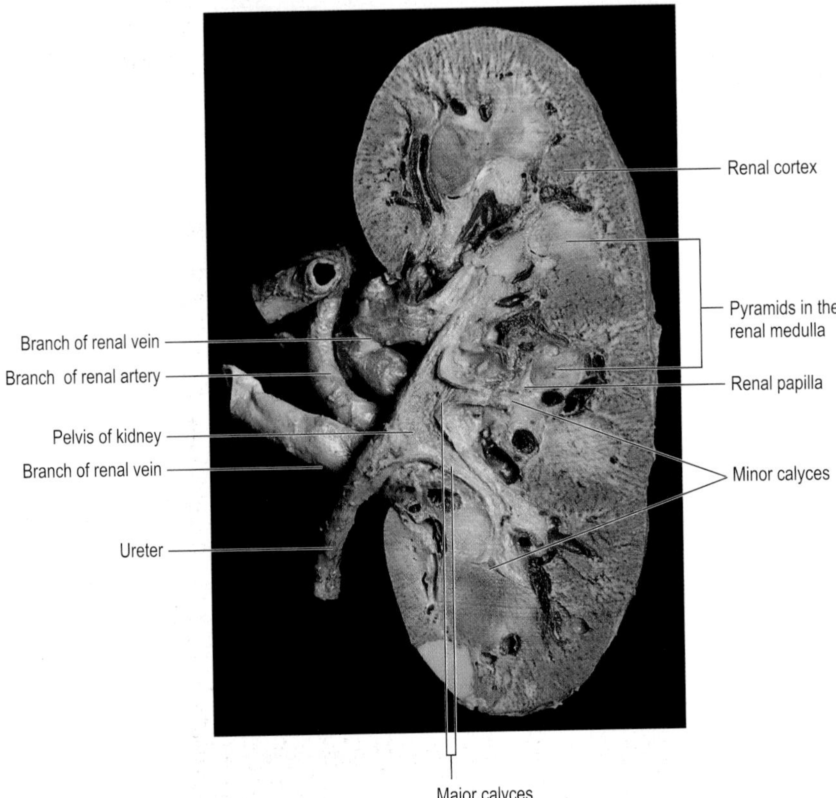


Fig. 4.72 Longitudinal section through the right kidney viewed from behind.

tributaries, with the exception of the gonadal veins, do not have valves.

## The common iliac arteries and veins

The common iliac artery from the bifurcation of the aorta passes downwards and laterally and bifurcates in front of the sacroiliac joint into external and internal iliac arteries – the former continues into the lower limb as the femoral artery and the latter divides into branches to supply the pelvis and perineum. ✪ The ureter crosses in front of the bifurcation of the artery. The apex of the sigmoid mesocolon also is related to this point. The common iliac and the external iliac arteries can be marked on the surface by extending the point of bifurcation of the abdominal aorta to a point midway between the anterior superior iliac spine and the pubic symphysis (the midinguinal point).

The common iliac veins formed by the union of external and internal iliac veins lie medial to the corresponding arteries at a deeper plane. The left vein is longer than the right as the inferior vena cava lies on the right side of the aorta. It crosses behind the right common iliac artery before joining the right vein to form the inferior vena cava (Fig. 4.63).

## The lumbar sympathetic trunk

The lumbar part of the sympathetic chain (see Fig. 4.63) lies along the anterolateral surface of the bodies of the lumbar vertebrae and along the medial border of the psoas. There are usually four ganglia in the lumbar region. The left lumbar sympathetic chain is overlapped by the aorta and the right by the inferior vena cava. Postganglionic fibres from the lumbar ganglia (grey rami) are distributed to the lumbar spinal nerves. The lumbar splanchnic nerves are

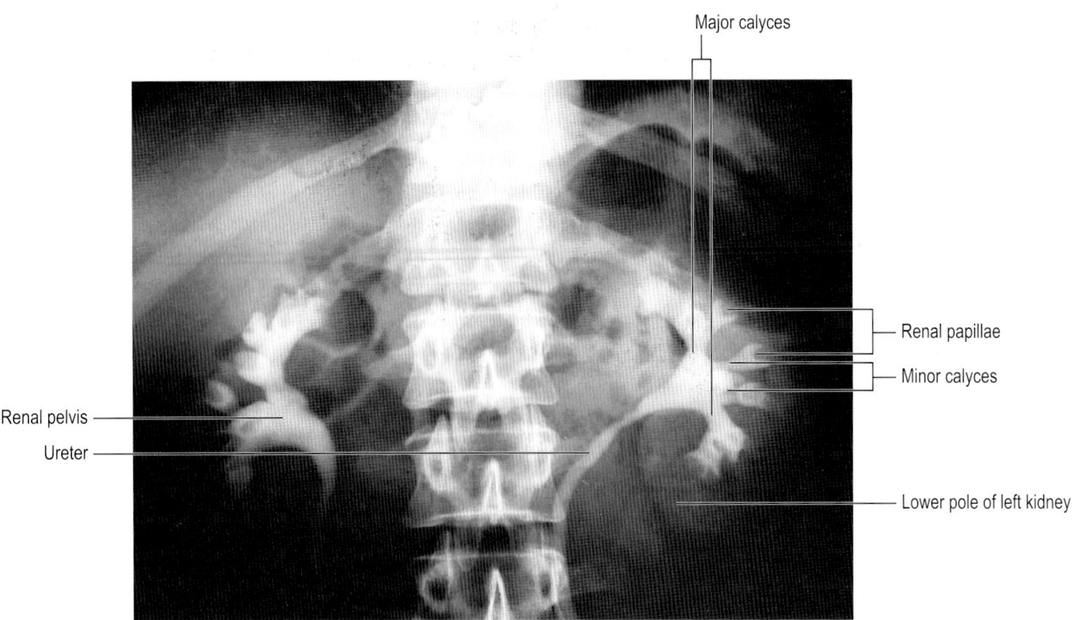


Fig. 4.73 Intravenous pyelogram (urogram).

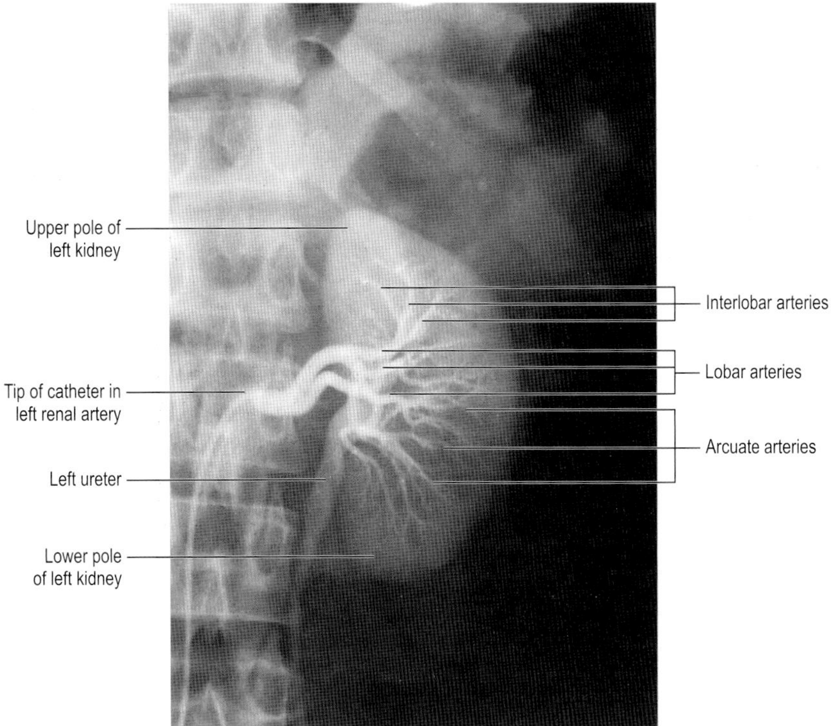


Fig. 4.74 Renal arteriogram.

preganglionic fibres connecting the ganglia to the aortic plexus (see Fig. 4.59). ✪ Lumbar sympathectomy is undertaken surgically or by producing neurolysis by injection of chemical agents such as phenol or alcohol. The procedure interrupts vasoconstrictor fibres and is undertaken in cases of peripheral vascular diseases of the lower limb.

## Kidneys

The kidneys (Figs 4.70–4.78) lie on the posterior abdominal wall behind the parietal peritoneum mostly covered by the costal margin. The right kidney is at a lower level compared with the left.

✪ The kidney has a fibrous capsule which is covered outside by the perirenal fat. Perirenal fat and the kidney are enclosed by the renal fascia which is formed by the splitting of transversalis fascia. These coverings, along with the renal vessels, anchor the kidney on the posterior abdominal wall. If the kidney ruptures the renal fascia distends and the swelling extends downwards into the pelvis.

The hilum of the kidney is in the transpyloric plane about 5cm from the midline, its upper pole lies 2.5cm and the lower pole 7.5cm away from the midline. Posteriorly, the

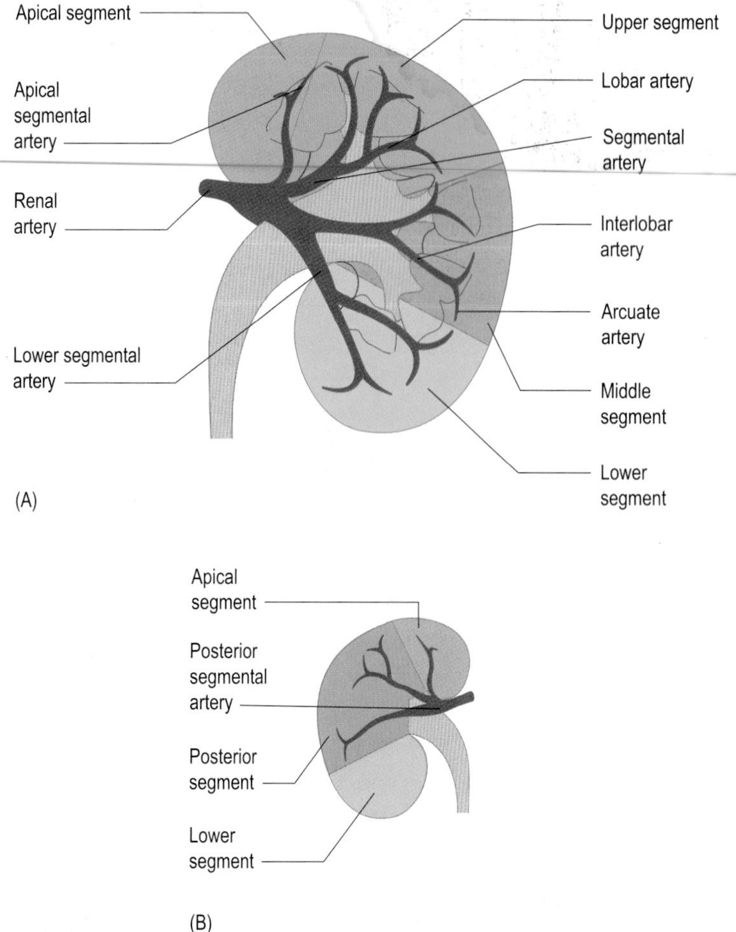


Fig. 4.75 The arterial supply of the kidney and the vascular segments: (A) anterior segments; (B) posterior segments.

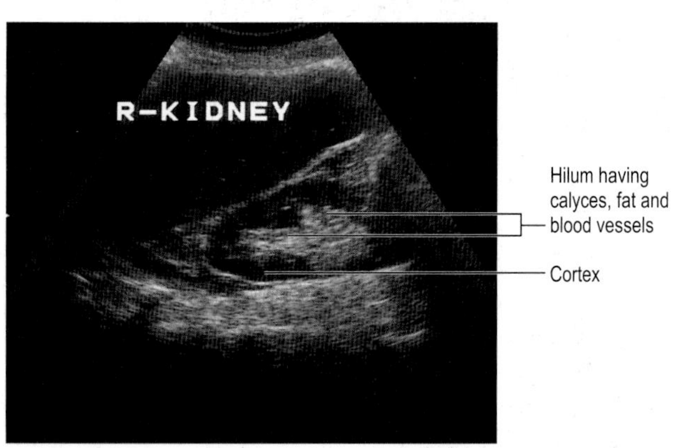


Fig. 4.76 Renal ultrasound.

kidneys lie on the diaphragm, the psoas major, the quadratus lumborum and the transversus abdominis. ✪ The costodiaphragmatic recess of the pleura, which is separated by the diaphragm, is an important posterior relation of the kidney.

The suprarenal gland on both sides sits on the upper pole of the kidney and overlaps onto its anterior surface (Fig. 4.70). Both kidneys are related to important regions of the peritoneal cavity. The right kidney lies behind the hepatorenal pouch (Fig. 4.49) whereas the left kidney lies behind the lesser sac. The anterior relations of the right kidney are the liver, the right suprarenal gland, the duodenum and the hepatic flexure of the colon. Similarly the stomach, spleen and the splenic flexure of the colon lie in front of the left kidney (Fig. 4.71).

✪ The hilum of the kidney has the renal vein, the renal artery and the pelvis of the ureter (renal pelvis). They lie in the order–vein, artery and ureter with the ureter posterior most. The renal pelvis, which is the commencement of the ureter, may be bifid. Also, the renal artery may give off branches and the renal vein may receive tributaries. These variations may create problems for the surgeon during dissection of the hilum.

In a longitudinal section of the kidney (Fig. 4.72) the renal cortex, which contains the glomeruli and the convoluted tubules, can be distinguished from the medullary pyramids, which has the loops of Henle, collecting ducts and collecting tubules. The apex of the pyramid projects into the minor calyx as renal papilla, one to three papillae opening into one minor calyx. The minor calyces unite together to form two or three major calyces which open into the renal pelvis (Figs 4.72, 4.73).

✪ At the hilum the renal artery typically divides into anterior and posterior branches from which five segmental arteries arise viz. apical, upper, middle, lower, and posterior. Vascular segments of the kidney are illustrated in Figure 4.75. Each segmental artery further divides into lobar arteries, one for each pyramid and the adjoining cortex. The lobar arteries divide into interlobar branches which give rise to arcuate arteries. There is virtually no anastomosis between branches of adjacent segmental arteries (Figs 4.74, 4.75). See Clinical boxes 4.17 and 4.18.

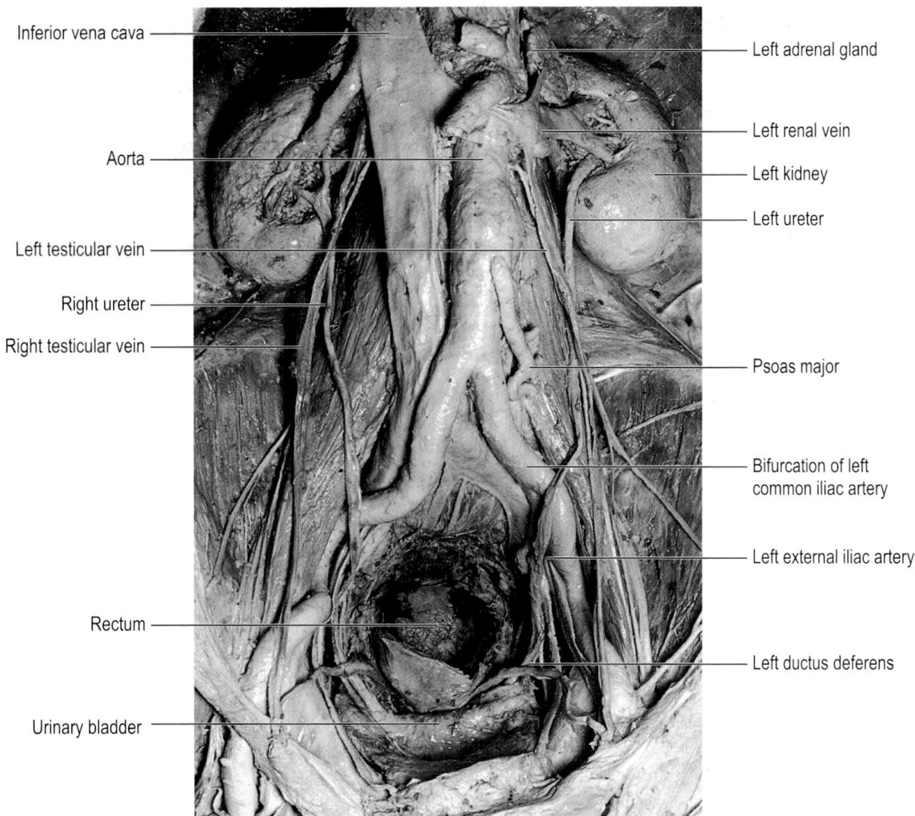


Fig. 4.77 The kidneys, ureters and the urinary bladder with the related structures. Dissection of the posterior abdominal wall.

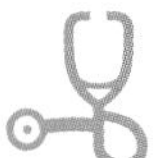

## *Clinical box 4.17*

### Surgical exposure of the kidney

This is done by a lumbar incision placed between the 12th rib and the iliac crest. Latissimus dorsi, external oblique, internal oblique and transversus muscles are encountered and divided. The peritoneum is pushed forward to expose the renal fascial capsule. The subcostal nerve (12th thoracic nerve) and vessels which lie on the posterior aspect of the upper part of the kidney are preserved. The bed of the 12th rib is dissected out taking care not to enter the pleural cavity, which is closely related to the medial part of the rib. Rupture of the pleura may occasionally happen leading to collapse of the lung. The pleura has to be sutured prior to re-inflation of the lung (by the anaesthetist).

✪ A normal kidney is not usually palpable. When enlarged, the swelling descends on inspiration. It is bimanually palpable and it may be possible to feel its upper border. Unlike the spleen, a notch is not felt on the renal swelling. These points are of importance to distinguish an enlarged left kidney from an enlarged spleen (see Clinical box 4.15).

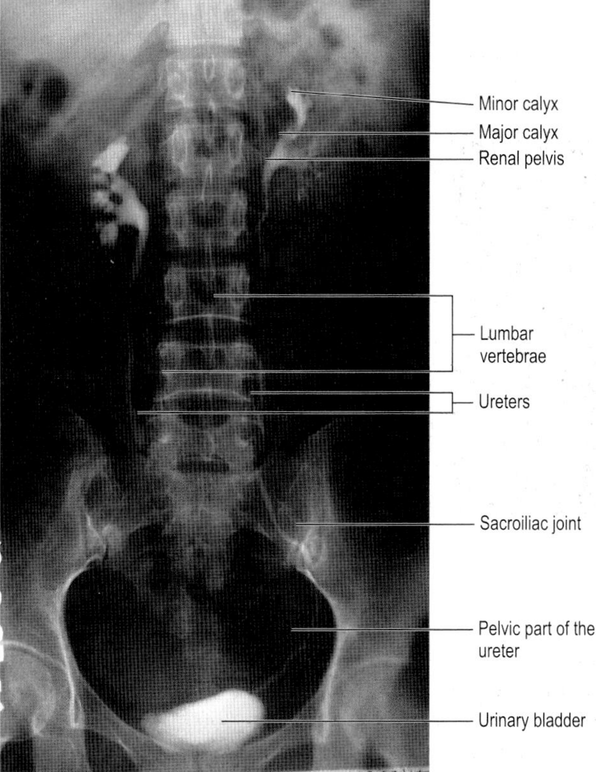


Fig. 4.78 Intravenous pyelogram (urogram) showing kidney, ureter and urinary bladder.

## The ureters

The ureter (Figs 4.77–4.79) lies on the psoas major muscle behind the parietal peritoneum. Its relations are clinically important. ✪ It is adherent to the peritoneum. On both sides the ureters cross the genitofemoral nerves and are crossed by the gonadal vessels. The right ureter lies behind the third part of the duodenum and as it descends is crossed by the ileocolic vessels and the root of the mesentery. The left ureter is crossed by the left colic vessels and at the pelvic brim it lies behind the apex of the sigmoid mesocolon. The

### Clinical box 4.18

**Congenital anomalies of the kidney**

The kidneys are developed in three successive stages, viz. the pronephros, mesonephros and metanephros. The pronephros mostly disappears. The adult kidney develops from two sources. The metanephros gives rise to the glomeruli, loops of Henle and the convoluted tubules. The collecting ducts, calyces, pelvis of the ureter and the ureter are derived from the ureteric bud from the mesonephric duct (duct of the mesonephros). The kidneys develop in the pelvis and ascend upwards to their lumbar position. As they do so they are supplied by arteries from different levels of the aorta. Some of these arteries may remain as aberrant arteries and they should be preserved and removed intact while removing kidney for transplantation and then anastomosed at the donor site to preserve the blood supply.

The kidney may fail to migrate cranially and remain as a pelvic kidney. The lower poles of the two kidneys which are close to each other while in the pelvis may fuse to become a horseshoe kidney which may get arrested during its ascent by one of the midline branches of the abdominal aorta.

The kidney may present with multiple cysts – the polycystic kidney. Though the actual cause of this is not known, it is speculated that it may be due to the failure of union between the metanephric and the mesonephric components.

The ureteric bud given off from the mesonephric duct may be double resulting in a double ureter, on one side or both. The original double ureter can fuse anywhere in their course. It can be bifid in its upper part or can open separately into the bladder.

psoas major separates the ureter from the transverse processes of the lumbar vertebrae. On a radiograph the ureter can be seen lying along the tips of the transverse processes and then in front of the sacroiliac joint. At operation it can be distinguished from nerves and vessels as a whitish non-pulsatile cord which is adherent to the peritoneum (moves with the peritoneum as the latter is pushed forward) and showing peristaltic activity when gently pinched with a forceps.

The ureter enters the pelvis by crossing anterior to the termination of the common iliac artery (Fig. 4.79). The pelvic part of the ureter lies on the side wall of the pelvis where it is related to the obturator nerve, obturator artery and other branches of the internal iliac artery. In the male the ductus deferens crosses the ureter before reaching the posterior surface of the bladder, whereas in the female the uterine artery crosses above the ureter (see Fig. 4.90) very near to the lateral fornix of the vagina (see also p. 118)

✪ The lumen of the ureter is not uniform throughout. It is narrower at the pelviureteric junction, where it crosses the bifurcation of the common iliac artery and where it enters the bladder. A renal stone passing through the ureter can be arrested at any of these sites. Pain sensation from the ureter is transmitted via sympathetic nerves to T11 to L1 segments and hence radiates from loin to groin and onto the medial part of the thigh.

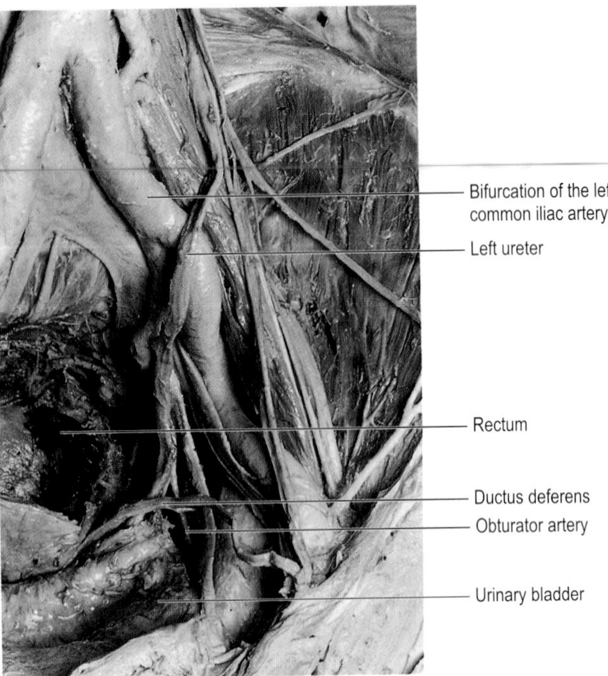


Fig. 4.79 Dissection of the lower part of the posterior abdominal wall and pelvis in the male to show the course of the left ureter. Sigmoid colon and the sigmoid mesocolon have been removed.

✪ The blood supply of the ureter is segmental by branches from the renal, gonadal, vesical and uterine arteries which anastomose on the adventitia covering its wall. The blood supply is therefore compromised if the ureter is stripped clean of its adventitia.

## Urinary bladder

See Figures 4.79–4.82. The empty bladder has a superior surface, two inferolateral surfaces and a base. The base faces posteriorly. The lower part of the bladder, which is continuous with the urethra, is known as the bladder neck. Only the superior surface is covered by peritoneum.

✪ The sigmoid colon rests on the superior surface of the bladder. Because of this relationship a colovesical fistula can occur in diverticular disease. The body of the uterus lies superior to the bladder in the female and the supravaginal cervix and the vagina separates the posterior surface from the rectouterine pouch and the rectum. The posterior surface of the bladder in the male is related to the seminal vesicle and the ductus deferens (lying below the rectovesical pouch), behind which lies the rectum.

The mucosa of the empty bladder is thrown into folds. These flatten as the bladder distends. The inner aspect of the posterior wall however is smooth. This is known as the trigone of the bladder and is bounded laterally by the opening of the two ureters and below by the urethra. In the male the trigone overlies the median part of the central zone of the prostate which, after middle age, projects above the internal orifice of the urethra as the uvula of the bladder.

✪ In the upper border of the trigone is the interureteric crest (interureteric ridge or bar) which extends between the two ureteric orifices. The interureteric crest can be seen during cystoscopy (examination of the interior of the bladder) and the two ureteric orifices can be seen discharging urine. The

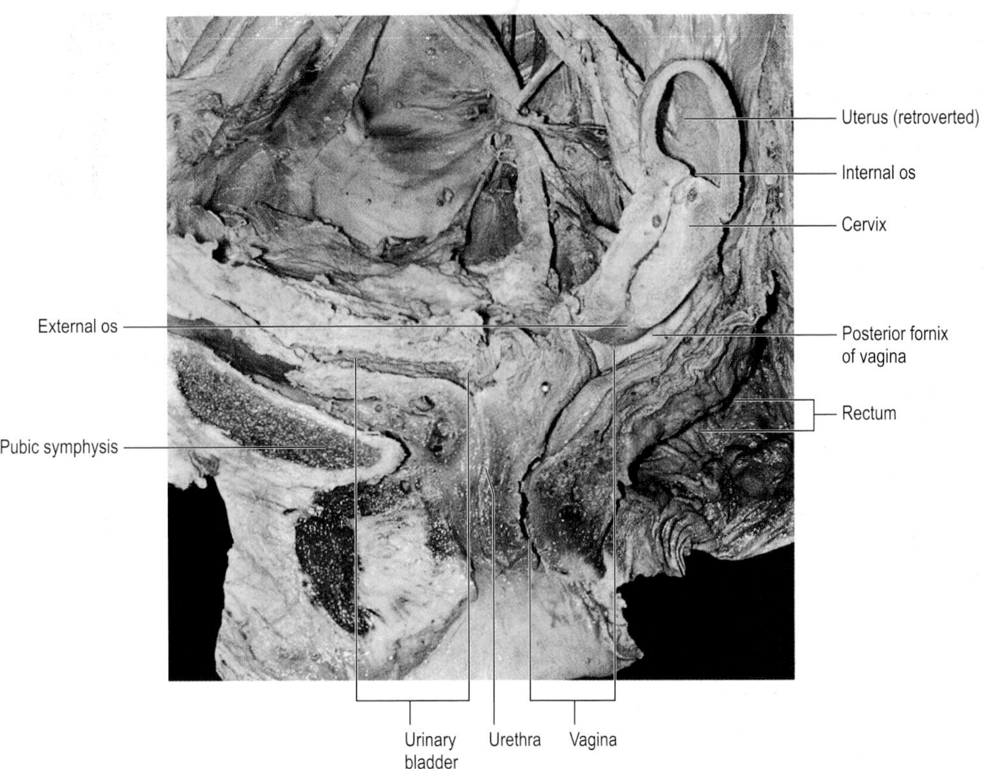


Fig. 4.80 Female pelvis and perineum – sagittal section, urinary bladder and the urethra.

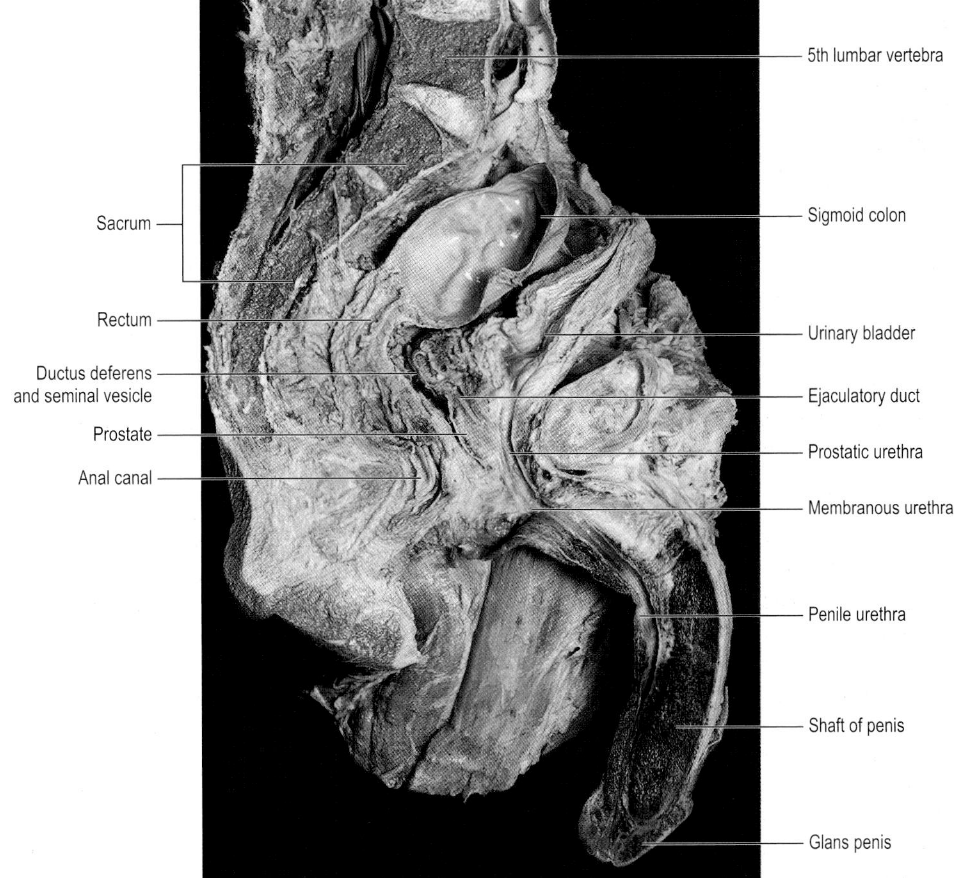


Fig. 4.81 Male pelvis and perineum – sagittal section, urinary bladder and the urethra.

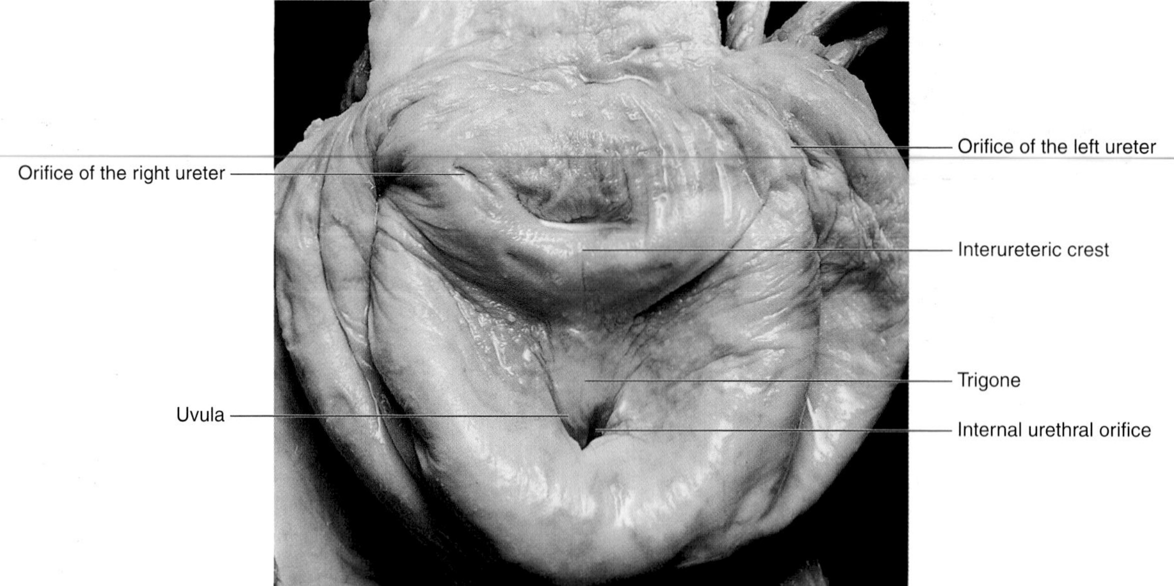


Fig. 4.82 The interior of the urinary bladder.

ureters lie obliquely in the bladder wall before their termination and have a valve-like mechanism which prevents reflux of urine during contraction of the bladder.

The mucosa of the bladder is lined by transitional epithelium which will not absorb urine. The underlying muscle is the detrusor muscle, the fibres of which run in different directions interlacing with each other.

✪ In urinary obstruction the detrusor muscle hypertrophies and the spaces in between the muscle fibres deepen to give rise to bladder diverticulae. Urine will collect in the diverticulae without draining, leading to infection of the bladder.

The muscle of the trigone is different from the detrusor. It extends into the lower part of the ureters and also into the urethra. At the bladder neck the trigonal muscle is circular in the male and forms the internal sphincter of the bladder. This prevents regurgitation of semen into the bladder during ejaculation. In the female urinary bladder, these fibres are longitudinal in direction and hence do not form a sphincter at the bladder neck.

✪ The bladder is innervated by sympathetic and parasympathetic nerves. The motor innervation of the bladder is by the parasympathetic nerves from S2, S3, S4 segments of the spinal cord (pelvic splanchnic nerves) except the trigonal muscle and the internal sphincter, which are supplied by the sympathetics. Sensation of bladder distension travels via the parasympathetic nerves whereas pain is transmitted by both para-sympathetics and sympathetics.

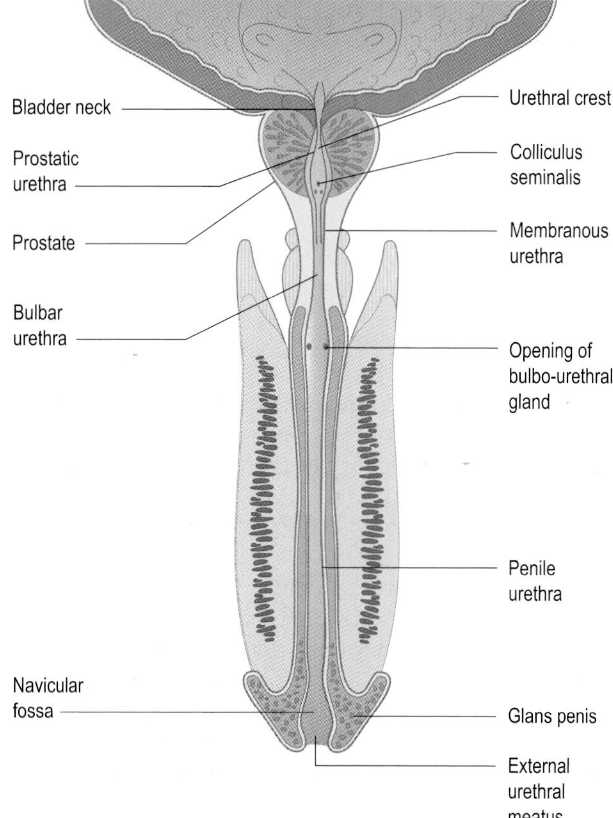


Fig. 4.83 The posterior wall of the male urethra.

## The male urethra

The male urethra (Figs 4.81, 4.83) is about 20cm long having three parts. It passes through the prostate (prostatic urethra), deep perineal pouch (membranous urethra) and then through the corpus spongiosum of the penis (penile urethra).

The prostatic urethra, which is about 2.5cm long, is the widest and the most dilatable part of the urethra. The posterior wall of this part has a linear bulge, the urethral crest, the widest part of which is the colliculus seminalis or verumontanum. Into the urethral crest opens the prostatic utricle, a small blind-ending sac which is the remnant of the paramesonephric duct. The two ejaculatory ducts, each formed by the union of the ductus deferens and the duct of the seminal vesicle, also open here. The gutter on either side of the urethral crest, the prostatic sinus, has the openings of the prostatic ducts from the peripheral zone of the prostate, whereas the central zone ducts open into the

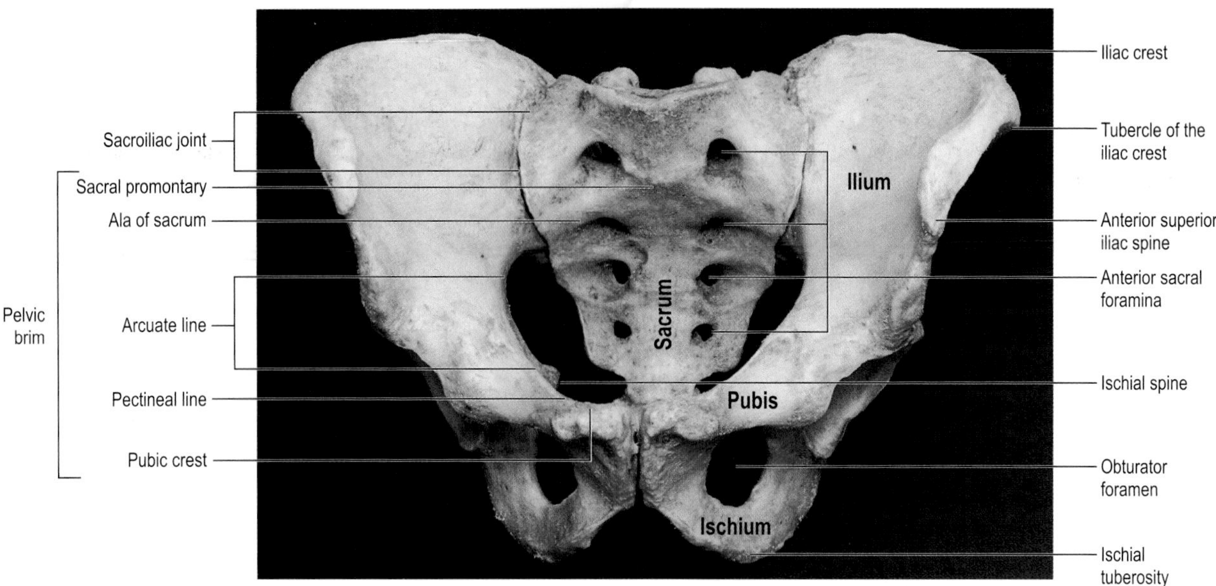


Fig. 4.84 Bony pelvis.

verumontanum around the orifices of the ejaculatory ducts (see description of prostate pgs 120, 121).

The membranous part, which is 1.5cm long, is short and narrow and is the least dilatable part of the male urethra. This part lying in the deep perineal pouch is surrounded by the external sphincter of the urethra.

The commencement of the penile urethra in the bulb of the penis is relatively fixed, whereas its continuation in the corpus spongiosum of the penis is mobile. In the glans penis it widens as the navicular fossa. ✪ The external urethral meatus, which is the narrowest part of the whole urethra, appears as a sagittal slit at the tip of the penis, helping to focus the urine as it comes through the dilatation of the navicular fossa.

The bulbourethral glands situated in the deep perineal pouch open into the bulbar part of the urethra. Besides this a number of mucous glands (of Littre) also open into the penile urethra with their orifices directed distally. ✪ These may get infected and also occasionally may cause confusion at the time of urethrography.

✪ There are two sphincteric mechanisms for the bladder and urethra. The internal sphincter at the bladder neck is not strong enough to maintain continence if the external sphincter is destroyed. Its main role is to prevent retrograde ejaculation into the bladder. It closes the bladder neck by sympathetic nerve stimulation during emission of semen into the prostatic urethra.

The external sphincter surrounds the membranous urethra. It maintains urinary continence and controls micturation. It has an internal component, lissosphincter, of smooth muscle, and an external component, rhabdosphincter, made of striated muscle. The external sphincter is innervated by sensory and motor fibres from the pudendal nerve (somatic) as well as by the autonomic nerves.

## Female urethra

The female urethra (Fig. 4.80) is about 4cm long, lies on the anterior wall of the vagina and opens in the vestibule between the anterior ends of the labia minora and the clitoris (see Fig. 4.95). ✪ The female urethra is more elastic and more easily distensible than that of the male. Hence catheterisation and instrumentation of the bladder and urethra in the female are more easily performed. As the short urethra opens into the vestibule urinary infection is more common in the female. The sphincter mechanism extends down the whole length of the urethra. Structurally the sphincter is similar to the external sphincter in the male with lissosphincter and rhabdosphincter components which are innervated by the pudendal and autonomic nerves. The sphincter is most well developed in the middle third of the urethra. Unlike in the male the female urethra does not have a well-defined sphincter at the bladder neck.

## The pelvic wall

The pelvis contains the terminal parts of the alimentary and urinary systems and also parts of the reproductive system.

The bony pelvis (Fig. 4.84) is made up of three bones: the two hip bones and the sacrum. The hip bones articulate with each other in front at the pubic symphysis and with the sacrum at the back through the two sacroiliac joints. Each hip bone has three components, the ilium, the pubis and the ischium, the three fusing together in the acetabulum.

Three pairs of muscles are seen on the walls of the pelvis. The side wall has the obturator internus muscle covering the obturator foramen. Posteriorly, taking origin from the sacrum and passing through the greater sciatic foramen is the piriformis muscle. The two levator ani muscles fuse in the midline to form a gutter in the floor of the pelvis (Figs 4.85, 4.86).

The levator ani takes origin from a line extending from the back of the pubis to the ischial spine and is described as having three parts: the pubococcygeus, the iliococcygeus and the ischiococcygeus. The iliococcygeus does not arise from the ilium but instead is attached to the fascia covering the obturator internus muscle.

The fibres of the levator ani run downwards medially and backwards. As they do so, the inner fibres of pubococcygeus are intimately related to the pelvic organs. The muscle is an

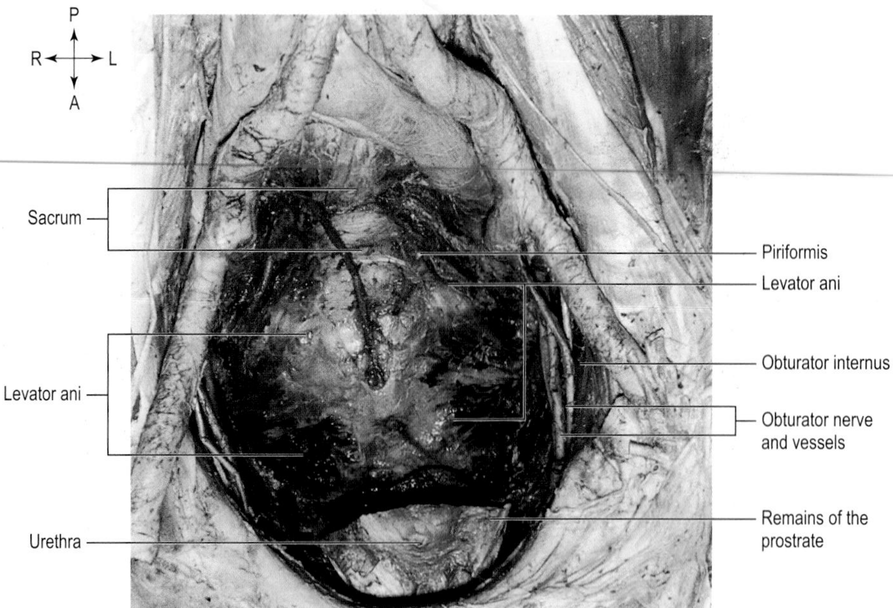


Fig. 4.85 The floor of the pelvis seen after removal of the pelvic organs.

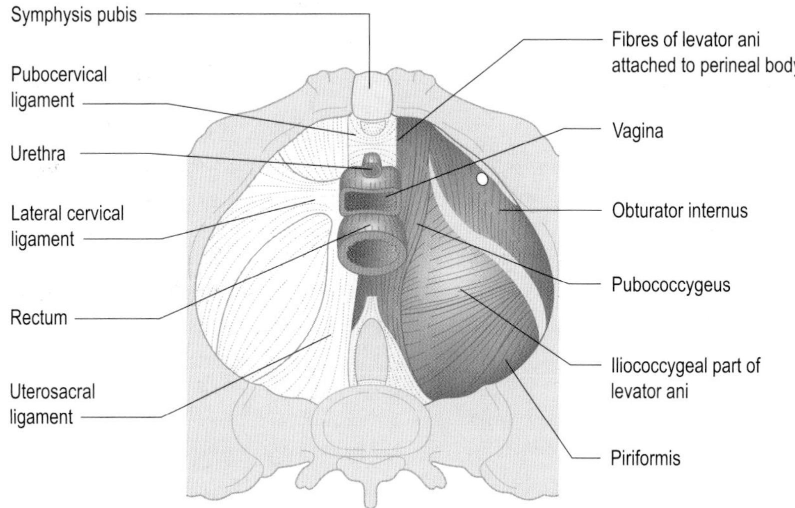


Fig. 4.86 Floor of the pelvis and muscles and ligaments supporting the uterus and vagina – superior view. Ligaments are shown on the left side and muscles on the right.

important structure maintaining the normal position of the pelvic organs. Fibres of the levator ani related to the prostate are known as the levator prostatae, those around the vagina form the sphincter vaginae. Behind these the fibres are inserted into a tough fibromuscular nodule, the perineal body, in front of the anorectal junction. A number of perineal muscles are also inserted into the perineal body. The perineal body together with the muscles attached to it prevent the pelvic organs from prolapsing into the perineum.

The pubococcygeus fibres of the levator ani around the anorectal junction is called the puborectalis muscle. The puborectalis fibres form a sling around the anorectal junction, i.e. fibres of one side become continuous with those of the opposite side. This sling maintains the forward angulation of the anorectal junction. Fibres of the sling also fuse with the deep part of the external sphincter of the anal canal and contribute to the formation of the anorectal ring. This forms an important part of the sphincteric mechanism at the anorectal region.

More lateral fibres of the levator ani fuse in a fibrous raphe behind the anorectal junction, the anococcygeal raphe.

## Female internal genital organs

See Figures 4.87–4.91.

### The ovary

The ovary is attached to the posterior leaf of the broad ligament by a double fold of peritoneum, the mesovarium. Continuation of the broad ligament (see below) from the ovary to the side wall of the pelvis is known as the suspensory ligament of the ovary. The ligament of the ovary, a thin fibrous cord, connects it to the uterus. This ligament then extends to the labium majus through the inguinal canal as the round ligament of the uterus. The ligament of the ovary and the round ligament of the uterus together can

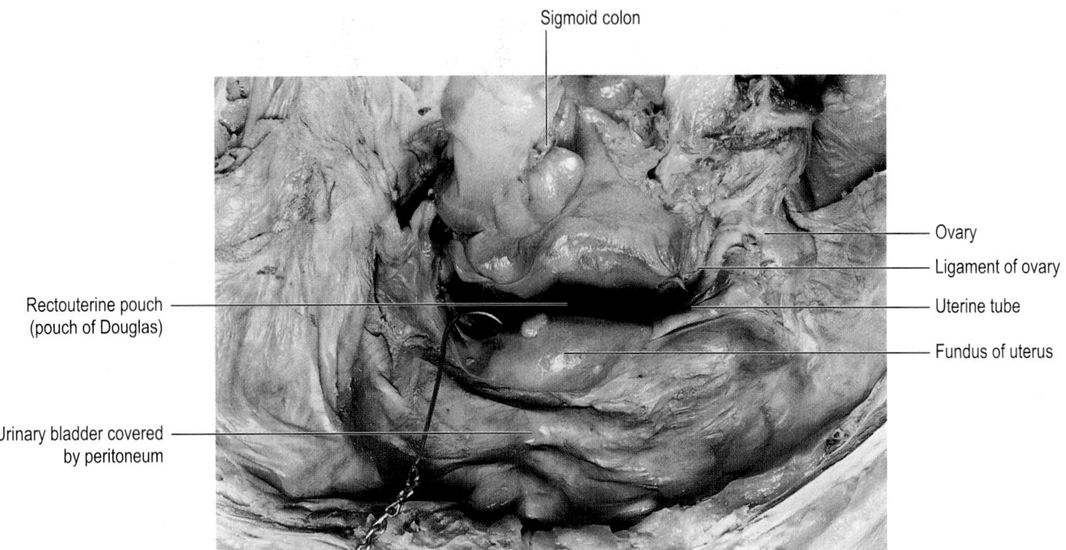


Fig. 4.87 Female pelvic organs seen from above.

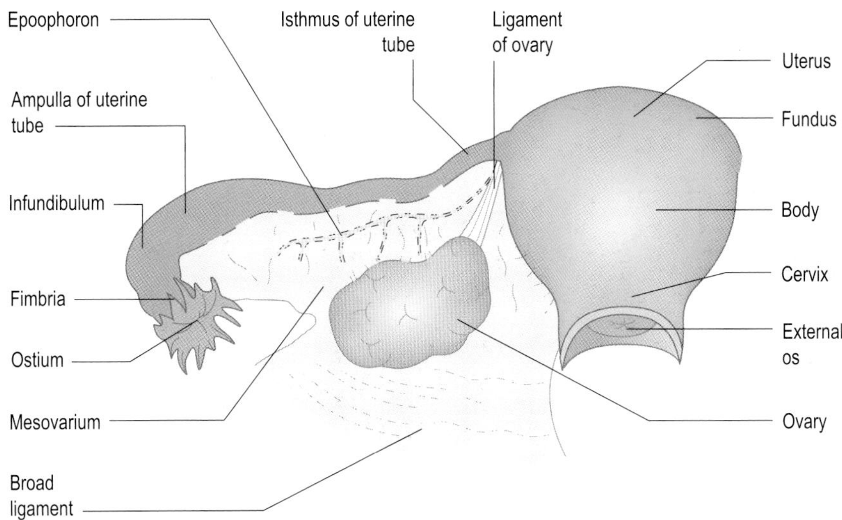


Fig. 4.88 Uterus, broad ligament and ovary – posterior view.

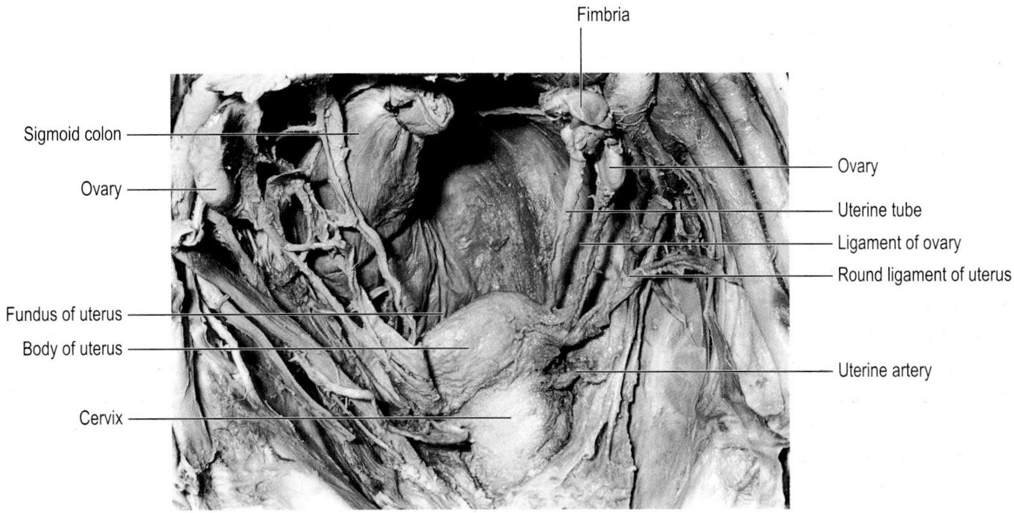


Fig. 4.89 Female pelvic organs after removal of peritoneum. Uterus is lifted up to show the anterior surface of cervix. Part of the sigmoid colon and coils of intestines have been removed.

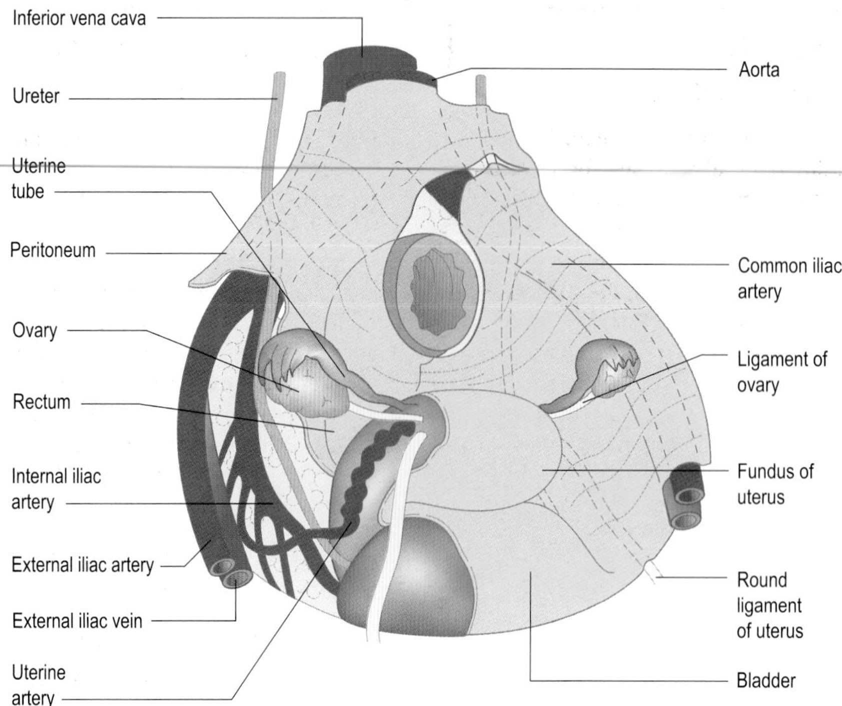


Fig. 4.90 The female pelvic organs seen from above (diagrammatic). The peritoneum on the right side has been partially removed.

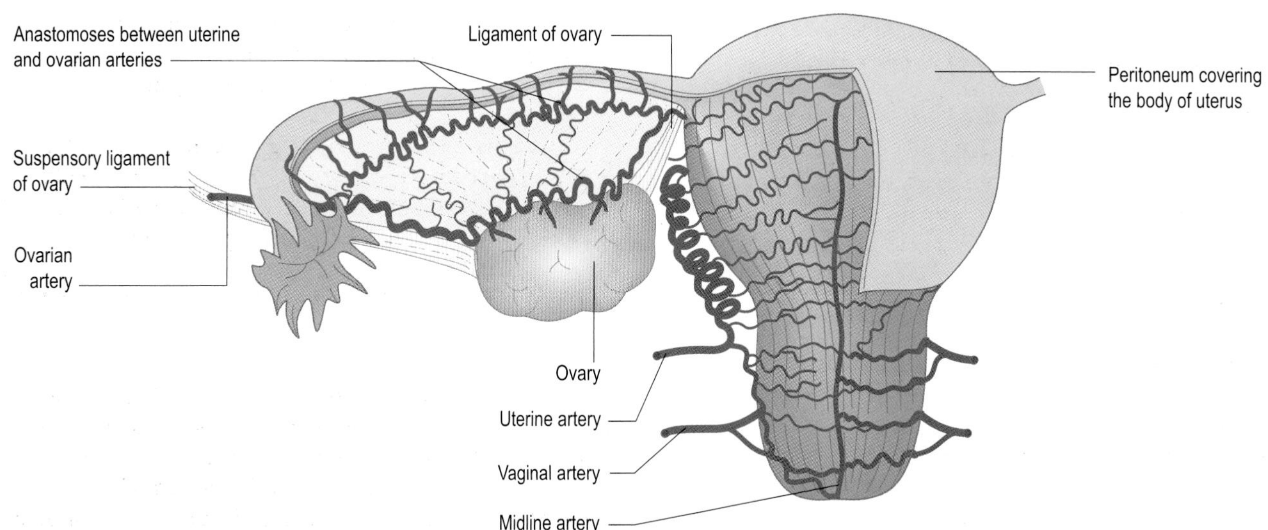


Fig. 4.91 Arterial supply of the ovary, uterine tube, uterus and vagina.

be considered to be homologous to the gubernaculum testis which connects the testis to the scrotal wall. The ovary lies on the side wall of the pelvis in the 'ovarian fossa' in the angle between the external and internal iliac vessels. ✪ The ureter lies close behind the ovary and has to be taken care of while ligating the ovarian vessels while doing an ovariectomy

✪ The ovary in its normal position may be just palpable by vaginal examination. It is laterally related to the obturator nerve. Inflammation of the ovary may cause pain along the distribution of the obturator nerve, along the medial aspect of the thigh.

The ovary is supplied by the ovarian artery given off just below the renal artery from the abdominal aorta. Veins form a plexus which eventually forms a single trunk. On the left side these drain into the renal vein and on the right side into the inferior vena cava. The lymphatics of the ovary drain into the para-aortic nodes. The blood supply of the ovaries and their lymphatic drainage are comparable to those of the testes.

## The uterus

Parts of the uterus are the fundus, body and the cervix (of the uterus) (Figs 4.87–4.91). The lower part of the cervix is inside the vagina. The lower part of the body, which is narrow, is known as the isthmus. The junction between the lumen of the body and that of the isthmus is the internal os.

The spaces around the cervix, inside the vagina, are the vaginal fornices. They are divided into anterior, posterior and lateral fornices according to their positions in relation to the vagina. The posterior fornix is deeper than the others. The opening of the cervix into the vagina is the external os.

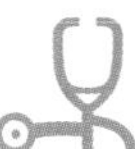

### *Clinical box 4.19*

**Innervation of the birth canal**

Knowledge of the sensory innervation of the birth canal is important in providing pain relief during childbirth. Pain from the body of the uterus is transmitted by the afferents accompanying the sympathetic nerves through the inferior and superior hypogastric plexuses into the lumbar sympathetic ganglia and then into lumbar and lower thoracic parts of the spinal cord. Pain from the cervix and the vagina is transmitted by the afferents accompanying the pelvic splanchnic nerves into the sacral part of the cord (S2, S3, S4). Pain caused by the dilatation of the vaginal orifice is transmitted by the sensory nerves of the vulva (external genitalia), the anterior part by the ilioinguinal nerves (L1) and the posterior part the pudendal nerves (S2, S3, S4). Also see epidural anaesthesia (p. 133).

In its normal position the uterus is angulated forward on the vagina (see Fig. 4.18). This is known as the anteverted position of the uterus and it is maintained by the levator ani (pelvic diaphragm) and the various ligaments connected to the uterus and vagina (Fig. 4.86).

Peritoneum covers the whole of the posterior surface and the upper third of the vagina and is reflected onto the rectum forming the rectouterine pouch (see Fig. 4.18).

✪ Anteriorly, the supravaginal part of the cervix and the isthmus are not covered by peritoneum. These parts enlarge during pregnancy and together become the lower segment of the uterus. It is the site of caesarean sections. The surgeon can thus open the uterus without entering the peritoneal cavity.

The uterine and the ovarian arteries supply the uterus. The uterine artery, a branch of the internal iliac artery, crosses above the ureter (water under the bridge!), adjacent to the lateral fornix, before ascending up in the broad ligament on the side of the uterus (Fig. 4.90). ✪ During hysterectomy (removal of uterus), while the surgeon ligates and cuts the uterine arteries, the ureters are in danger of being clamped or cut inadvertently. The ovarian artery, supplying the fundus, runs along the uterine tube and anastomoses with the uterine artery (Figs 4.90, 4.91).

✪ Lymphatic drainage is important in relation to the spread of carcinoma of the uterus. The lymph vessels from the fundus follow the ovarian vessels and drain into the para-aortic nodes whereas those from the body drain into the external iliac nodes. Lymphatics of the cervix drain into the external iliac, internal iliac as well as the sacral nodes. Some lymphatics from the fundus and the upper part of the body may accompany the round ligament of the uterus to drain into the superficial inguinal nodes. See Clinical box 4.19.

## Vagina

From the uterine end the vagina is directed downwards and forwards as it passes between the pubovaginalis part of the levator ani, the deep perineal pouch, to open in the vestibule, which is the space between the two labia minora in the vulva (external genitalia). Urethra also opens here. The urethral orifice is anterior to the vaginal orifice. The vagina is highly stretchable having the benefit of being supplied by a number of arteries with a rich anastomosis on its wall (Fig. 4.91).

✪ A number of structures can be felt by vaginal examination which include cervix of the uterus and fornices of the vagina. Anteriorly the urethra, bladder and symphysis pubis and posteriorly the rectum, as well as collection of fluid and malignant deposits in the pouch of Douglas, can also be felt. The body of the uterus, ovaries and the uterine tubes may be felt with pressure applied to the lower abdominal wall. See Clinical box 4.20.

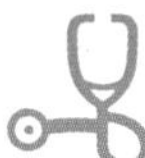

### *Clinical box 4.20*

**Perineal tear**

Injury to the vaginal wall and the pubococcygeus part of the levator ani (pelvic floor) can occur due to excessive stretching during childbirth. The severity of the injury is graded as 1–4. In Grade 1 only the vaginal mucosa is torn whereas a grade 4 tear injures the vaginal wall, the anal canal and also the rectum, with associated damage of the pubococcygeus. The tear of the pelvic floor may alter the position of the bladder neck and urethra causing stress incontinence in which there is dribbling of urine when the intra-abdominal pressure is raised during coughing and sneezing.

## The uterine tube

The uterine tube consists of from medial to lateral intramural part (in the uterine wall), isthmus, ampulla and the infundibulum or fimbriated end with a number of finger-like processes, the fimbriae, one of them applied to the ovary. It ends laterally near the ovary by opening into the peritoneal cavity. The opening is called the ostium. The tube lies inside the broad ligament (Fig. 4.88).

✪ The patency of the tube is essential for normal pregnancy. Infection of the tube (salpingitis) may result in scarring and closure of the tubes. In tubal sterilisation the uterine tubes are cut to prevent future pregnancies. See Clinical box 4.21.

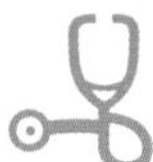

### *Clinical box 4.21*

**Ectopic pregnancy**

Fertilisation of the ovum normally occurs in the ampulla of the uterine tube. From there it migrates to the uterus to implant in the mucosa of the body of the uterus. In tubal ectopic pregnancies the fertilised ovum may implant in the uterine tube instead of passing into the uterus. The tube, however, cannot accommodate the growing fetus and the placenta and it will rupture into the peritoneal cavity resulting in bleeding and peritonitis.

Occasionally as the embryo enlarges it may enter the abdominal cavity where it may survive for a short while causing an abdominal pregnancy. Pain and peritonitis caused by the rupture of a tubal pregnancy on the right side can be misdiagnosed as appendicitis.

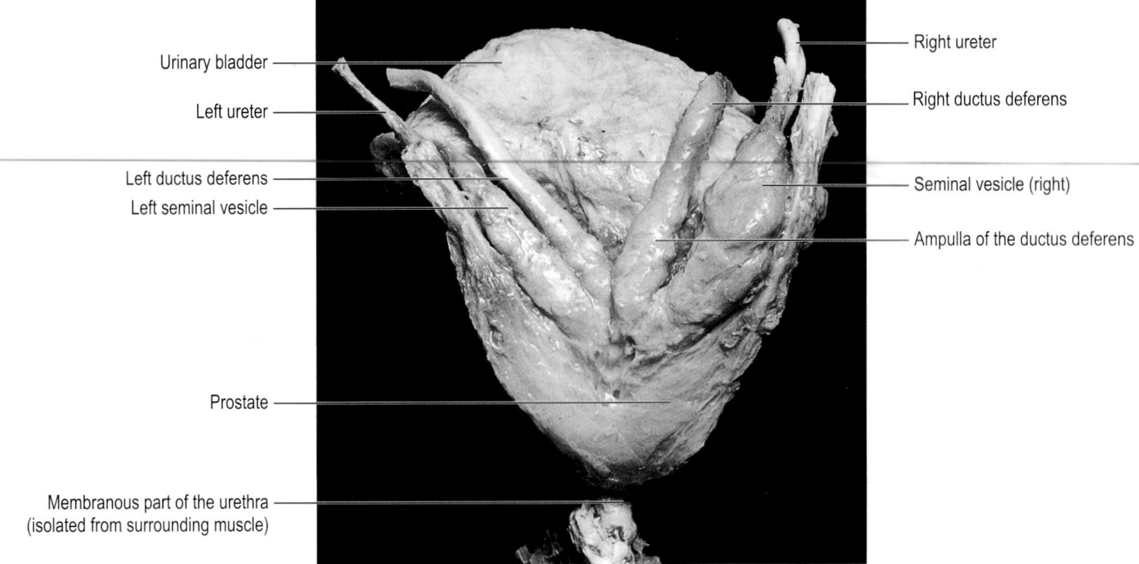


Fig. 4.92 Posterior aspect of the male urinary bladder and related urogenital organs.

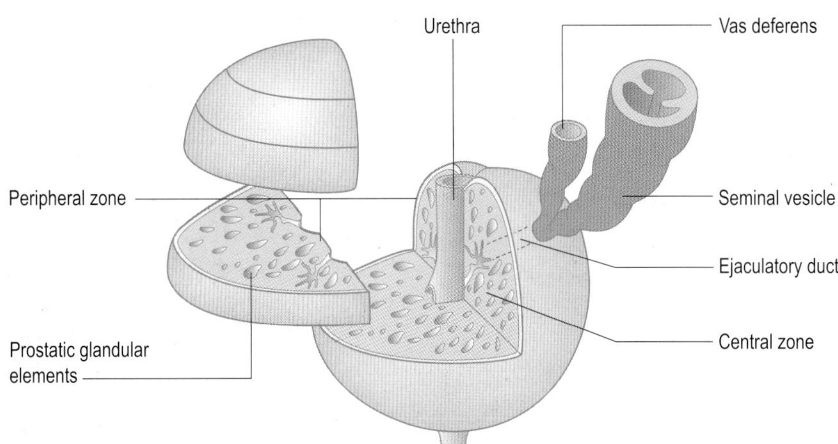


Fig. 4.93 The prostate and the ejaculatory duct.

## Male internal genital organs

The ductus deferens (vas deferens) which transports spermatozoa to the urethra starts at the inferior pole of the testis as a continuation of the epididymis. It passes through the inguinal canal and the deep inguinal ring before reaching the posterior surface of the bladder. The dilatation just before its termination is the ampulla of the vas deferens. The ductus terminates by joining the duct of the seminal vesicle to form the ejaculatory duct. The ejaculatory ducts open into the prostatic part of the urethra.

✪ The seminal vesicles secrete the bulk of the seminal fluid. Rarely the seminal vesicle may become infected and the tenderness may be felt during rectal examination. Normal seminal vesicles are not palpable per rectum.

### Prostate gland

The prostate (Figs 4.92, 4.93; see also Fig. 4.81) lies below the bladder. The urethra and the two ejaculatory ducts pass through the prostate. The ejaculatory ducts drain into the prostatic part of the urethra. The prostate has a base and an apex – the base, which is the upper surface, is fused with the bladder neck and the blunt apex projects downwards. ✪ The posterior surface of the prostate has a groove which is normally felt on rectal examination. When the prostate enlarges this groove disappears. Veins of the prostate drain into the prostatic venous plexus around the gland. This in turn is connected to the vertebral venous plexuses (Batson's veins). There are no valves in these connections. Malignant tumours of the prostate spread through these veins into the vertebral column.

The prostate contains fibromuscular tissues and glands which open into the urethra. The prostate has a central and a peripheral zone which respectively have approximately 25% and 75% of the glandular tissue each. The wedge-shaped central zone which forms the base of the gland contains small glands which are not coiled. The ducts of the central zone open at apex on the verumontanum (see prostatic urethra, p. 114). The peripheral zone forming the lower part of the gland surrounds the central zone but does not reach the upper part of the gland. Glands of the peripheral zone are long and tortuous and the ducts open into the prostatic sinuses. Prostatic secretion added to the seminal fluid is important for the survival of spermatozoa.

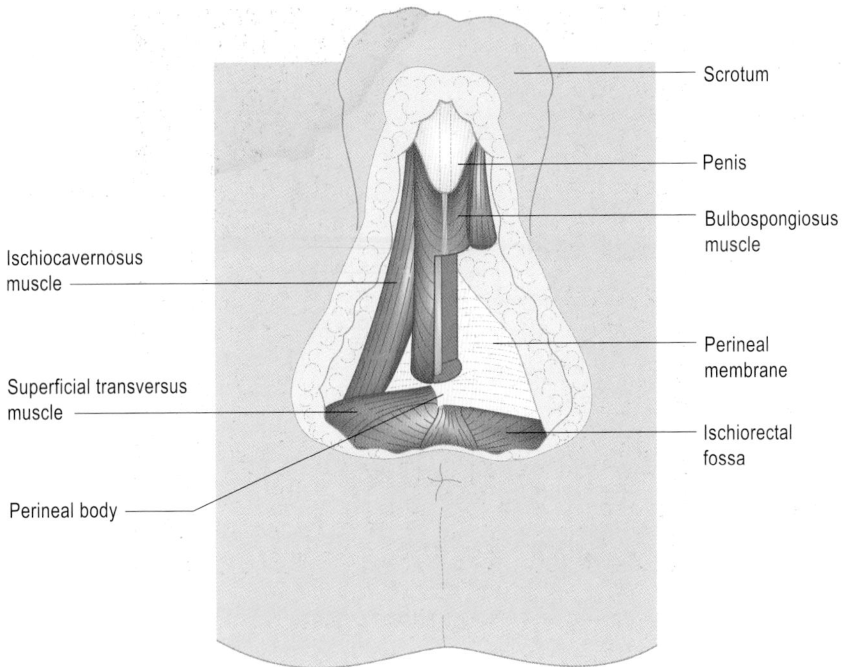


Fig. 4.94 The superficial perineal pouch muscles of the male perineum and the perineal membrane – inferior view. The superficial muscles and part of the penis have been removed on the left side of the perineum to show the perineal membrane (scrotum and the penis are lifted up).

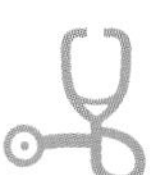

### *Clinical box 4.22*

**Surgical approach to prostate**

Operation for benign hyperplasia of the prostate is usually done by the transurethral route (transurethral resection of prostate or TURP) with a resectoscope. Resection is confined to the region above the verumontanum to avoid damage to the external urethral sphincter. This sphincter is important for maintaining urinary continence. The internal sphincter at the bladder neck may be damaged in this procedure. As the internal sphincter prevents retrograde ejaculation (see prostatic urethra pgs 114, 115) this function may suffer after the surgery. Total removal of the prostate can be done by a suprapubic approach or through the perineal route.

✪ Benign hyperplasia/hypertrophy of the prostate is extremely common in men above the age of 60. It is the central zone of the prostate which is usually affected by benign hypertrophy. The peripheral zone is almost exclusively the site of origin of carcinoma of the prostate. See Clinical box 4.22.

## Perineum

The space below the pelvic diaphragm is defined as the perineum (Figs 4.94–4.96). For descriptive purposes the perineum is divided by an imaginary line connecting the two ischial tuberosities into the anal triangle, which contains the anal canal and the two ischiorectal fossae, and the urogenital triangle, containing the urethra and the external genitalia.

### Urogenital triangle

This part of the perineum has the superficial and the deep perineal pouches separated by the perineal membrane, a

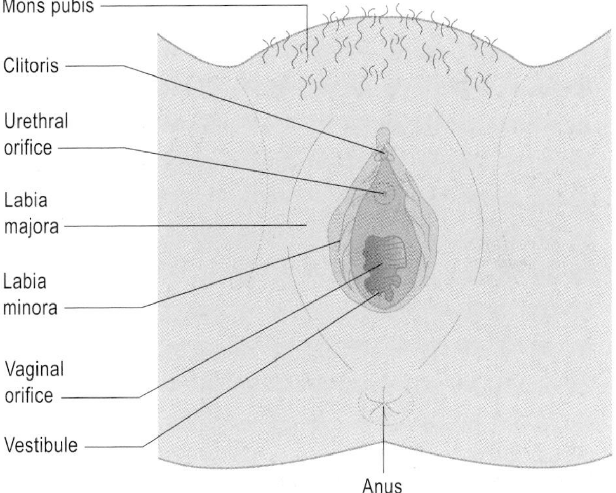


Fig. 4.95 Female perineum showing the external genitalia.

triangular sheet of fibrous tissue extending between the two ischiopubic rami.

### The superficial perineal pouch

This space is superficial to the perineal membrane and is bounded externally by the membranous layer of the superficial fascia (Colles' fascia) which is an extension of the fascia from the anterior abdominal wall into the perineum. The superficial perineal pouch hence is continuous with the space under the membranous layer of the superficial fascia in the anterior abdominal wall. Extension of Colles' fascia to the scrotum and the penis make them communicate with the superficial perineal pouch.

In the male, the superficial perineal pouch contains the erectile tissues contributing to the formation of the penis and the thin muscles covering them. The urethra passes through the corpus spongiosum of the penis (Figs 4.94, 4.97). ✪ If the urethra is ruptured urine and blood will accumulate in the superficial pouch and spread upwards

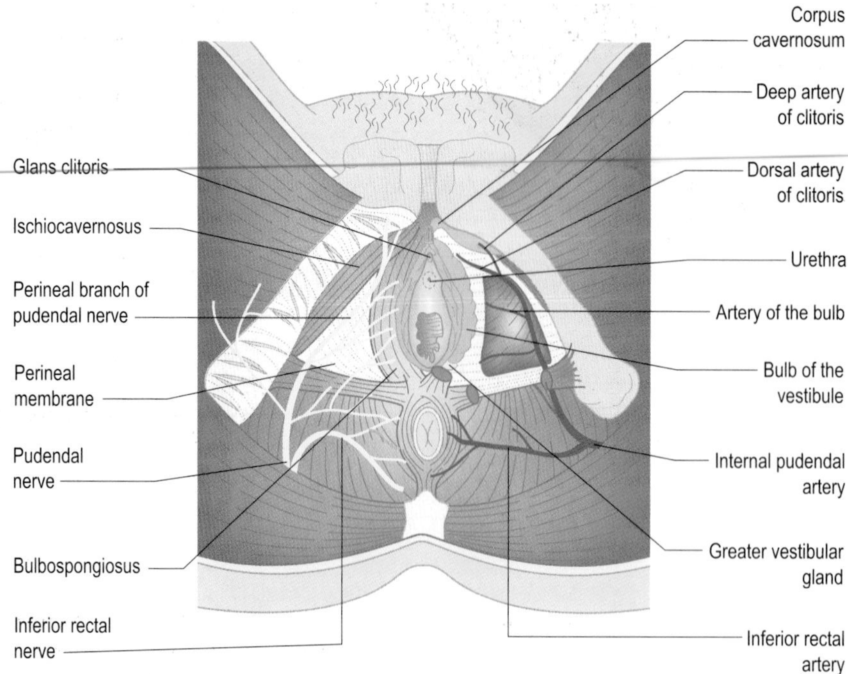


Fig. 4.96 Dissection of the female perineum. Arteries are shown on the left and nerves on the right. The superficial muscles have been removed on the left to show the bulb of the vestibule and the greater vestibular gland.

into the space extending up the anterior abdominal wall and also into the scrotum and penis.

In the female, as in the male, the superficial perineal pouch contains the erectile tissues. These are the two crura forming the clitoris and a paired structure on either side of the vestibule, the bulb of the vestibule. These erectile tissues also (as those in the male) are covered by thin muscles.

The perineum is supplied by the internal pudendal artery and the pudendal nerve. These leave the pelvis through the greater sciatic foramen and enter the perineum through the lesser sciatic foramen. The anterior part of the skin is supplied by the ilioinguinal nerve.

### The deep perineal pouch

This space deep to the perineal membrane contains the deep transversus perineii muscle. The middle part of the muscle surrounds the urethra, forming the external sphincter of the male urethra, and exerts a prolonged tone on the urethra to keep it closed (see page 115). This part of the urethra is called the membranous part of the urethra. In the female, the deep transversus perineii muscle is pierced by the urethra and the vagina. The external sphincter is similar in structure to that in the male but it extends through the whole length of the urethra.

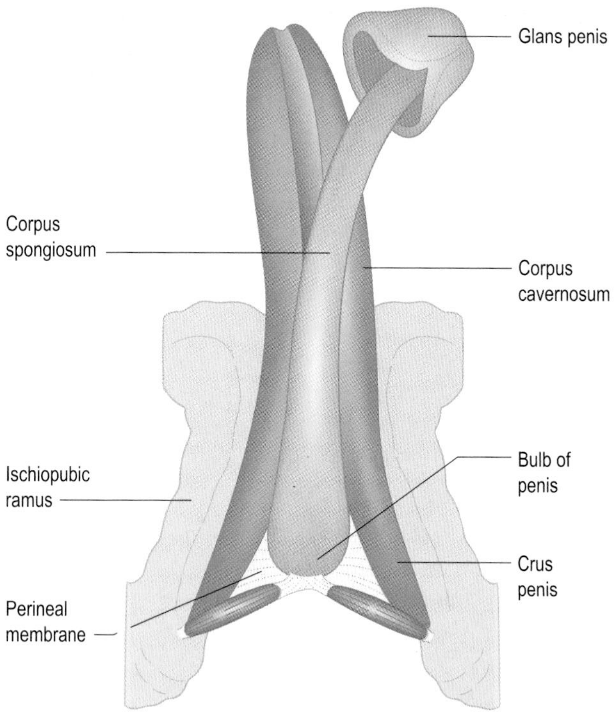


Fig. 4.97 Roots of the penis in the superficial perineal pouch.

## The penis

See Figures 4.97 and 4.98. The attached parts of the penis known as the roots of the penis consist of a crus on either side and the bulb in the midline, the former attached to the ischiopubic ramus and the perineal membrane and the latter to the perineal membrane. The crus continues forward as the corpus cavernosum and the bulb as the corpus spongiosum. The two corpora cavernosa are bound together on the dorsal aspect of the corpus spongiosum, all three contributing to the body or shaft of the penis. The corpus spongiosum extends beyond the anterior end of the corpora cavernosa and expands to become the glans penis. The penile urethra enters the bulb and traverses the whole length of corpus spongiosum to open at the external urethral meatus at the end of the glans penis. The skin of the penis is hairless and at the tip it folds on itself over the glans penis as the prepuce. The prepuce is attached to the neck of the glans. The frenulum, an extension of the skin

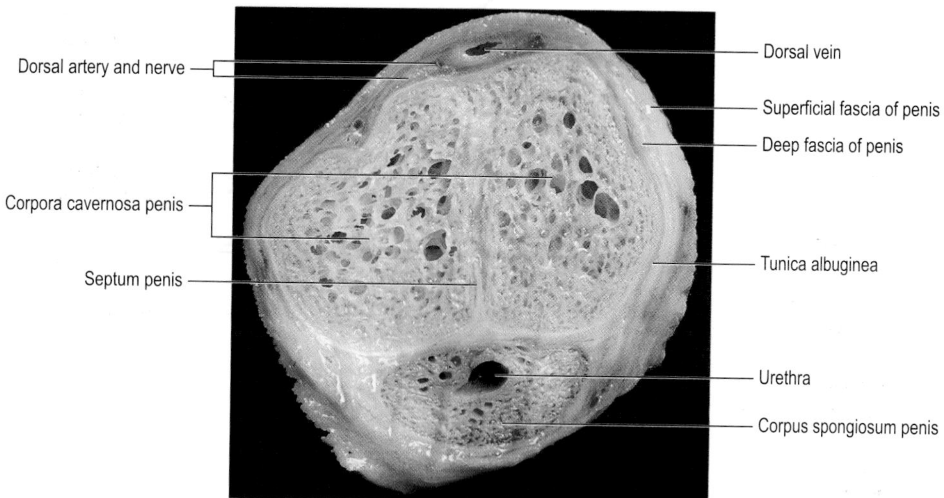


Fig. 4.98 Transverse section of penis.

from the prepuce to the undersurface of the glans, extends to the urethral orifice.

## Blood supply

Three pairs of arteries, all branches of the internal pudendal artery, supply the penis. The artery to the bulb supplies the bulb, the corpus spongiosum and the glans. The deep artery of the penis supplies the corpus cavernosum. The dorsal artery of the penis supplies the skin, fascia and glans and anastomoses with the artery to the bulb. The venous drainage is partially through veins accompanying the arteries into the internal pudendal vein but mostly through the deep dorsal vein of the penis which pierces the suspensory ligament (connection of deep fascia to the pubic symphysis), and, passing in the gap between the pubic symphysis and the perineal membrane, enters the pelvis to join the vesicovenous plexus. The dorsal skin is drained by the superficial dorsal vein which joins the superficial external pudendal vein, a tributary of the long saphenous vein.

## Nerve supply

The skin of the penis is supplied by the scrotal nerves and the dorsal nerves of the penis, all branches from the pudendal nerve. The dermatome involved mainly is S2, with a small area of supply of the proximal part by L1 via the ilioinguinal nerve. ✪ The increased blood flow essential for erection is facilitated by parasympathetic stimulation whereas ejaculation is initiated by sympathetic stimulation (many students remember this as 'Point' and 'Shoot'!).

# Chapter 5
# Vertebral column and the spinal cord



## Vertebral column

The vertebral column consists of: seven cervical vertebrae, twelve thoracic, five lumbar, the sacrum consisting of five fused vertebrae and the coccyx formed by the fusion of four or more rudimentary vertebrae (Fig. 5.1).

The vertebral column transmits the body weight on to the lower limbs through the sacroiliac joints. The spinal cord and its coverings and the spinal nerves are contained inside the vertebral canal.

### Curvatures

The thoracic and sacral part of the vertebral column is concave forward whereas it is convex forward (lordotic) in the cervical and lumbar regions (Fig. 5.1). The sinusoidal shape of the vertebral column is developed after birth. In the fetus the vertebral column is 'C'-shaped with the concavity facing anteriorly. After birth secondary curvatures with convexity develop in the cervical region when the child holds up its head and also in the lumbar region when the legs start weight bearing.

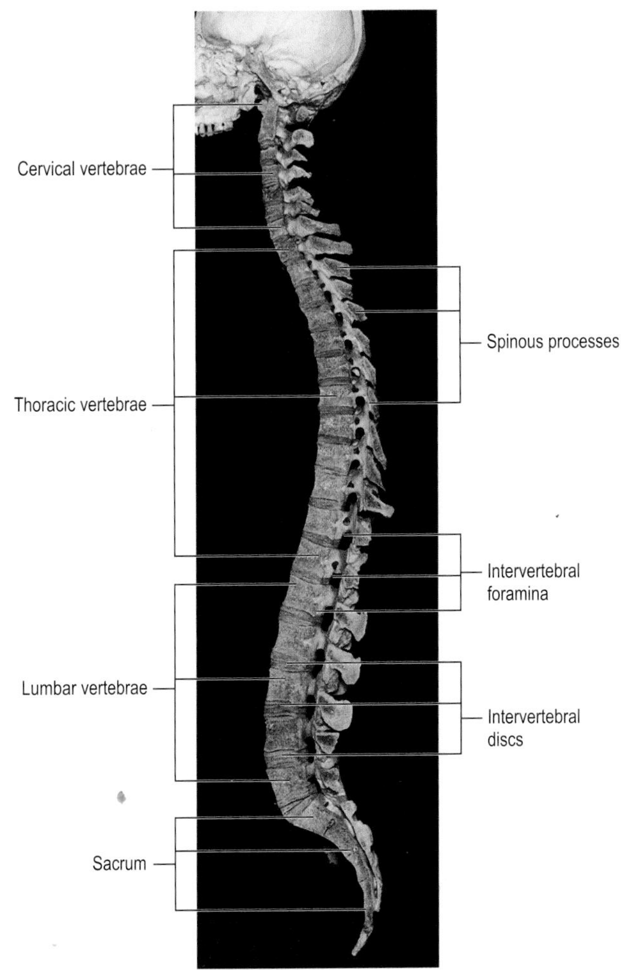


Fig. 5.1 Sagittal section of the vertebral column viewed from the side.

## Individual vertebrae

Each individual vertebra (Figs 5.1–5.4) consists of a body and a neural arch surrounding the vertebral foramen. The neural arch consists of a pedicle and a lamina on either side. The two laminae fuse to form the spinous process. The arch also has two transverse processes and a pair of superior and inferior articular processes for articulation with the adjacent vertebrae.

The cervical vertebrae can be distinguished from lumbar and thoracic vertebrae as they have small bodies, small and bifid spines (except C7) and the foramen transversarium in their transverse processes. The atlas (C1) has no body but has two lateral masses connected by the anterior and posterior arches (Fig. 5.4). The atlas articulates above with the occipital bone and below with the axis (C2). Nodding and lateral flexion movements take place at the atlanto-occipital joints. Projecting upwards from the body of axis is the odontoid process (dens) which articulates with the anterior arch of the atlas. Rotation of the head occurs in the atlantoaxial joints. An individual thoracic vertebra can be identified by noting the presence of articular facets on the body and on transverse processes (except T11 and T12). Lumbar vertebrae are massive to withstand body weight. The lumbar vertebrae and the intervening discs contribute 25% of the total length of the column.

### Surface anatomy

✪ The uppermost spinous process which is palpable is that of the seventh cervical vertebra, known as the vertebra prominence as it has a long and non-bifid spine. The highest point of the iliac crest is in line with the interval between L3 and L4 spines. See Clinical box 5.1.

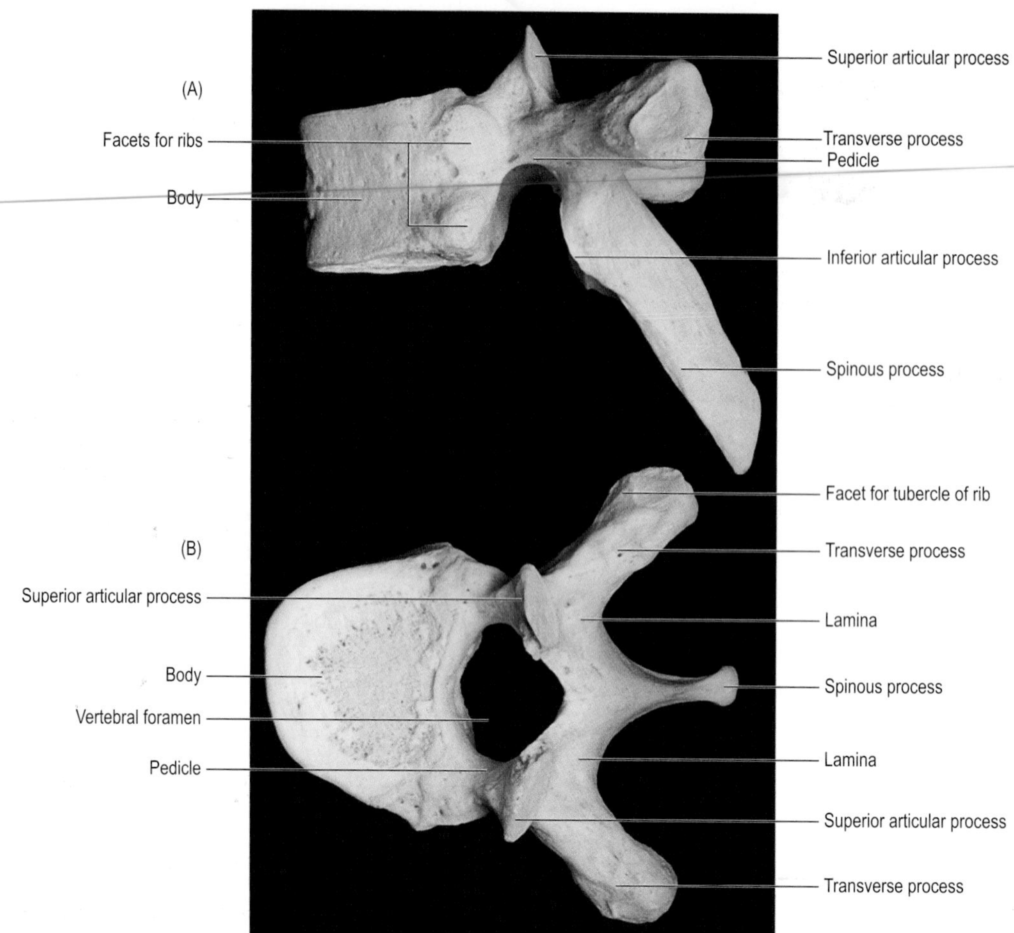


Fig. 5.2 Thoracic vertebra: (A) lateral view, (B) superior view.

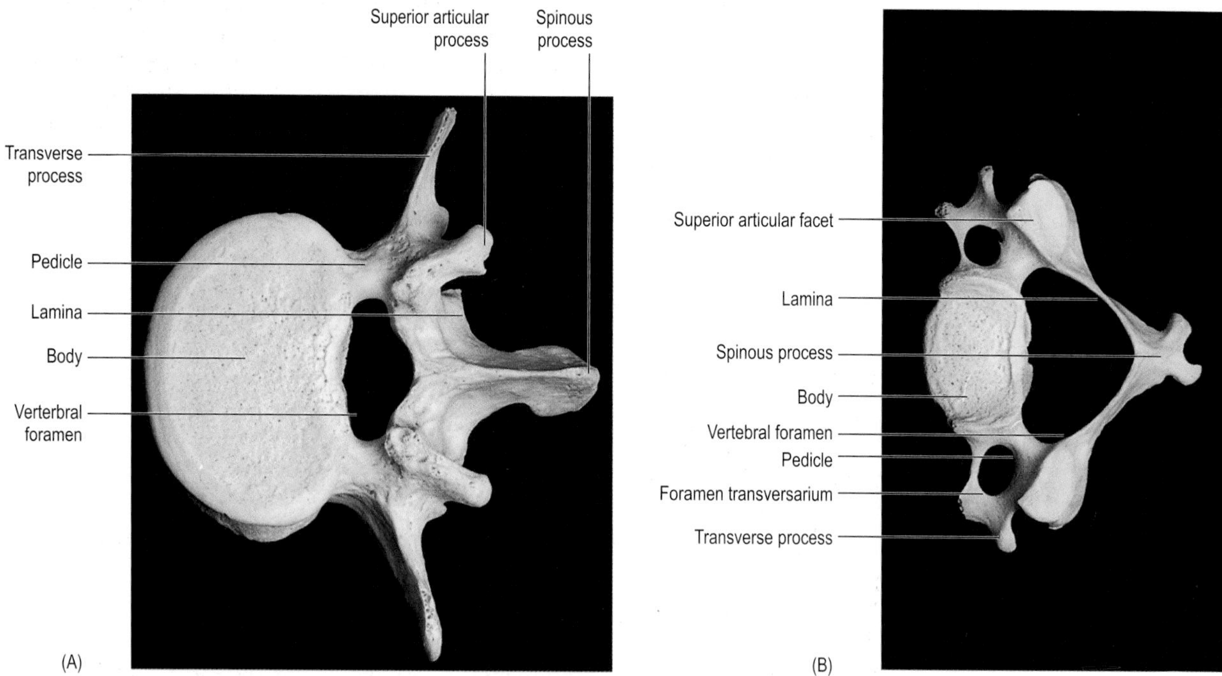


Fig. 5.3 Superior views: (A) lumbar vertebra, (B) cervical vertebra.

## Joints between the vertebrae

The bodies of the adjoining vertebrae are joined by the intervertebral disc whereas the facet joints (zygopophyseal joints), which are synovial joints, link the articular processes (Figs 5.5–5.7). The major longitudinal ligaments connecting the vertebrae are the anterior and posterior ligaments connecting the bodies of the vertebrae, ligamentum flavum in between the adjacent laminae, and supraspinous and interspinous ligaments connecting the spines. These joints

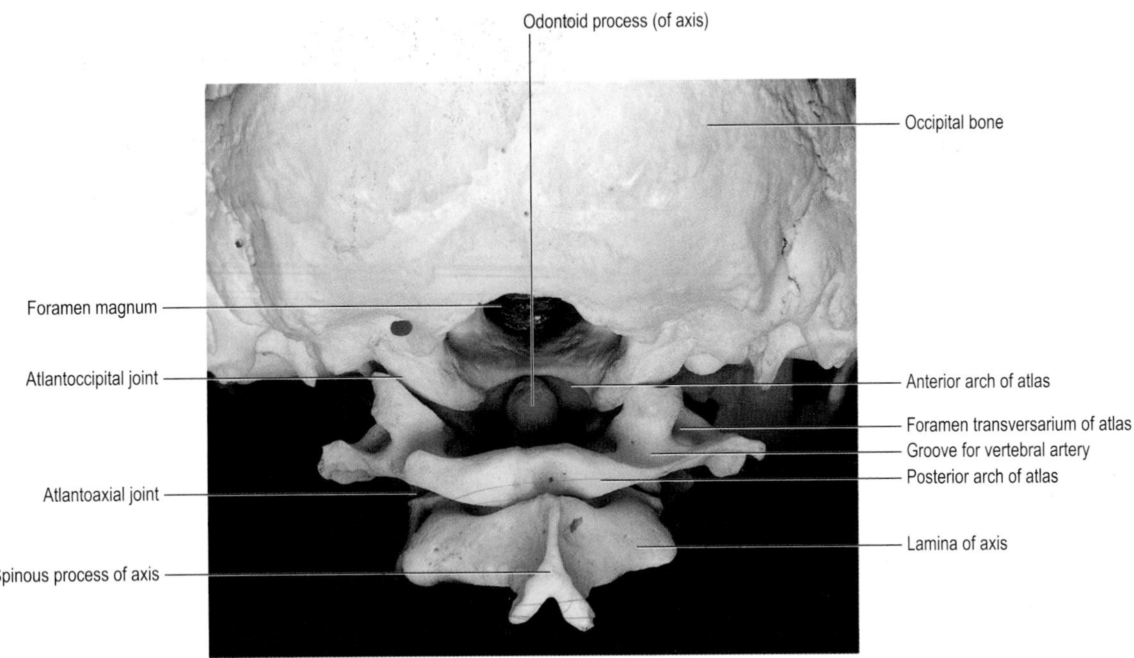


Fig. 5.4 Atlas, axis and the occipital bone – viewed from behind.

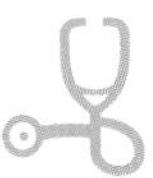

## *Clinical box 5.1*

### Injuries to the vertebrae and vertebral column

Individual vertebra can be fractured, often by a compression force on the vertebral column as occurs by falling from a height or by a weight landing on the shoulder. The T12, L1 and L2 are commonly affected. If this occurs with a force in the anteroposterior direction the fractured vertebra may dislocate. A displaced fracture can injure the spinal cord. As the articular surfaces of the facet joints in the cervical region are nearly horizontal the cervical vertebrae can dislocate without fracture. This can happen in a motor car accident where this part of the column suddenly jerks forward with tremendous force.

A whiplash injury of the neck can occur due to a rear-end collision of a motor vehicle. In this the upper cervical vertebrae and the head flex forward and then recoil backwards forcefully causing a hyperextension injury. Flexion of the head is limited by the chin hitting the chest. But extension has no anatomical limitation. Ligaments, facets joints and nerve roots can be damaged causing neck pain, paraesthesia (pins and needles) in the upper limbs and other neurological signs and symptoms.

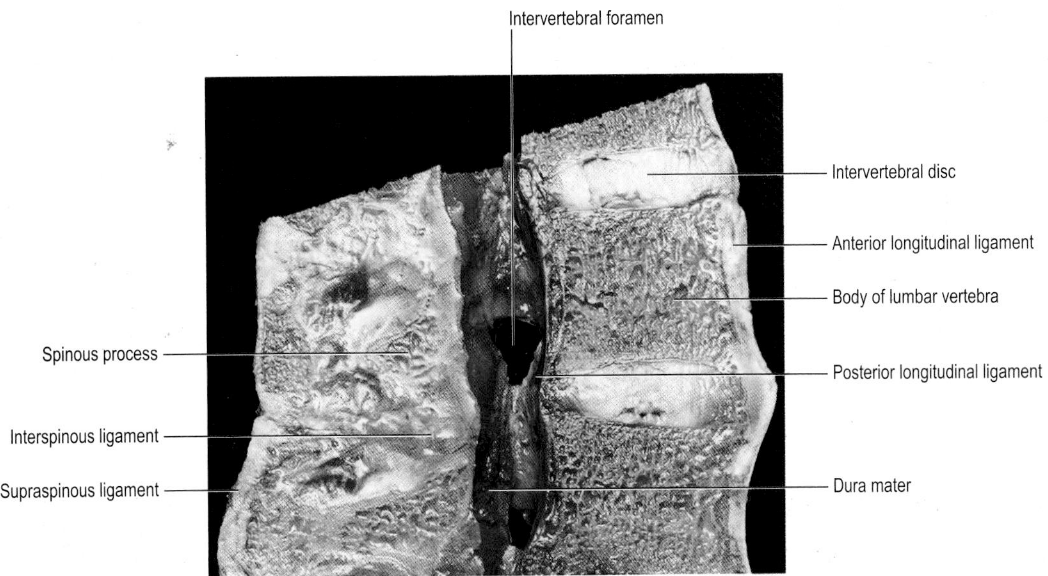


Fig. 5.5 Sagittal section through lumbar vertebrae – lateral view.

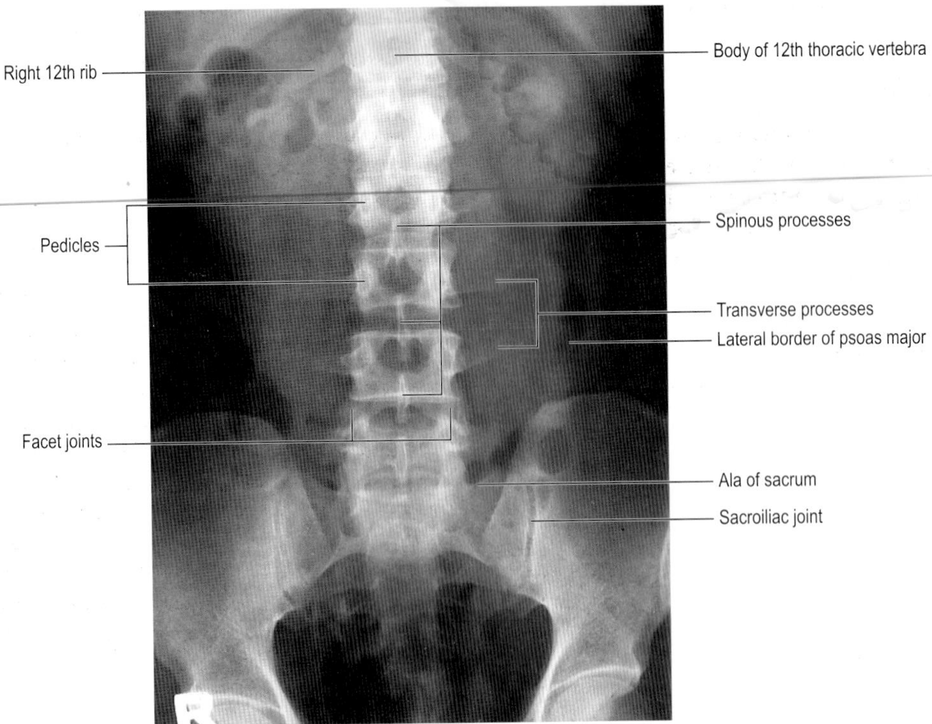


Fig. 5.6 Anteroposterior radiograph of the lumbar spine and the sacroiliac joint.

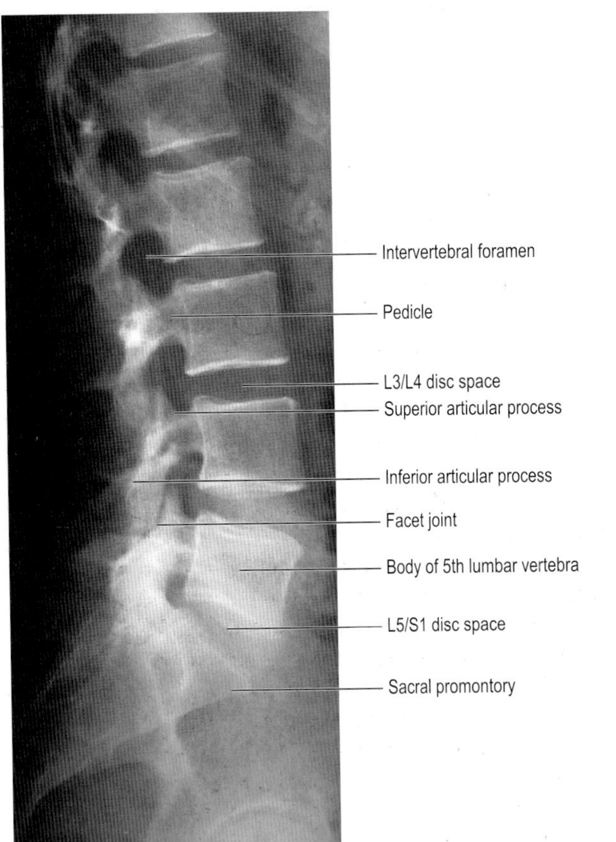


Fig. 5.7 Lateral view of the lumbar spine.

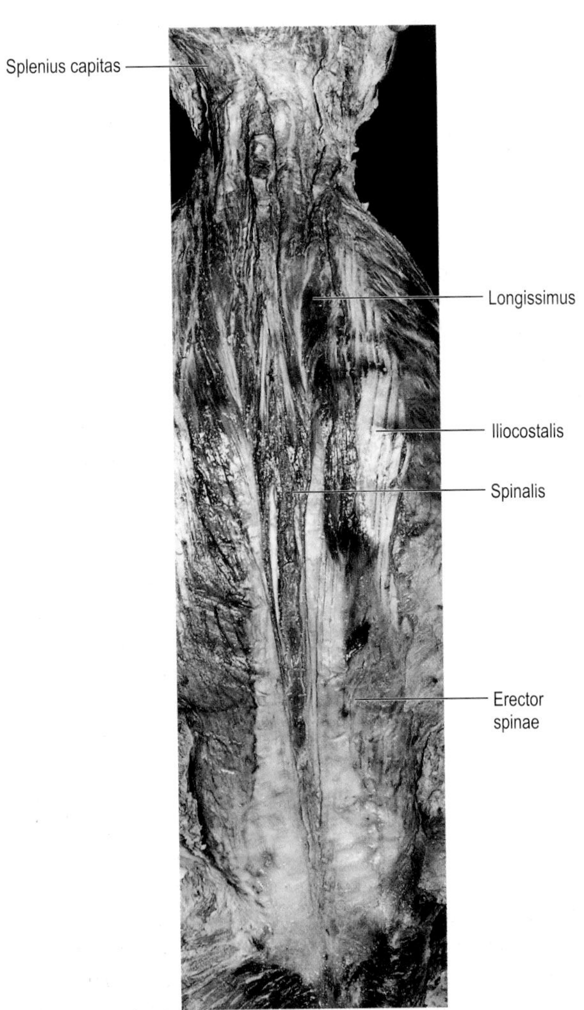


Fig. 5.8 Deep muscles of the back. Erector spinae and its three parts (spinalis, longissimus and iliocostalis) exposed after removal of superficial muscles of the back.

and ligaments, as well as the muscles of the back (Fig. 5.8), stabilise the vertebral column.

### The intervertebral foramen

The intervertebral foramina which transmit the spinal nerves and the accompanying radicular arteries (which

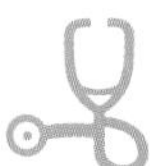

*Clinical box 5.2*

**Back pain**

Low back pain is a very common cause of chronic disability in the western world. One in five individuals in the 30–60 age group suffers from back pain. Though the causes of backache are many, in the majority of cases it is associated with some abnormality of the intervertebral discs at the L4/L5 and L5/S1 levels.

As one gets older the intervertebral disc gradually dries out. The water-holding capacity of the nucleus pulposus decreases, and what was once a thick turgid gel now thins out to become a desiccated, brittle structure. The annulus fibrosus develops fissures mostly in its posterior aspect. Internal derangement of the disc without herniation causes back pain as the periphery of the annulus fibrosus and the posterior longitudinal ligament are innervated by pain fibres.

Disc herniation into the vertebral body causes reactive bone formation, producing osteophytes. Flattening of the disc and abnormal bone formation in the vertebral margin are characteristic features of the condition known as spondylosis. As a result of narrowing of the disc space, caused by the thinning of the disc, the facet joints get slightly displaced causing osteoarthritis of the joints. Osteoarthritis of the joints and the osteophytes on the vertebrae narrow the intervertebral foramen causing nerve compression and pain.

An acute disc herniation or prolapse is less common. Compression of the disc by lifting a weight in the flexed position of the spine is often the precipitating cause. It often happens at the L4/L5 or L5/S1 level. It almost always happens in individuals in whom the hydrophilic nature of the disc is already disturbed. When the nucleus pulposus loses its water-holding capacity and degenerates it can bulge through and even break through the annulus to produce nerve compression. As the nucleus is situated more towards the posterior aspect of the disc it herniates posterolaterally into the intervertebral foramen causing nerve compression. A straight posterior herniation is often prevented by the firm attachment of the disc to the posterior longitudinal ligament. More commonly herniation happens in the lumbar part of the vertebral column and can cause back pain or pain radiating to the leg (sciatica) by compression of the nerve roots. When a particular disc herniates it usually affects the nerve below, i.e. when the disc between L4 and L5 herniates, the L5 nerve root is affected and the L4 nerve, being above the disc, escapes injury.

supply the spinal cord) are on the lateral aspect of the vertebral column. Each foramen lying between the pedicles of the adjoining vertebrae is bounded anteriorly by the vertebral bodies and the disc and posteriorly by the facet joints (Fig. 5.7). In the lumbar region, where nerve root compression is more common, the nerves increase in size from above downwards whereas the intervertebral foramen diminishes in size. Discs losing height over the years narrow the foramen.

✪ Herniation of the disc, arthritis of the facet joints as well as bony irregularities in the pedicle or vertebral body can narrow the intervertebral foramen and cause nerve root compression.

### The intervertebral disc

The intervertebral discs are fibrocartilagenous structures which are strong to withstand compression forces but are also flexible to allow movements between the vertebrae. Each disc has two parts, a nucleus pulposus surrounded by annulus fibrosus. The former is a well-hydrated gel having proteoglycan, collagen and cartilage cells. The annulus fibrosus is made of 10–12 concentric layers of collagen whose obliquity alters in successive layers. Peripherally the annulus fibrosus is attached to the vertebral bodies as well as to the posterior longitudinal ligament. The annulus resists the expansion of the nucleus pulposus. The fluid content of the intervertebral discs is determined by the proteoglycans (e.g. GAGs), which are highly hydrophilic molecules. Diurnal fluctuations in fluid content occur as the loading, placed on the spine by gravity, forces some of the fluid from the discs. During sleep, when pressure on the spine is reduced, water is drawn back into the discs. Such cycles help to provide the cartilagenous tissue with nutrients, which naturally has a poor vascular supply.

The forces placed upon the intervertebral discs at any one time can be quite substantial. Posture and different activities cause various pressure changes within the discs. Pressure while standing is substantially more compared to that while lying supine. Lifting a weight, especially in the flexed position of the spine, increases the pressure. If these are combined with a twisting action then internal forces will increase further.

✪ Movements of the vertebral column are forward flexion (40°), extension (15°), lateral flexion (30°) and rotation (40°). Rotation is maximum at the thoracic region whereas it is very limited in the lumbar spine. Flexion and extension on the other hand is limited in the thoracic region due to the presence of the rib cage. Movements are based on orientation of articular surfaces of the facet joints. In the thoracic region the surfaces are almost in the coronal plane whereas in the lumbar region they are in the sagittal plane. In the cervical they are more horizontal making them more prone to dislocation (see Clinical box 5.1).

As there are eight cervical nerves and only seven cervical vertebrae the spinal nerves emerge through the intervertebral foramen in the following order. C1–C7 spinal nerves exit above their corresponding vertebrae. C8 nerve passes through the foramen between C7 and T1 vertebrae. All subsequent nerves emerge below their corresponding vertebrae. Thus the intervertebral foramen between L4 and L5 vertebrae transmits the L4 spinal nerve. See Clinical box 5.2.

## The sacroiliac joint

The sacroiliac joint is a synovial joint through which the body weight is transmitted from the sacrum to the hip bone.

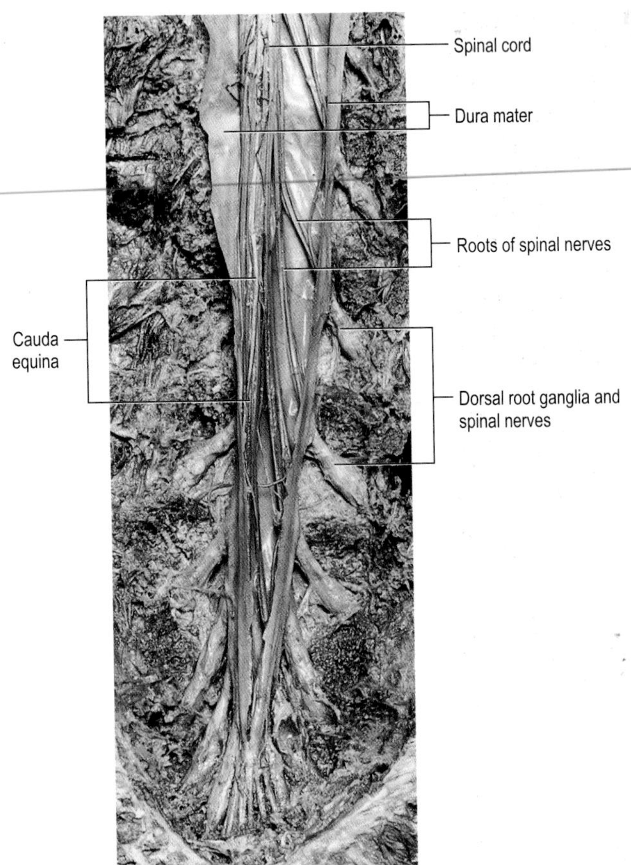


Fig. 5.9 Vertebral canal and the sacral canal opened up from the back to show the cauda equina.

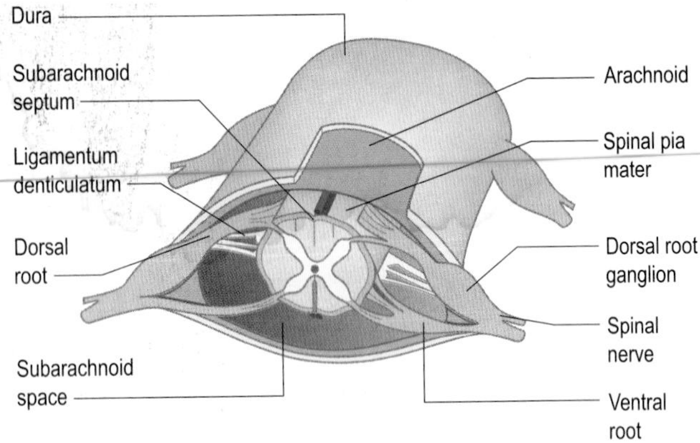


Fig. 5.10 Spinal cord and meninges.

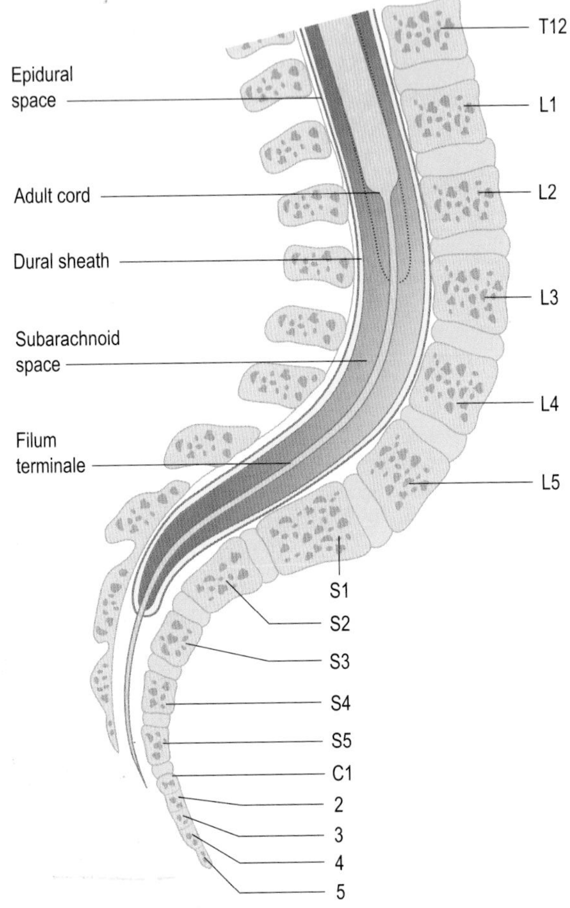


Fig. 5.11 The termination of the spinal cord in the adult, showing its variation. This also shows the termination of the dural sheath.

The articular surface of the sacrum and the corresponding surface on the ilium are irregular and they fit together closely. ✪ The reciprocal irregularities of the joint surfaces and the strong ligaments of the joint make this a stable joint. However strain and arthritis of the joint causes back pain as one gets older.

## Spinal cord and meninges

The spinal cord (Figs 5.9–5.13) extends from the lower end of the medulla oblongata at the level of the foramen magnum to the lower border of the first or the upper border of the second lumbar vertebra. The lower part of the cord is tapered to form the conus medullaris from which a prolongation of pia mater, the filum terminale, extends downwards to be attached to the coccyx. In the third month of intrauterine life, the spinal cord fills the whole length of the vertebral canal but from then on the vertebral column grows more rapidly than the cord. At birth the cord extends as far as the third lumbar vertebra and eventually reaches its adult level gradually.

The three layers of the meninges envelop the spinal cord. The dura mater which is continuous with that of the brain extends up to the second sacral vertebra. The arachnoid mater lines the inner surface of the dura and pia mater is adherent to the surface of the cord. The subarachnoid space with the cerebrospinal fluid extends up to the level of the second sacral vertebra. The epidural space (Figs 5.12, 5.13) outside the dura contains fat and the components of the vertebral venous plexus.

The spinal cord is suspended in the dural sheath by the denticulate ligaments. This ligament, which has a serrated lateral edge, forms a shelf between the dorsal and ventral roots of the spinal nerves.

The cord has on its surface a deep anterior median fissure and a shallower posterior median sulcus. It also has, on either side, a posterolateral sulcus along which the dorsal roots of the spinal nerves are attached.

The area of the spinal cord from which a pair of spinal nerves are given off is defined as a spinal cord segment. The cord has 31 pairs of spinal nerves and hence 31 segments – eight cervical, twelve thoracic, five lumbar, five sacral and one coccygeal.

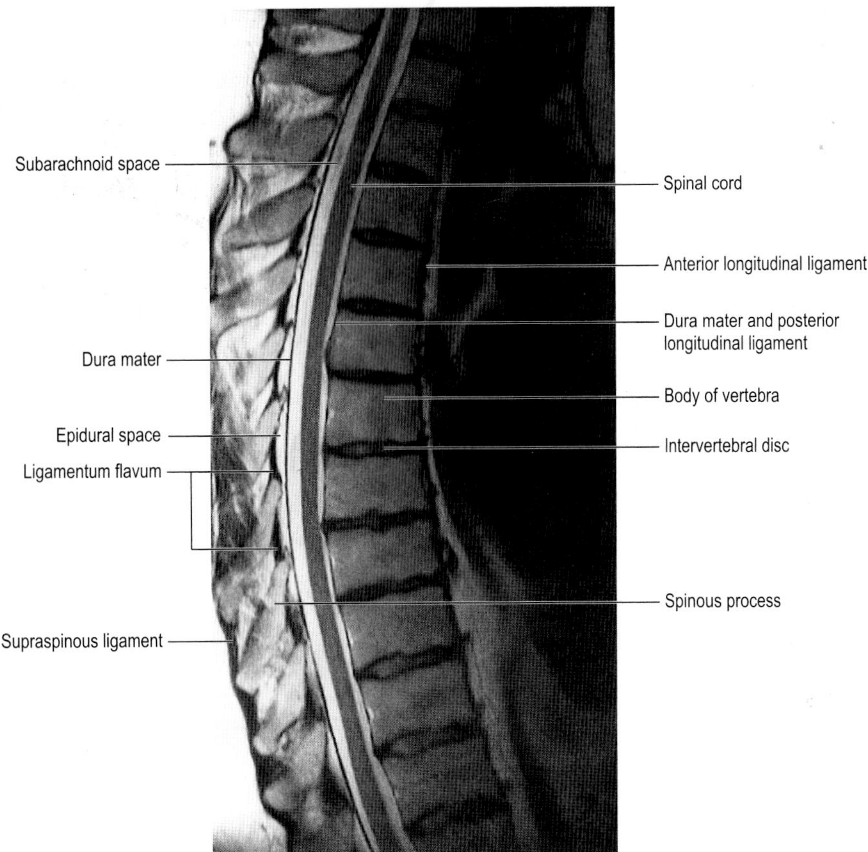


Fig. 5.12 Sagittal MRI scan of the thoracic spine.

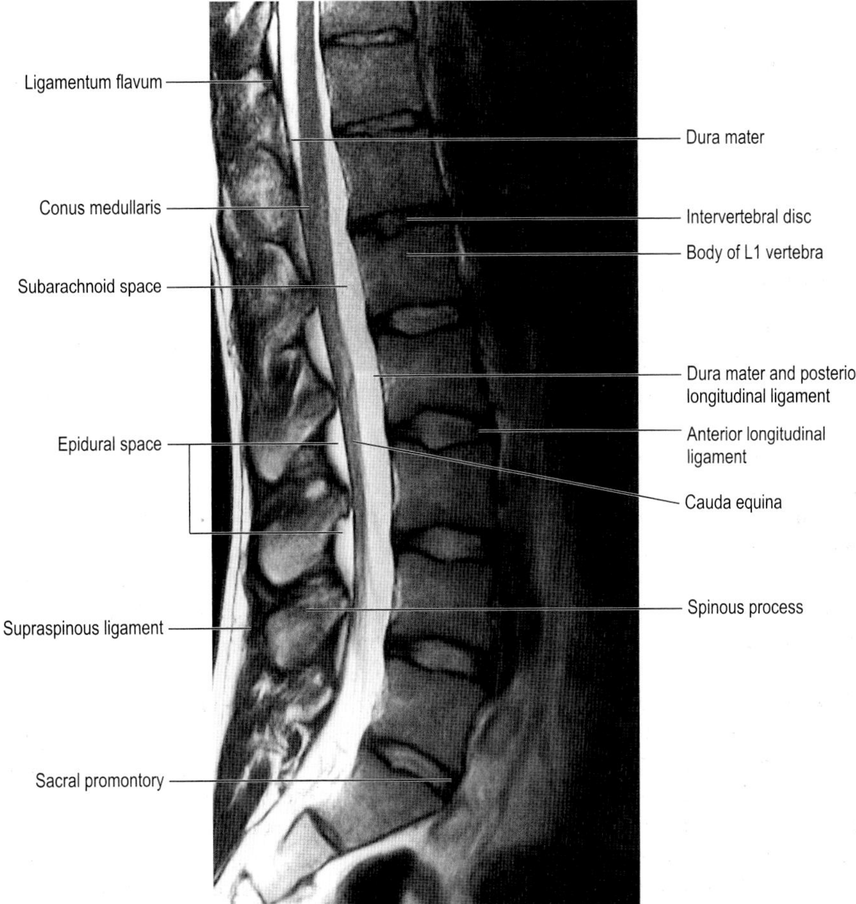


Fig. 5.13 Sagittal MRI scan of the lumbar spine.

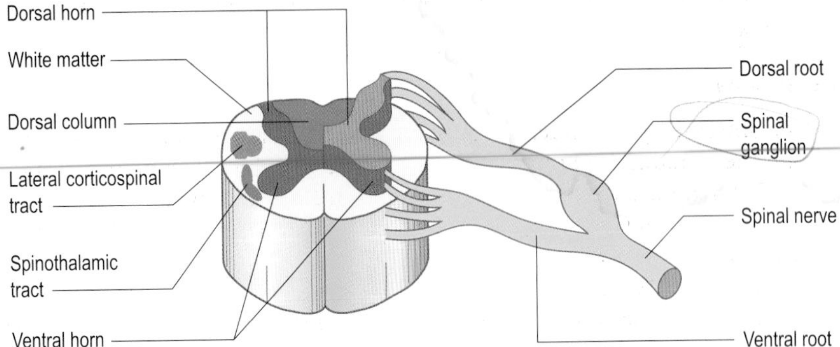


Fig 5.14 Structure of the spinal cord.

The dorsal root of the spinal nerve which carries sensory fibres has a dorsal root ganglion (spinal ganglion) which has the cells of origin of the dorsal root fibres. The ventral (anterior) root, which is motor, emerges on the anterolateral aspect of the cord on either side. The anterior and posterior roots join together at the intervertebral foramen to form the spinal nerve, which on emerging from the foramen divides immediately into the anterior and posterior rami, each containing both motor and sensory fibres. The length of the nerve roots increases progressively from above downwards. The lumbar and sacral nerve roots below the termination of the cord form the cauda equina.

### Blood supply of the spinal cord

The blood supply of the spinal cord is derived from the anterior and posterior spinal arteries. The anterior spinal artery is a midline vessel lying in the anterior median fissure and is formed by the union of a branch from each vertebral artery. It supplies the whole of the cord in front of the posterior grey column. The posterior spinal arteries, usually one on either side posteriorly, are branches of the posterior inferior cerebellar arteries or arise directly from the vertebral arteries. They supply the posterior grey columns and the dorsal columns on either side.

✪ The spinal arteries are reinforced at segmental levels by radicular arteries from the vertebral, ascending cervical, posterior intercostal, lumbar and sacral arteries. The radicular arteries enter the vertebral canal through the intervertebral foramina accompanying the spinal nerves and their ventral and dorsal roots. These arteries may be compromised in resection of segments of the aorta in surgery of aneurysms. (Also see p. 67).

### Internal structure of the spinal cord

The grey matter containing the sensory and motor nerve cells are surrounded by the white matter with the ascending and descending tracts. In a transverse section the grey matter is seen as an 'H'-shaped area containing in its middle the central canal. The central canal is continuous above with the fourth ventricle. The posterior (dorsal) horn of the grey matter has the termination of the sensory fibres of the posterior (dorsal) root. The larger anterior (ventral) horn contains motor cells which give rise to fibres of the anterior (ventral) roots. In the thoracic and upper lumbar regions there are lateral horns which have the cells of origin of the preganglionic sympathetic fibres.

The white matter is divided into the dorsal, lateral, and ventral columns, each containing a number of ascending and descending fibre tracts. The dorsal column (Fig. 5.14) contains fibres subserving fine and discriminative tactile sensation as well as proprioception. A major tract in the lateral column is the lateral corticospinal tract. The corticospinal tracts control skilled voluntary movements and motor power and consist of axons of neuron in the frontal and parietal lobes of the contralateral cerebral hemisphere. They form synaptic connections with motor neurons in the spinal cord. The spinothalamic tracts, which

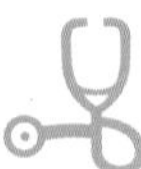

*Clinical box 5.3*

**Spinal cord injuries**

Over 80% of spinal cord injuries result from road traffic accidents. A complete section of the cord causes loss of movements and sensation distal to the level of lesion.

In an incomplete injury, some function may be present below the site of lesion. In the anterior cord syndrome caused by damage to the anterior half of the cord, the spinothalamic tracts (pain and temperature) and the corticospinal tract (motor control and power) are damaged sparing the posterior column (proprioception). There is loss of power and reduction in pain and temperature sensation below the level of the lesion. Touch and proprioception are not affected as the dorsal column remains intact. The injury can occur due to fracture and dislocation of the vertebral body damaging the anterior part of the cord. Bone fragments can directly injure the spinal cord. The trauma can also injure the anterior spinal artery resulting in ischaemia of the anterior part of the cord. A posterior cord syndrome, commonly seen in hyperextension injuries fracturing the posterior elements of the vertebrae, affects proprioception below the level of the lesion. Patients have good motor power and sensation for pain and temperature below the level of the lesion. They have an unsteady gait (ataxia) due to loss of proprioception. A hemisection of the cord (Brown–Sequard syndrome) can occur due to a penetrating injury. This results in loss of motor power and proprioception on the affected side below the lesion. As the spinothalamic tract perceives pain and temperature sensation from the opposite side of the body these sensations are preserved on the affected side but are lost on the opposite side. The uninjured side, unlike the injured side, has good motor power but loss of sensation to pin prick and temperature.

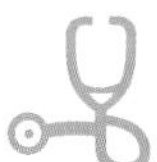

## *Clinical box 5.4*

### Epidural anaesthesia

Regional anaesthesia can be obtained by introducing local anaesthetic agents into the extradural space. It blocks the nerve roots outside the dura causing analgesia. The patient can breathe spontaneously if the block does not extend above the midthoracic level. The procedure is done by introducing a large needle (16–18G) into an interspinous space, usually at the L3/L4 level, after infiltrating the tissues with a local anaesthetic agent. The patient can be in the sitting position or in the lateral position (lying on one side). As it proceeds inwards the needle encounters skin, subcutaneous tissue, supraspinous ligament and interspinous ligament before reaching the epidural space. Loss of resistance (caused by the ligaments) will be an indication that the needle is in the epidural space. As there are blood vessels in the epidural space it is prudent to aspirate before injecting. Blood on aspiration will require another attempt a space above. The anaesthetic agents used are usually 1% lidocaine and 0.25–0.5% bupivacaine. The anaesthesia lasts for 1–2 hours. Addition of adrenaline can prolong the duration to 6–7 hours. Introduction of a plastic catheter through the needle into the epidural space allows repeated injections, especially when the length or extent of surgery is uncertain.

The procedure is commonly used for pain relief during childbirth. Blocking up to T12 or T11 levels relieves pain from the birth canal (see Clinical box 4.19, p. 119). If Caesarean section has to be done the level should be raised to T6 to anaesthetise the anterior abdominal wall and the parietal peritoneum.

If the anaesthetic solution is introduced into the subarachnoid space it is known as spinal anaesthesia or subarachnoid or intradural block. The needle used for this is thinner (22–26G) than that for epidural. The volume of anaesthetic agent used also will be smaller.

Spinal anaesthesia can cause postoperative headache. Both spinal and epidural anaesthesia can cause hypotension. Hence they should not be done without having an indwelling intravenous drip in place.

lie more towards the anterior part of the cord, conduct pain and temperature sensation from the opposite side of the body. See Clinical box 5.3.

✪ The epidural space is the interval between the vertebrae and the dura mater of the spinal cord (Figs 5.12, 5.13). It contains the small arteries which supply the spinal cord and the vertebral venous plexuses. Veins in these plexuses (Bateson's veins) contain no valves.

Metastases from malignant tumours in the breast and the prostate can reach the vertebrae through the vertebral venous plexuses which are connected to the veins draining these organs. ✪ Introduction of analgesic solutions into the epidural space in the lumbar region (epidural anaesthesia) is commonly performed to relieve pain during childbirth. See Clinical box 5.4.

✪ A sample of cerebrospinal fluid can be obtained by doing a lumbar puncture. This is done by introducing a trochar and cannula into the subarachnoid space between the spinous processes of L3 and L4, which is at the level of the highest point of the iliac crest. As the spinal cord terminates higher up this procedure will not damage the cord.

# Chapter 6
# Lower limb



## Introduction

The general plan of the lower limb (Figs 6.1–6.3) is similar to that of the upper limb. It consists of the thigh, leg and foot which correspond to the arm, forearm and hand of the upper extremity. The gluteal region or the buttock lies behind the pelvis and hip above the back of the thigh. The boundary between the anterior abdominal wall and the thigh is the inguinal ligament, which extends between the anterior superior iliac spine and the pubic tubercle. The femoral artery pulsation can be felt at the midinguinal point on palpation against the head of the femur. The structures in the thigh are arranged in three compartments – anterior or extensor, medial or adductor and posterior or flexor. The anterior or ventral position of the extensors and the posterior or dorsal position of the flexors are opposite to those seen in the upper limb. This is because the lower limb rotated medially during development unlike the lateral rotation which occurred in the upper limb. The leg also has three compartments – anterior or extensor, lateral or peroneal and posterior or flexor. The foot has dorsal and plantar aspects.

The function of the lower limb is to support the body weight and to propel it forward during locomotion. For this purpose it is constructed with large bones, massive muscles and stable joints.

The hip bone or the innominate bone connects the femur to the vertebral column at the sacrum. The thigh contains the femur, which in turn connects the hip joint to the knee joint. The leg, which extends from the knee to the ankle, has the tibia and fibula. The foot contains the tarsal bones, the metatarsals and the phalanges.

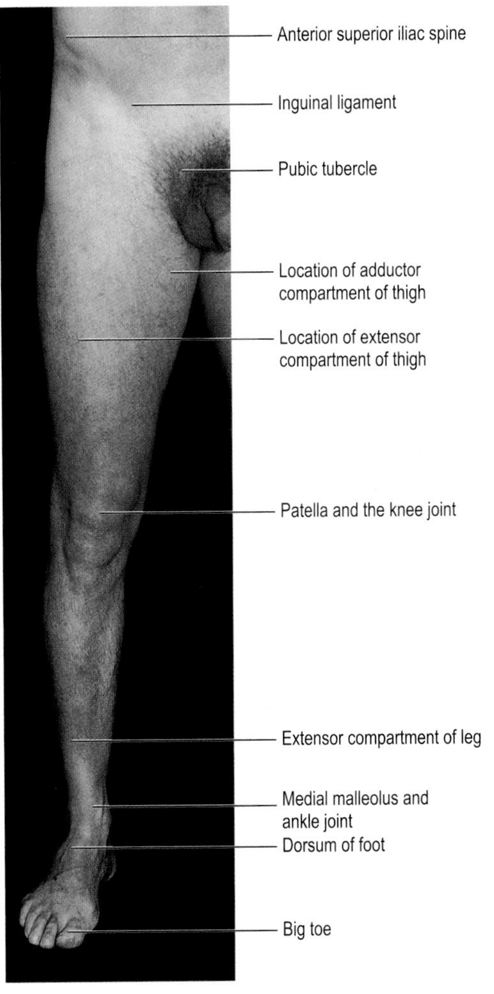


Fig. 6.1 Parts of the lower limb viewed from the front.

✪ The body weight in erect standing is transmitted from the vertebral column to the femur via the hip bone and from there through the tibia to the tarsal bones. The fibula, therefore, is a non-weight-bearing bone.

The lower limb is innervated by nerves arising in the lumbar and sacral plexuses. The arterial supply is through the femoral artery and its continuation as the popliteal and anterior and posterior tibial arteries. As in the upper limb the venous drainage is via a superficial and deep set of veins. The lymph is drained into the inguinal group of lymph nodes.

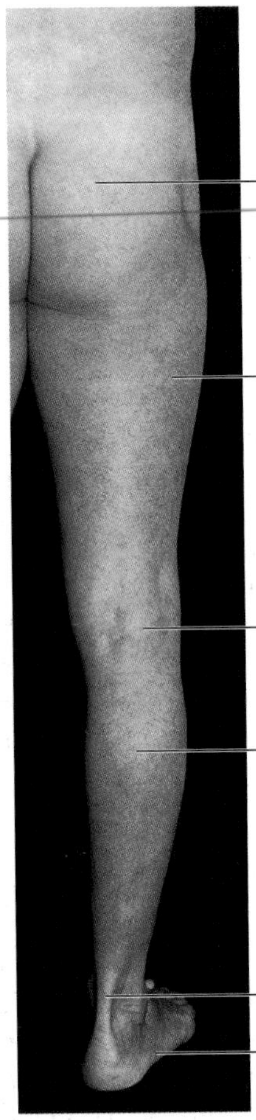

Fig. 6.2 Parts of the lower limb viewed from behind.

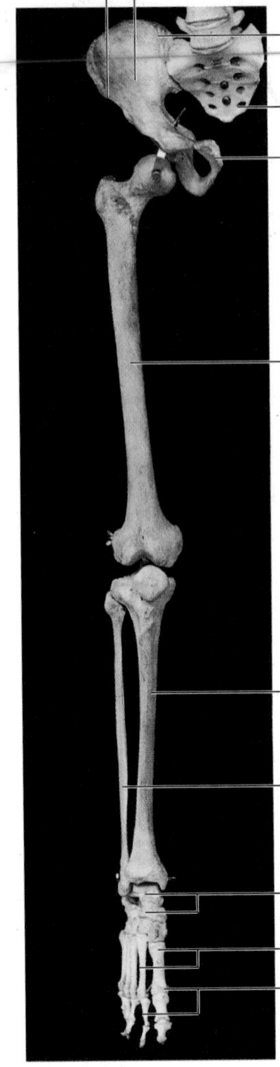

Fig. 6.3 The bones of the lower limb.

## Bones of hip and thigh

### Hip bone

The hip bone (Figs 6.3, 6.4) consists of a superior part, the ilium, a posteroinferior part, the ischium, and an anteromedial part, the pubis. All three contribute to the

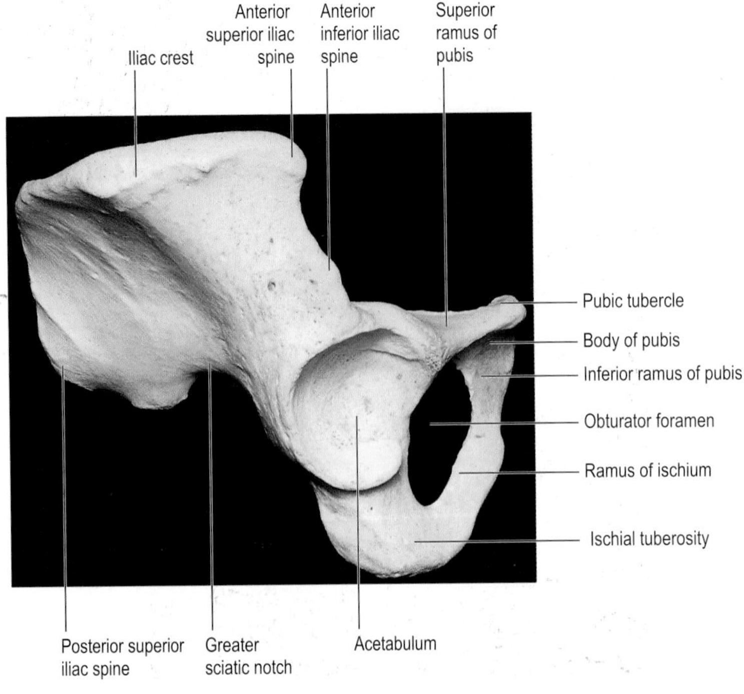


Fig. 6.4 The hip bone – external aspect.

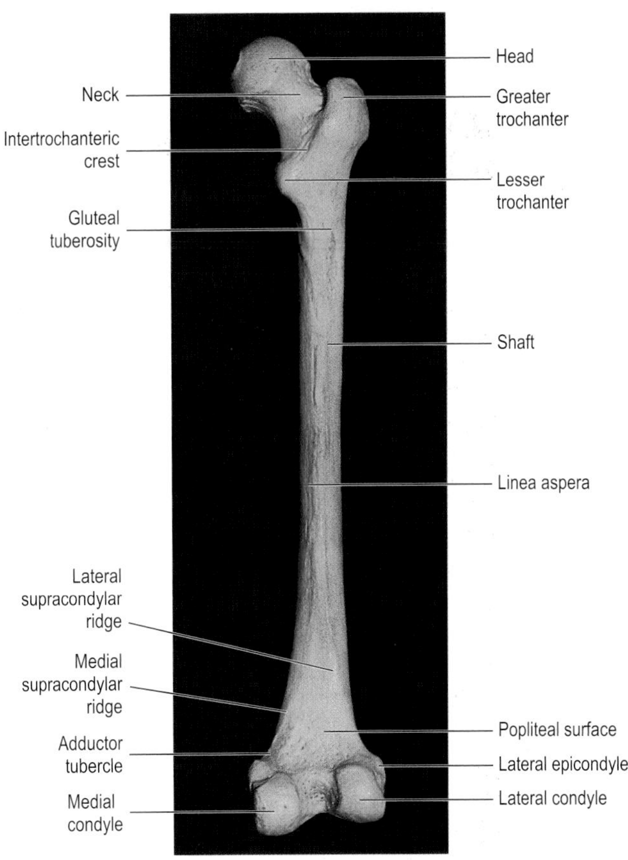


Fig. 6.5 Femur – posterior aspect.

formation of the acetabulum where there is a triradiate cartilage separating the three components until 15–17 years of age. This fuses completely in the adult. The acetabulum articulates with the head of the femur. The iliac crest, posterior superior iliac spine, anterior superior iliac spine, pubic tubercle and the ischial tuberosity are palpable and are important landmarks in surface anatomy. The rest of the hip bone is covered by large muscles, and hence not palpable.

### Femur

The neck of the femur (Fig. 6.5) projects upwards and medially and also slightly forwards from the shaft, forming an angle of 115–140° with the shaft. When the angle is less than normal the condition is known as coxa vara and when more coxa valga. ✪ A fracture of the neck of femur, common in the elderly, can cause avascular necrosis of the head of the femur as the blood supply to the head reaches it through the neck. The greater trochanter is the only part which is palpable at the upper end of the femur. A number of major muscles are attached to the greater and lesser trochanters.

✪ The shaft of the femur is related to a chain of arterial anastomoses. Severe haemorrhage occurs in a fracture of the shaft when these arteries are torn. A large number of muscles are attached to the linea aspera which is a sharp ridge at the posterior aspect of the femur.

## Femoral triangle

The femoral triangle (Figs 6.6, 6.7) is in the upper part of the front of the thigh and it is bounded laterally by the medial border of sartorius, medially by the medial border of the adductor longus and above by the inguinal ligament. The muscles forming the floor from medial to lateral are the adductor longus, pectineus, the psoas major and the iliacus.

The femoral triangle contains from medial to lateral the femoral vein, the femoral artery and the femoral nerve.

✪ The femoral artery, the continuation of the external iliac artery, and the femoral vein, which continues into the abdomen as the external iliac vein, are enclosed inside the

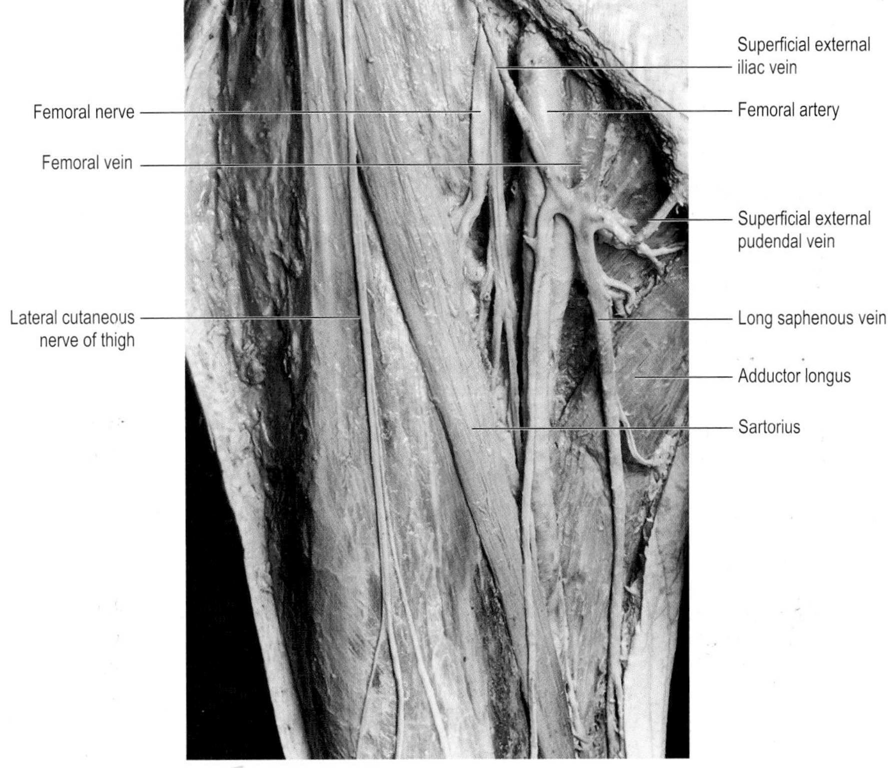


Fig. 6.6 The femoral triangle. Contents of the femoral triangle – femoral artery, femoral vein and femoral nerve.

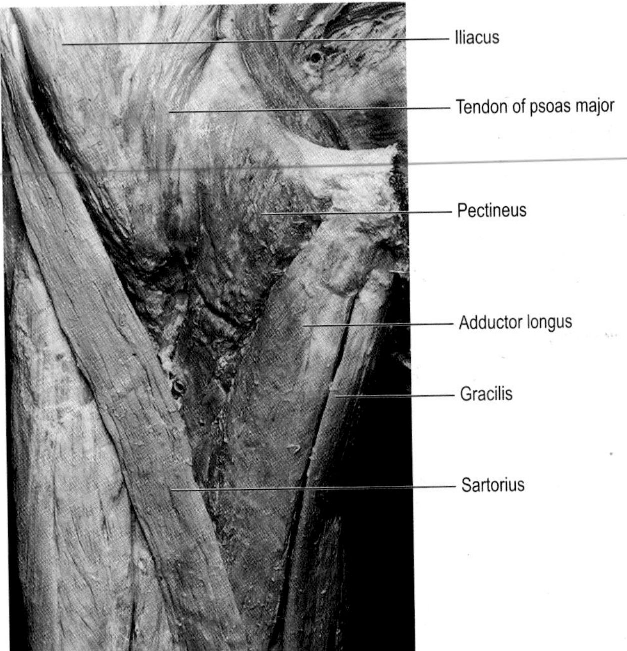


Fig. 6.7 Floor of the femoral triangle.

femoral sheath, which has a potential space medial to the vein, the femoral canal. This communicates with the abdominal cavity through the femoral ring. A femoral hernia can pass through the femoral ring into the femoral canal. See Clinical box 6.1.

✪ The femoral artery enters the thigh at a point midway between the anterior superior iliac spine and the pubic symphysis (midinguinal point) where its pulsation can be felt easily. The artery can be cannulated at this point to place an arterial line.

✪ The position of the vein in the living can be found by feeling the femoral artery pulsation. The vein is immediately medial to the artery just below the inguinal ligament. The long (great) saphenous vein receives a number of tributaries corresponding to the superficial branches of the femoral artery just before it joins the femoral vein (Fig. 6.6). This is an identification point to distinguish it from the femoral vein at operation. The femoral vein here has only one tributary, the long saphenous vein.

✪ The femoral nerve is lateral to the artery but is at a deeper plane compared with the artery and sometimes even posterior to the artery. It divides into its branches as soon as it enters the thigh. These anatomical variations make it a difficult nerve to block by injection of local anaesthetic agents. The nerve supplies the pectineus, the sartorius and the four parts of the quadriceps femoris, i.e. the rectus femoris, the vastus lateralis, the vastus intermedius and the vastus medialis. Its sensory branches are the medial and the intermediate cutaneous nerves of the thigh and the saphenous nerve. See Clinical box 6.2.

### Sartorius

The sartorius muscle (Fig. 6.7) extends from the anterior superior iliac spine to the medial condyle of the tibia. The sartorius is supplied by the femoral nerve. It is a flexor of the hip and knee and also, along with other long muscles connecting the hip bone to the leg, balances the hip bone on the femur.

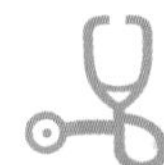

### *Clinical box 6.1*

#### Femoral hernia

The femoral triangle contains, from medial to lateral, the femoral vein, the femoral artery and the femoral nerve. The femoral artery and vein are enclosed inside the femoral sheath. The femoral sheath has a potential space medial to the vein, the femoral canal. Normally this contains a lymph node, Cloquet's node, which drains deep tissues of the lower limb as well as the glans penis. The femoral canal communicates with the abdominal cavity through the femoral ring. A femoral hernia can pass through the femoral ring into the femoral canal. The femoral ring is bounded laterally by the femoral vein, medially by the lacunar ligament (Gimbernat's ligament) which is a prolongation of the inguinal ligament on to the pubic bone, anteriorly by the inguinal ligament, and posteriorly by the pectineal ligament (of Ashley Cooper) which is a continuation of the lacunar ligament on to the posterior border of the pectineal surface of the superior pubic ramus. The boundaries of the ring are unyielding and hence the femoral hernia emerging through it can get obstructed and strangulated.

Unlike the indirect inguinal hernia the femoral hernia is not congenital. Relation to the pubic tubercle is important in distinguishing a femoral hernia from an inguinal hernia. The neck of the femoral hernia lies below and lateral to the pubic tubercle (position of the femoral ring), whereas the inguinal hernia is above and medial to the pubic tubercle. As the femoral hernia enlarges, it emerges through the saphenous opening and projects upwards to lie above the inguinal ligament. There are several well known approaches for the repair of a femoral hernia. In the lower approach, there is a possibility of bleeding from the abnormal obturator artery which is an enlarged pubic branch of the obturator artery. This often lies lateral to the pectineal ligament causing no harm but occasionally may be very close to it, producing bleeding while stitching the ligament.

### The quadriceps femoris

This major muscle (Figs 6.8–6.10) – consisting of the rectus femoris, the vastus lateralis, the vastus intermedius and the vastus medialis – extends the knee joint. The rectus femoris, taking origin from the hip bone, is also a flexor of the hip joint. The other three components take origin from the femur and as such can act only on the knee.

✪ To test the muscle the patient is asked to extend the knee against resistance. The muscle can be seen and felt as contracting. The four parts of the quadriceps are supplied by branches from the femoral nerve.

The three vasti and the rectus femoris are inserted into the patella through the quadriceps tendon (Fig. 6.11). They then insert into the tibial tuberosity through the patellar tendon or the ligamentum patellae. The quadriceps tendon, patella and the ligamentum patellae together form the extensor mechanism of the knee. A thin sheet of the quadriceps tendon passes across the front of the patella into the ligamentum patellae and the retinacula. The patellar retinacula are expansions of the quadriceps tendon connecting the patella to the tibial condyles.

## Clinical box 6.2

### Block dissection of the inguinal lymph nodes

The inguinal lymph nodes are classified as superficial and deep. The superficial nodes are arranged in horizontal and vertical chains, the former along the inguinal ligament and the latter along the long saphenous vein. The horizontal group drain structures in the perineum whereas the vertical group receive lymph from most of the superficial tissues of the lower limb. The deep nodes lie in the femoral canal and at the saphenofemoral junction. They drain the deep tissues of the limb as well as the glans penis. The superficial nodes also drain into the deep nodes.

Squamous cell carcinomas of the skin of the leg and carcinoma of the penis metastasise into the inguinal nodes. Removal of the nodes along with the adjoining tissues and structures as a block is a successful treatment of these conditions. Superficial and deep fascia over the femoral triangle, the long saphenous vein and its tributaries are all removed, along with the lymph nodes and fat in the femoral triangle. Only the femoral artery, femoral vein and femoral nerve are left intact. The inguinal ligament is often incised to expose the external iliac vessels and nodes around them are also removed.

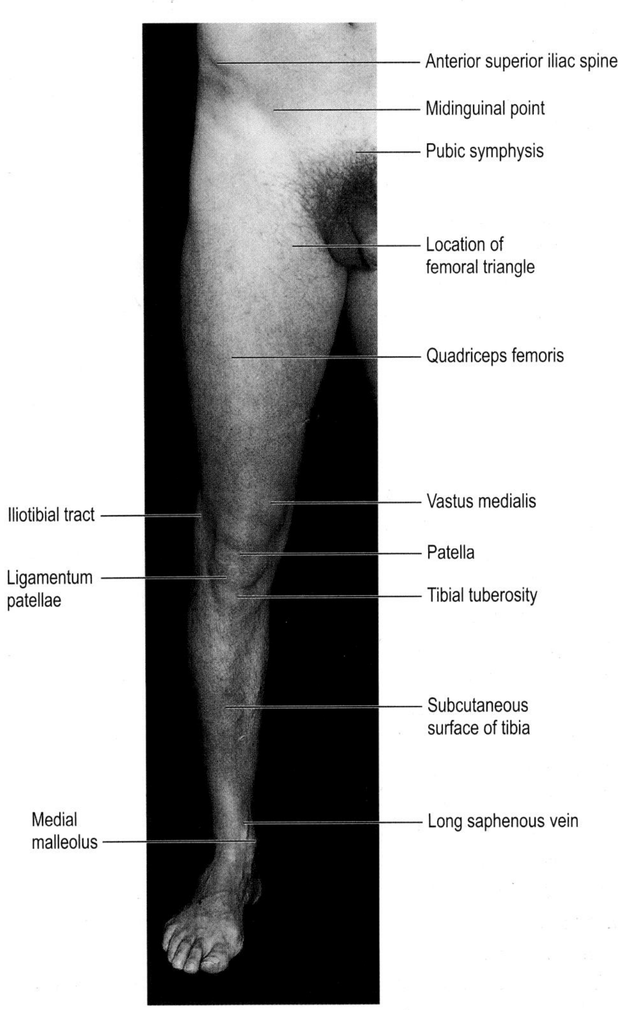


Fig. 6.8 Surface anatomy of front of thigh, leg and foot. Location of femoral triangle and midinguinal point.

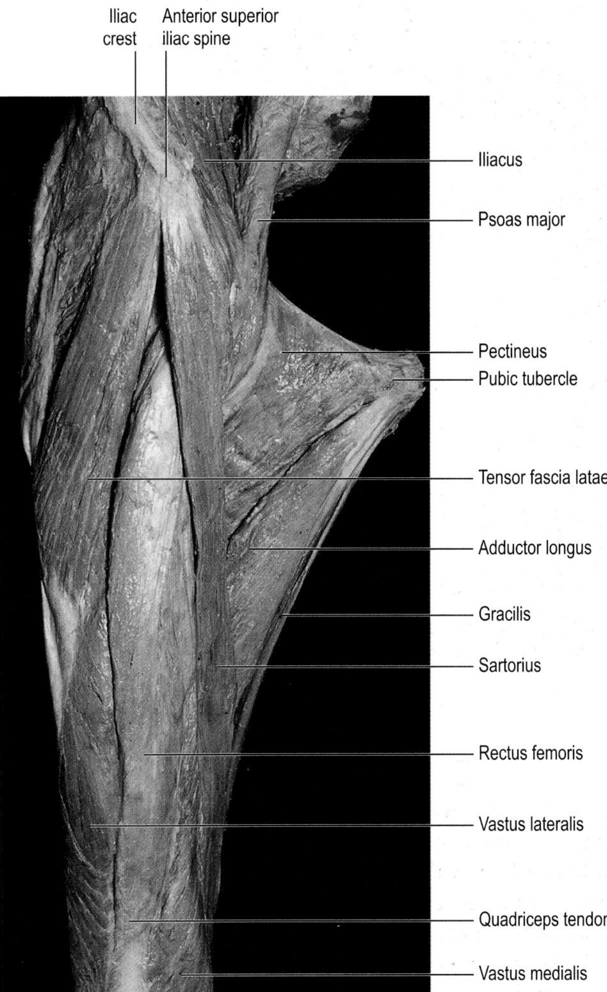


Fig. 6.9 Muscles in the anterior and medial aspects of thigh. The quadriceps femoris.

The vastus lateralis and vastus medialis mostly take origin from the linea aspera of the femur. The vastus intermedius arises from the anterior surface of the femur deep to the rectus femoris. Unlike the other members of the quadriceps, the vastus medialis is fleshy at its lower end and these fibres lie horizontally as they attach to the patella. It can be seen on the surface in a muscular person (Fig. 6.8).

✪ The long axis of the shaft of femur is not vertical but slants downwards and medially. Therefore when the quadriceps contracts its direction of pull is upwards and lateral, causing the patella to move in the same direction. The patella thus has a tendency for dislocating upwards and laterally. Pull of the lower horizontal fibres of the vastus medialis is an important factor preventing such dislocation.

✪ The quadriceps via the extensor mechanism (quadriceps tendon, patella, and the ligamentum patellae) extends the knee joint. Quadriceps contraction is an important factor in stabilising the knee joint. Without that the knee tends to flex when it is weight-bearing. Persons with quadriceps paralysis tend to press the thigh to counteract the flexion of the knee whilst walking.

### Iliotibial tract

The deep fascia of the thigh, the fascia lata, has a thick lateral aspect. This is the iliotibial tract (Fig. 6.12) which extends from the iliac crest to the lateral condyle of the tibia. Along with the quadriceps muscle, the iliotibial tract to which the

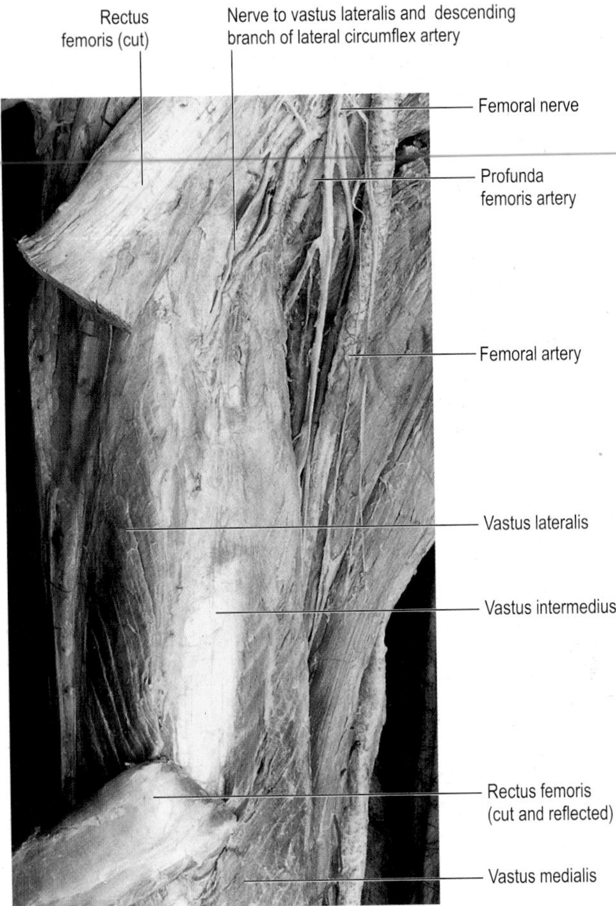


Fig. 6.10 Vastus intermedius.

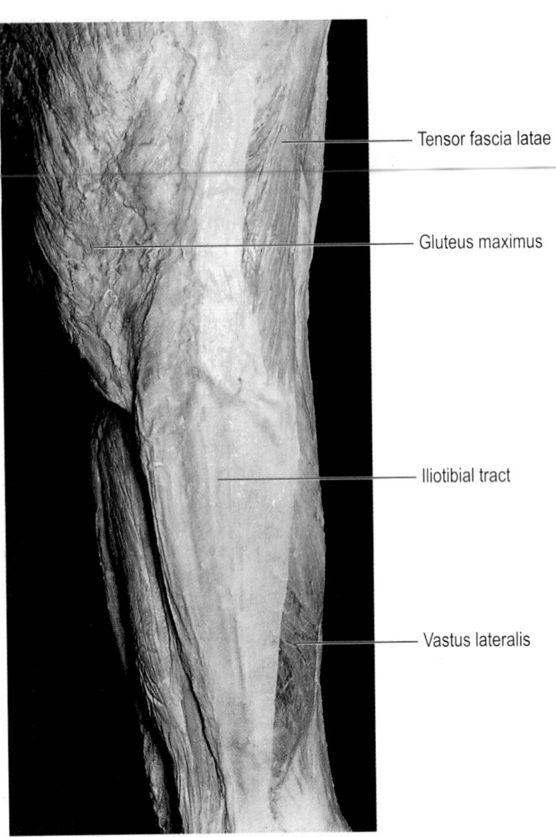


Fig. 6.12 Lateral aspect of thigh. Iliotibial tract and the insertion of gluteus maximus and tensor fascia latae (right side).

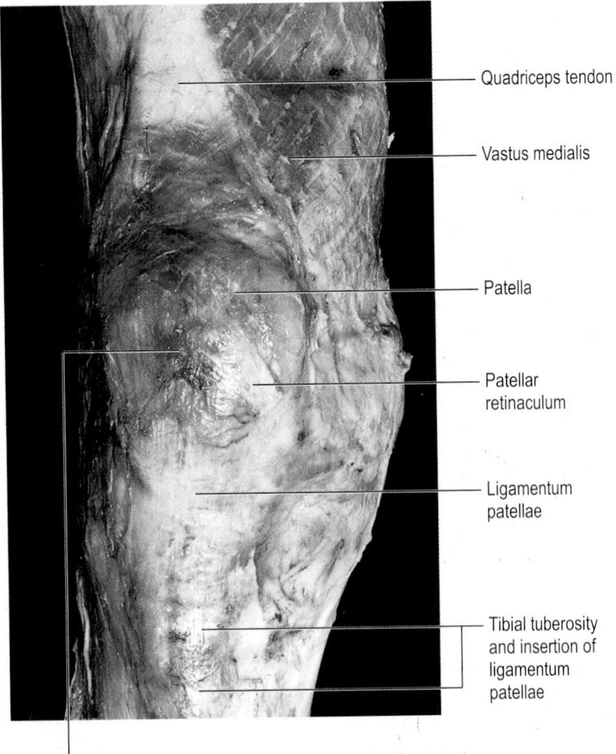


Fig. 6.11 Quadriceps tendon, patella and ligamentum patellae.

gluteus maximus and the tensor fascia latae are attached is an important structure in stabilising the knee joint. It may be visible on the surface when the knee is extended (Fig. 6.8).

## The adductor compartment or the medial compartment of the thigh

The adductor compartment (Figs 6.13–6.16) is separated from the anterior compartment by the medial intermuscular septum and contains: the adductors longus, brevis, magnus, gracilis and the obturator externus. All these muscles are supplied by the obturator nerve.

The adductors are inserted into the linea aspera of the femur. ✪ The adductor longus (Fig. 6.9) has a tendinous origin from just below the pubic tubercle. Its tendon can be palpated in the living by adducting the thigh against resistance. The gracilis is a slender muscle connecting the pubic bone to the medial condyle of the tibia.

The adductor brevis (Fig. 6.13) lying deep to the adductor longus but anterior to the adductor magnus takes origin from the body of the pubis. It is inserted to the linea aspera behind the insertion of the adductor longus.

✪ 'Groin strain', a common sports injury among sprinters and footballers, usually results from abnormal stretching or tearing of the upper attachment of the adductor muscles.

Adductor magnus has adductor and hamstring components. The adductor component takes origin from the ramus of the pubis and its extensive insertion is into the linea aspera behind that of the adductor brevis. The hamstring part arises from the ischial tuberosity, and is inserted to the adductor tubercle of the femur and is

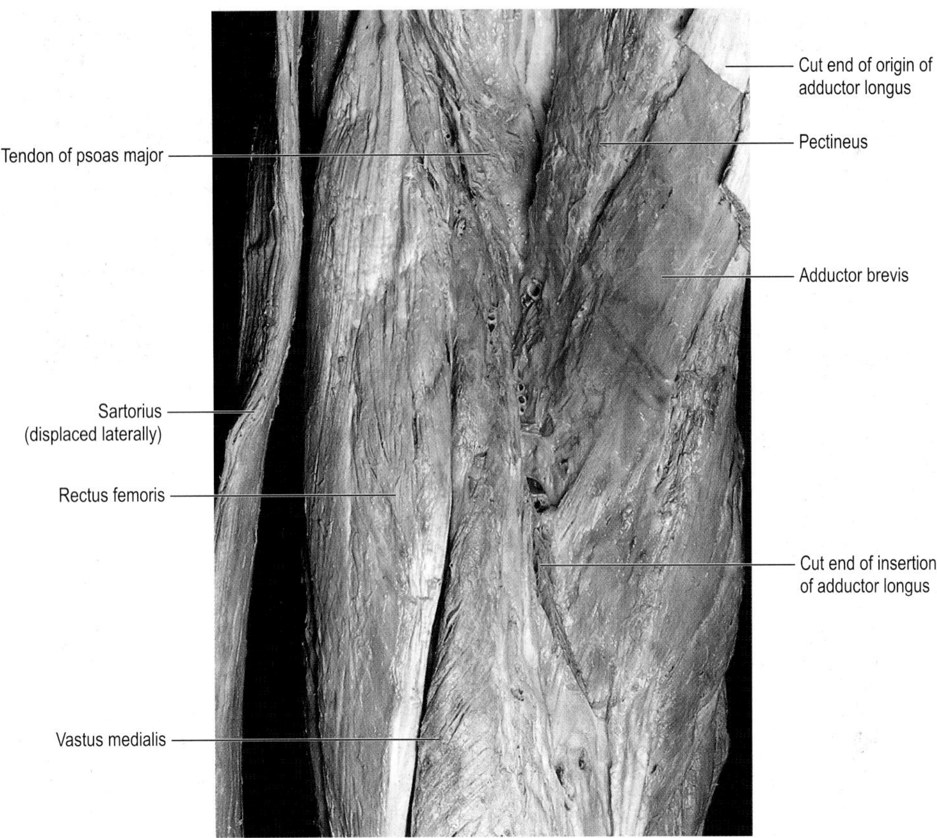


Fig. 6.13 The medial aspect of thigh. The adductor brevis seen after removal of adductor longus.

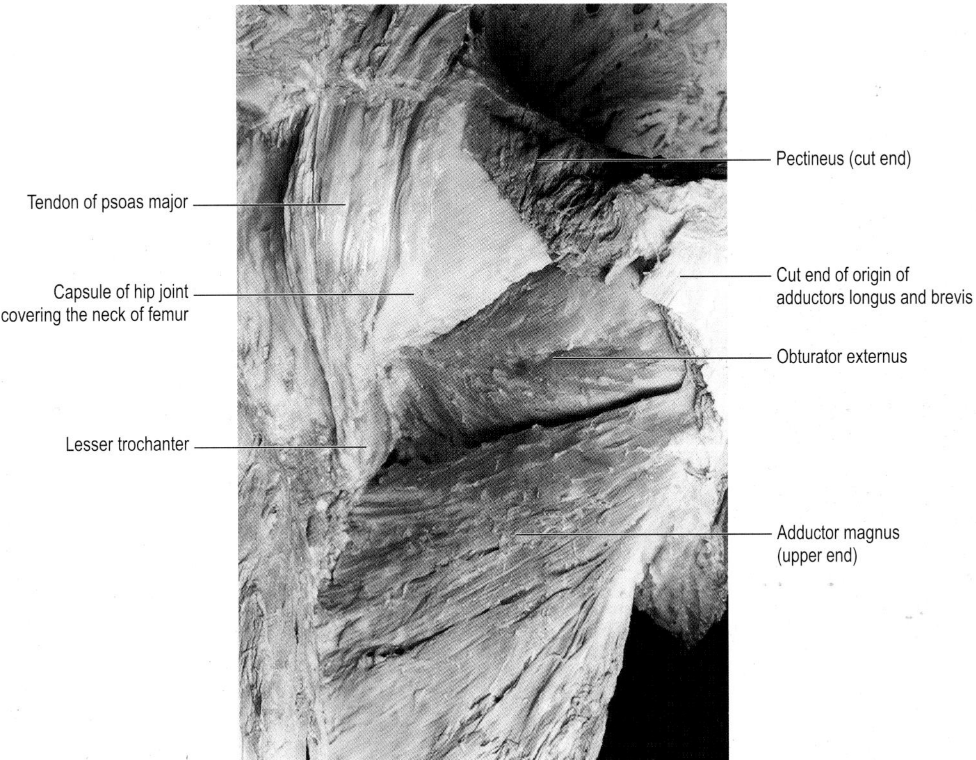


Fig. 6.14 Upper part of the medial aspect of thigh. Obturator externus.

supplied along with the rest of the hamstring muscles by the sciatic nerve. Its aponeurosis above the insertion has a hiatus through which the femoral vessels enter the popliteal fossa.

The obturator externus (Fig. 6.14) is a muscle covering the external aspect of the obturator foramen. It spirals posteriorly and laterally round the neck of the femur to its tendinous insertion to the trochanteric fossa of the femur.

### Action of the adductors

✪ As their names imply the three adductor muscles move the thigh towards the midline at the hip joint (as you settle

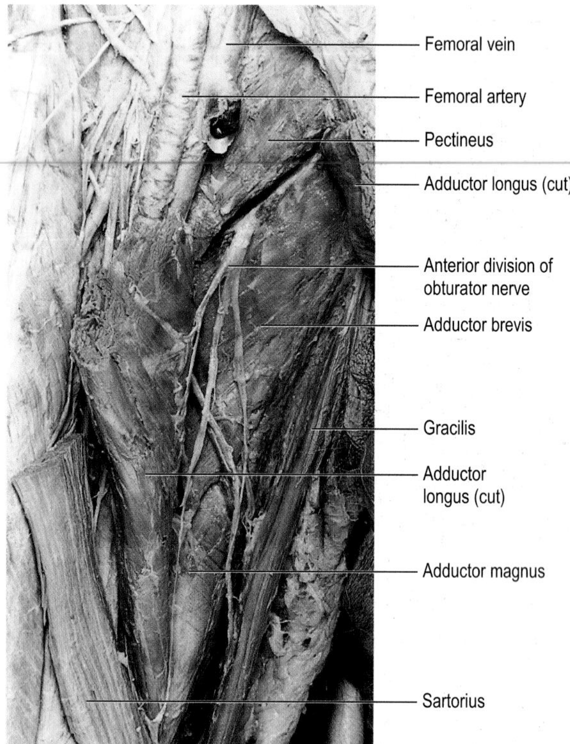


Fig. 6.15 Medial aspect of thigh. Obturator nerve – anterior division.

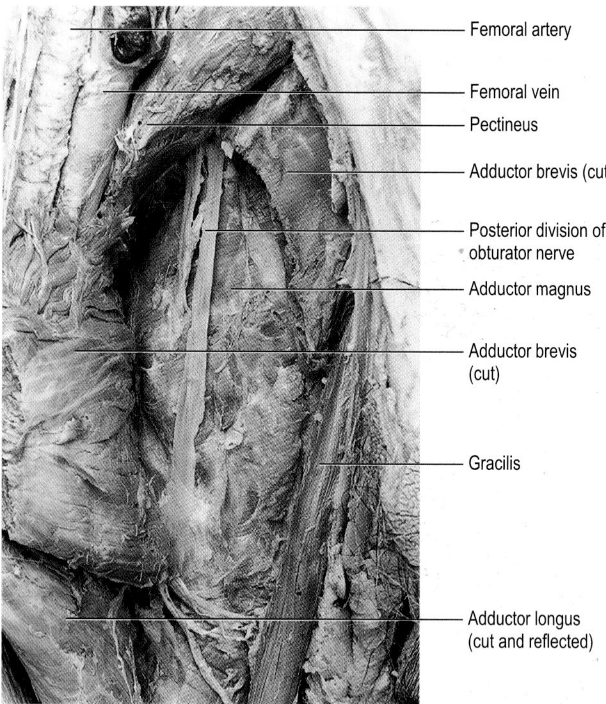


Fig. 6.16 Medial aspect of thigh. Posterior division of obturator nerve after reflection of adductor longus and adductor brevis.

down on a car seat). They are also important in balancing while standing, preventing abduction. The adductor longus and brevis can also act as medial rotators of the thigh (prevent lateral rotation while standing). The part of the adductor magnus originating from the ischial tuberosity, along with the other hamstring muscles, extend the hip joint. The obturator externus is one of the many lateral rotators of the hip joint.

### Obturator nerve

The obturator nerve (Figs 6.15, 6.16) supplies all the muscles in the medial compartment of the thigh. It enters the thigh by passing through the obturator foramen accompanied by the obturator artery. As it goes through the foramen it divides into anterior and posterior branches. The anterior division of the obturator nerve, lying deep to the adductor longus on the surface of the adductor brevis, gives branches to the adductor longus, adductor brevis and the gracilis and the skin of the medial part of the thigh. The posterior division of the obturator nerve emerges through the obturator externus after supplying it to lie on the adductor magnus. It supplies the adductor magnus and gives a branch which accompanies the femoral artery into the popliteal fossa to supply the capsule of the knee joint.

✪ Articular branches of the obturator nerve supply the hip and knee joints and hence pain produced in one joint can manifest as referred pain in the other. Similarly pelvic inflammation involving the obturator nerve can produce referred pain along the medial aspect of the thigh.

### Obturator artery

The obturator artery, a branch of the internal iliac artery, emerges through the obturator foramen and divides into branches which encircle the obturator foramen. Its branches anastomose with the medial circumflex artery. It gives a small articular branch to the hip joint.

### Adductor canal

The subsartorial or the adductor canal (Fig. 6.17) is the space containing the femoral artery and the vein below the femoral triangle. It is known as Hunter's canal because John Hunter first described the exposure and ligation of the femoral artery for treatment of popliteal aneurysm.

It is a gutter-shaped groove bounded laterally by the vastus medialis and medially by the adductor longus above and the adductor magnus below. Its contents are the femoral artery, the femoral vein, the nerve to vastus medialis and the saphenous nerve.

The femoral artery as it descends in the canal crosses from the lateral to the medial side of the femoral vein. The saphenous nerve crosses from the lateral side of the artery to its medial side. The femoral artery and vein pass into the popliteal fossa from the adductor canal by passing through a hiatus in the adductor magnus. The saphenous nerve leaves the canal by passing along the posterior border of the sartorius and then accompanies the long saphenous vein as it descends in the leg.

## Gluteal region

### Surface anatomy and osteology

The gluteal region (Fig. 6.18) or the buttock lies above the hip joint on the posterior aspect of the pelvis and it extends from the iliac crest above to the gluteal fold below. ✪ The iliac crest (Fig. 6.19) is palpable throughout. The highest point of the iliac crest (Fig. 6.18) is at the level of the spinous process of the fourth lumbar vertebra, the level often used in examination of the vertebral column and for doing a lumbar puncture. It is also the level of bifurcation of the abdominal aorta. The iliac crest terminates posteriorly as the posterior superior iliac spine. Its position is often indicated by a depression on the surface and it is at the level of the second

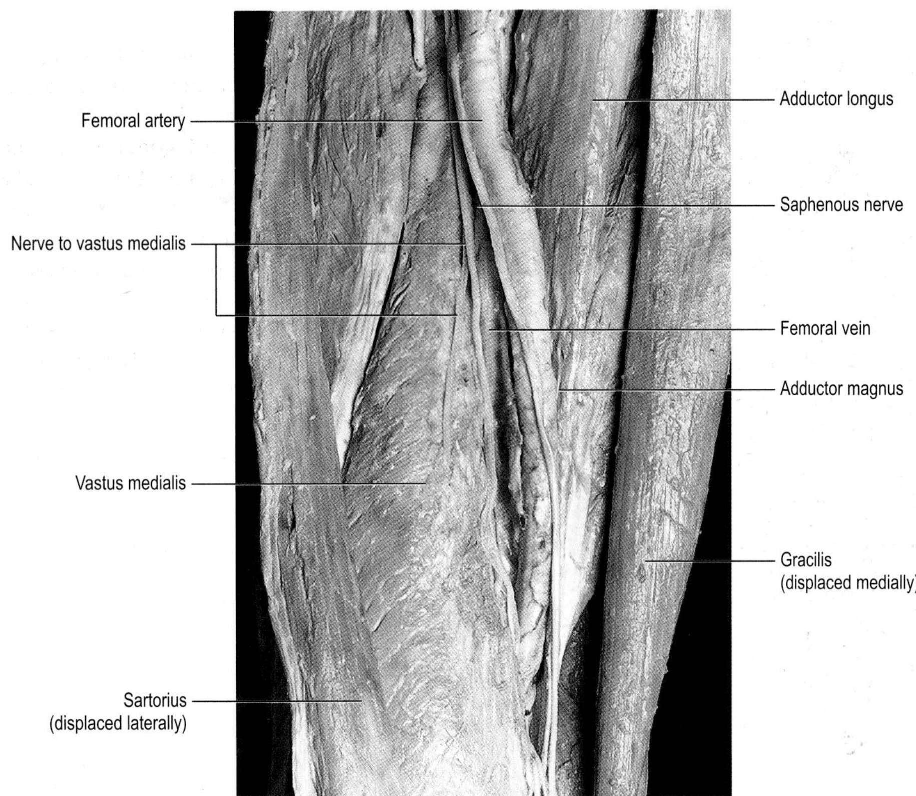


Fig. 6.17 Adductor canal.

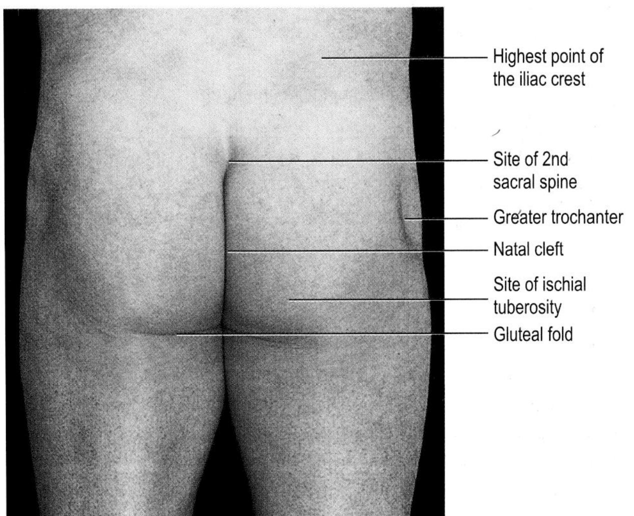


Fig. 6.18 Surface anatomy of the gluteal region.

segment of the sacrum. ✪ A hand's breadth below the middle of the iliac crest is the greater trochanter, which can be seen and felt in front of the hollow on the side of the hip. It is the only part of the femur which is palpable at its upper end. ✪ The ischial tuberosity is palpated at the lower part of the buttock (Fig. 6.18). It is covered by the gluteus maximus while standing whereas while sitting the muscle rises and uncovers the bone. Hence the ischial tuberosity which supports the body weight while sitting down is more easily felt in that position.

The prominence of the buttock is contributed by the gluteus maximus and the overlying fat. The natal cleft separates the buttocks. Its upper end corresponds to the third sacral spine. ✪ The gluteal region is a common site for

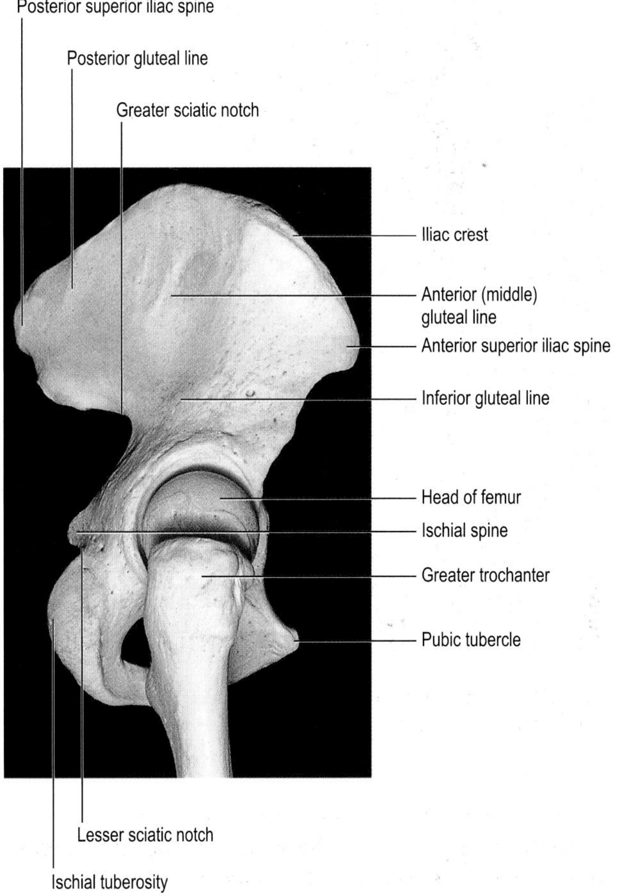


Fig. 6.19 The hip bone and the upper end of femur – lateral view.

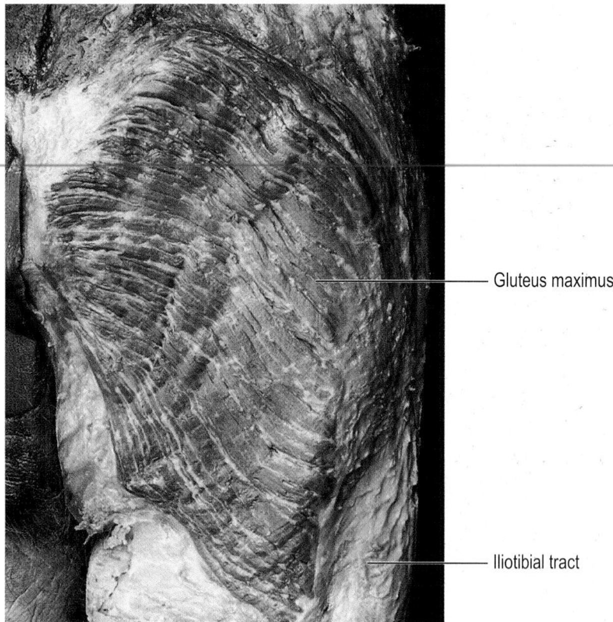


Fig. 6.20 Gluteus maximus.

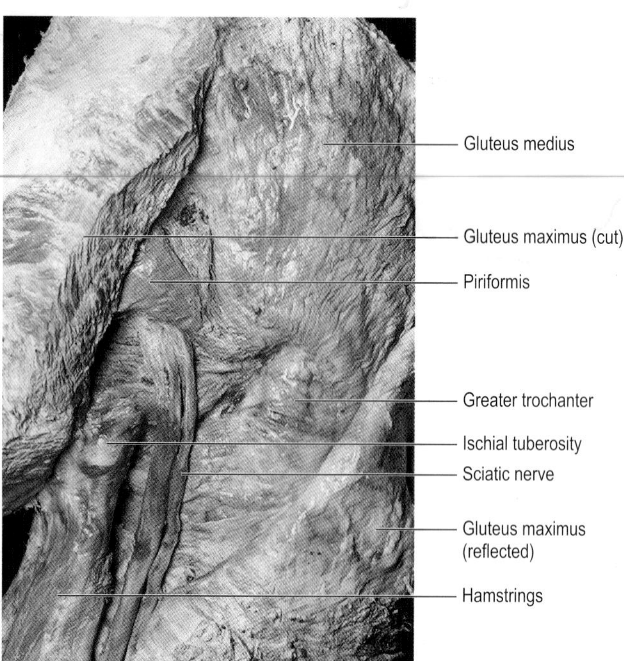


Fig. 6.21 Structures deep to the gluteus maximus. The gluteus medius.

intramuscular injections. These are given in the upper outer quadrant to avoid damage to the sciatic nerve.

### Gluteus maximus

Figure 6.20 shows the gluteus maximus. It takes origin from the ilium behind the posterior gluteal line, the sacrum and the sacrotuberous ligament, a thick ligament extending from the ischial tuberosity to the sacrum.

Major part of the muscle is inserted into the iliotibial tract (p. 139). The deeper portion is inserted into the gluteal tuberosity of the femur (p. 137). Its nerve supply is by the inferior gluteal nerve.

*Action* The muscle is a powerful extensor of the hip joint as in running and climbing stairs. It acts as an antigravity muscle controlling flexion as in sitting down from the standing posture. It is also a lateral rotator of the hip. Through the iliotibial tract it can extend as well as stabilise the knee joint.

### Gluteus medius

This muscle (Fig. 6.21) takes origin from the gluteal surface of the ilium between anterior and posterior gluteal lines. It is inserted on the lateral surface of the greater trochanter and is innervated by the superior gluteal nerve.

### Gluteus minimus

This lies deep to the medius. Its origin is from the gluteal surface of the ilium between the anterior and inferior gluteal lines. Insertion of the muscle is on the anterior aspect of the greater trochanter. The muscle is innervated by the superior gluteal nerve.

*Action* ✪ The gluteus medius and minimus abduct the hip joint. When standing on one leg, gluteus medius and minimus of the supporting side prevent the hip from tilting to the unsupported side (it prevents adduction). When the muscles are paralysed, the tendency for tilting the pelvis to the unsupported side will be compensated by arching the trunk towards the supporting side.

### The short lateral rotators of the hip

These consist of the piriformis, the obturator internus, the gemelli and the quadratus femoris (Fig. 6.22). The obturator internus lies on the lateral wall of the pelvis. Its tendon emerges through the lesser sciatic foramen to be inserted on the greater trochanter. The two gemelli arise from the margin of the lesser sciatic notch and accompany the tendon of the obturator internus before inserting on the greater trochanter. The quadratus femoris takes origin from the ischial tuberosity and is inserted to the greater trochanter. Besides laterally rotating the thigh these muscles help to do the fine adjustment and stabilise the hip joint.

### Sciatic nerve

This, the largest nerve in the body, is formed in the sacral plexus (L4, L5, S1–3). It emerges from the pelvis through the greater sciatic notch lying below the piriformis (Fig. 6.22). ✪ In the gluteal region it is closely related to the posterior aspect of the hip joint separated only by the short lateral rotators of the thigh and hence is vulnerable in hip joint surgery and in posterior dislocation of the thigh. It can also be damaged in intramuscular injections when misplaced. It supplies the muscles of the posterior compartment of the thigh and those of the leg and foot. Its cutaneous branches supply the skin of the leg and foot except the skin along the medial border, which is supplied by the saphenous nerve. The sciatic nerve in the lower third of the back of the thigh divides into the common peroneal and the tibial nerves. However these two divisions of the nerve can remain separate almost throughout their course.

✪ Surface marking of the sciatic nerve – draw a line connecting the posterior superior iliac spine and the ischial tuberosity. The junction between the lower and middle third of this line is the point of entry of the nerve into the gluteal region. Join this to the midpoint between the greater trochanter and the ischial tuberosity and extend it vertically down to the lower third of the thigh. This marks the whole course of the nerve in the thigh.

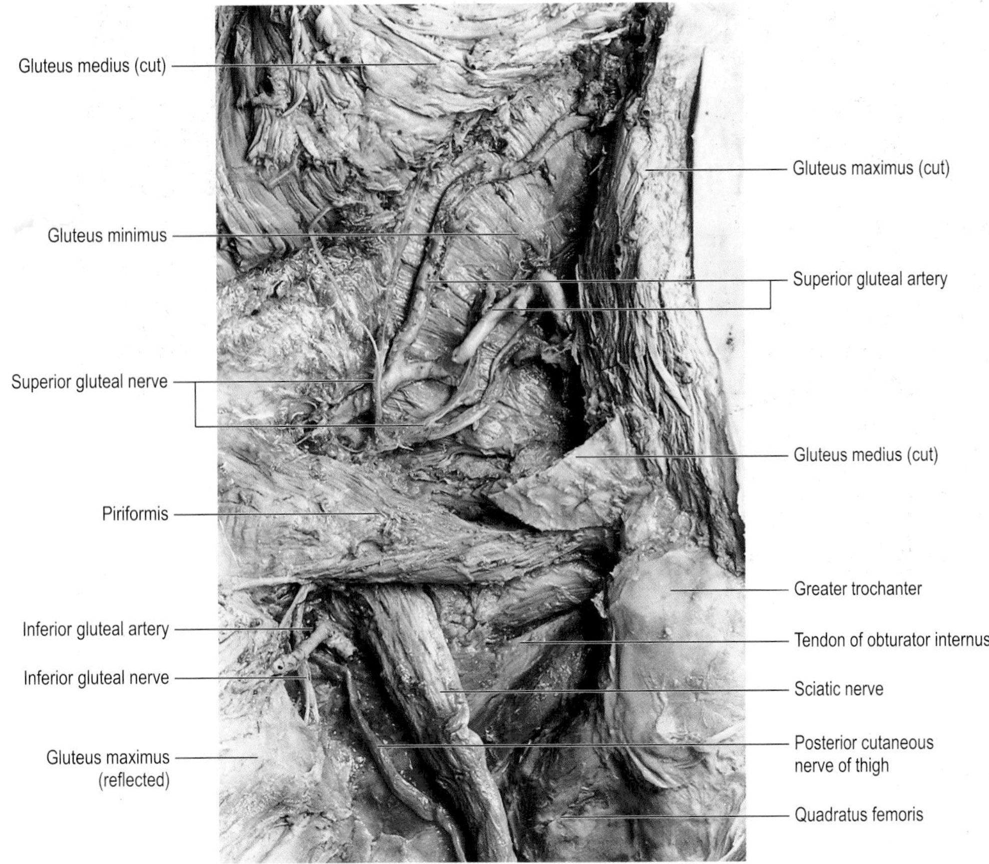


Fig. 6.22 Structures of the gluteal region seen after reflection of gluteus maximus and gluteus medius.

**Posterior cutaneous nerve of the thigh (S2, S3)**

Posterior cutaneous nerve of the thigh (Fig. 6.22) supplies the back of the thigh and upper half of the back of the leg. It is derived from the same nerve root as the pelvic splanchnic nerve which supplies the pelvic viscera (p. 114). ✪ Referred pain may sometimes be felt in pelvic inflammation along the back of the thigh and leg because of the common root value.

## Back of thigh

### The hamstrings

The hamstrings muscle group (Fig. 6.23) consists of the biceps, the semitendinosus, the semimembranosus and the hamstring part of adductor magnus.

*Origin* Common origin from the ischial tuberosity. The short head of the biceps takes origin from the linea aspera of the femur.

*Insertion* The biceps on the head of the fibula, the semitendinosus and the semimembranosus on to the medial condyle of the tibia, the adductor magnus into the adductor tubercle on the femur just above its medial condyle.

*Nerve supply* The sciatic nerve.

*Action* ✪ They are flexors of the knee joint. When the knee is straight they limit flexion of the hip. They also have an extensor action on the hip joint, especially when the position of the hip is intermediate between full flexion and full extension. This extensor action is important in walking. The semitendinosus and the semimembranosus can medially rotate the flexed knee and the biceps can act as a lateral rotator.

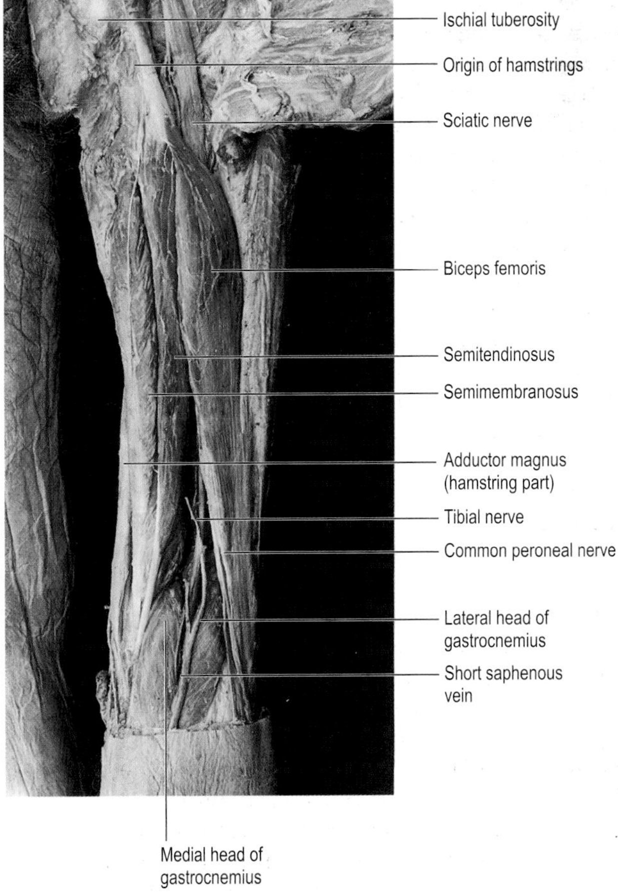


Fig. 6.23 Posterior compartment of thigh and the popliteal fossa.

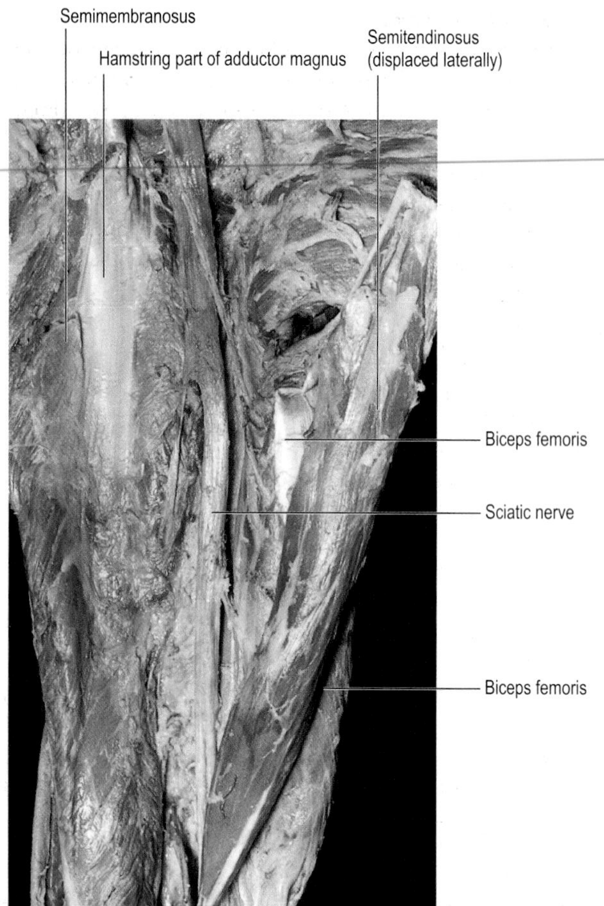


Fig. 6.24 Sciatic nerve in the posterior compartment of thigh.

✪ 'Pulled hamstrings' is a common injury in athletes and footballers caused by tearing of the attachments of the muscles to the ischial tuberosity.

### Sciatic nerve (L4, L5, S1–3)

The sciatic nerve runs vertically down lying between the hamstrings (Fig. 6.24). About a hand's breadth or more above the knee joint, at the apex of the popliteal fossa, the nerve divides into common peroneal and tibial nerves. This division may occur at a higher level or the two components may emerge separate from the pelvis as they are formed separately in the sciatic plexus. ✪ The surface marking of the nerve is indicated by a line connecting the midpoint between the ischial tuberosity and the greater trochanter to the apex of the popliteal fossa (see also p. 144).

## The popliteal fossa

This space behind the knee joint (Figs 6.25–6.28) is bounded above by the tendon of the biceps laterally, the semitendinosus and semimembranosus medially, and below by the lateral and medial heads of the gastrocnemius. It contains the tibial and the common peroneal branches of the sciatic nerve, the popliteal artery and the popliteal vein.

### Common peroneal nerve

The common peroneal nerve (Figs 6.25, 6.27, 6.28) lies along the posterior border of the tendon of the biceps and gives off a number of branches in the popliteal fossa.

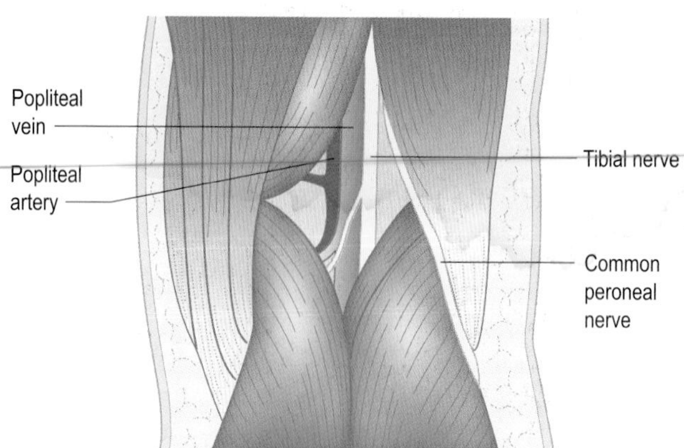


Fig. 6.25 Popliteal artery, popliteal vein and the nerves in the popliteal fossa.

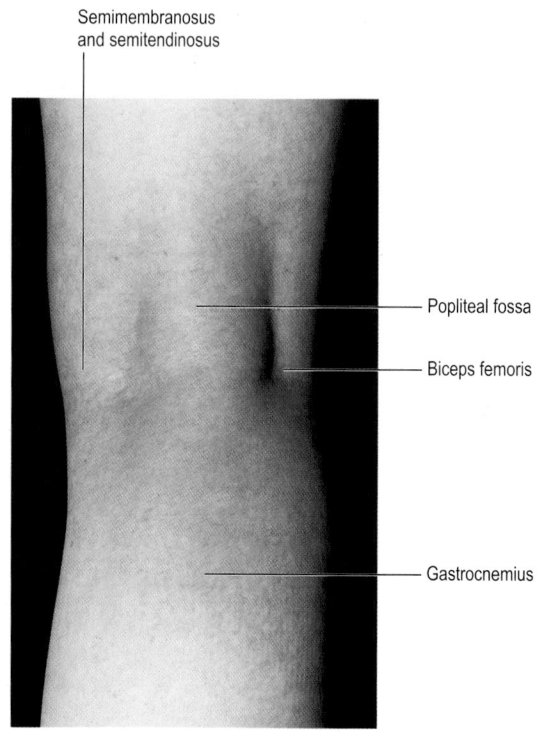


Fig. 6.26 Surface anatomy of the popliteal fossa.

Sural (peroneal) communicating branch – joins the sural nerve in the leg to supply the lateral border of the foot. Lateral cutaneous nerve of the calf supplies the front and lateral aspect of the leg in its upper part. Superior and inferior lateral genicular branches accompany the corresponding arteries to supply the capsule and the lateral ligament of the knee joint.

### The tibial nerve

The tibial nerve (Figs 6.25, 6.27, 6.28) lies in the midline and disappears after passing deep to the two heads of the gastrocnemius. It supplies all the muscles which take origin in the popliteal fossa, i.e. two heads of the gastrocnemius, plantaris, soleus and popliteus. The sural nerve which accompanies the short saphenous vein supplies skin of the lateral border of the foot. The tibial nerve gives off three genicular branches.

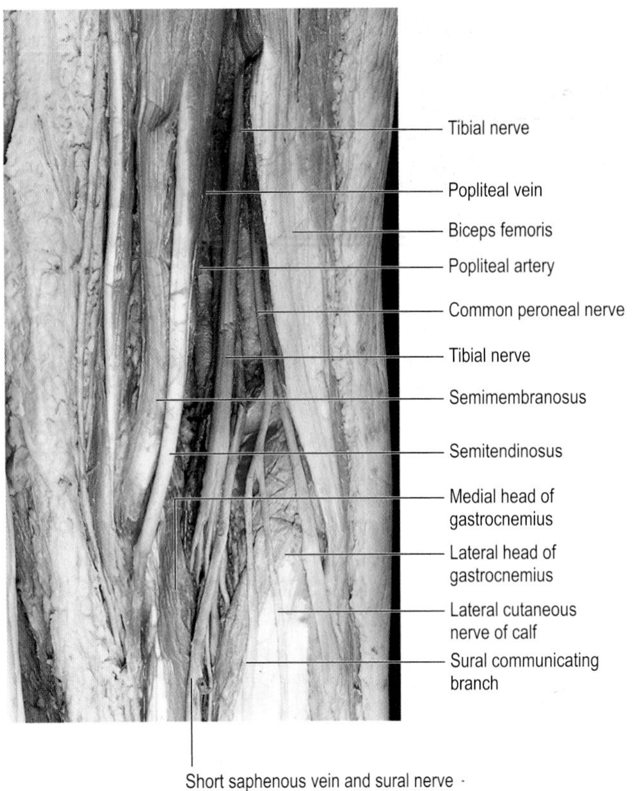


Fig. 6.27 The popliteal fossa, boundaries and contents.

## The popliteal artery

The popliteal artery (Figs 6.25, 6.27) and vein lie at a deeper plane compared with the nerves. The popliteal vein, formed by the venae comitantes of the anterior and posterior tibial arteries, is often joined by the short saphenous vein.

The popliteal artery is the continuation of the femoral artery after it has passed through the hiatus in the adductor magnus which is about a hand's breadth above the knee joint. It lies deep in the popliteal fossa and is separated from the tibial nerve by the popliteal vein. In the lower part of the popliteal fossa the artery bifurcates to form the anterior and posterior tibial arteries. ✪ Vascular surgeons normally describe the upper part of the latter as the tibioperoneal trunk. It is normally about 2cm long and bifurcates into the posterior tibial and peroneal arteries.

✪ The popliteal artery pulsation can be felt on deep palpation after the knee is flexed to relax the muscles and the deep fascia.

✪ The popliteal artery may be damaged in supracondylar fracture of the femur, especially if there is displacement of the lower fragment by the pull of the gastrocnemius.

✪ The artery can be surgically exposed through posterior, medial or lateral approaches. The posterior approach is through the interval between the two heads of the gastrocnemius, avoiding the nerves and the popliteal vein. In the medial approach the medial head of gastrocnemius is detached from its femoral attachment after retracting the semimembranosus and semitendinosus medially. In the lateral approach, which passes behind the iliotibial tract and the lateral intermuscular septum, the biceps is displaced backwards.

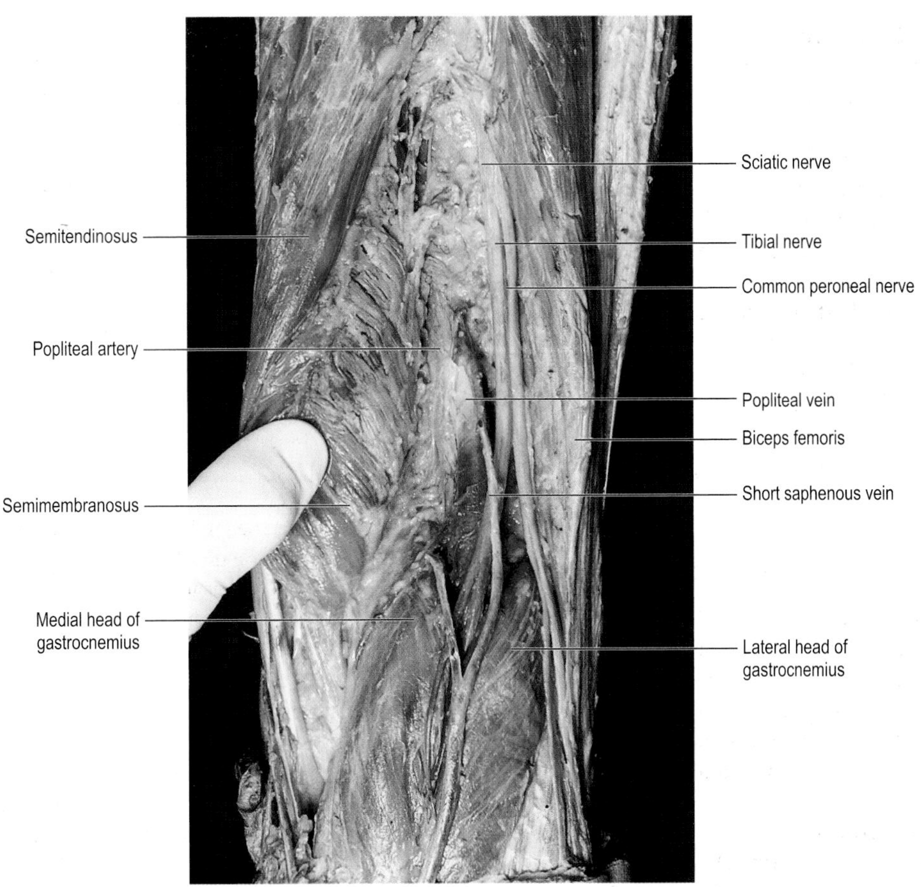


Fig. 6.28 Structures in the popliteal fossa (tibial nerve displaced slightly laterally to show the popliteal vein and artery).

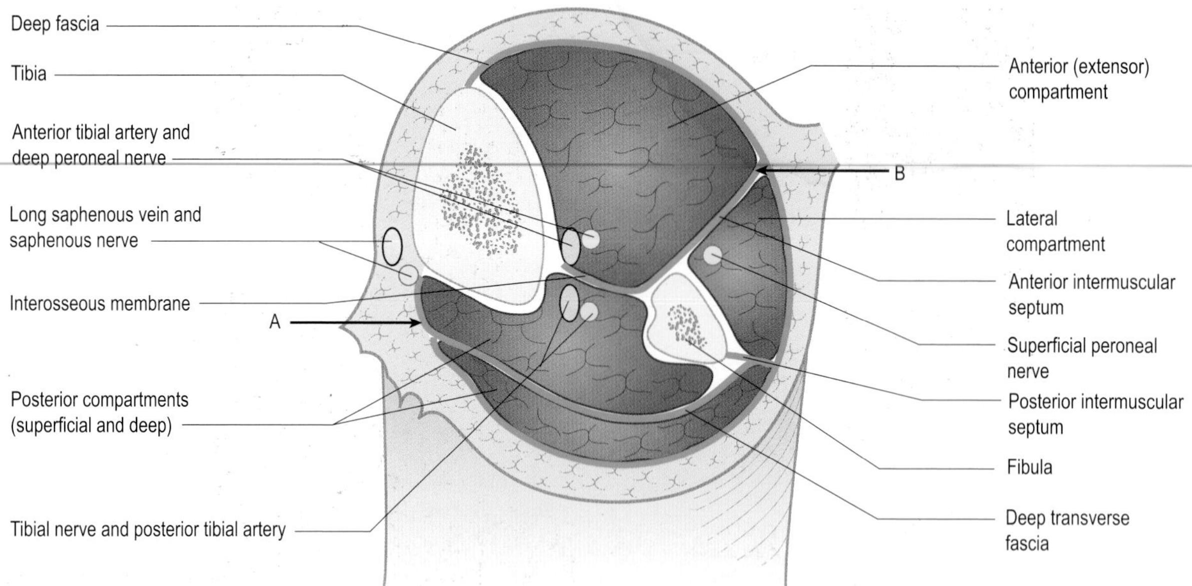


Fig. 6.29 Cross-section of the leg showing compartments of the leg. Arrows A and B show the regions incised for fasciotomy.

## Leg

Structures in the leg are arranged in four compartments bounded by unyielding deep fascia, intermuscular septae, the interosseous membrane and bones (Fig. 6.29). The four compartments are the anterior (extensor), lateral (peroneal) and posterior (flexor), which is further divided into superficial and deep compartments. As each compartment is bounded by unyielding tissues, bleeding into the compartment and/or swelling of the muscles will increase the compartmental pressure as there is no room for expansion. This in turn will compromise the blood supply to the muscles resulting in ischaemic changes. The condition is known as compartment syndrome. See Clinical box 6.3.

## Front of leg and dorsum of foot

The front of the leg has the subcutaneous medial surface of the tibia (Fig. 6.30) on the medial side and the extensor (anterior) compartment of the leg containing the dorsiflexors on the anterolateral side (Fig. 6.31).

### The extensor compartment

This compartment occupies the space between the tibia and fibula in front of the interosseous membrane (Fig. 6.29). It contains the tibialis anterior, extensor hallucis longus, extensor digitorum longus and peroneus tertius muscles, along with the deep peroneal nerve and the anterior tibial vessels. ✪ This is a tight space bounded by unyielding bones, deep fascia, intermuscular septae and the interosseous membrane and hence is a site where neurovascular structures can be compressed by haematoma or muscle oedema, causing compartment syndrome.

The deep fascia in the lower part is thickened to form the superior and the inferior extensor retinacula which holds the tendons of the muscles against the ankle joint and prevents them from bowstringing.

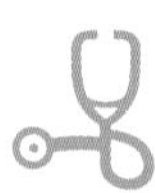

### *Clinical box 6.3*

**Compartment syndrome**

Bleeding and swelling of muscles in any one compartment of the leg can increase the compartment pressure. Increased pressure reduces the capillary blood flow causing ischaemia of the muscles in the compartment. This in turn will cause more swelling and further increase in pressure. Prolonged ischaemia causes necrosis of muscles and nerves. Nerve changes may be reversible in the early changes but muscle necrosis can lead on to fibrosis and development of contractures.

The compartment syndrome can be a complication of tibial fractures, especially closed fractures. It may occur as a complication of ischaemia reperfusion injuries after embolectomy as a result of muscle swelling. Any condition causing swelling of the leg, including muscle hypertrophy following prolonged exercise and even swelling of the leg inside a plaster cast are all possible causes. Pain more severe than the trauma sustained is characteristic of the condition. The main artery need not be occluded and the pulse may be still present. Dorsiflexion of the toes increases the severity of pain (stretching the muscles). As a diagnostic test a small catheter can be inserted to the compartment to measure the pressure. The compartment pressure should normally be about 30mmHg less than the diastolic pressure. Anything more than that should warrant a fasciotomy where the deep fascia is cut longitudinally to lay open the compartment. Usually this is done by two incisions which can lay open all the four compartments (Fig. 6.29). The extensor and peroneal compartments are opened by a long incision in line with the anterior intermuscular septum which is attached to the anterior border of the tibia. The two posterior compartments can be opened by a long incision behind the medial border of the tibia. The long saphenous vein and the saphenous nerve are close to the incision and should be preserved.

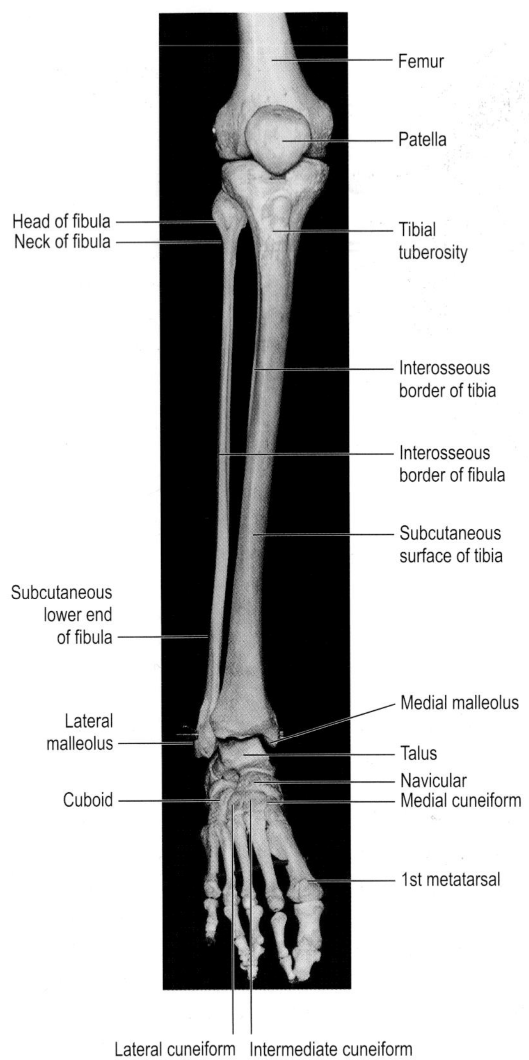


Fig. 6.30 Bones of the leg and foot.

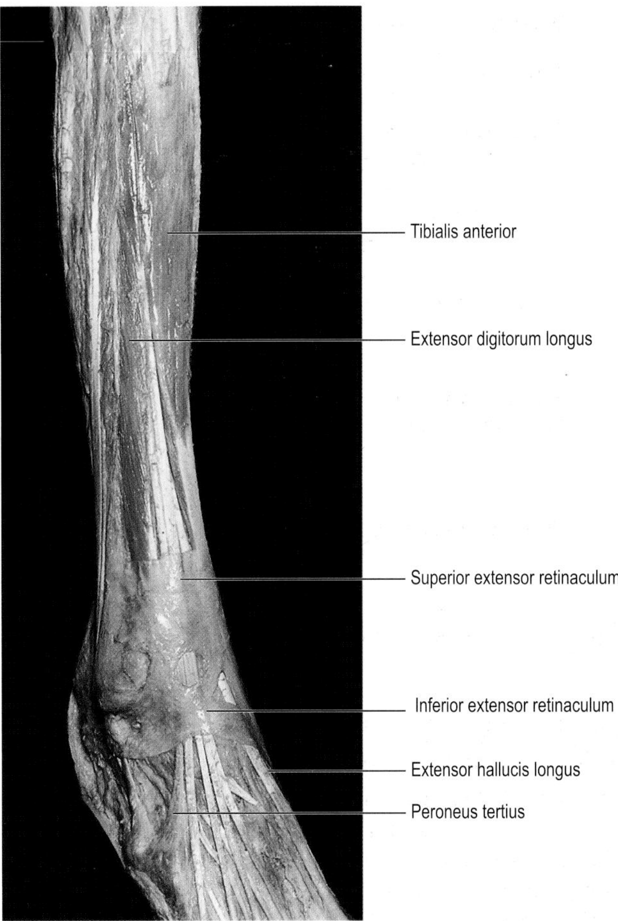


Fig. 6.31 Muscles of the extensor compartment of leg.

### Tibialis anterior

This takes origin from anterolateral surface of the tibia and the interosseous membrane and is inserted into the medial cuneiform and the adjoining first metatarsal bone (Fig. 6.31). It dorsiflexes the ankle and inverts the foot.

*Test* By feeling the tendon at the ankle when the foot is dorsiflexed against resistance.

### Extensor hallucis longus

The origin of the muscle is from the fibula and the interosseous membrane. Its tendon (Figs 6.32, 6.33) is inserted on the distal phalanx of the big toe. It is a dorsiflexor of the big toe and the ankle joint.

*Test* By dorsiflexing the big toe against resistance.

### Extensor digitorum longus

Takes origin from the extensor surface of the fibula, interosseous membrane as well as a small area on the lateral condyle of the tibia.

*Insertion* It has four tendons (Figs 6.32, 6.33) which are inserted to the terminal phalanges of the lateral four toes. Their mode of insertion is similar to that of the extensor digitorum of the hand, as these tendons contribute to the dorsal extensor expansion over the proximal phalanges.

*Action* ✪ The muscle dorsiflexes the lateral four toes and the tendons can be seen and felt as this is done against resistance.

### Peroneus tertius

This arises from the lower third of the fibula and is inserted to the base of the fifth metatarsal bone with an extension of the insertion on its dorsal surface. It is an evertor of the foot.

### The deep peroneal nerve and the anterior tibial artery

All the muscles in the front of the leg are supplied by the deep peroneal nerve which accompanies the anterior tibial artery. These lie between the extensor hallucis longus and the tibialis anterior in front of the interosseous membrane (Fig. 6.34). The nerve lies lateral to the artery and is one of the terminal branches of the common peroneal nerve. As it descends the nerve crosses over to the medial side of the artery but crosses back again to the lateral side in the lower part of the leg. The deep peroneal nerve emerges in the space between the big toe and second toe to supply the skin on its adjacent surfaces. Extensor digitorum brevis having tendons reaching the toes is a muscle arising from the dorsal surface of the calcaneum. The part going to the big toe separates off early from the main muscle mass and is known as the extensor hallucis brevis. Extensor digitorum brevis is also supplied by the deep peroneal nerve.

The anterior tibial artery enters the extensor compartment after it branches off from the popliteal artery by crossing over the interosseous membrane. The

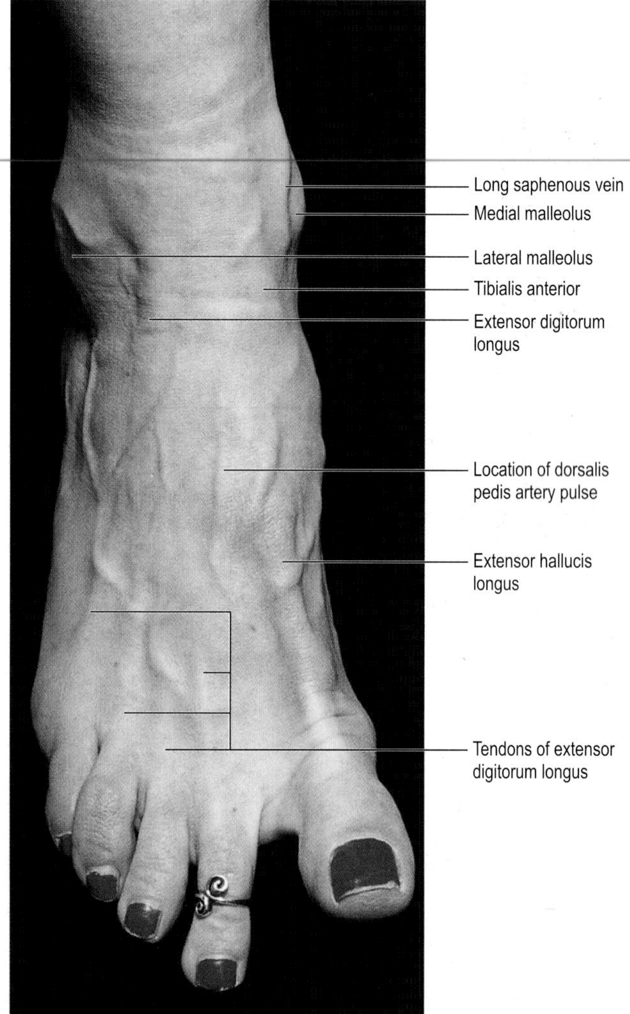


Fig. 6.32 Surface anatomy of the dorsum of the foot.

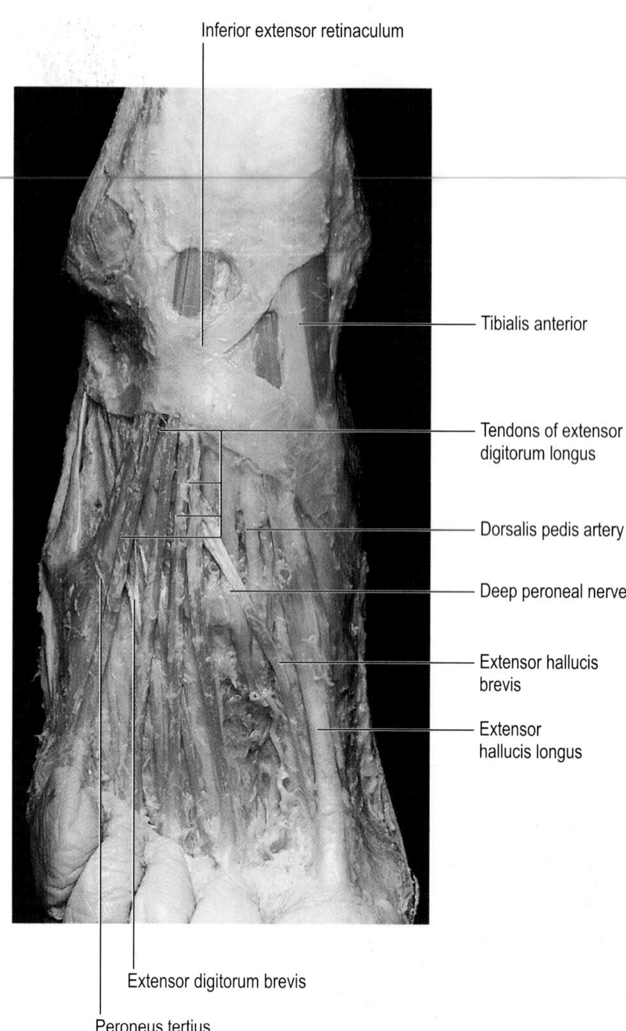


Fig. 6.33 Structures on the dorsum of the foot.

continuation of the artery on the dorsum of the foot is known as the dorsalis pedis artery.

✪ The dorsalis pedis artery pulsation can be felt on the dorsum of the foot lateral to the tendon of the extensor hallucis longus against the navicular and medial cuneiform bones. This artery may be replaced by a perforating branch of the peroneal artery, the pulsation of which may be palpable in front of the lateral malleolus.

## Lateral compartment of the leg

This muscular compartment which lies on the lateral aspect of the leg contains the peroneus longus and peroneus brevis muscles as well as the superficial peroneal nerve which supplies them (Figs 6.29, 6.35, 6.36). Peroneus longus takes origin from the upper two-thirds of the fibula and its tendon passes behind the lateral malleolus to enter the sole of the foot. It then crosses obliquely across to the medial aspect of the sole of the foot to be inserted to the medial cuneiform bone and the base of the first metatarsal. Peroneus brevis arises from the lower two-thirds of the lateral surface of the fibula and its tendon, lying in front of that of the peroneus longus behind the lateral malleolus, is inserted to the tubercle of the base of the fifth metatarsal bone. The peroneus longus and brevis are evertors of the foot. The two peronei tendons are bound down to the lateral malleolus by the superior and inferior peroneal retinacula. The superficial

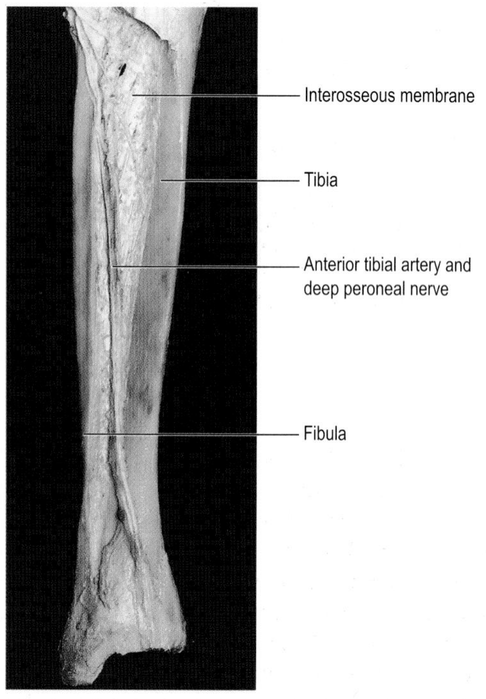


Fig. 6.34 Interosseous membrane – anterior aspect.

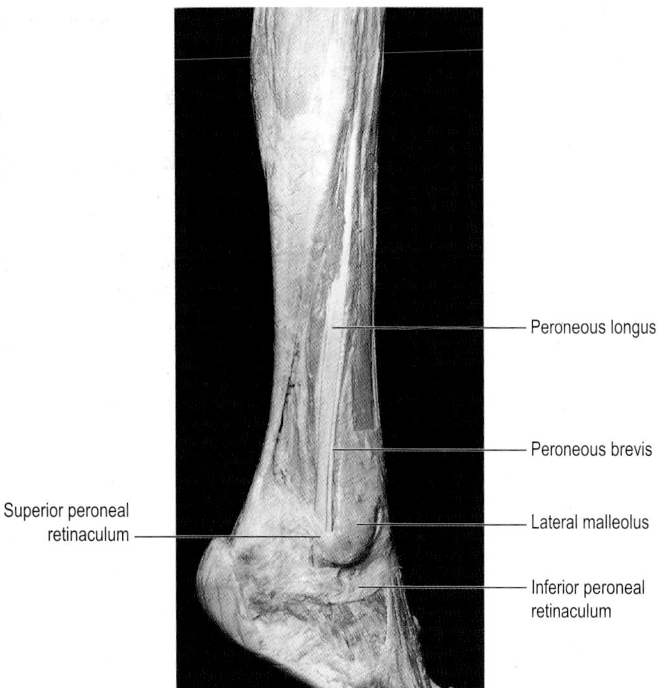


Fig. 6.35 Lateral compartment of the leg.

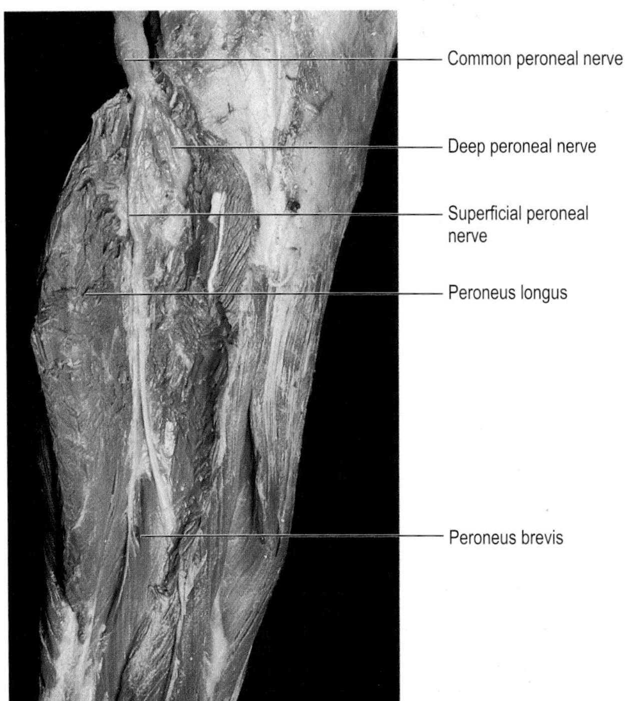


Fig. 6.36 Lateral compartment of the leg. Common peroneal nerve and its divisions.

peroneal nerve begins in the substance of the peroneus longus at the division of the common peroneal nerve. It supplies the two peronei muscles as well as the skin of the lower part of the front of the leg and that of the dorsum of the foot.

✪ The common peroneal nerve winds round the neck of the fibula and divides into superficial peroneal and deep peroneal nerves (Fig. 6.36). It is very superficial as it lies on the neck of the fibula and can easily be damaged in injuries of this region causing a foot drop as a result of paralysis of the dorsiflexors.

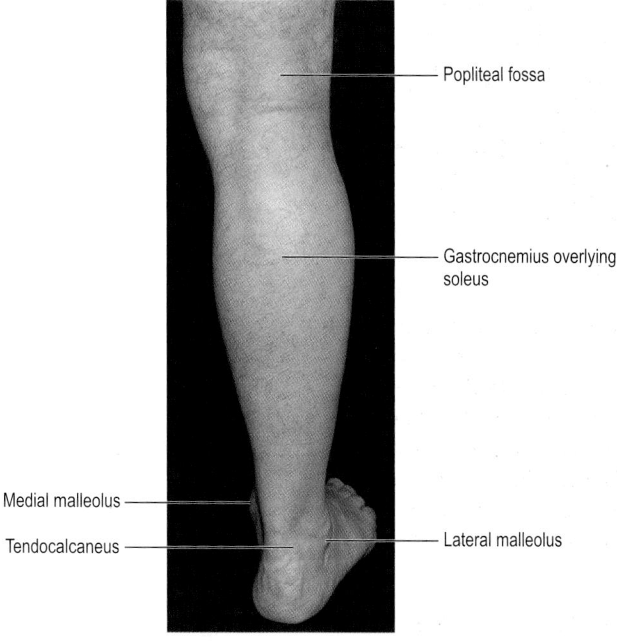


Fig. 6.37 Surface anatomy of the back of the leg.

## Posterior compartments of the leg

The superficial muscles produce the bulge at the back of the leg (Figs 6.37, 6.38). ✪ The short saphenous vein (Fig. 6.38) from the lateral aspect of the dorsal venous arch ascends behind the lateral malleolus to reach the back of the leg. It pierces the deep fascia anywhere between the middle of the calf and the roof of the popliteal fossa to drain into the popliteal vein. The vein, which has several communications with the great saphenous vein, is accompanied by the sural nerve.

The muscles of the calf which are the plantar flexors of the foot and of the toes are arranged in superficial and deep compartments (Fig. 6.29) separated by the thick deep transverse fascia.

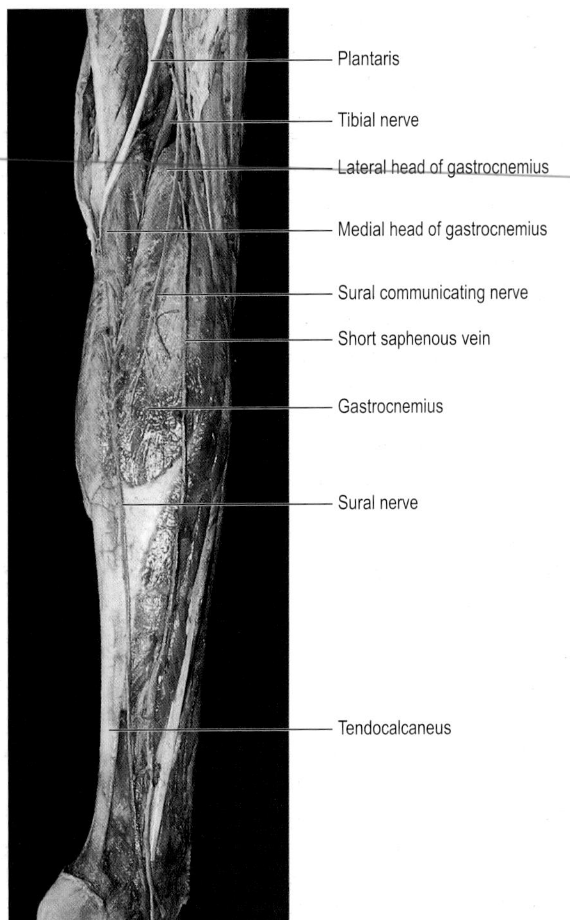


Fig. 6.38 Superficial structures of the back of the leg.

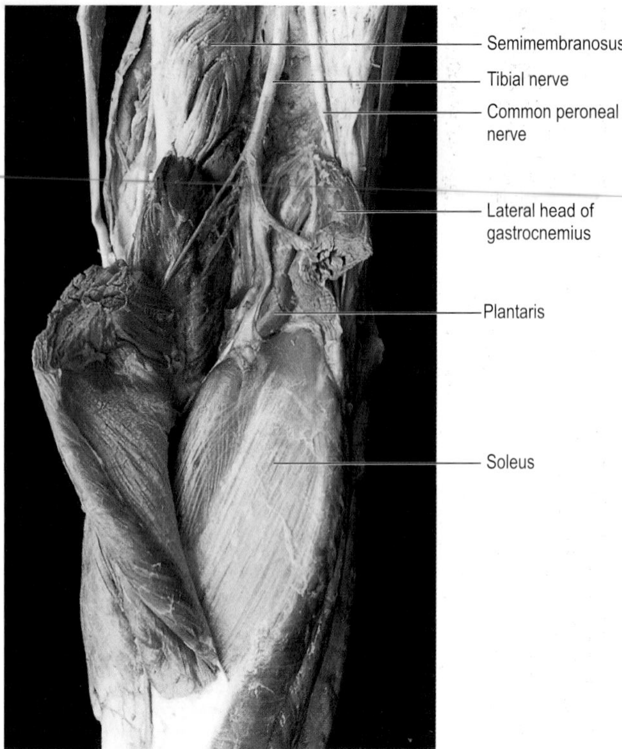


Fig. 6.39 Back of the leg. Structures under the gastrocnemius.

## Superficial compartment

The superficial muscles which are the main plantar flexors of the foot consist of the gastrocnemius, soleus and plantaris, the tendons of which converge to form the tendo calcaneus or Achilles' tendon (Figs 6.38, 6.39, 6.40). The tendoachilles is attached to the posterior surface of the calcaneus. ✪ Rupture of this large tendon can happen in sports injuries. As the tendon is easily palpable a gap is felt on it after it ruptures. Plantar flexion of the foot is weak (there will be some plantar flexion by the deep flexors). The patient is unable to stand on tiptoe.

The gastrocnemius arises by two heads from the lateral and medial femoral condyles (Fig. 6.39). ✪ The plantaris, with a small belly and a long slender tendon, originates from the lateral supracondylar ridge of the femur. Its tendon can be harvested for tendon grafting. However the muscle is absent in about 10% of subjects. The soleus takes origin from the upper third of the back of the fibula, the soleal line of the tibia and from a fibrous arch connecting these two origins. ✪ The muscle contains a venous plexus and the perforating veins connecting the superficial and deep groups of veins pass through it. Contraction of the soleus (soleal pump) aids venous return and stagnation of venous blood here can produce deep vein thrombosis and pulmonary embolism.

## Deep compartment

This is separated from the superficial compartment by the deep transverse fascia. The deep group of muscles contains the flexor digitorum longus, flexor hallucis longus and the tibialis posterior (Fig. 6.40). Flexor digitorum longus takes origin from the posterior surface of the tibia. The flexor

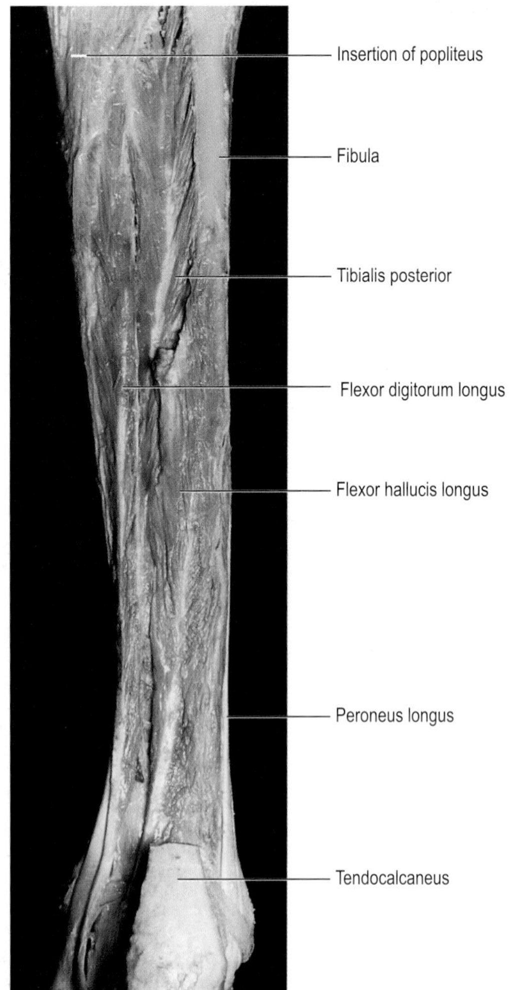


Fig. 6.40 Origin of deep muscles of the posterior compartment of the leg.

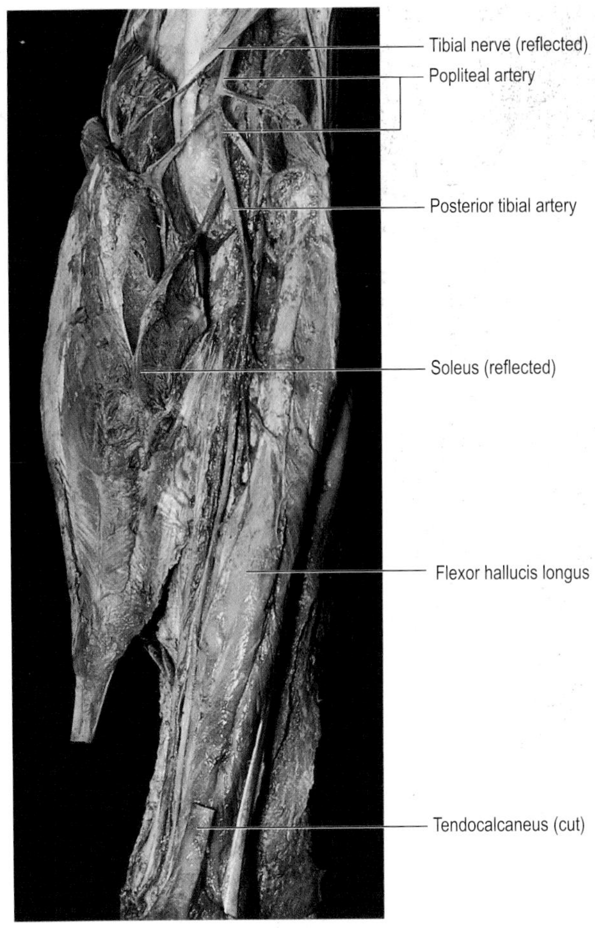


Fig. 6.41 Deep structures of the back of the leg.

hallucis longus, the bulkiest of the three deep flexor muscles, takes origin from the fibula and the interosseous membrane (Figs 6.41, 6.42). It is fleshy until the heel and is known as the 'beef of the heel'. The tibialis posterior is the deepest muscle in the calf and its fibres arise from the back of the fibula and tibia and the interosseous membrane. The tendons of these three muscles pass deep to the flexor retinaculum to enter the sole of the foot. Their further course is described under 'The sole of the foot' below. The flexor retinaculum is a thickening of the deep fascia extending between the medial malleolus and the medial tubercle of the calcaneus. ✪ This roofs the tarsal tunnel (Fig. 6.42) in which lies, from anterior to posterior, the tendons of tibialis posterior, flexor digitorum longus, posterior tibial artery, tibial nerve (which divides here to form the medial and lateral plantar nerves) and the tendon of flexor hallucis longus.

All the muscles in both the posterior compartments are supplied by the tibial nerve. The artery of the posterior compartment is the posterior tibial artery, a terminal branch of the popliteal artery.

### The tibial nerve

This supplies all the muscles in the two posterior compartments. It lies deep to the soleus along with the posterior tibial artery. Its cutaneous branch, the sural nerve, often joined by the sural communicating branch from the common peroneal nerve, supplies the lateral border of the foot. At the lower part of the leg the tibial nerve passes deep to the flexor retinaculum, where it divides into the lateral and medial plantar nerves, to supply the sole of the foot.

### Posterior tibial artery

The posterior tibial artery commences at the lower border of the popliteus as one of the two terminal branches of the popliteal arteries, the other being the anterior tibial artery. It

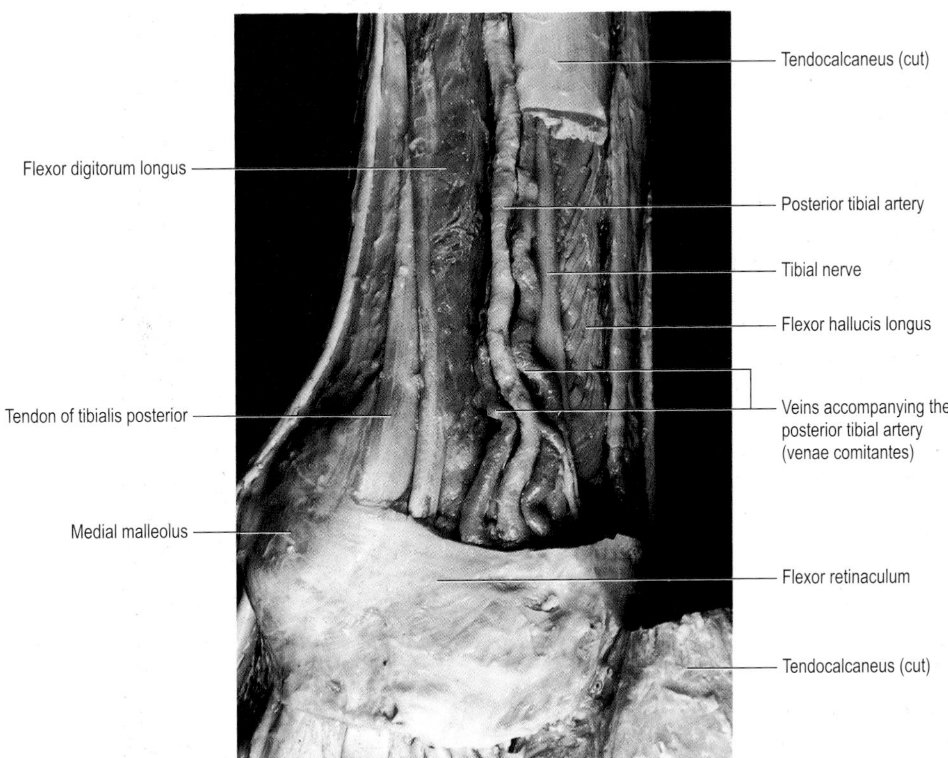


Fig. 6.42 Deep dissection of the lower part of the back of the leg. Structures entering the tarsal tunnel. Right side – seen from the medial aspect.

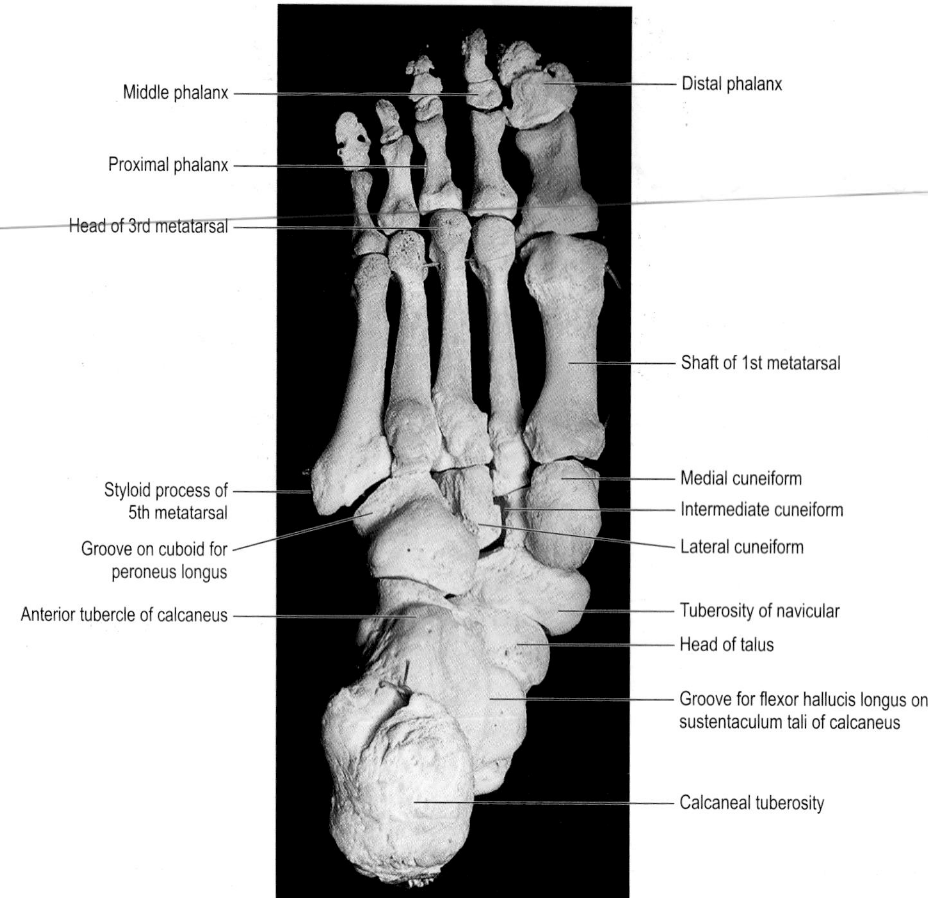


Fig. 6.43 Bones of the foot, plantar aspect.

supplies the back of the leg, i.e. the two posterior compartments and the sole of the foot. Near its commencement the artery gives off the peroneal artery which supplies the deep muscles of the calf and the muscles in the lateral compartment and descends along the medial border of the fibula. The peroneal artery pierces the interosseous membrane to enter the extensor compartment and may replace or supplement the dorsalis pedis artery. The posterior tibial artery enters the sole of the foot by passing deep to the flexor retinaculum. ✪ Its pulsation can be felt midway between the medial malleolus and the medial border of the tendocalcaneus. The pulsation of the peroneal artery is felt in front of the lateral malleolus at its medial border.

### Skeleton of the foot

The skeleton of the foot (Fig. 6.43) consists of seven tarsal bones, five metatarsal bones and the phalanges of the toes. The tarsal bones are the calcaneus, talus, navicular, cuboid and the three cuneiforms. The largest tarsal bone is the calcaneus. Superiorly it articulates with the talus and distally with the cuboid. The talus from distal to proximal has a head, neck and body. The head of the talus articulates with the navicular. The medial, intermediate and lateral cuneiform bones articulate proximally with the navicular and distally with the medial three metatarsal bones. The lateral two metatarsal bones articulate proximally with the cuboid. The metatarsal bones have expanded bases proximally and rounded heads at their distal ends. The first metatarsal is shorter and thicker than the others. The fifth metatarsal bone has a pointed process (styloid process) laterally at its base for the attachment of the peroneus brevis tendon. The big toe has only two phalanges, proximal and distal, whereas each of the remaining four has a proximal, middle and distal phalanx. The skeleton of the foot can be compared with that of the hand. See Clinical boxes 6.4, 6.5.

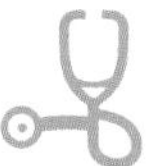

*Clinical box 6.4*

**Avascular necrosis of talus**

A fracture of the talus through its neck (the constriction proximal to the head), often caused by a violent dorsiflexion of the ankle, may cause avascular necrosis of the talus. This is because the talus has a precarious blood supply. As most surfaces of the talus contribute to joints they are lined by hyaline cartilage which is avascular. The only part where there is periosteum (and hence blood vessels) besides the nutrient vessels is the neck of the talus. Vessels enter here and travel proximally to the body and distally to the head.

## The sole of the foot

The muscles of the sole of the foot are arranged in four layers and are covered by the plantar aponeurosis, which is a thickening of the deep fascia. The plantar aponeurosis and the muscles of the sole of the foot, extending from the

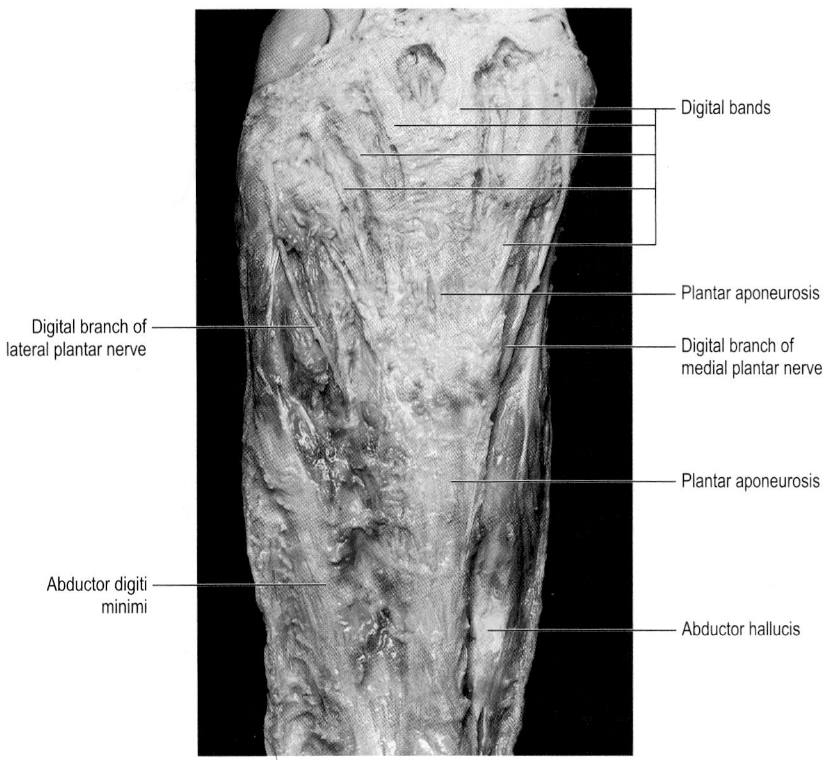


Fig. 6.44 Plantar aponeurosis.

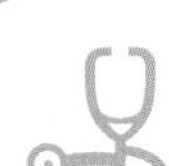

### *Clinical box 6.5*

**Fractures of the metatarsal bones**

Metatarsal bones can fracture by compression, as when a heavy object falls on the foot. Shaft of the metatarsals can also fracture when the foot loses balance and when it is turned suddenly, a type of injury common in footballers and dancers. The styloid process of the fifth metatarsal can be avulsed by the pull of the peroneus brevis in a severe inversion injury of the foot. Metatarsal bones can also fracture due to fatigue (March fracture).

proximal part of the foot to its distal part, act like tie beams or bowstrings, to maintain the longitudinal arches of the foot.

## Plantar aponeurosis

This is the thickened middle portion of the deep fascia which is attached proximally to the medial process of the calcanean tuberosity (Fig. 6.44). Distally it divides into five slips, one to be attached to the fibrous flexor sheath on each toe as well as to the deep transverse metatarsal ligaments which connect the heads of the metatarsal bones.

### Muscles of the first layer

These are shown in Figure 6.45.

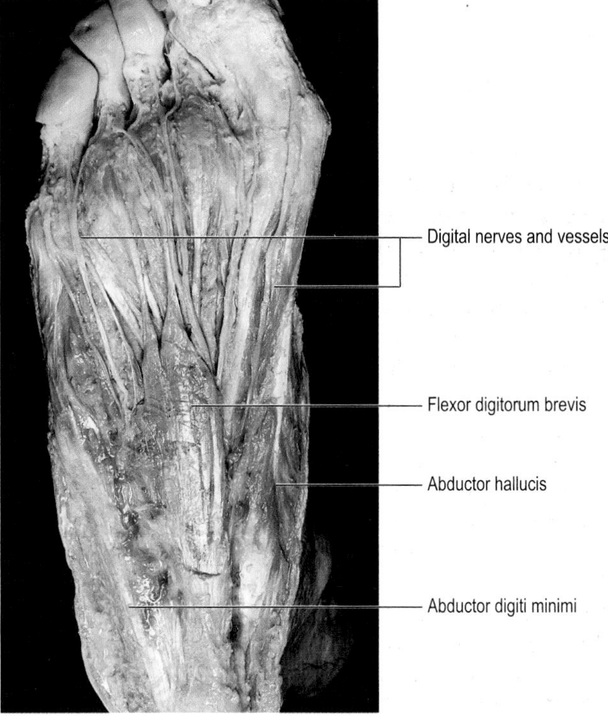


Fig. 6.45 Sole of the foot, first layer.

*Abductor hallucis*

*Origin* Medial process of calcanean tuberosity, flexor retinaculum.

*Insertion* Medial side of base of proximal phalanx of big toe.

*Flexor digitorum brevis*

*Origin* Medial process of calcanean tuberosity, plantar aponeurosis. Gives off four tendons, one for each toe.

*Insertion* Middle phalanges of lateral four toes. Tendon splits for passage of tendons of flexor digitorum longus.

*Abductor digiti minimi*

*Origin* Medial and lateral processes of calcanean tuberosity.

*Insertion* Lateral side of the base of the proximal phalanx of the little toe along with the flexor digiti minimi brevis.

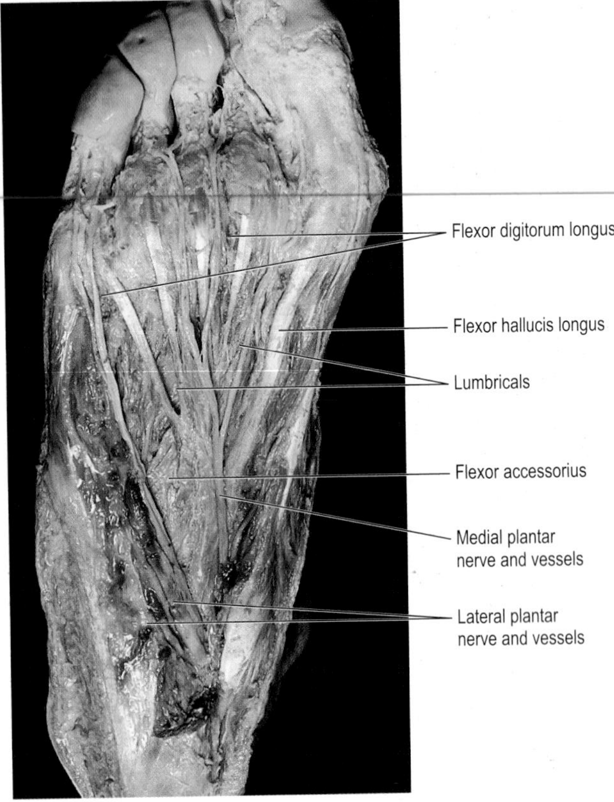


Fig. 6.46 Sole of the foot, second layer. Medial and lateral plantar nerves and vessels.

### The second layer

See Figure 6.46.

*Tendon of flexor hallucis longus*
Lies along the medial border of the foot like a bowstring maintaining the medial longitudinal arch and is crossed inferiorly by the tendon of the flexor digitorum longus. The tendon lies between the two sesamoid bones at the base of the big toe and is finally inserted to the base of the distal phalanx of the big toe.

*Tendon of the flexor digitorum longus*
Proximally in the sole of the foot it divides into four tendons for the lateral four toes as it crosses the tendon of the hallucis longus. The four lumbricals take origin from these. The flexor accessorius is inserted to the digitorum longus tendon. The four tendons for the digits lie deep to those of the digitorum brevis until they reach the plantar surface of the toes where they pierce the brevis tendons to be inserted to the base of the distal phalanges. The arrangement of the lumbricals is similar to those in the palm of the hand.

*The lateral and medial plantar nerves and arteries*
The medial plantar nerve supplies the abductor hallucis, flexor hallucis brevis, flexor digitorum brevis and the first lumbrical. All the remaining intrinsic muscles including the adductor hallucis are supplied by the lateral plantar nerve. The cutaneous branches of the lateral plantar nerve supply the lateral third of the skin of the sole and the lateral one and a half digits. The sensory supply of the remaining skin is by the medial plantar nerve. Thus, the distribution of the two plantar nerves in the sole of the foot resembles the distribution of the median and the ulnar nerves in the palm of the hand – the lateral plantar is similar to the ulnar nerve and the medial plantar to the median.

### The third layer

See Figure 6.47.

*Flexor hallucis brevis*
*Origin* Cuboid, tendon of tibialis posterior.
*Insertion* Splits into two parts to be inserted to the lateral and medial sides of the proximal phalanx of the big toe along with abductor hallucis and adductor hallucis respectively. Small sesamoid bone in each tendon.

*Adductor hallucis*
*Origin* Oblique head from tendon of peroneus longus and metatarsals 2–4. Transverse head from deep transverse ligament and capsules of four metatarsophalangeal joints.
*Insertion* Lateral aspect of proximal phalanx of big toe along with lateral part of flexor hallucis brevis.

*Flexor digiti minimi brevis*
*Origin* Base of fifth metatarsal.
*Insertion* Lateral side of base of proximal phalanx of little toe.

### The fourth layer

The peroneus longus tendon lies in the groove of the cuboid bone before reaching its insertion to the medial cuneiform and the first metatarsal bone. The tibialis posterior tendon is inserted into the tuberosity of the navicular bone and also into all the tarsal bones except the talus. There are two sets of interossei in this layer, three plantar and four dorsal (Figs 6.48, 6.49). Toes 3–5 receive plantar interossei. They are arranged in such a way that they produce adduction of the toes by moving them towards the second toe. The dorsal interossei are abductors of the toes, i.e. moving the toes away from the axis of the movement going through the middle of the second toe. The second toe thus has two dorsal interossei, one on either side. The other two are for toes 3 and 4. The arrangement of the interossei is comparable with those in the palm of the hand.

The long plantar ligament covers the undersurface of the calcaneus and distally is attached to the cuboid and the central three metatarsal bones. It converts the groove on the cuboid into a tunnel in which the tendon of the peroneus longus lies.

### Plantar calcaneonavicular (spring) ligament

The spring ligament extends from the sustentaculum tali to the navicular bone. The head of the talus rests on its upper surface, which forms part of the capsule of the subtalar joint.

## The hip joint

The hip joint (Figs 6.50–6.55) is a ball-and-socket type of synovial joint between the head of the femur and the acetabulum of the hip bone (innominate bone) (Fig. 6.54). As the joint supports the body weight in standing and also propels the trunk forward in locomotion it has to be stable and very mobile. Stability is achieved by a number of factors including its thick capsule and strong ligaments. The mobility is due to the long femoral neck which joins the shaft at an angle.

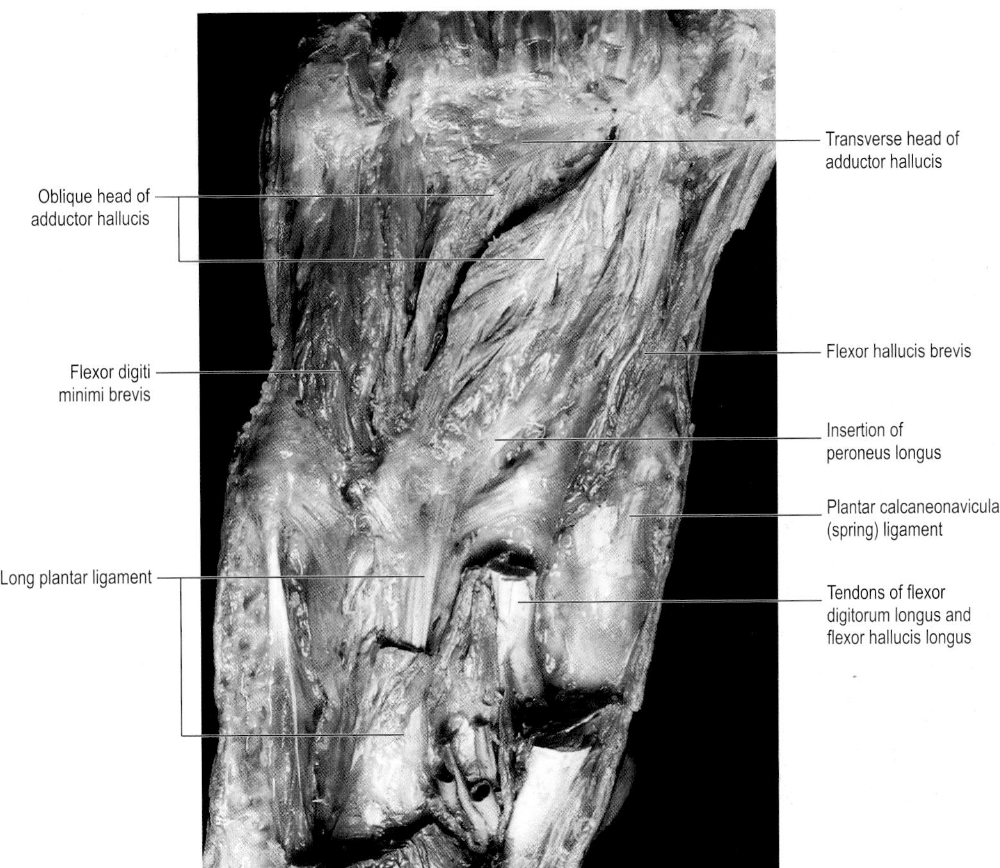


Fig. 6.47 Sole of the foot, third layer.

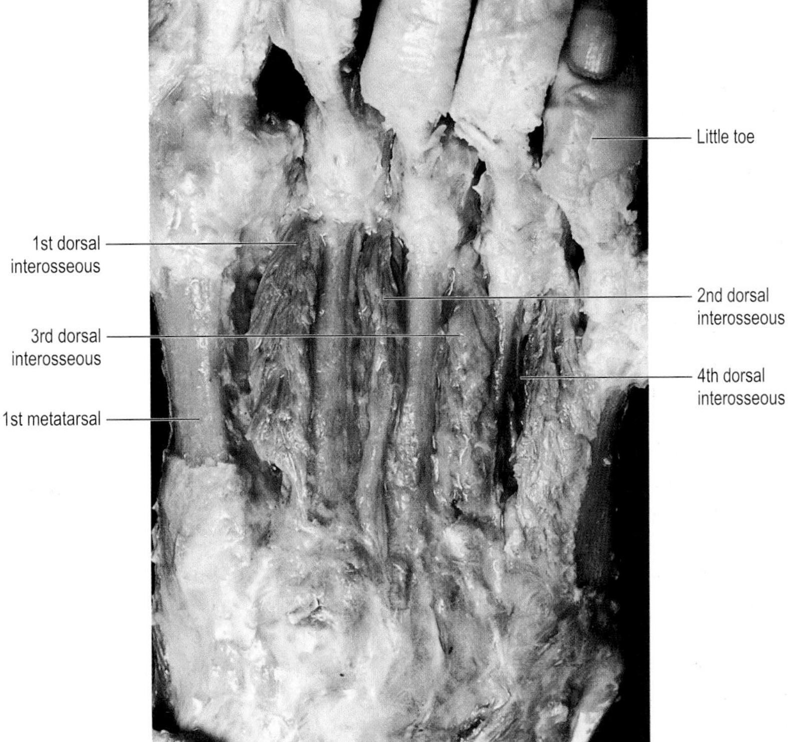


Fig. 6.48 The four dorsal interossei seen from the dorsal aspect of the foot.

## Bony components

The acetabulum has a 'C'-shaped articular surface (Fig. 6.50), the lunate surface, which is lined by hyaline cartilage. The rim of the acetabulum is lined with a fibrocartilagenous acetabular labrum, part of which bridges across the acetabular notch as the transverse acetabular ligament. The deeper part of the acetabulum is non-articular and is occupied by the Haversian pad of fat. The head of the femur is mostly covered by articular cartilage (hyaline). The head has a pit (fovea) which is non-articular and receives the

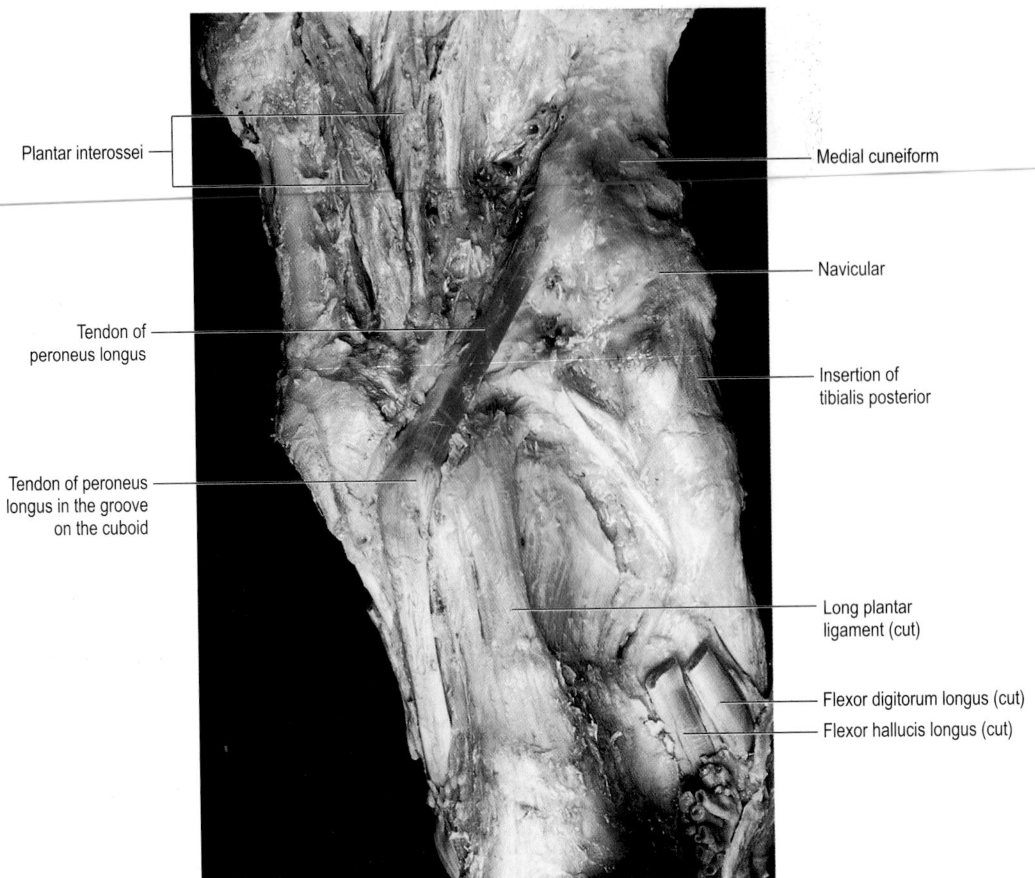


Fig. 6.49 Fourth layer of sole of the foot and the course of peroneus longus tendon.

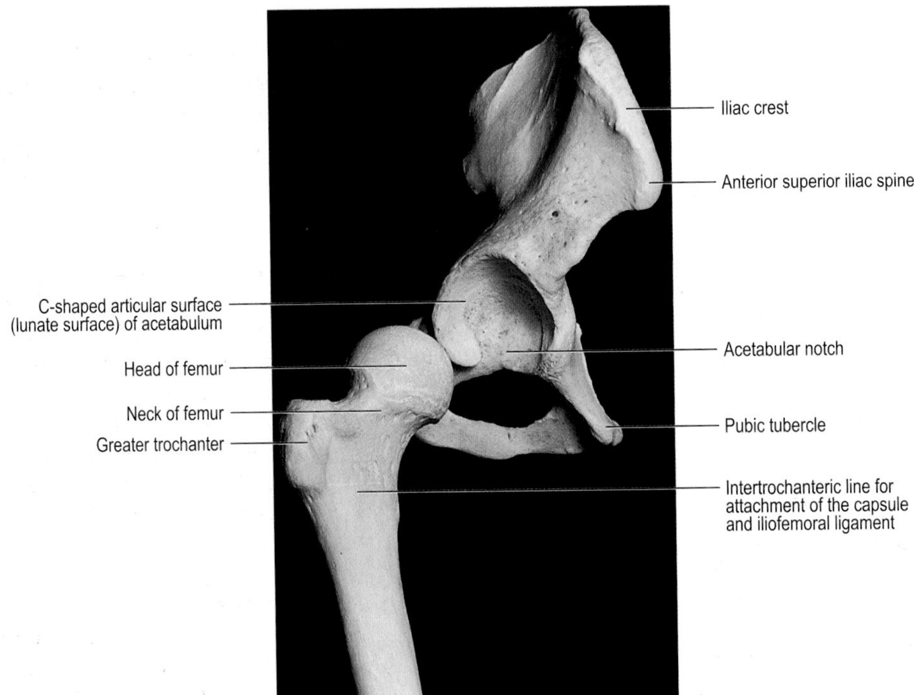


Fig. 6.50 Hip bone and the upper end of femur.

attachment of the ligament of the head of femur which extends to it from the transverse acetabular ligament.

### Capsule

The fibrous capsule (Fig. 6.51) is strong, having its acetabular attachment around its margin just beyond the labrum and transverse ligament. The femoral attachment is on the intertrochanteric line anteriorly and about halfway down the neck posteriorly. The distal half of the posterior aspect of the neck is therefore extracapsular. From its attachment to the femoral neck, fibres of the capsule are reflected back along the neck as retinacular fibres (Fig. 6.52). The blood

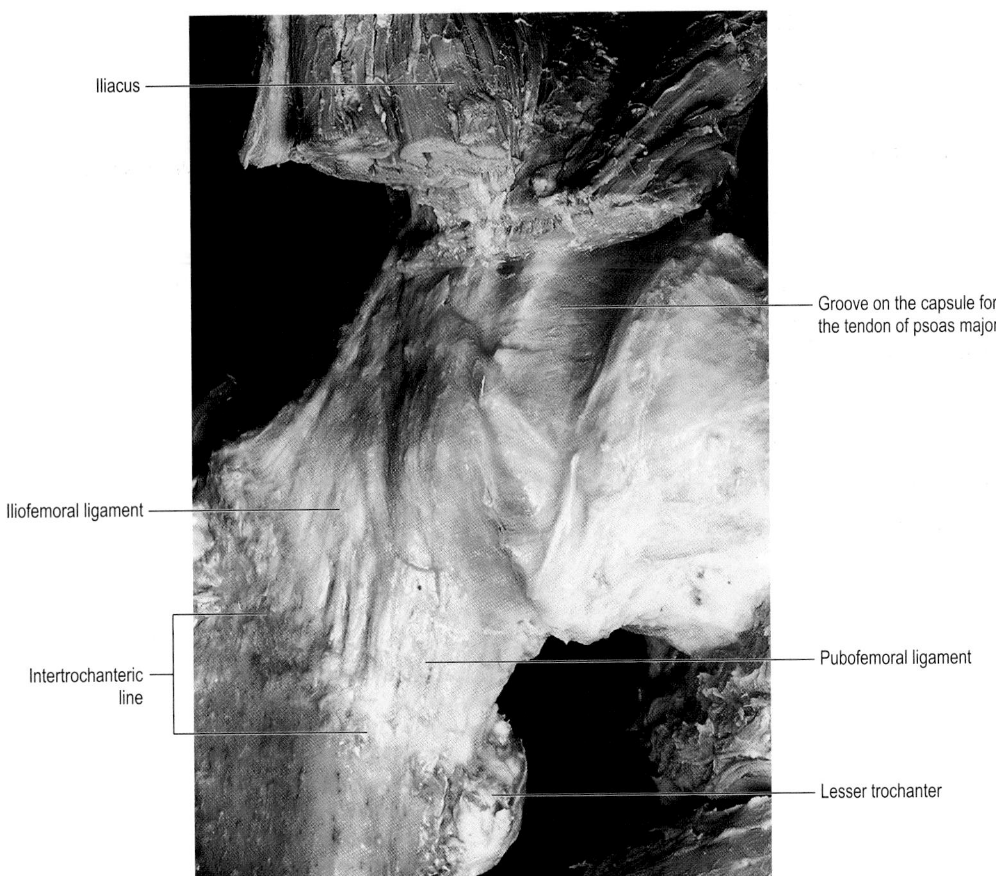


Fig. 6.51 The capsule and ligaments of the hip joint – anterior aspect.

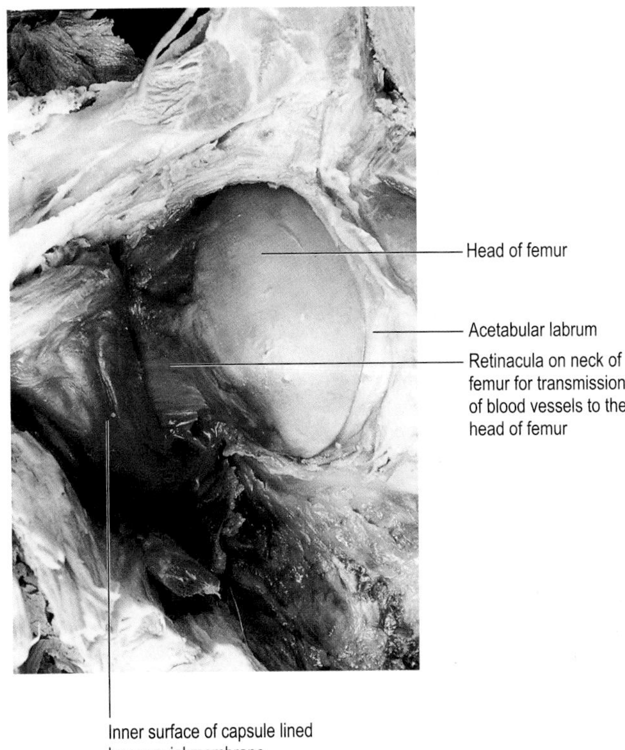


Fig. 6.52 Interior of the hip joint – anterior view.

vessels supplying the femoral head lie deep to these.
✪ Intracapsular fracture of the neck of femur, which is a common injury in the elderly, can result in avascular necrosis of the head of the femur due to rupture of the retinacular fibres and the blood vessels underneath.

## Ligaments

The fibrous capsule is reinforced by three strong extracapsular ligaments. The iliofemoral ligament (ligament of Bigelow) reinforces the anterior aspect of the capsule. The ligament limits extension of the hip joint. The pubofemoral ligament blends with the capsule and the medial part of the iliofemoral ligament. The ischiofemoral ligament spirals on the femoral neck posteriorly. The ligament of the head of femur which extends from the transverse acetabular ligament and the fovea on the head of femur is intracapsular (Fig. 6.53).

## Synovial membrane

The synovial membrane lines the capsule and all intracapsular structures except the articular cartilage in the acetabulum and on the femoral head. The synovial cavity often communicates with the iliac bursa through a gap in the capsule.

## Relations

From medial to lateral the joint is covered anteriorly by the pectineus, tendon of psoas and the iliacus (Fig. 6.7). The obturator externus (Fig. 6.55) spirals downwards and laterally on the inferior aspect of the joint. The pectineus separates the joint from the femoral vein and the psoas tendon separates it

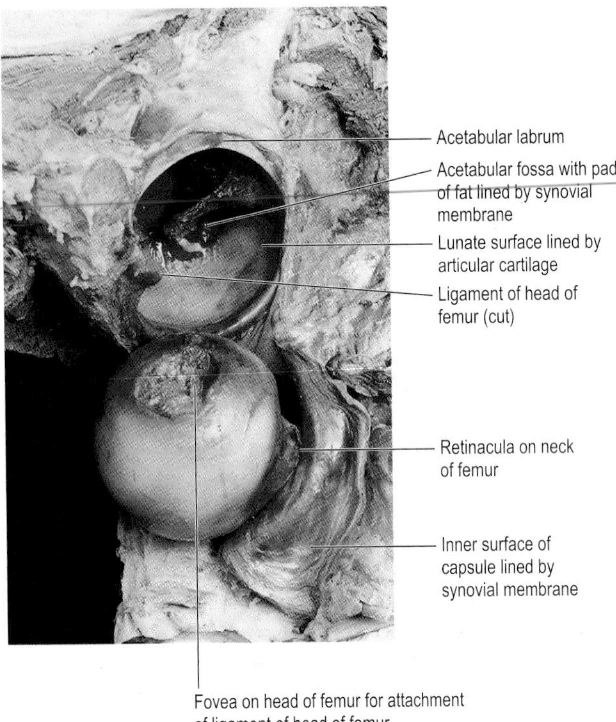


Fig. 6.53 Interior of the acetabulum after dislocation of head of femur.

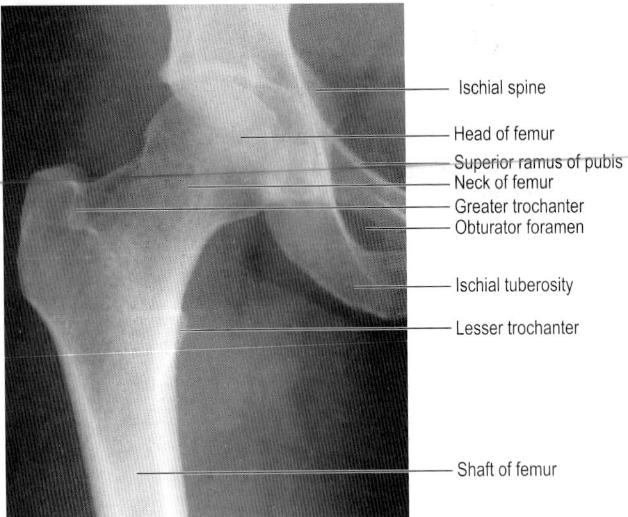


Fig. 6.54 Radiograph of the anteroposterior view of the hip joint.

from the femoral artery. The iliac bursa lies between the iliacus and the joint capsule. The piriformis, the obturator internus tendon, the two gemelli and the sciatic nerve are the immediate posterior relations (Fig. 6.22). The joint is laterally related to the iliotibial tract and medially to the structures in the pelvic cavity. As the acetabular fossa forms the lateral wall of the pelvis, the ovary in the female is separated from the joint only by obturator internus and the lining parietal peritoneum.

✪ Trochanteric bursa, inflammation of (bursitis) which causes hip pain, lies over the lateral aspect of the greater trochanter deep to the gluteus medius. There is also a bursa over the ischial tuberosity, inflammation of which is also painful and is known as the 'weaver's bottom'.

### Movements

✪ In flexion, the head of the femur rotates about a transverse axis up to about 120° when the knee is flexed. It is more

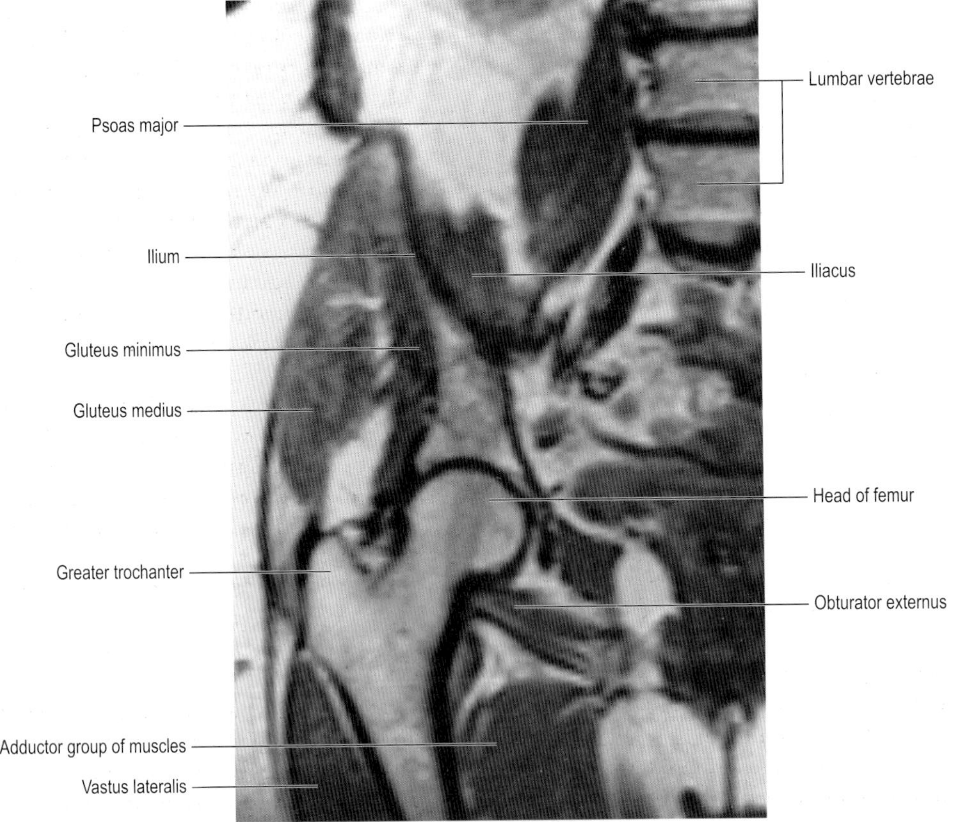


Fig. 6.55 Coronal MRI of the hip region.

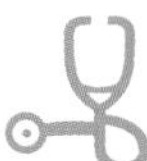

### *Clinical box 6.6*

**Fracture neck of femur**

Though there is a high incidence of fracture of the neck of the femur in elderly females it can occur in any age group and in either sex. Elderly ladies are relatively unsteady on their feet, often also suffer from poor eyesight, and hence tend to trip and fall. The classical finding on examination is a shortening and lateral rotation which is caused by excessive pull by the psoas major muscle. Normally the psoas flexes the hip – when the neck of the femur is broken it pulls the limb forward and rotates it laterally.

The fracture neck of femur is classified as intracapsular or extracapsular, which is also known as intertrochanteric fracture. The intracapsular can be subcapital or transcervical. Orthopaedic surgeons use Garden's classification based on displacement to grade intracapsular fractures. In Garden grade 1 the displacement is minimal whereas it is very marked in grade 4.

The main arterial supply of the head is through the neck of the femur and hence delay in treatment can result in avascular necrosis of the head of the femur where the head crumbles and collapses due to ischaemia. In an intertrochanteric fracture (extracapsular), some blood supply to the head is spared and hence the chance of avascular necrosis is less. The treatment very often is surgical. The procedure varies depending on the age and the type of the fracture. In an elderly person with an intracapsular fracture, the head and neck will be replaced by a prosthesis, a procedure known as hemiarthroplasty. If the acetabulum is very badly worn out, the acetabulum and the femoral head and neck will be replaced by doing a total hip replacement. In a younger person with an intracapasular fracture internal fixation is done by using cannulated hip screws over guide wires under fluoroscopic control. The screws will hold the head and neck together.

Though an extracapsular fracture may heal well with conservative treatment these too are treated by internal fixation as prolonged recumbency may cause problems such as lung infection and deep vein thrombosis. A dynamic hip screw which holds the head and neck together and which in turn is fixed to the shaft of the femur is used for internal fixation.

limited when the knee is extended due to tension in the hamstrings. Flexion is achieved by the psoas major and the iliacus assisted by the sartorius, the rectus femoris and the pectineus. The movement is limited by the tension of the hamstrings. Extension, the reverse of flexion, is possible to a range of about 20° produced by gluteus maximus at the extremes of movements and hamstrings in the intermediate ranges. Tension of the iliofemoral ligament limits extension. During abduction the head of femur rotates about an anteroposterior axis up to about 60°. The movement is produced by gluteus medius and minimus assisted by tensor fasciae latae and sartorius. Tension of the adductors and the pubofemoral ligament limits abduction. Adduction, the opposite of abduction, is by adductors longus, brevis and magnus, aided by the pectineus and the gracilis. In lateral rotation the femoral head rotates about a vertical axis passing through the centre of head to the medial condyle. The femoral neck swings backward about this axis. Due to the angle between the neck and the shaft this axis of rotation does not pass though the shaft of the femur. The piriformis, the obturator internus, the superior and inferior gemelli, the quadratus femoris, the obturator externus, assisted by gluteus maximus and sartorius are lateral rotators. Anterior fibres of the gluteus medius and minimus assisted by tensor fasciae latae act as medial rotators.

✪ Contraction of the abductors is essential in one-leg standing, in walking and running, to prevent adduction of the hip. When the neck of the femur is fractured rotation takes place about an axis passing through the shaft of the femur. The psoas and the iliacus then laterally rotate the femur which is characteristic of a fractured femoral neck.

✪ The hip joint can dislocate due to violent trauma as in a road traffic accident. Posterior dislocation is more common than anterior and central (where the head of the femur breaks through the acetabulum into the pelvis) dislocations. The sciatic nerve is prone to injury in posterior dislocations. See Clinical boxes 6.6, 6.7, 6.8.

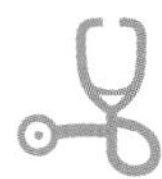

### *Clinical box 6.7*

**Dislocation of hip**

The hip joint is very stable unlike the shoulder. It has a deep socket in the form of acetabulum in which the head of the femur makes a good fit. The fibrous capsule is strong and tight and is reinforced by strong ligaments, especially in front of the joint. The strong muscles moving the joint also adds to its stability. In spite of its strong construction the hip joint can dislocate as it is susceptible to severe traumatic forces, especially in road traffic accidents (RTAs). It can dislocate anteriorly, posteriorly or centrally (into the pelvis by breaking the acetabulum). The posterior dislocation is the commonest. Majority of posterior dislocation occurs when a severe force is directed upwards along the femur when it is flexed and adducted. This happens in a RTA when the knee strikes the dashboard. As the sciatic nerve lies immediately behind the joint it may be damaged.

The treatment is usually by reduction under general anaesthesia. Following this traction will be applied to the limb for about 6 weeks to allow healing of the capsule. If the dislocation is associated with fracture of the acetabulum an open reduction and internal fixation may be necessary.

## The knee joint

In this, the largest synovial joint in the body, the condyles of the femur articulate with those of the tibia and the patella articulates with the femur. It is a modified hinge joint where besides flexion and extension there is a certain amount of rotation possible when the joint is flexed. Structures related to the knee joint can be seen in Figures 6.56–6.69.

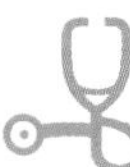

## *Clinical box 6.8*

### Surgical exposure of the hip joint

The hip joint can be exposed using different approaches. Being a deep-seated joint surgical exposure is likely to encounter a number of structures surrounding it. In the posterior approach the gluteus maximus is split and the underlying gluteus medius and minimus are detached. The sciatic nerve is retracted medially. The obturator internus tendon and the two gemelli are cut to expose the capsule.

The anterior approach is through the gap between the sartorius medially and the gluteus medius and minimus laterally. The reflected head of the rectus femoris which lies over the anterior aspect of the capsule is cut to expose the joint.

The anterolateral approach is between the tensor fasciae late and the gluteus medius. Anterior fibres of the gluteus medius and minimus are retracted or detached from their attachment to the greater trochanter. The superior gluteal nerve is vulnerable in this approach. Bleeding can occur from the branches of the lateral circumflex artery.

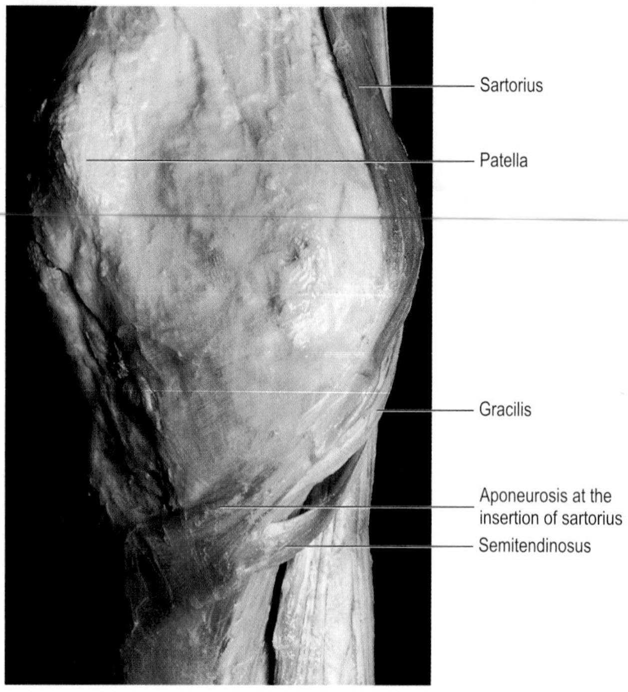


Fig. 6.57 Structures related to the medial aspect of the knee joint. Sartorius, gracilis and semitendinosus.

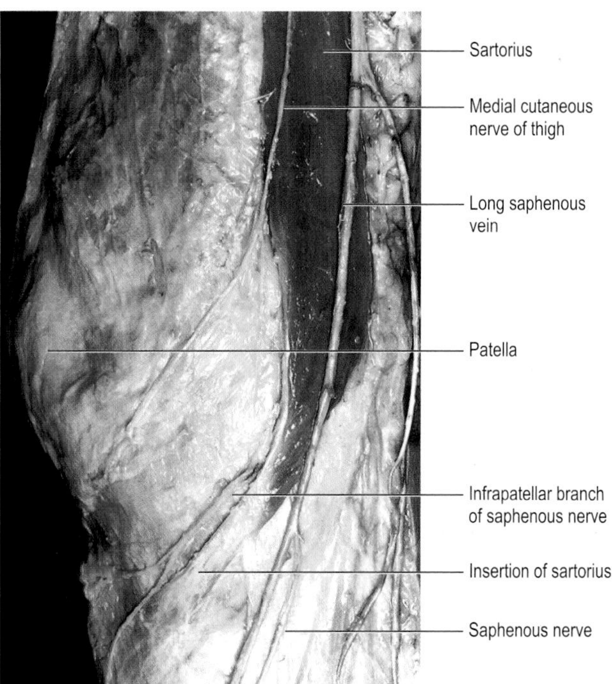


Fig. 6.56 Structures related to the medial aspect of the knee joint. Long saphenous vein and saphenous nerve.

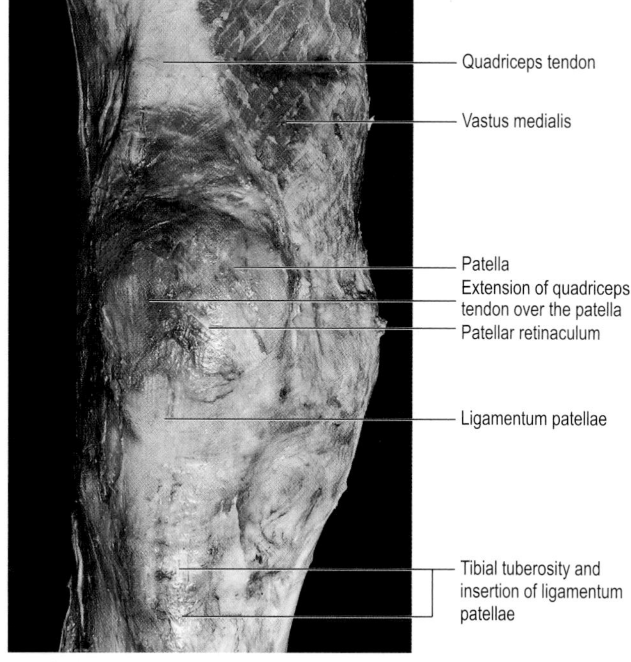


Fig. 6.58 Anterior aspect of the knee joint.

The knee joint has on its medial aspect the medial (tibial) collateral ligament and on its lateral aspect the lateral (fibular) collateral ligament, posteriorly the oblique popliteal ligament and the popliteus muscle, and anteriorly the tendon of the quadriceps, patella and the ligamentum patellae. (Fig. 6.58).

The quadriceps tendon, the patella and the ligamentum patella in the anterior aspect of the joint forming the extensor mechanism of the knee has been described already (p. 138).

### Tibial collateral ligament

This ligament (Fig. 6.61) is broad and extends from the medial epicondyle of the femur to the medial surface of the tibia. It is crossed by the tendons of the sartorius, the gracilis and the semimembranosus with a bursa intervening. The ligament blends with the capsule of the knee joint and it is also posteriorly attached to the medial meniscus. ✪ Rupture of the ligament due to a blow on the lateral aspect of the joint can cause tearing of the medial meniscus. The medial inferior genicular vessels and nerves and an extension of the semimembranosus tendon insertion are deep to the distal part of the ligament.

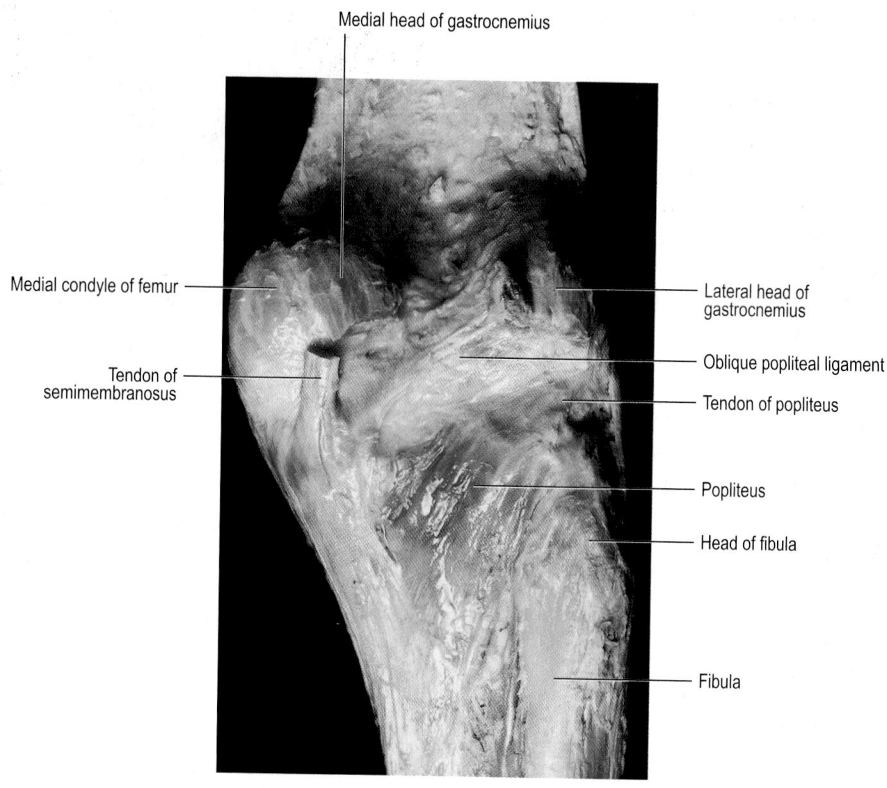


Fig. 6.59 Posterior aspect of the knee joint. Oblique popliteal ligament.

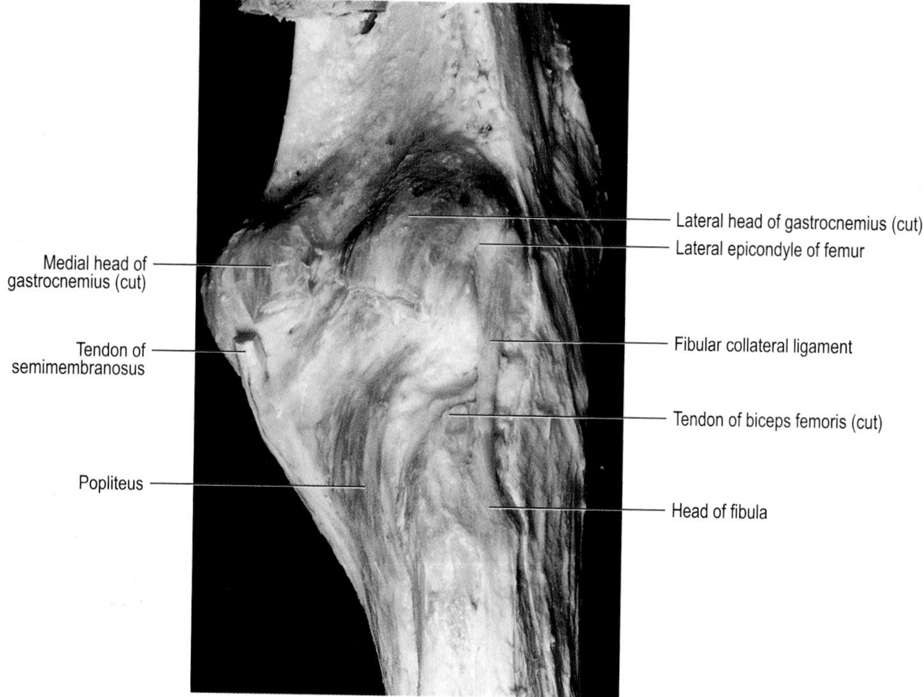


Fig. 6.60 Posterolateral aspect of the knee joint. Fibular collateral ligament.

## Fibular collateral ligament

This is a cord-like ligament which is attached to the lateral epicondyle of the femur above and to the head of the fibula below (Fig. 6.60). It is covered by the tendon of the biceps. Unlike the medial ligament it is not attached to the capsule of the joint or to the lateral meniscus.

## Oblique popliteal ligament

This ligament (Fig. 6.59), which blends with the posterior aspect of the capsule of the joint, is an extension of the insertion of the semimembranosus from the posterior aspect of the medial tibial condyle upwards and laterally to the lateral condyle of the femur. The popliteal artery lies on it and the genicular nerves and vessels pierce it.

## Cruciate ligaments

The two cruciate ligaments which lie within the capsule maintain the anteroposterior stability of the joint. They are named after their tibial attachments, the anterior cruciate ligament being attached to the anterior aspect of the

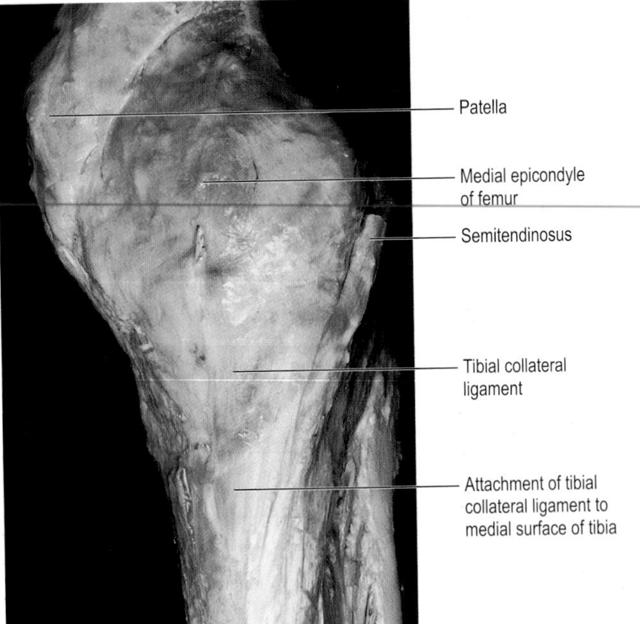


Fig. 6.61 Medial aspect of the knee joint. Tibial collateral ligament.

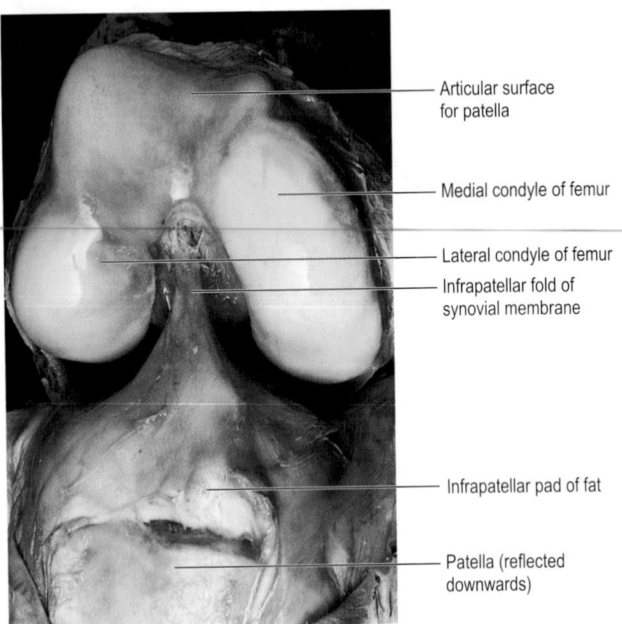


Fig. 6.62 Knee joint opened from the front after reflection of the quadriceps tendon and the patella.

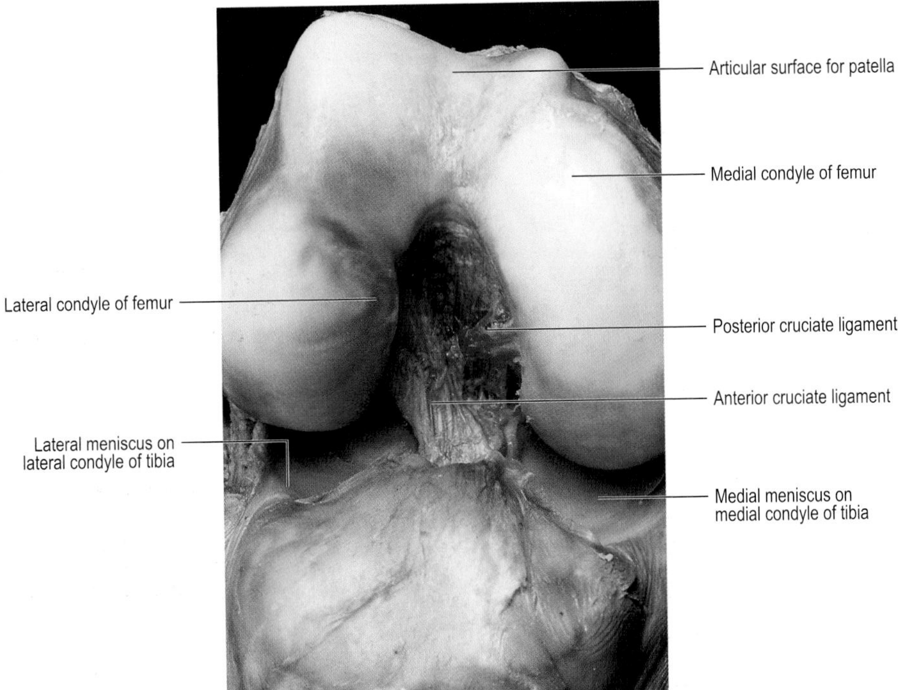


Fig. 6.63 Interior of the knee joint seen from the front – the cruciate ligaments.

intercondylar area of the tibia and the posterior cruciate ligament to the smooth impression on the posterior aspect. They are extrasynovial and when they cross the anterior cruciate is anterolateral to the posterior ligament.

✪ The anterior cruciate ligament (Fig. 6.63) from its tibial attachment between the anterior horns of the medial and lateral menisci ascends posterolaterally to be attached to the lateral femoral condyle at its posteromedial aspect.

✪ The posterior cruciate ligament is the most posterior structure in the intercondylar area of the tibia and its attachment extends on to the posterior surface of the shaft (see Fig. 6.69). From there it ascends to its femoral attachment to the anterolateral aspect of the medial condyle. It is shorter and stronger than the anterior cruciate ligament.

✪ The anterior cruciate ligament resists excessive forward glide of the tibia on the femur or backward glide of the femur on the tibia. The posterior cruciate ligament resists excessive posterior glide of the tibia on the femur or anterior glide of femur on tibia. They can be tested by bending the knee to 90° and rocking the tibia forward and backward (the drawer test).

✪ The menisci (Figs 6.64, 6.65) are tough avascular fibrocartilages whose anterior and posterior ends are anchored to the intercondylar area of the tibia. They deepen the concavity of the tibial surface and also help to spread the

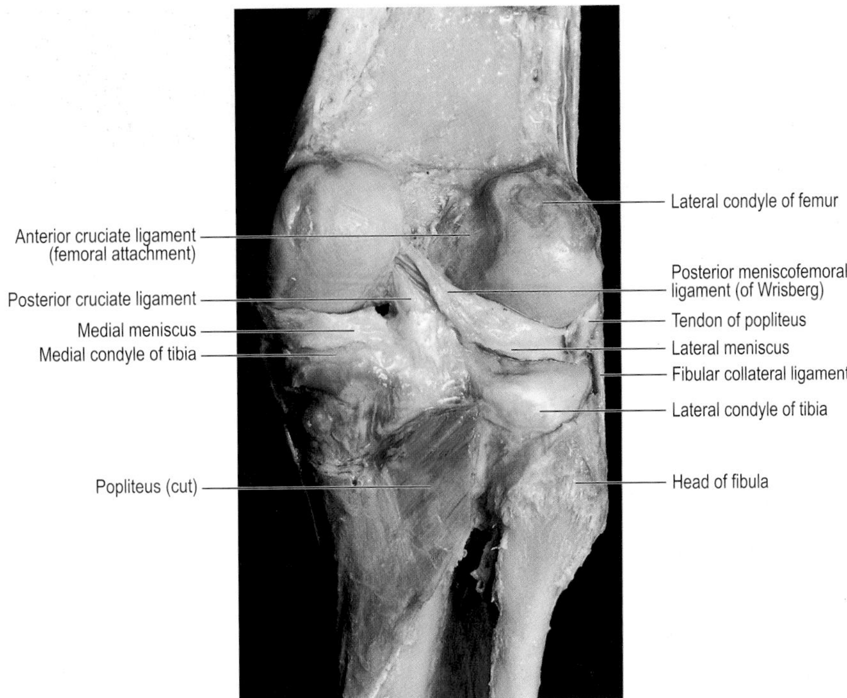


Fig. 6.64 Interior of the knee joint viewed from behind.

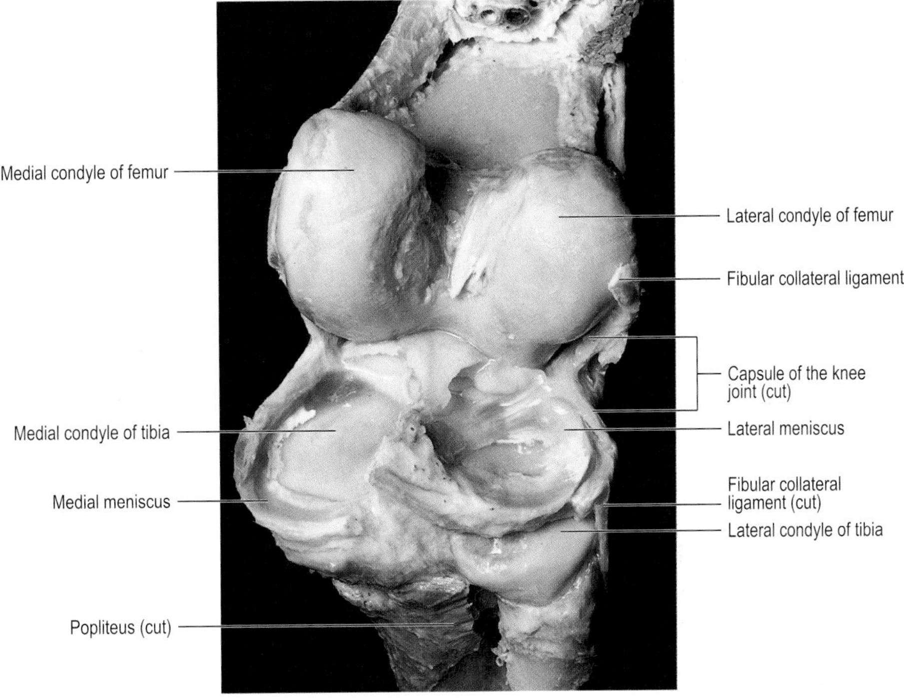


Fig. 6.65 Interior of the knee joint viewed from behind – lateral and medial menisci.

synovial fluid. The medial meniscus is less mobile than the lateral meniscus and hence is more prone to injury. Its mobility is markedly restricted by its attachment to the tibial collateral ligament. The anterior horn of the meniscus is attached to the intercondylar area in front of the anterior cruciate ligament whilst its posterior horn is similarly attached in front of the posterior cruciate ligament. The meniscus is broader posteriorly. The lateral meniscus is more circular and is attached to the popliteus which makes it more mobile and less prone to injury. Its anterior horn is attached behind the anterior cruciate ligament in front of the intercondylar tubercle of the tibia, whilst the posterior horn attachment is behind the tubercle but in front of the attachment of the posterior horn of the medial meniscus.

From the posterior aspect of the lateral meniscus the anterior and posterior meniscofemoral ligaments (of Humphry and Wrisberg) (Fig. 6.64) extend upwards and medially to the medial femoral condyle. The anterior meniscofemoral ligament lies in front of the posterior cruciate ligament and the posterior ligament behind. See Clinical boxes 6.9, 6.10.

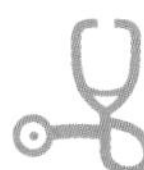

## Clinical box 6.9

### Meniscal tears of the knee

This commonly occurs in professions where the knee is susceptible to a twisting force while weight-bearing. It is common in footballers and miners. The medial meniscus is more commonly torn than the lateral meniscus. When the flexed knee is abducted and externally rotated forcefully the medial meniscus gets split between the grinding surfaces of the medial condyles of the femur and tibia. The knee will be painful and it will be swollen because of effusion. The knee locks because the torn segment of the meniscus gets lodged between the tibia and femur blocking extension. **McMurray's test** will be positive. In this a flexed knee is rotated while extending. If the movement causes a painful click the test is positive. Treatment is meniscectomy by arthroscopy followed by exercises for strengthening the quadriceps as it might have wasted following the injury.

✪ The synovial membrane of the joint is extensive. The suprapatellar bursa, an extension of the synovial cavity, extends upwards under the quadriceps (Figs 6.68, 6.69). The infrapatellar fold of synovial membrane (Fig. 6.62) extending from that covering the infrapatellar pad of fat is attached to the intercondylar area of the femur.

✪ A number of bursae are associated with the knee joint besides the suprapatellar bursa. There are two subcutaneous bursae anteriorly, subcutaneous infrapatellar bursa and the prepatellar bursa, in front of the tibial tubercle and the patella respectively. The deep infrapatellar bursa lies deep to the patellar ligament. Laterally there is a bursa between the fibular collateral ligament and the biceps femoris and another one deep to the fibular collateral ligament. Medially there is a bursa between the sartorius and the gracilis tendons and the tibial collateral ligament. The semimembranosus bursa is between that muscle and the medial head of gastrocnemius and may communicate with the joint cavity via a bursa which is deep to the gastrocnemius. Similarly the bursa under the popliteus also communicates with the joint cavity. The suprapatellar bursa under the lower part of the quadriceps is an upward extension of the synovial cavity of the knee joint.

✪ Inflammation of the bursae or bursitis causes swelling around the knee. Leaning forward on the knees produces friction between the prepatellar bursa and the bone causing prepatellar bursitis or housemaid's knee. The infrapatellar bursitis, which is also known as clergyman's knee, is more distally placed. A painless swelling at the back of the knee medially may be a semimembranosus bursa. Swelling of the joint by fluid collection in the synovial cavity may be masked by its extension into the suprapatellar bursa deep to the quadriceps

AP and lateral views of radiological images of the knee are shown in Figures 6.66 and 6.67. MRI scans of the joint can be seen in Figures 6.68 and 6.69.

### Movements

✪ Flexion and extension are the main movements of the knee joint. When the knee is fully extended the posterior part of the capsule and all the ligaments except the posterior cruciate ligament are taut converting the leg and thigh into a rigid column – the knee is 'locked'. Flexion and extension of the tibia is accompanied by rotation – medial rotation of the femur during extension and lateral rotation during flexion. During flexion the popliteus will rotate the femur laterally loosening the ligaments to 'unlock' the joint. The popliteus, which has a tendinous origin from the lateral condyle of the

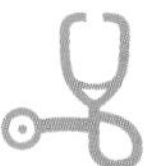

## Clinical box 6.10

### Ligament injuries of the knee

**Anterior cruciate ligament**

Rupture of the anterior cruciate ligament (ACL) is a common injury. It causes bleeding into the joint (haemarthrosis). The anterior cruciate ligament normally limits forward movement of the tibia on the femur. In sporting activities a force pushing the upper end of the tibia forward, especially when associated with a twisting force, can avulse the ligament. Integrity of ACL is tested by the **anterior drawer test** and **Lachman's test**. In the former the flexed tibia is drawn forward on the femur by holding its upper end with both hands. If positive (i.e. when the ligament is torn) the tibia moves forward. In the Lachman's test with the knee more or less straight the lower end of the femur is held firmly with one hand while the upper end of the tibia is moved anteriorly with the other. Normally there is only very minimal movement. If the ACL is torn the tibia will freely glide forward. A ruptured ACL, if left untreated, will make the knee unstable and it is likely to give way periodically while walking. Reconstruction of the ligament is done by using part of patellar ligament or hamstring tendon.

**Posterior cruciate ligament**

The posterior cruciate ligament may be injured by a force pushing the tibia excessively backwards on the femur. A positive posterior drawer test where the flexed tibia can be pushed backwards may be elicited.

**Collateral ligaments**

Medial collateral ligament ruptures more frequently than lateral. Injury is caused by a violent abduction force on the tibia. The medial collateral injury may be part of a triad along with a tear of the medial meniscus and rupture of the anterior cruciate ligament.

**Rupture of the extensor mechanism**

Rupture of the quadriceps tendon, fracture of the patella or rupture of the patellar tendon may happen by resisted extension of the knee. It happens while stumbling on a chair or when the foot is caught by an obstacle while running or jumping and also while kicking a muddy football. Location of the injury varies with age. In young people the patellar tendon ruptures, in the middle aged the patella fractures, whereas in the elderly it is usually the quadriceps tendon which ruptures.

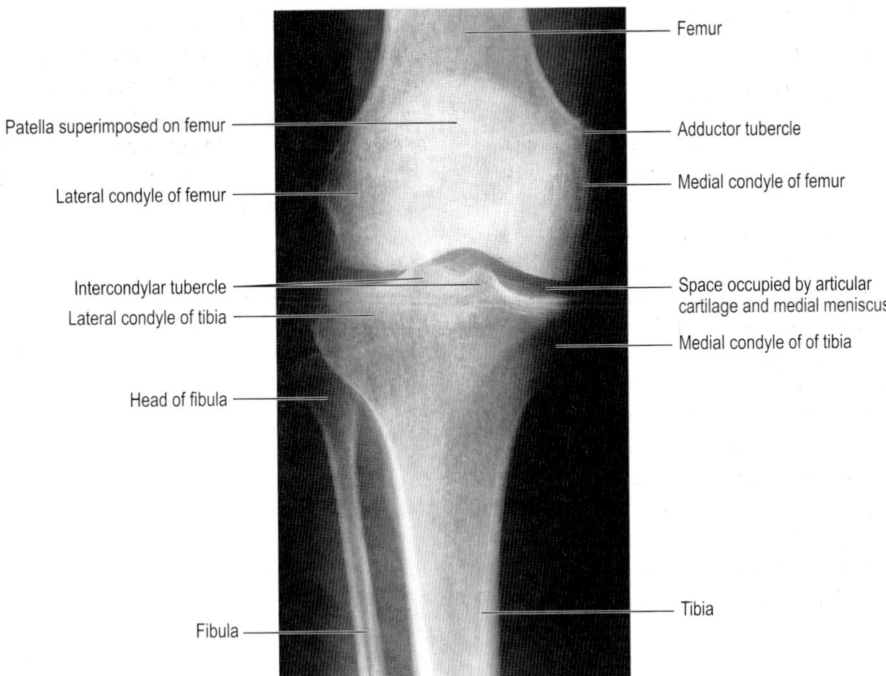


Fig. 6.66 Anteroposterior radiograph of the knee joint.

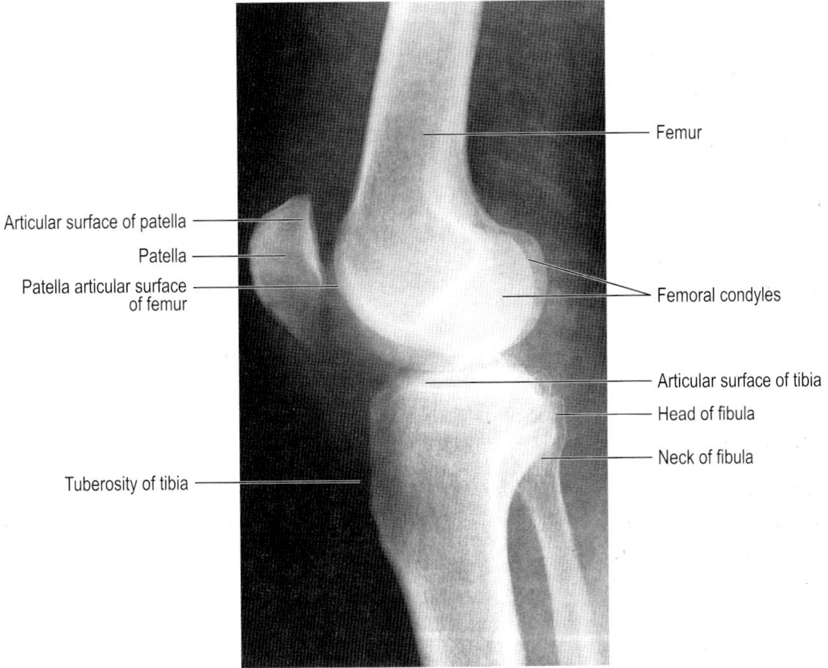


Fig. 6.67 Lateral radiograph of the knee joint.

femur inside the joint, is inserted to the upper part of the posterior surface of the tibia.

Medial and lateral rotation can take place independently of flexion and extension in a flexed joint. The sartorius, the semitendinosus, the gracilis and the semimembranosus rotate the tibia medially and the biceps rotate it laterally.

✪ The patella moves upwards during extension with a tendency for lateral displacement because of the pull of the quadriceps upwards and laterally parallel to the obliquity of the femur. Lateral dislocation of the patella is prevented by the prominence of the lateral condyle of the femur and by the horizontal fibres of the vastus medialis, which are inserted to the medial surface of the patella.

## Ankle joint

The tibia and fibula are connected to each other by the superior and the inferior tibiofibular joints as well as by the interosseous membrane (see Fig. 6.34). The inferior tibiofibular joint is a syndesmosis (fibrous joint) where the two bones are bound together by the strong interosseous tibiofibular ligament or the inferior tibiofibular ligament.

The synovial joint between the lower ends of the tibia and fibula and the talus is the ankle joint (Figs 6.70–6.75). Plantar flexion and dorsiflexion of the foot are the main movements in this joint. The deep socket formed by the tibia and fibula with the medial and lateral malleoli gripping the sides of the

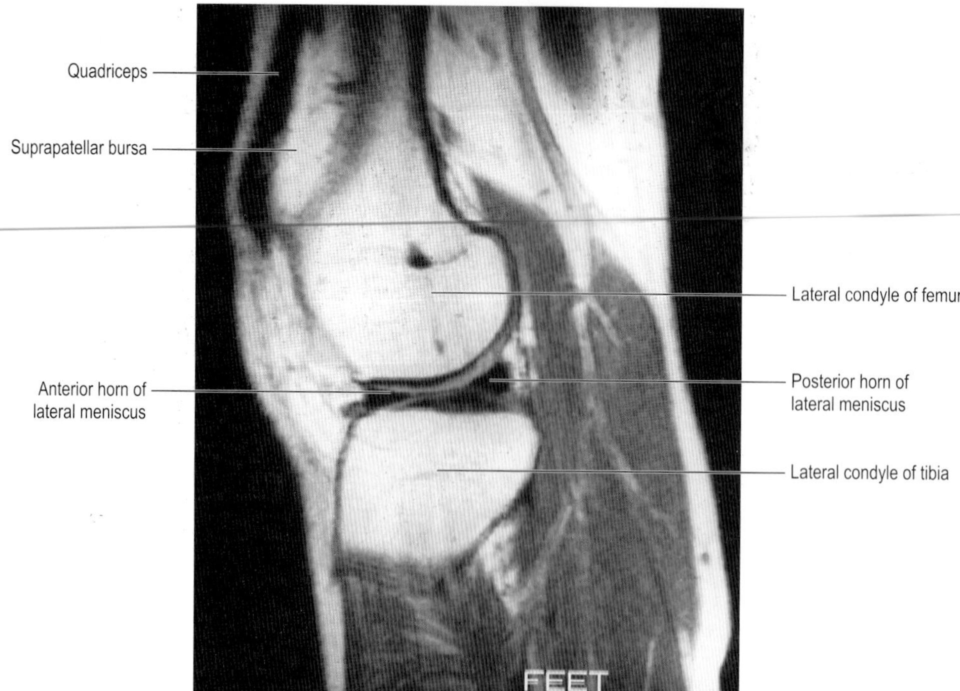


Fig. 6.68 Sagittal MRI through the lateral part of right knee joint.

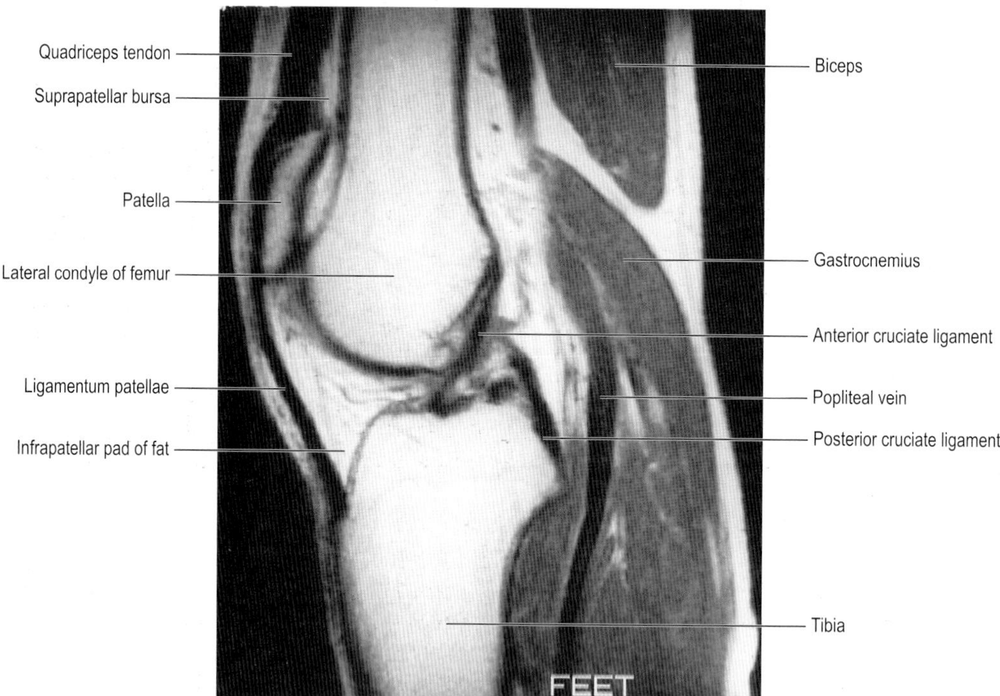


Fig. 6.69 Sagittal MRI of right knee joint showing attachments of anterior cruciate ligament. Section through medial aspect of lateral femoral condyle.

talus along with the ligaments and the muscles crossing the joint stabilise the ankle joint. ✪ The lower end of the tibia and fibula forming the socket for the talus is held together by the tibiofibular syndesmosis, injury to which makes the ankle joint very unstable

## Osteology

The lower ends of the tibia and fibula along with the two malleoli form the tibiofibular mortise into which the talus is received. The medial surface of the lateral malleolus articulates with the lateral surface of the talus, the inferior surface of tibia with the superior articular surface (trochlear surface) of the talus, and the lateral surface of the medial malleolus with the medial surface of the talus (Figs 6.70–6.73). The posterior border of the tibia, often known as the posterior malleolus, also contributes to the tibiofibular mortise which grip the talus. The joint is most stable in dorsiflexion when the broad end of the trochlear surface (Fig. 6.74) fills the tibiofibular mortise.

## Capsule and ligaments

The fibrous capsule is thin in front and behind but is reinforced on either side by ligaments.

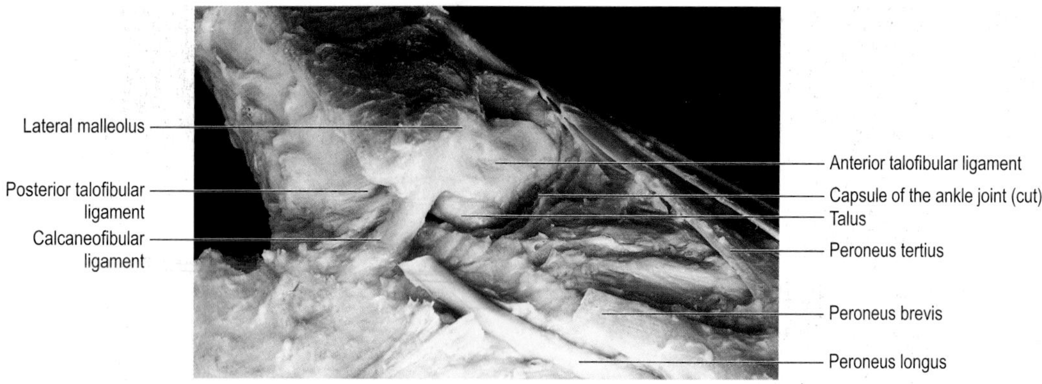


Fig. 6.75 Lateral aspect of the ankle

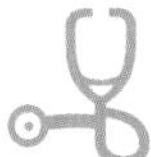

*Clinical box 6.11*

**Ankle injuries**

A wide variety of fractures can occur at the ankle often associated with ligament injuries. Fracture of the medial malleolus, lateral malleolus and posterior malleolus can occur. Ligaments often injured are the deltoid ligament, the anterior talofibular ligament, the calcaneofibular ligament and the interosseous (inferior) talofibular ligament. Commonest injury is a sprained ankle where the anterior talofibular and/or the calcaneofibular ligament are partially torn. It is caused by a sudden inversion of the foot while it is in plantar flexion.

More serious injuries at the ankle are sustained by a forceful inversion of the foot associated with external rotation of the talus. As the talus rotates laterally the lateral malleolus is fractured. This should still leave a stable ankle. However if the force is more violent the rotation of the talus can fracture the posterior and medial malleoli and tear the deltoid ligament. In a very severe external rotation injury the inferior tibiofibular joint is disrupted, making the tibia and fibula separate from each other. This will make the ankle very unstable.

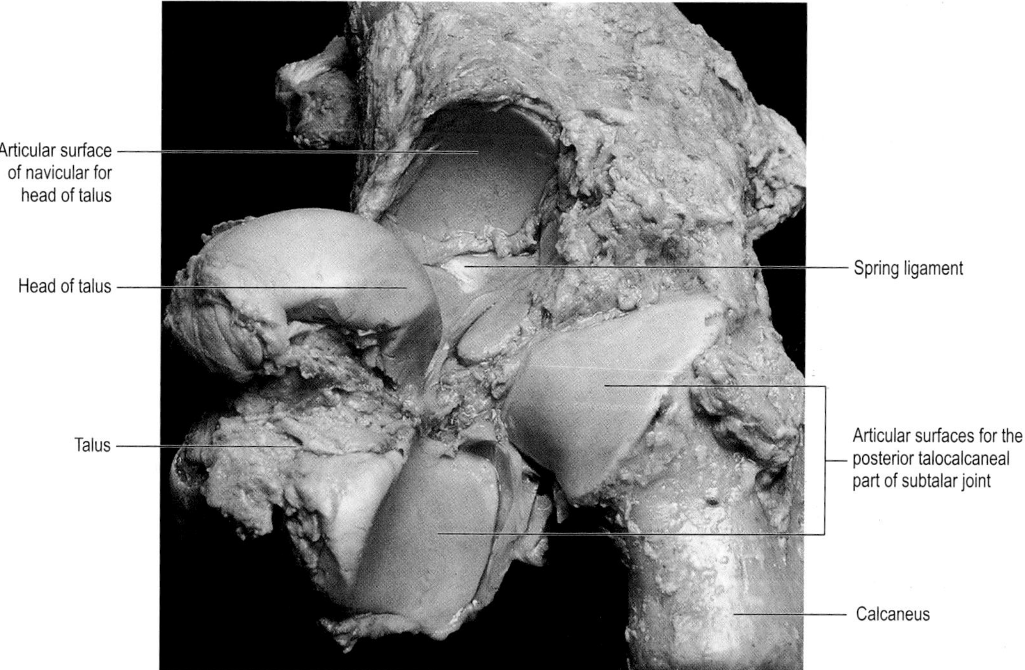


Fig. 6.76 Subtalar joint opened up.

main evertors. As the muscles involved are attached beyond the midtarsal joint, in the early part of inversion and eversion the midtarsal joint also moves. In inversion the midtarsal joint adducts and in eversion it abducts.

When the foot is on the ground, adduction of the forefoot is masked by lateral rotation of the leg. Similarly, eversion of a fixed foot is accompanied by medial rotation of the leg.

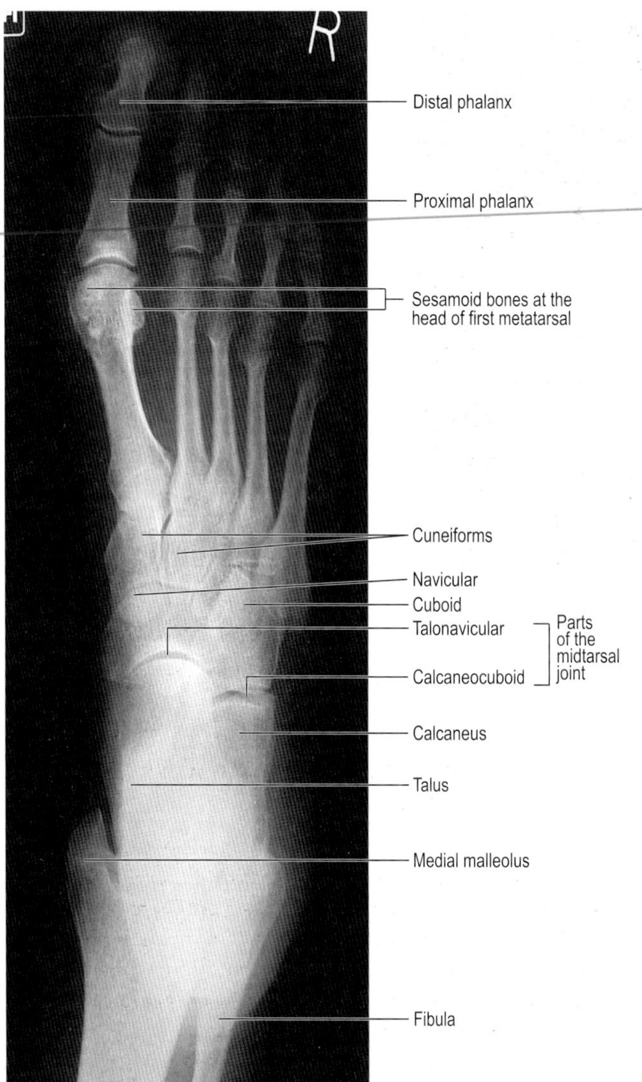


Fig. 6.77 Radiograph of the foot. Dorsiplantar view. Parts of the midtarsal joint.

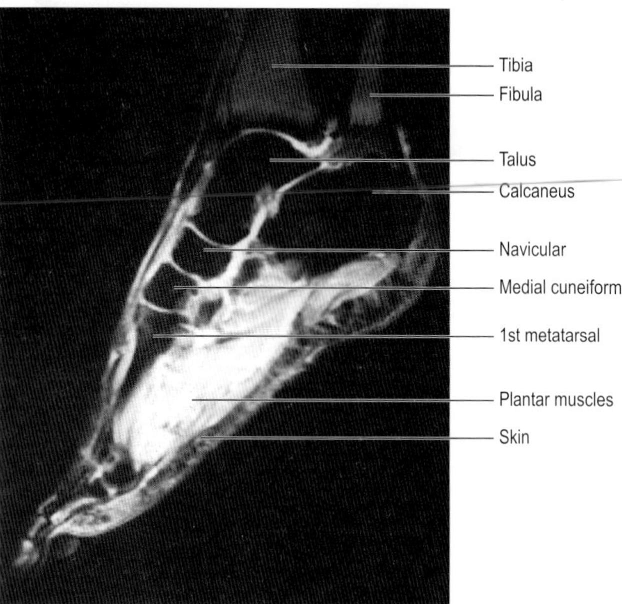


Fig. 6.78 Sagittal MRI of the foot. Components of the medial longitudinal arch.

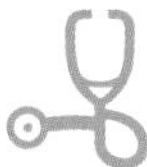

## *Clinical box 6.12*

**Hallux valgus**

In this condition the first metatarsal deviates medially and the big toe laterally. A bulge contributed by a bunion will be present in the region of the first metatarsophalangeal joint. The big toe may overlap or under-ride the second toe. The condition is often familial and the incidence is higher in females.

The foot is one of the most dynamic parts of the body. It provides physical contact with the ground and supports the body weight. Yet the foot is flexible and resilient, enabling it to absorb shocks transmitted to it. The foot also provides the spring and lift during walking, running and jumping. All these functions are achieved by the segmented but arched configuration of the foot. ✪ For descriptive purposes the arches of the foot are divided into the medial (Fig. 6.78) and lateral longitudinal arches and the transverse arch. Each arch consists of a number of bones and joints and is supported by muscles and ligaments. The arches are maintained by the shapes of the bones, the ligaments connecting them, the plantar aponeurosis as well as the muscles of the foot. The tendon of the flexor hallucis longus (Fig. 6.79) is the most important muscular structure supporting the medial longitudinal arch. See Clinical box 6.12.

## Blood supply of the lower limb

### Arterial supply of the lower limb

Arteries of the lower limb are illustrated in Figure 6.80. The femoral artery is the continuation of the external iliac artery beyond the midinguinal point. Its upper part is in the femoral triangle and the lower part in the adductor canal. After the first inch (2.5cm) a major branch is given off from its lateral aspect, the profunda femoris (Figs 6.80, 6.81). ✪ A branch of the profunda vein crosses the artery near its origin. Ligation and division of the vein exposes the profunda femoris artery. ✪ The main stem of the artery is also known as the common femoral, the profunda femoris as the deep femoral, and the continuation of the main artery beyond the profunda as the superficial femoral – the terms mostly used by radiologists and vascular surgeons. The pulsation of common femoral is easily palpable at the midinguinal point, which is the midpoint of a line connecting the anterior superior iliac spine to the pubic symphysis (the joint between the two pubic bones). ✪ The artery can be easily catheterised in this part for the purpose of angiography and angioplasty. It is also a convenient site for taking samples to estimate blood gases.

✪ The profunda femoris through its branches supplies the muscles of the thigh. Lateral and medial circumflex femoral arteries are two of its major branches. There is a network of anastomoses (Fig. 6.80) between the branches of the profunda and those of the anterior and posterior tibial arteries (see below). When the superficial femoral is blocked these anastomoses will open up and act as a collateral channel.

✪ The popliteal artery (Fig. 6.82) whose pulsation is palpable in the popliteal fossa (p. 147) is the continuation of

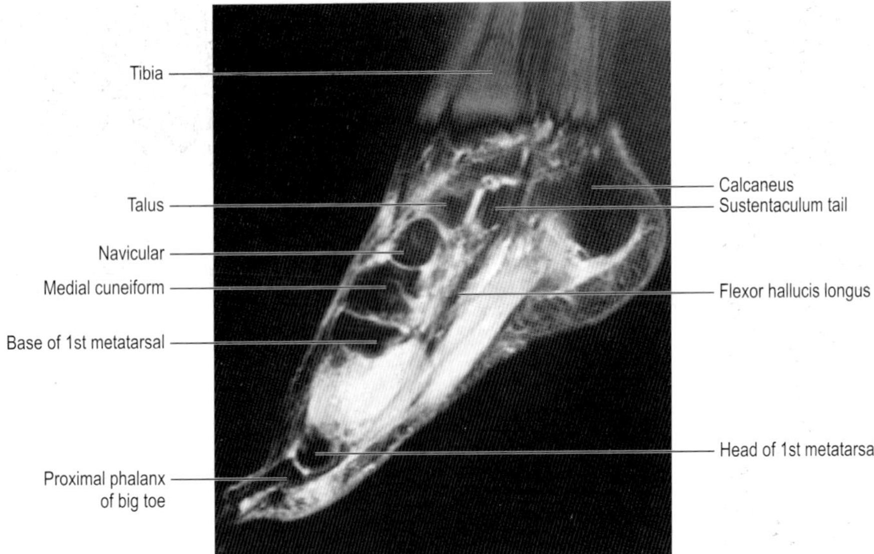


Fig. 6.79 Sagittal MRI of the foot. Tendon of flexor hallucis longus.

the femoral artery beyond the adductor hiatus. At the lower border of the popliteus muscle it divides into anterior and posterior tibial arteries. The former enters the anterior compartment by passing over the upper border of the interosseous membrane. The latter continues in the posterior compartment of the leg as the tibioperoneal trunk (Fig. 6.82) for about 2cm and bifurcates into posterior tibial and peroneal arteries.

The anterior tibial artery from the anterior compartment of the leg continues on to the foot as the dorsalis pedis artery (Fig. 6.83) from which the arcuate artery and the dorsal metatarsal arteries arise (see also pgs 149, 150).

✪ The posterior tibial artery descends in the posterior compartment of the leg and enters the sole of the foot by passing deep to the flexor retinaculum. The peroneal artery, though small, is important as it is usually not affected by atherosclerosis especially in diabetics (see also pgs 153, 154). See Clinical box 6.13.

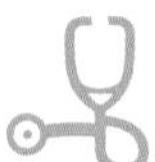

### *Clinical box 6.13*

**Locating the arterial pulsations in the lower limb**

Palpating the various arterial pulsations in the lower extremity is an important part of clinical examination, especially in patients with cardiovascular diseases.

The femoral artery pulsation is felt at the midinguinal point located halfway between the anterior superior iliac spine and the pubic symphysis. The femoral artery is a continuation of the external iliac artery.

The popliteal artery pulsation is located in the middle of the popliteal fossa behind the knee on deep palpation. Patient is in the prone position with the leg flexed to relax the deep fascia over the popliteal fossa (clinically this is often difficult to feel!).

The posterior tibial is felt midway between the medial malleolus and the medial tubercle of the calcaneus.

Pulsation of the dorsalis pedis, the continuation of the anterior tibial artery, is felt in the first interosseous space on the dorsum of the foot. It may normally be absent in about 30% of cases.

The peroneal artery pulsation is felt on the anterior surface of the lateral malleolus.

## The veins of the lower limb

A superficial and deep groups of veins drain the lower limb, the long saphenous and the short saphenous being the major ones in the former group.

### The long (great) saphenous vein

This, the longest vein in the body, starts in the medial aspect of the dorsum of the foot. ✪ It crosses the ankle in front of the medial malleolus (Figs 6.84–6.87), a constant relationship which is useful in an emergency to do a cut-down for venous access. As it ascends it lies about a hand's breadth behind the medial border of the patella (Figs 6.56, 6.88). About 3.5cm below and lateral to the pubic tubercle, the vein goes through an opening in the deep fascia, the saphenous opening (Figs 6.84, 6.89), to join the femoral vein. The vein is closely related to the saphenous nerve below the knee. ✪ Damage to the nerve while stripping the vein may cause numbness or paraesthesia along the medial border of leg and foot. In the treatment of varicose veins the long saphenous vein is usually stripped above the knee to avoid damage to the saphenous nerve (see also p. 177).

### The short saphenous vein

Commencing from the lateral aspect of the dorsal venous arch the short saphenous vein ascends behind the lateral malleolus accompanied by the sural nerve (Fig. 6.91). ✪ The nerve damage which may occur during stripping of the vein causes numbness or paraesthesia along the lateral border of the foot. The small saphenous vein perforates the deep fascia at a variable point between the middle of the calf and the roof of the popliteal fossa and usually ends in the popliteal vein.

### Deep veins

These are named after the arteries they accompany (Fig. 6.90) and are present as venae comitantes in the lower part

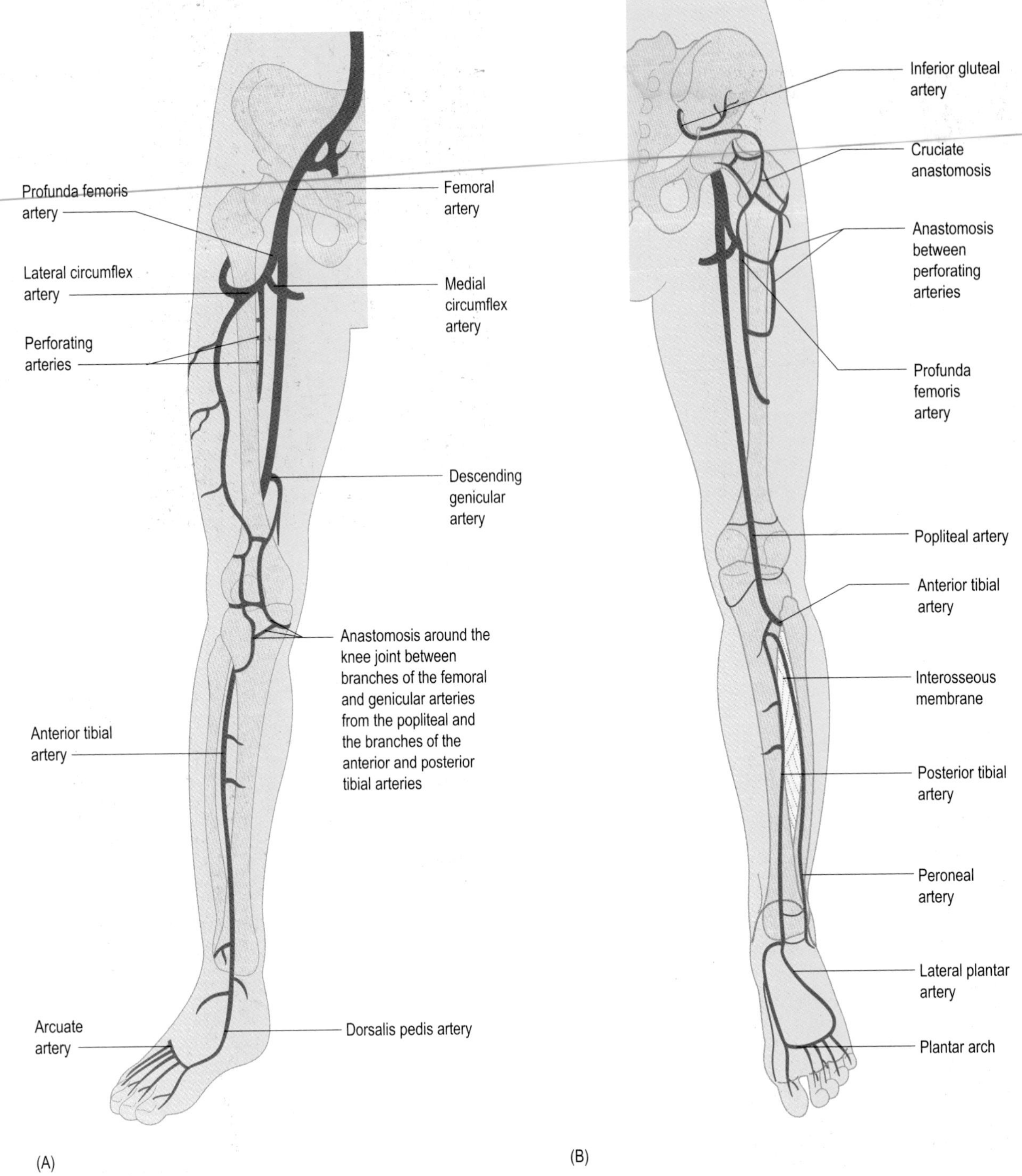


Fig. 6.80 Summary diagrams showing the arteries of the lower limb: (A) anterior view, (B) posterior view.

of the leg. Higher up, the popliteal and femoral veins accompany the relevant arteries. The femoral vein continues into the pelvis as the external iliac vein.

### Perforating veins

These connect the superficial veins to the deep veins and are seen at different levels. There is a valve close to where the perforating vein perforates the deep fascia. ✪ Common sites for the perforators are in the lower half of the medial aspect of calf, one just below the middle of the calf and another in the lower thigh. The lower perforators are joined by a longitudinal trunk, the posterior arch vein which usually joins the long saphenous vein below the knee. ✪ Blood flows from the superficial to the deep veins through the perforating veins. Flow in the opposite direction is prevented by the valves, the incompetence of which causes varicose veins and venous ulcers. See Clinical box 6.14.

## Segmental and cutaneous innervation

✪ The dermatomes of the lower limb (Figs 6.92, 6.93) lie in a numerical sequence downwards at the front of the limb and upwards on its posterior aspect. The myotomes are: at the hip – L2, L3 flexors, L4, L5 extensors; knee – L3, L4 extensors, L5, S1 flexors; ankle – L4, L5 dorsiflexors, S1, S2

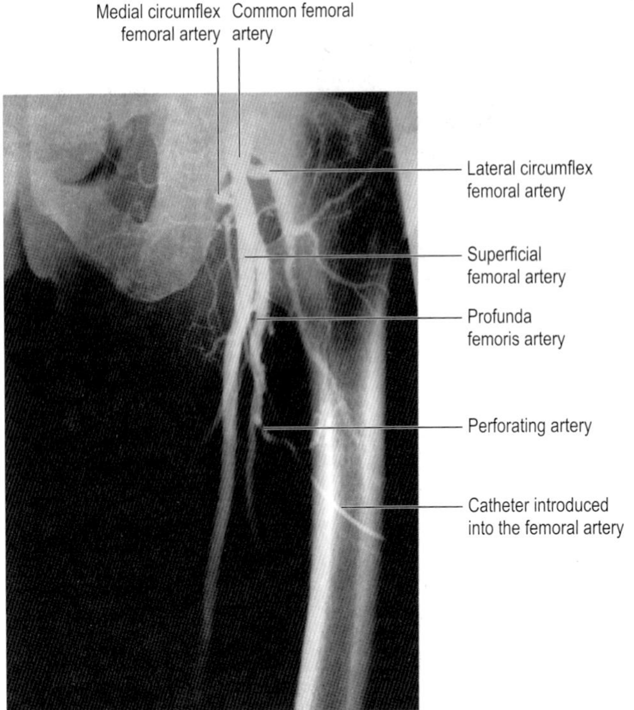


Fig. 6.81 Angiogram of the femoral artery.

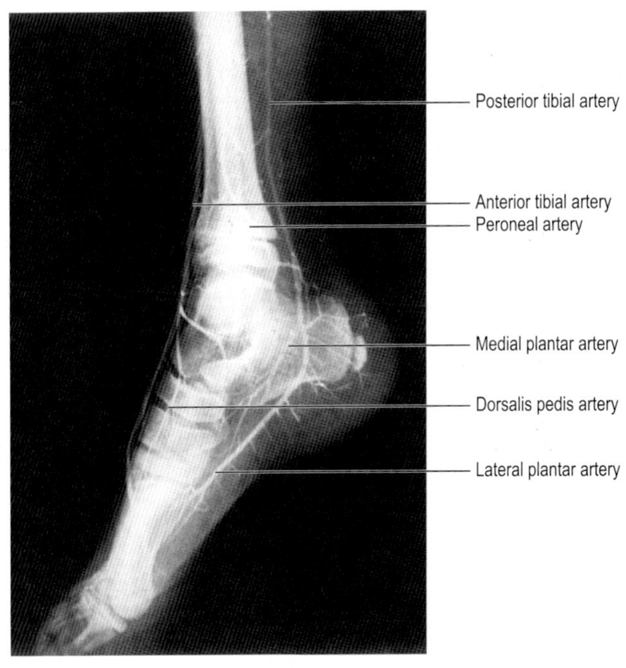


Fig. 6.83 Foot angiogram. Lateral view.

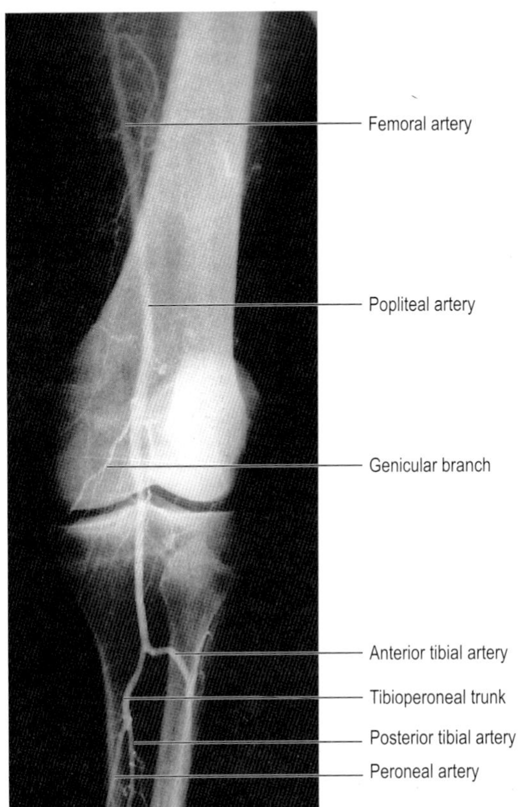


Fig. 6.82 Popliteal artery and branches – angiogram.

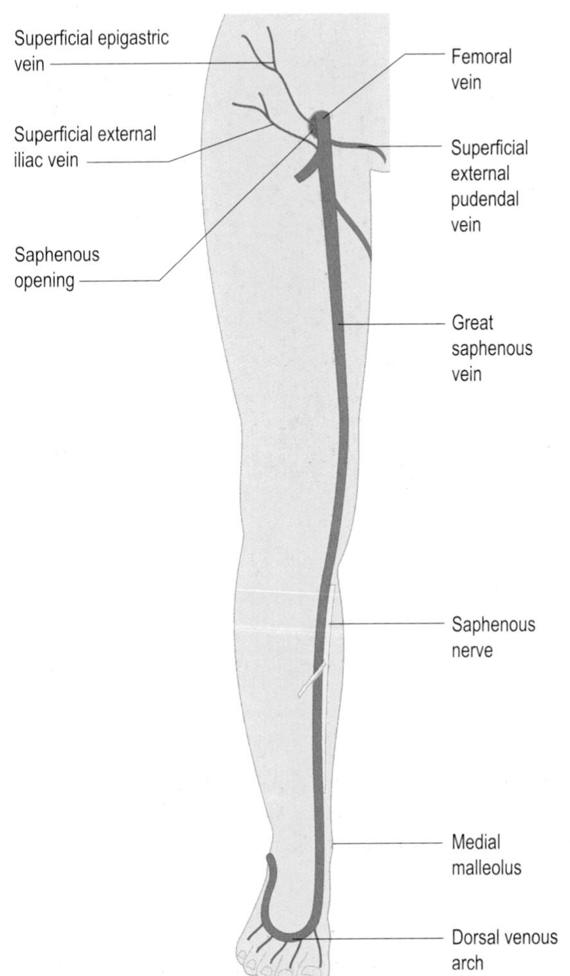


Fig. 6.84 The great saphenous vein.

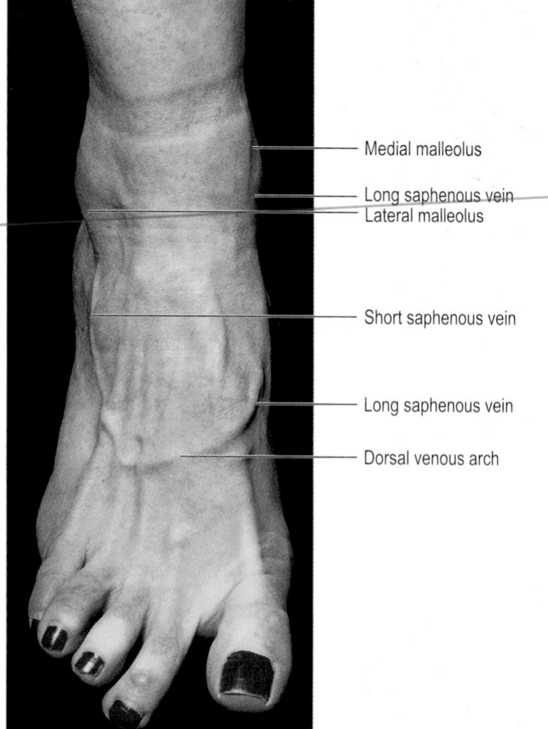


Fig. 6.85 Surface anatomy of the veins on the dorsum of foot.

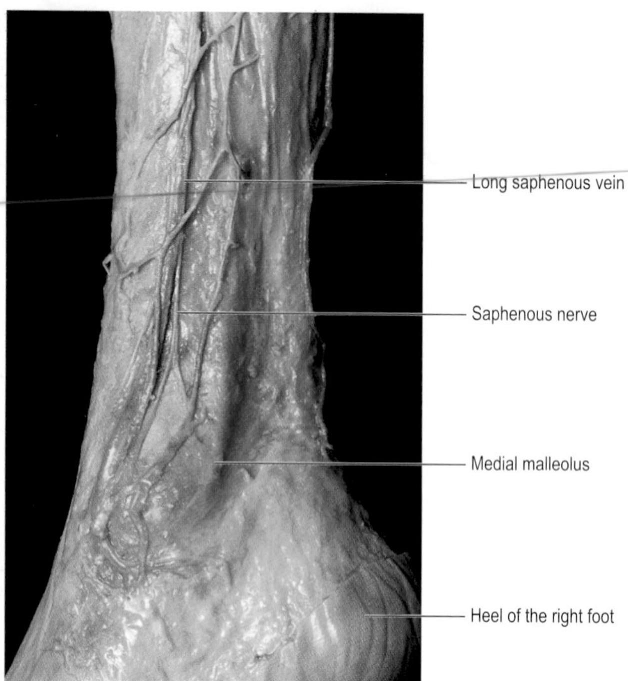


Fig. 6.87 Long saphenous vein and the saphenous nerve in front of the medial malleolus.

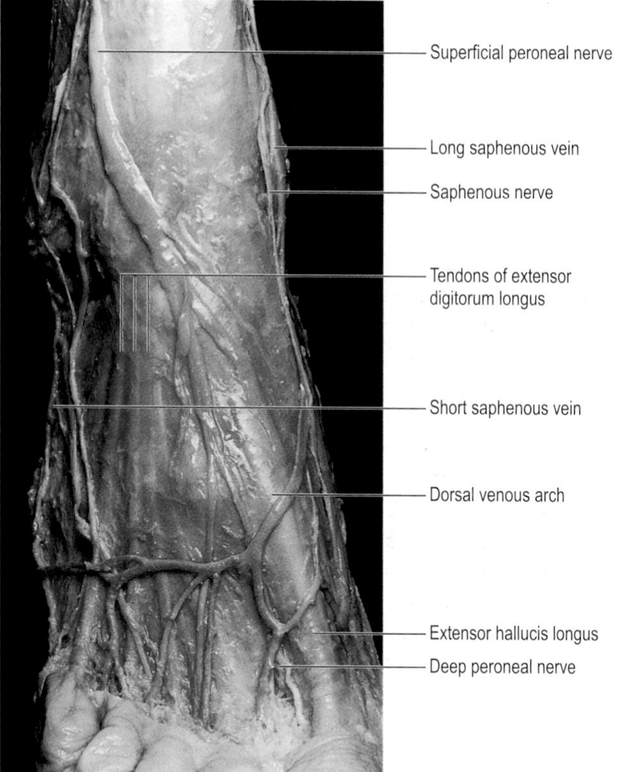


Fig. 6.86 Superficial veins on the dorsum of the foot.

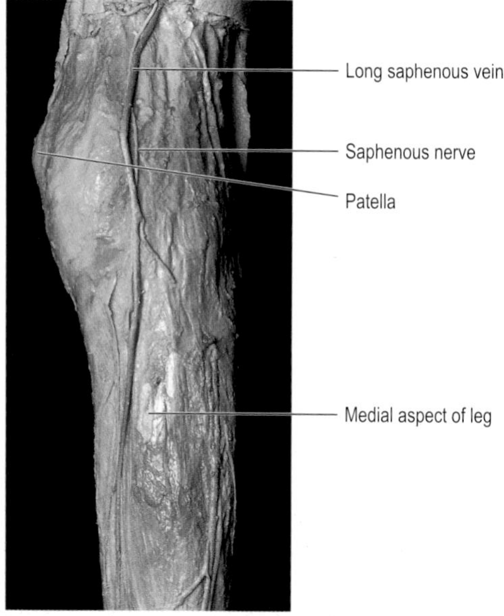


Fig. 6.88 Medial aspect of leg and knee joint. Long saphenous vein and saphenous nerve behind the patella.

plantar flexors. Hence the segments tested by the knee jerk are L3, L4 and the ankle jerk S1, S2.

## Cutaneous nerves

See Fig. 6.94.

✪ The ilioinguinal nerve (L1) emerges through the superficial inguinal ring to supply the root of the penis, anterior third of the scrotum and vulva, and an adjoining small area in the upper part of the thigh.

The genitofemoral nerve (L1, L2) divides into a genital and a femoral branch; the latter, containing L1 fibres, enters the thigh accompanying the femoral artery and pierces the femoral sheath to supply the skin overlying the femoral triangle (Fig. 6.94). (The genital branch containing L2 fibres is a content of the spermatic cord and it supplies the cremaster, tunica vaginalis and the scrotal skin.)

The medial and intermediate femoral cutaneous nerves (L2, L3) are cutaneous branches of the femoral nerve, and they supply the medial and the anterior aspects of the

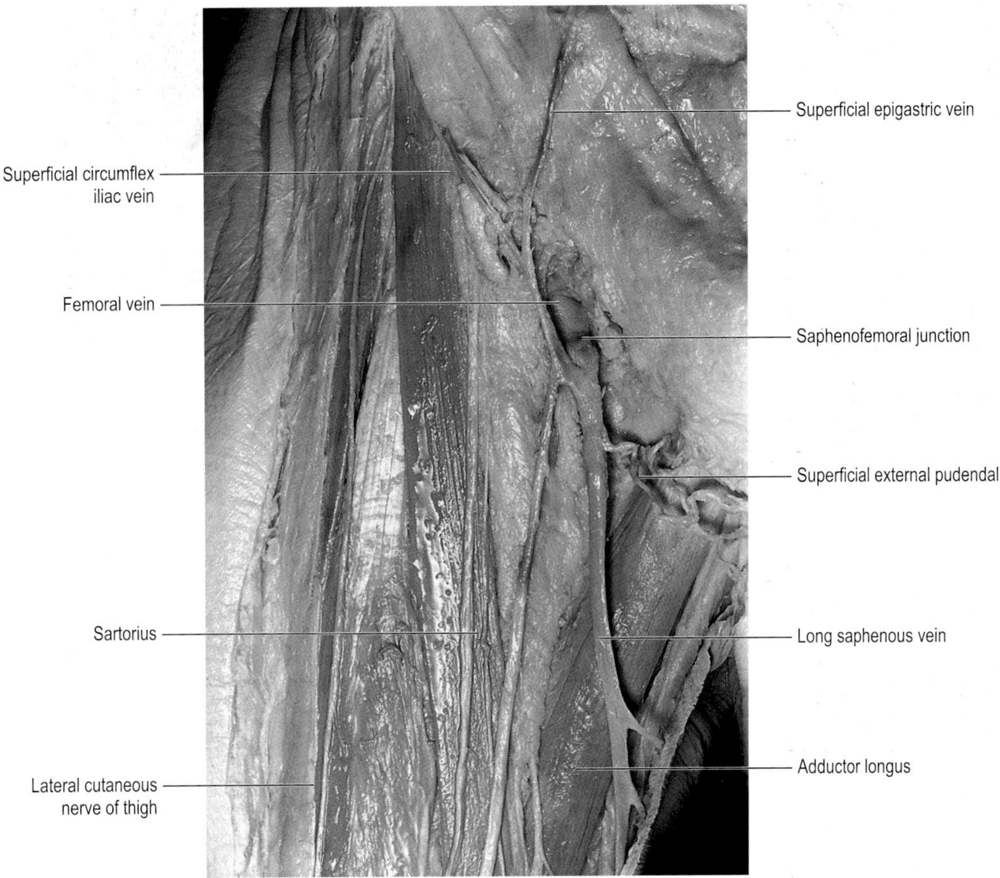


Fig. 6.89 Long saphenous vein and the saphenofemoral junction.

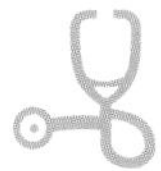

## *Clinical box 6.14*

### Varicose veins

In this condition the veins become dilated and tortuous, often due to incompetence of valves. Increased venous pressure caused by compression of the major veins by a tumour, venous thrombosis or even pregnancy can cause varicose veins. It is more common in the lower extremity in an age group mostly 50 and over. About 10–20% of the population, both men and women, can get varicose veins. Obesity, prolonged dependent position of the legs (as with jobs that involve sitting or standing still for long periods of time) and a family history of varicose veins are all predisposing factors. The vein commonly affected is the great saphenous vein, with incompetence at the saphenofemoral junction. Varicosity of the vein from this level will extend downwards. Short saphenous vein varicosity, due to incompetence of valves of the perforating veins, is also common. Complications of varicose veins are thrombophlebitis, haemorrhage, venous pigmentation of the skin, and venous stasis of the skin leading on to varicose ulcers. When there is venous stasis the skin is poorly nourished and it easily breaks down to become an ulcer. This happens more frequently in the anteromedial aspect of the lower end of tibia as the venous drainage there is normally precarious. A varicose ulcer, if left untreated, can turn malignant to become a Marjolin's ulcer.

thigh respectively. The saphenous nerve is the only branch of the femoral nerve to supply the leg and foot. It gives a cutaneous innervation to the medial surface of the leg and the medial border of the foot. In the leg it is closely related to the great saphenous vein and it can be rolled under the fingers where it lies over the medial condyle of the tibia about a hand's breadth behind the medial border of the patella (Fig. 6.56).

The lateral femoral cutaneous nerve (L2, L3) pierces the inguinal ligament 1cm medial to the anterior superior iliac spine to supply the lateral aspect of the thigh.

✪ Compression of the lateral cutaneous nerve of the thigh at the point where it pierces the inguinal ligament or more proximally as it traverses the iliac fascia causes pain and a tingling sensation along the lateral aspect of the thigh, a condition known as meralgia paraesthetica.

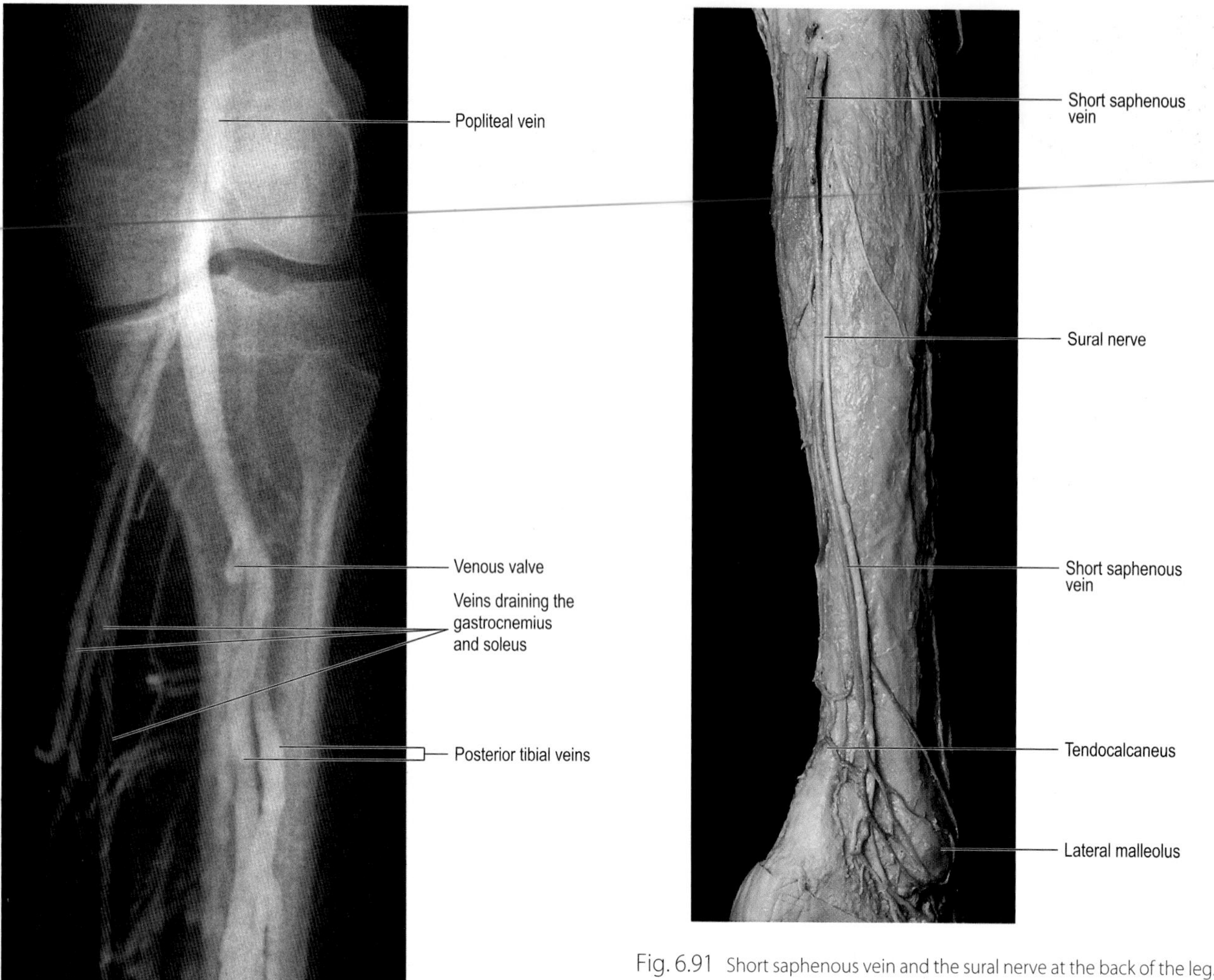


Fig. 6.90 Deep veins of the leg – venogram.

Fig. 6.91 Short saphenous vein and the sural nerve at the back of the leg.

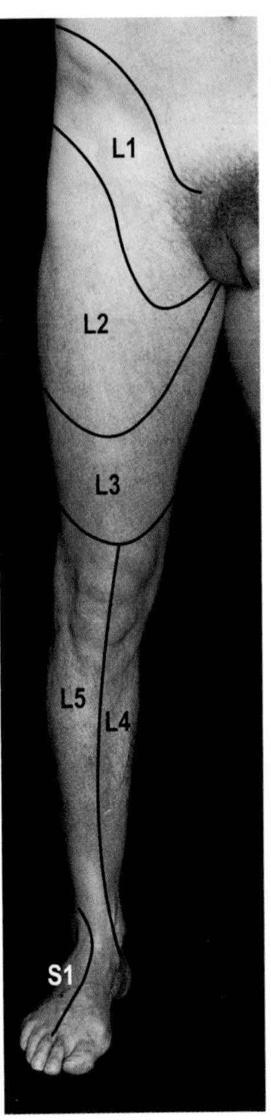


Fig. 6.92 Dermatomes of the lower limb – anterior aspect.

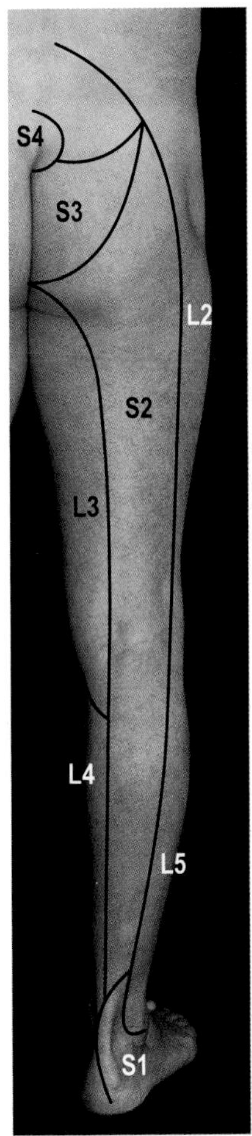


Fig. 6.93 Dermatomes of the lower limb – posterior aspect.

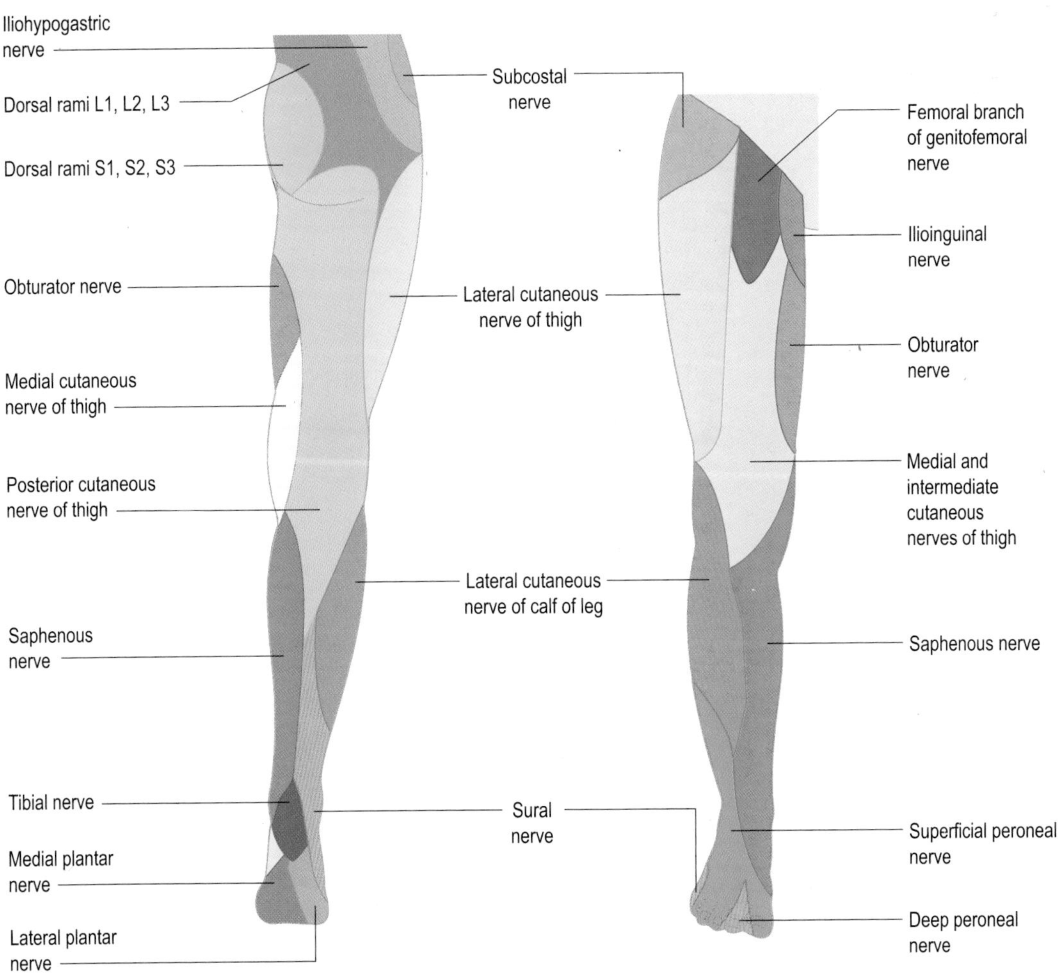


Fig. 6.94 The territories of supply of the cutaneous nerves of the lower limb: (A) posterior view, (B) anterior view.

# Chapter 7
# Head and neck



A thorough knowledge of anatomy is required to diagnose and treat a number of clinical conditions affecting the neck. The sternocleidomastoid muscle divides the neck into two large triangles, the anterior triangle between sternocleidomastoid and the midline and the posterior triangle between it and the trapezius.

## The front of the neck

The front of the neck, or the anterior triangle, has the thyroid gland, the carotid sheath and the infrahyoid muscles (Figs 7.1–7.8).

### Surface anatomy

In the midline, from above downwards, the mandible, the hyoid bone, the thyroid cartilage, the cricoid cartilage, the tracheal rings and the suprasternal notch can be felt (Fig. 7.1). The movement of the thyroid cartilage up and down with swallowing is easily visible. The two sternocleidomastoid muscles can be seen and felt by turning the head against resistance to the opposite side. In the middle of the neck, at the anterior border of the sternocleidomastoid, the pulsation of the common carotid artery is palpable. The internal jugular vein lies lateral to the artery with the vagus nerve between the two vessels.

The lower border of the cricoid, which is at the level of the sixth cervical vertebra, is an important level in the neck and it corresponds to:

- the junction of the larynx with the trachea
- the junction of the pharynx with the oesophagus
- the site at which the carotid artery can be compressed against the carotid tubercle of the transverse process of the C6 vertebra.

### Superficial structures

The superficial fascia contains the platysma (Fig. 7.2), a striated muscle, which extends from the region of the clavicle, pectoralis major, and the deltoid to the mandible

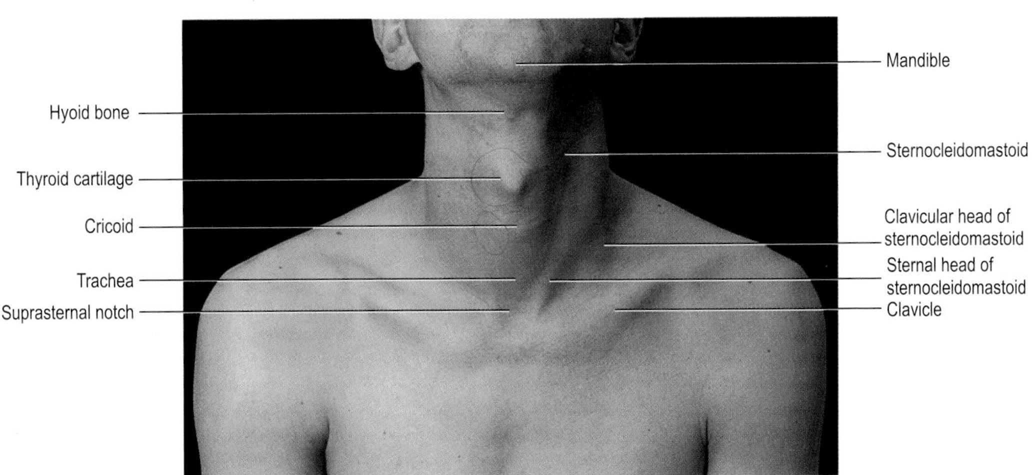


Fig. 7.1 Surface anatomy of the front of the neck.

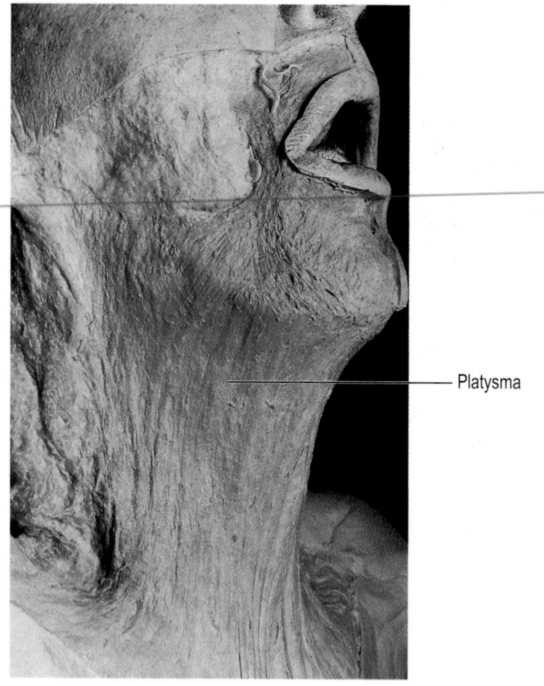


Fig. 7.2 The platysma.

above. ✪ To prevent retraction of the severed muscle contributing to a broad scar platysma is sutured with the skin when neck wounds are sutured. The muscle has good vascularity. Hence when skin flaps are raised platysma is included to maintain a good blood supply. The platysma is supplied by the cervical branch of the facial nerve.

### Infrahyoid muscles

The sternohyoid, sternothyroid and thyrohyoid connect the sternum, hyoid bone and thyroid cartilage (Fig. 7.3). The omohyoid extends between the hyoid and the scapula. These are known as the infrahyoid muscles or the strap muscles. They are supplied by the ansa cervicalis (C1, C2, C3) which is a nerve loop on the internal jugular vein. The branches to the muscles enter in their lower half. ✪ During exposure of a large goitre the strap muscles are cut in their upper half to preserve the nerve supply from the ansa cervicalis.

### The common carotid artery

The right common carotid artery is a branch of the brachiocephalic trunk and the left is a direct branch from the arch of the aorta. At the upper border of the thyroid cartilage the common carotid artery divides into the external and the internal carotid arteries. ✪ The bifurcation can be at a higher level: a surgeon ligating the external carotid should be aware of this to avoid an inadvertent ligation of the common carotid. The common carotid and the internal carotid arteries are enclosed by the carotid sheath, in which the internal jugular vein lies lateral to the arteries, with the vagus nerve in between the vein and the artery (Fig. 7.4).

### The internal jugular vein

This is the major vein in the neck (Figs 7.4, 7.6, 7.8) draining the pharyngeal veins, the facial vein and the thyroid veins. It starts at the base of the skull as a continuation of the sigmoid venous sinus and terminates behind the sternoclavicular joint by joining the subclavian vein to form the brachiocephalic vein. Its tributaries are shown in Figure 7.8.

✪ Internal jugular vein cannulation is carried out at the middle of the anterior border of the sternocleidomastoid, immediately lateral to the carotid pulse or in a lower approach near the apex of the triangular gap between the sternal and the clavicular heads of the sternocleidomastoid (Fig. 7.3).

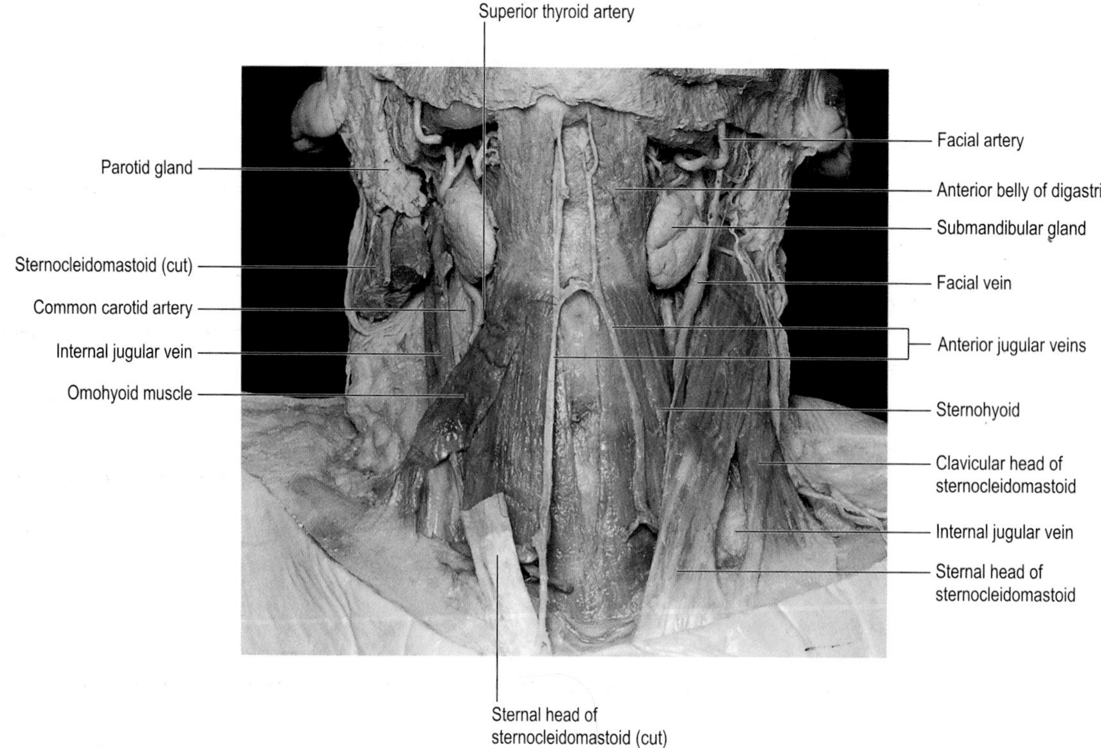


Fig. 7.3 Superficial dissection of the anterior aspect of the neck.

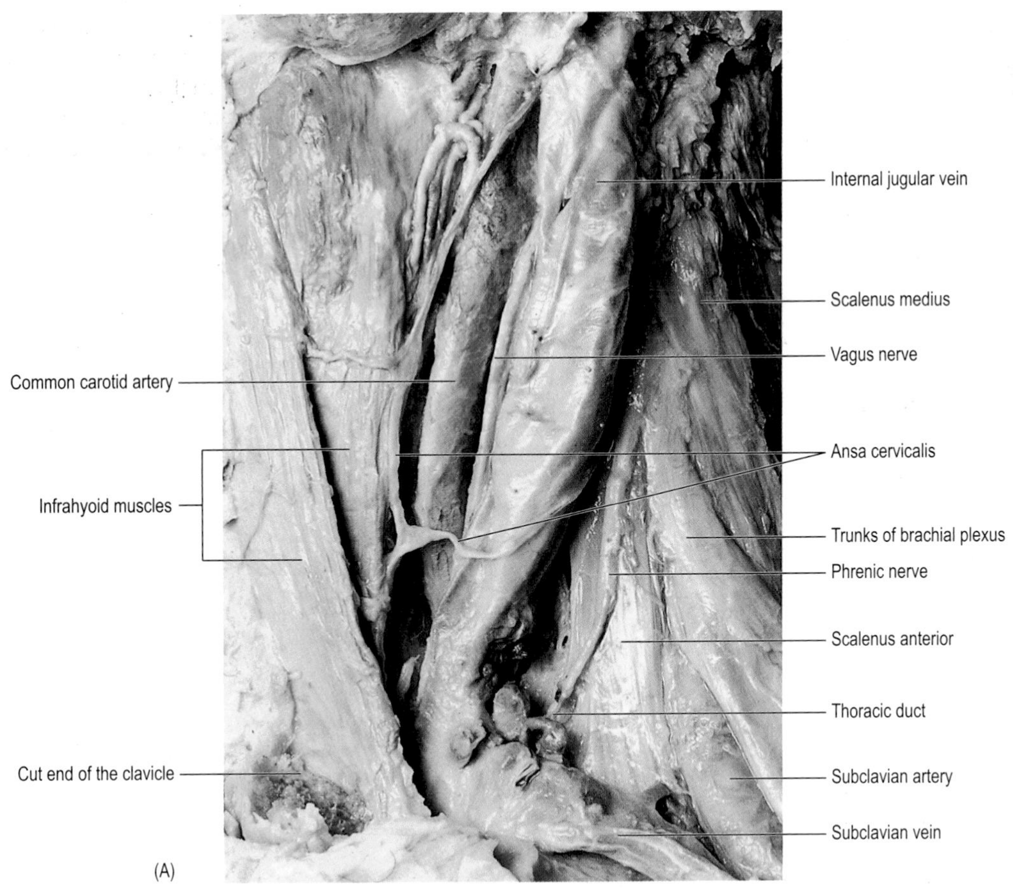


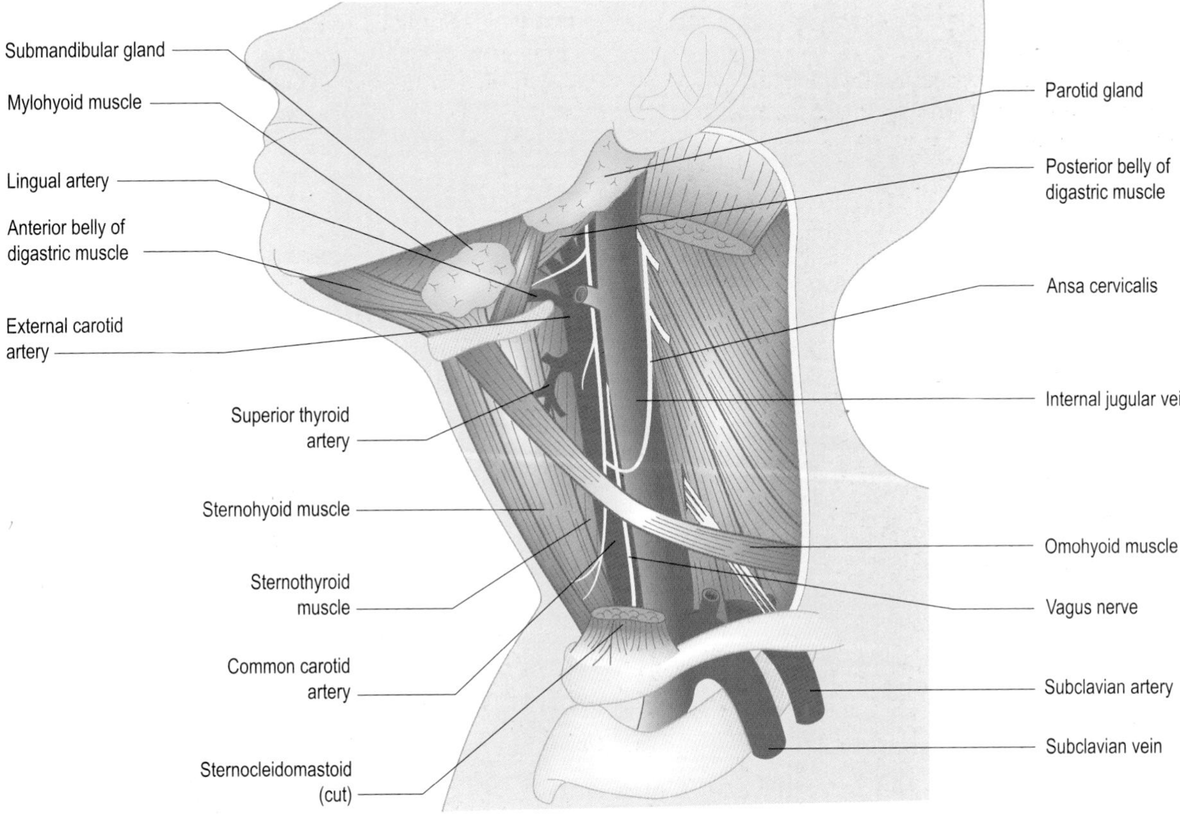


Fig. 7.4 (A) Structures deep to the sternocleidomastoid on the left side. Left clavicle and sternocleidomastoid have been removed. (B) Carotid arteries and internal jugular vein.

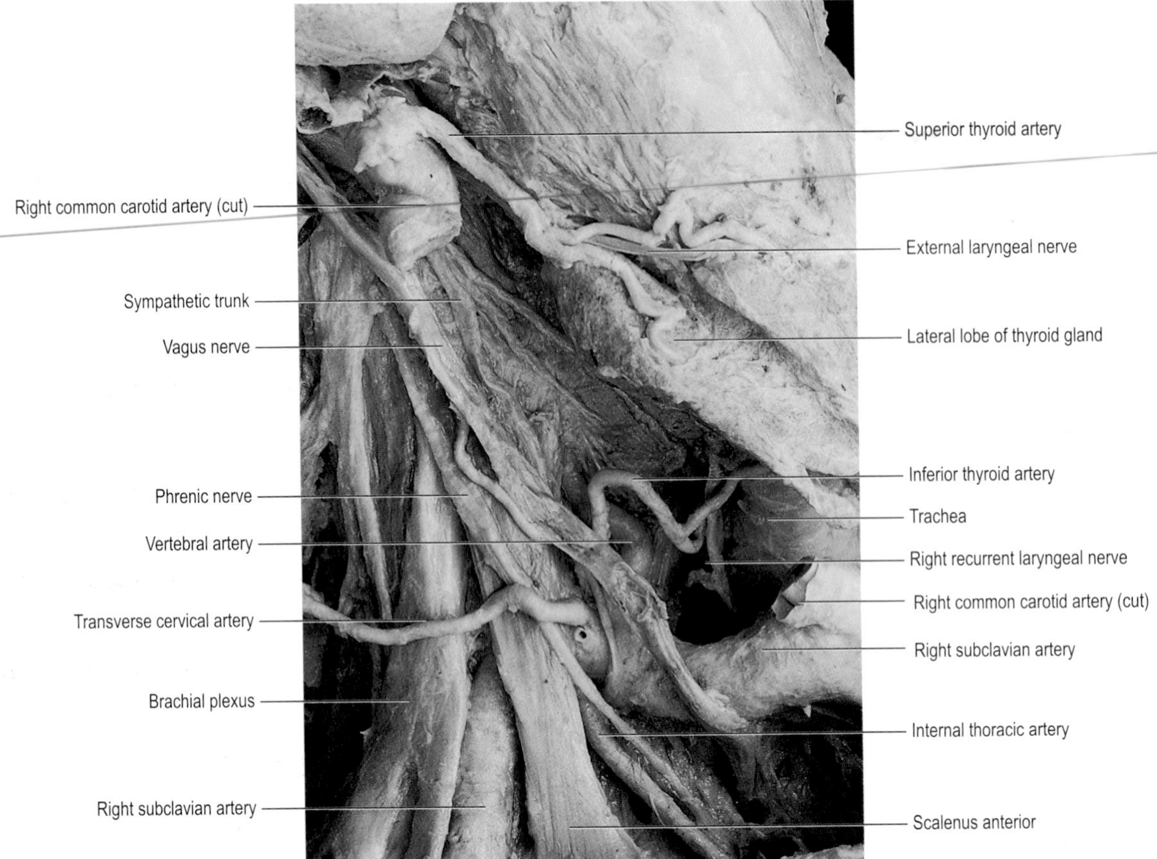


Fig. 7.5 Deep dissection of the lower half of the right side of the neck after removal of the clavicle and the right sternocleidomastoid showing branches of the subclavian artery and the structures related to the scalenus anterior. The common carotid artery and the internal jugular vein have also been removed.

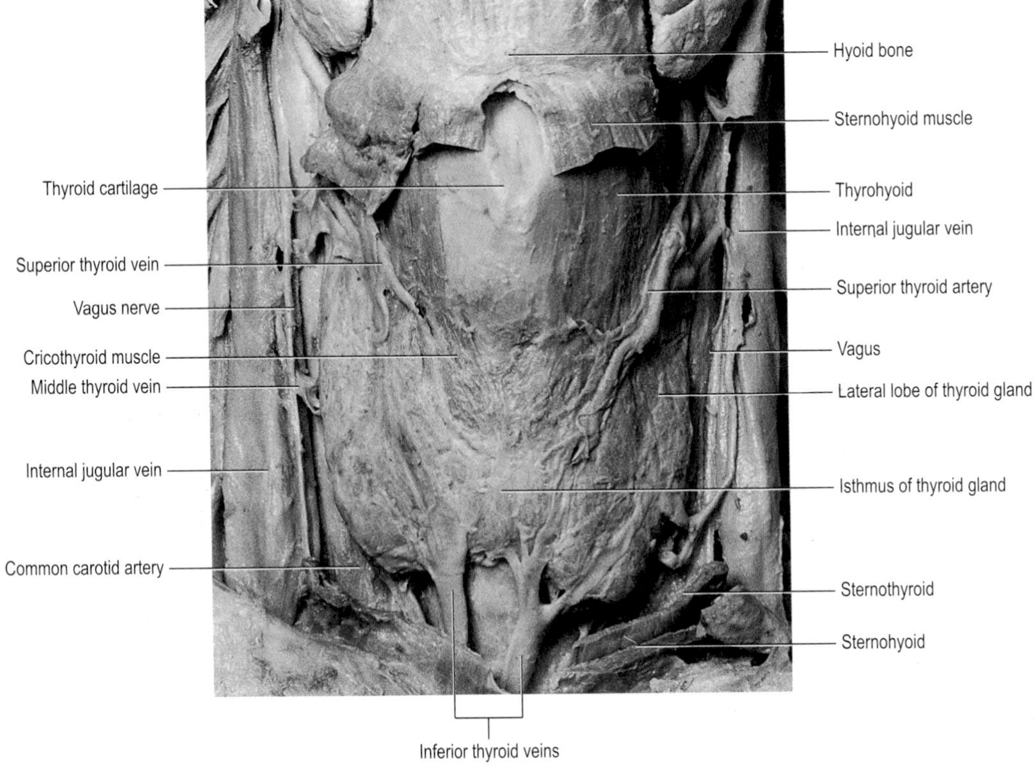


Fig. 7.6 Anterior view of the thyroid gland and its blood supply seen after removal of the sternocleidomastoid and the infrahyoid muscles.

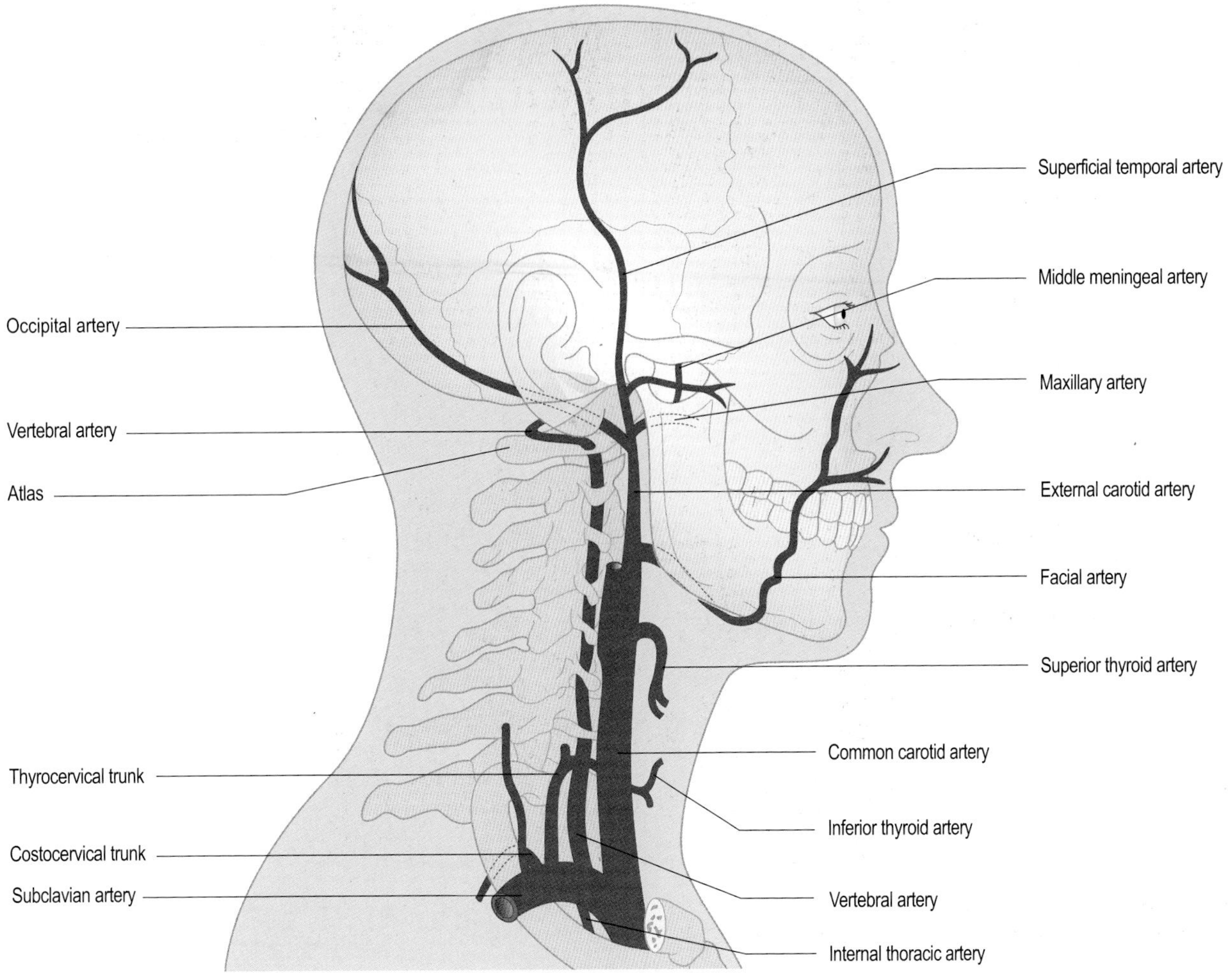

Superficial temporal artery
Middle meningeal artery
Occipital artery
Maxillary artery
Vertebral artery
Atlas
External carotid artery
Facial artery
Superior thyroid artery
Common carotid artery
Thyrocervical trunk
Inferior thyroid artery
Costocervical trunk
Subclavian artery
Vertebral artery
Internal thoracic artery

Fig. 7.7 The subclavian and the carotid arteries.

Inferior petrosal sinus
Pharyngeal veins
Internal jugular vein
Common facial vein
Lingual vein
Superior thyroid vein
Middle thyroid vein
Subclavian vein
Brachiocephalic veins
Superior vena cava

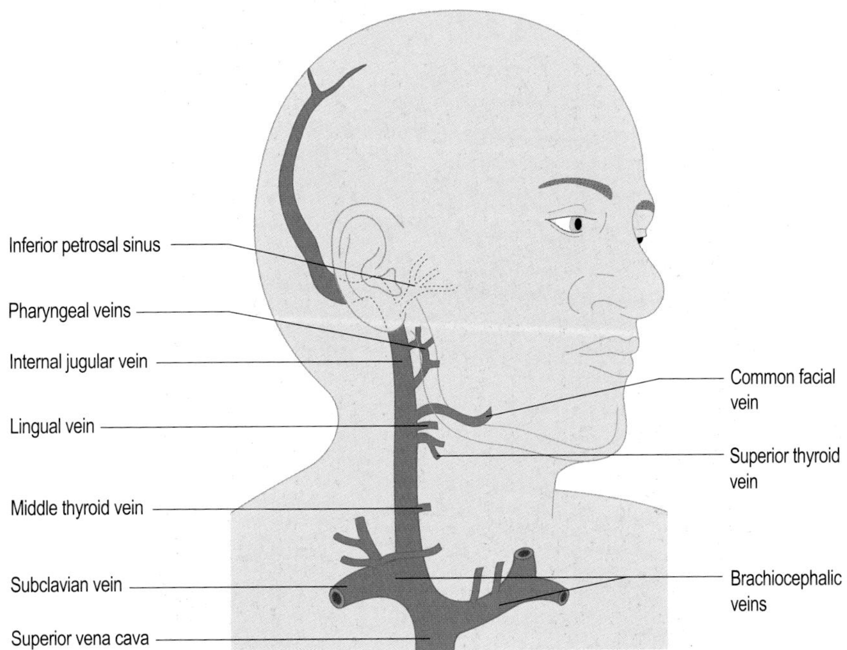

Fig. 7.8 The internal jugular vein and its tributaries.

## The thyroid gland

The thyroid gland has two lateral lobes connected by a midline isthmus (Fig. 7.6). ✪ The gland is firmly bound to the larynx and trachea by the pre-tracheal fascia and hence moves with them during swallowing. The isthmus lies in front of the second, third and fourth tracheal rings. A pyramidal lobe, a remnant of the thyroglossal duct, is sometimes seen as a midline extension of the isthmus upwards over the thyroid cartilage. The parathyroid glands are embedded in the posterior surface of the lateral lobes. The thyroid gland is covered anteriorly by the infrahyoid muscles.

The thyroid gland has a rich blood supply. The superior thyroid artery, a branch of the external carotid, enters the upper pole of the gland. The inferior thyroid artery (Figs 7.5, 7.7), a branch of the thyrocervical trunk of the subclavian, enters the middle of the posterior aspect. The inferior thyroid artery also supplies the parathyroid glands. ✪ Bilateral ligature of the inferior thyroid artery in thyroid surgery can cause ischaemia of the parathyroids. The venous drainage is extensive and variable. The superior thyroid vein accompanies the artery and drains into the internal jugular vein (Fig. 7.8). The inferior thyroid veins are many and they drain into the subclavian or brachiocephalic veins. The middle thyroid veins are variable in number and may drain into the superior and inferior veins or by a short trunk into the internal jugular vein. ✪ Because the vein is short its careless handling may tear the internal jugular vein causing serious haemorrhage during thyroid surgery. The recurrent laryngeal nerve crosses the inferior thyroid artery very close to the thyroid gland (see Fig. 7.33). The nerve is usually deep to the artery but may be superficial to it or pass through its branches. It lies in the groove between the trachea and the oesophagus before reaching the inferior pole of the thyroid gland. The recurrent laryngeal nerves supply the muscles of the larynx. ✪ A malignant tumour of the thyroid gland may compress the recurrent laryngeal nerve, affecting the movements of the vocal cords and resulting in a change in the voice. The nerve is also prone to damage in thyroid surgery because of its close relation to the inferior thyroid artery. The external laryngeal branch of the superior laryngeal nerve is related to the superior thyroid vascular pedicle. Damage to the nerve paralyses the cricothyroid muscle causing a voice change. See Clinical box 7.1.

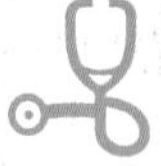

### *Clinical box 7.1*

**Embryology and developmental anomalies of the thyroid gland**

The thyroid gland develops in the floor of the pharynx migrating in front of the developing trachea to its permanent site in the base of the neck. First differentiation of the thyroid begins at about 4 weeks and its development and migration is completed by about 6 months. The track associated with thyroid migration is called the thyroglossal duct. It lies in the midline extending from the foramen caecum in the tongue via the hyoid bone to its usual position in the neck. Remnants of the duct persist as the foramen caecum of the tongue, the pyramidal lobe of the thyroid and a fibrous cord – sometimes known as the 'levator glandulae thyroidiae'.

The thyroid may fail to migrate and remain embedded within the tongue – the lingual thyroid. A lingual thyroid bleeds and may ulcerate. The patient is usually hypothyroid. The migration can extend beyond the neck into the mediastinum. Occasionally this may cause a mediastinal goitre causing pressure effects on mediastinal structures due to compression of major veins, trachea, oesophagus and the left recurrent laryngeal nerve.

Epithelial remnants of the thyroglossal duct may proliferate and become cystic to give rise to thyroglossal cyst or sinus. This is a midline swelling. Removal of the sinus involves dissection of the whole tract, including removal of the middle of the hyoid bone because of its intimate relation to the thyroglossal duct.

## The parathyroid glands

There are usually four glands, two on each side of the neck. The glands generally lie deep to the thyroid gland. They develop from the third and fourth branchial pouches, migrating down into the neck during development. The glands from the fourth pouch become the superior or upper parathyroids and those from the third pouch become the inferior glands. ✪ The surgeon generally recognises the superior and inferior glands in their relationship to the inferior thyroid artery – those lying cephalad being the superior parathyroids and those caudally placed being the inferior glands. The blood supply of the glands is usually derived from the inferior thyroid artery.

The position of the glands is very variable. Whilst the upper one is normally just above the inferior thyroid artery and the inferior normally towards the deep aspect of the lower pole of the thyroid gland, the glands can in fact lie in many positions in the neck as well as in the mediastinum. Not infrequently the inferior glands may be found in the thymus. Not only is the position of the glands very variable, their number also varies. In a few people only three glands are present whilst around 6% of the population will have five glands and about 0.5% will have six.

## The trachea

The trachea (see also Chapter 3) lies in front of the oesophagus in the midline. In front it is related to the infrahyoid muscles and the isthmus of the thyroid gland. Posteriorly lies the oesophagus with the recurrent laryngeal nerves in the groove between the two. ✪ Tracheostomy is an operation done to keep the airway patent. In this, a hole is made in the trachea at the level of the second or third tracheal ring and a tracheostomy tube is introduced. In a dire emergency an opening can be made through the cricothyroid ligament in the midline to maintain the airway (see Larynx – p. 206, Fig. 7.38b).

## Root of the neck

✪ Knowledge of anatomy of the root of the neck is essential to perform procedures such as subclavian vein catheterisation, brachial plexus block and to understand the effects of a Pancoast tumour (Pancoast syndrome).

The root of the neck is the junctional area between the thorax and the neck and contains all the structures going from the thorax to the neck and vice versa (Fig. 7.9).

The apex of the lung and the apical pleura project into the neck from the thorax. This is covered by a fascia known

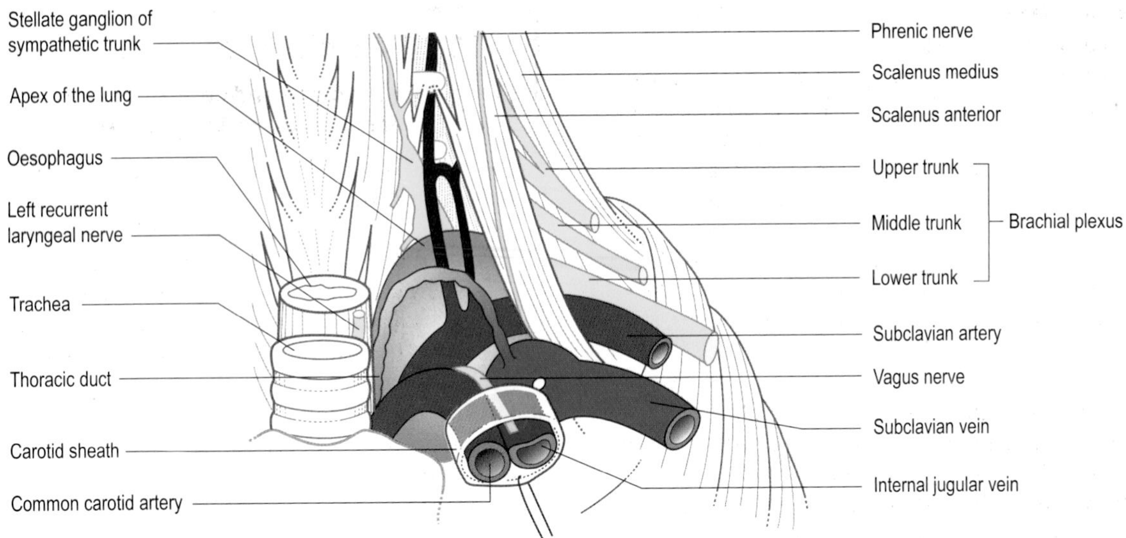


Fig. 7.9 Root of the neck. The carotid sheath and its contents are cut and reflected to show the deep structures of the left side of the root of the neck.

as the suprapleural membrane or Sibson's fascia. Sibson's fascia is attached to the inner border of the first rib and to the transverse process of the sixth cervical vertebrae. ✪ It functions to prevent the lung and pleura rising further into the neck during respiration. The subclavian artery and vein and the brachial plexus lie on the suprapleural membrane.

✪ At the lower part of the neck (root of the neck) the scalenus anterior muscle lies in between the subclavian artery and subclavian vein (Figs 7.4, 7.6, 7.9). The phrenic nerve lies on the scalenus anterior. As the right vagus crosses the subclavian artery to enter the thorax it gives off the right recurrent laryngeal nerve which winds round the artery to reach the groove between the trachea and the oesophagus. ✪ On the left side the thoracic duct arches laterally, lying between the carotid sheath and the vertebral artery, and enters the junction between the internal jugular and the subclavian veins. Inadvertent puncture or laceration of the thoracic duct will cause escape of lymph into the surrounding tissue and occasionally chylothorax.

## The subclavian artery

See Figures 7.4, 7.5 and 7.7. The right subclavian artery is a branch of the brachiocephalic trunk and the left arises directly from the arch of the aorta. It lies posterior to the insertion of the scalenus anterior on the first rib. The subclavian vein runs parallel to the artery but in front of the scalenus anterior slightly at a lower level. The roots and the trunks of the brachial plexus lie behind the subclavian artery on the first rib between the scalenus anterior and the scalenus medius muscles. The artery beyond the first rib continues into the axilla as the axillary artery.

✪ The subclavian artery pulsations can be felt at the medial third of the clavicle near the lateral border of the sternocleido-mastoid on deep palpation against the first rib.

The branches of the subclavian artery are the vertebral artery, the internal mammary (thoracic) artery, the thyrocervical trunk and the costocervical trunk (Fig. 7.7).

The vertebral artery is the first branch of the subclavian artery. It enters the foramen transversarium at the sixth cervical vertebra, ascends through the foramina transversaria of the sixth to the first cervical vertebrae and enters the cranial cavity and branches to supply the brain and spinal cord. The internal thoracic (mammary) artery passes vertically downwards a finger's breadth lateral to the sternum. In the sixth intercostal space it divides into the musculophrenic artery and the superior epigastric artery. The thyrocervical trunk is a branch of the subclavian artery medial to the scalenus anterior. It divides into the inferior thyroid artery, the transverse cervical and the suprascapular arteries. The inferior thyroid artery lies behind the carotid sheath and ascends in front of the scalenus anterior. At the level of the transverse process of the sixth cervical vertebra the artery arches medially and enters the posteromedial aspect of the capsule of the thyroid gland at its lower third. The recurrent laryngeal nerve is closely related to the artery and its branches near the lower pole of the thyroid gland.

## The subclavian vein

The subclavian vein (Figs 7.4, 7.8, 7.9) follows the course of the subclavian artery in the neck, but lies in front of the scalenus anterior on the first rib. Veins accompanying the branches of the subclavian artery drain into the external jugular, the subclavian vein or its continuation, the brachiocephalic vein (formed by the union of the subclavian and the internal jugular veins). ✪ Subclavian venepuncture can be carried out by inserting the needle below the clavicle at the junction of its middle and medial thirds and advanced upwards and medially behind the clavicle towards the sternoclavicular joint. There is the risk of pneumothorax and an inadvertent puncture of the subclavian artery in this procedure as the vein lies on the apex of the lung in front of the artery (Fig. 7.9).

## Thoracic duct (see also p. 69)

This duct carries lymph from the whole body except that from right side of thorax, right upper limb, and right side of head and neck. It arises in the abdomen, passes through the thorax and enters the neck lying on the left side of the oesophagus (Fig. 7.9). At the root of the neck it arches laterally, lying between the carotid sheath and the vertebral artery, and enters the junction between the internal jugular and the subclavian veins. ✪ Inadvertent puncture or laceration of the thoracic duct will cause escape of lymph into the surrounding tissue and occasionally chylothorax.

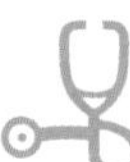

*Clinical box 7.2*

**Pancoast's tumour and Horner's syndrome**

Interruption of the head and neck supply of sympathetic nerves will result in Horner's syndrome, characterised by constriction of pupil, slight ptosis and anhydrous on the side of the lesion. This can be caused by any condition causing pressure on the cervical part of the sympathetic chain.

Pancoast's tumour is a carcinoma of the apical part of the lung which spreads locally to involve structures at the root of the neck. Involvement of the brachial plexus and cervical sympathetic chain causes severe pain in the shoulder region radiating toward the axilla and scapula along the ulnar aspect of the muscles of the hand, atrophy of hand and arm muscles and Horner's syndrome.

### Stellate ganglion

The sympathetic trunk is continued into the neck from the thorax. There are three cervical ganglia: superior, middle, and inferior. The sympathetic trunk lies embedded on the posterior wall of the carotid sheath. The superior ganglion lies at the level of C2 & C3, the middle at the level of C6, and the inferior ganglion at the neck of the first rib behind the vertebral artery (see Fig. 7.33). Often the inferior ganglion is fused with the first thoracic ganglion to form the stellate ganglion (Fig. 7.9). Grey rami from this reach the upper limb through the roots of the brachial plexus, mostly through C7 and C8. The preganglionic input to the cervical ganglia (including the stellate) are from the upper thoracic white rami. ✪ In sympathectomy to denervate the upper limb the T2–T4 ganglia and the white rami are severed preserving the T1 connection and the stellate ganglion to avoid Horner's syndrome. The thoracic part of the sympathetic chain (p. 70) can be seen lying on the heads of the upper ribs through a thoracoscope after deflating the lung. Resection of T2–T4 segment is carried out to produce a dry hand in patients suffering from hyperhidrosis. See Clinical box 7.2.

### Brachial plexus

The anterior primary ramus of C5 and C6 join to form the upper trunk of the brachial plexus, C7 forms the middle trunk and the C8 and T1 join to form the lower trunk. The nerves lie sandwiched between the scalenus anterior and the medius above and lateral to the subclavian artery. See Clinical boxes 7.3 and 7.4.

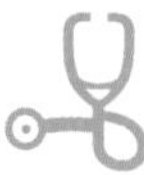

*Clinical box 7.3*

**Brachial plexus blocks**

A number of approaches are described to block the brachial plexus in the supraclavicular region. In the supraclavicular perivascular method the needle is inserted at the middle of the clavicle just lateral to the subclavian artery pulsation and directed backwards, downwards and inwards. Pneumothorax and or haematoma are complications.

In the interscalene approach the needle is inserted at a higher level at the level of the cricoid cartilage and advanced towards the transverse process of the sixth cervical vertebra. The local anaesthetic is injected deep to the prevertebral fascia (the plane containing the nerves). The risk of pneumothorax is less in the interscalene approach. Phrenic nerve paralysis, recurrent laryngeal nerve paralysis, and Horner's syndrome due to paralysis of the stellate ganglion and inadvertent injection into the vertebral artery are complications.

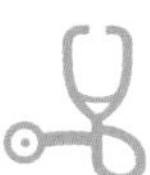

*Clinical box 7.4*

**Cervical rib**

This is a condition in which an extra rib or part of a rib may develop as a prolongation of C7 transverse process. It can be bony, fibrous, or partly fibrous and partly bony; and if complete will extend up to the scalene tubercle of the first rib. The components of the brachial plexus which normally lie on the first rib get displaced upwards by the extra rib, leading to compression of the lower trunk (C8, T1). In addition the subclavian vessels may also be stretched, giving rise to Raynaud's phenomenon in the hand.

Diagnosis of the cervical rib is not difficult as it is seen on x-ray if it is bony. But when it is a fibrous band, diagnosis depends on the absence of any cervical spine abnormality and the presence of vascular and neuritic symptoms.

### Lymph nodes of the head and neck

The lymph nodes of the head and neck can be classified in to a superficial and a deep group.

#### The superficial nodes

The few nodes which lie superficial to the deep fascia are in two subgroups:

- the anterior cervical nodes along the anterior jugular vein
- the superficial cervical nodes along the external jugular vein.

Afferents to these nodes are from the superficial tissues of the regions corresponding to those drained by the veins along which they lie.

Efferents from the superficial nodes join the deep cervical nodes.

#### The deep lymph nodes of the head and neck

✪ Most of the deep lymph nodes are arranged roughly in a vertical chain along the internal jugular vein. The deep cervical nodes form the terminal group for all lymphatics in the head and neck. All tissues in the head and neck drain into intermediary groups and then into the deep cervical nodes. The deep cervical nodes lie covered by the fascia of the carotid sheath, closely related to the internal jugular vein. They are subdivided into:

- the superior deep cervical nodes
- the inferior deep cervical nodes.

✪ The superior group lies in the region where the posterior belly of the digastric crosses the internal jugular vein and hence, nodes here are also known as the

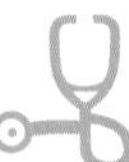

## Clinical box 7.5

**Block dissection of the neck**

In this all the lymph nodes in the anterior and posterior triangles of the neck along with the associated structures are removed en-bloc. It extends from the mandible above to the clavicle below and from the midline anteriorly to the anterior border of the trapezius posteriorly. All the structures from the platysma to the pretracheal fascia are removed, leaving only the carotid arteries, the vagus nerve, the sympathetic trunk, and the lingual and the hypoglossal nerves. The sternocleidomastoid, the posterior belly of the digastric and the omohyoid are all removed along with the internal jugular and the external jugular veins, the submandibular gland and the lower part of the parotid gland. The accessory nerve, to which lymph nodes are related in the posterior triangle, is also sacrificed.

jugulodigastric nodes. This group is closely related to the spinal accessory nerve. They drain the tonsil and the tongue and the efferents go to the lower deep cervical nodes and/or to the jugular trunk.

✪ The lower group lies where the omohyoid crosses the internal jugular vein and hence are called the jugulo-omohyoid group. These drain the tongue, oral cavity, trachea, oesophagus, and the thyroid gland.

✪ A few nodes in the deep cervical group extend into the posterior triangle and lie along the course of the accessory nerve. There are also few nodes in the root of the neck – the supraclavicular nodes which enlarge in late stages of malignancies of thorax and abdomen. A classical example is Virchow's node associated with gastric carcinoma (Troisier's sign). See Clinical box 7.5.

## Posterior triangle

The posterior triangle (Figs 7.10–7.12) or the side of the neck contains the accessory nerve, external jugular vein, the cervical plexus and proximal parts of the brachial plexus of nerves supplying the upper limb.

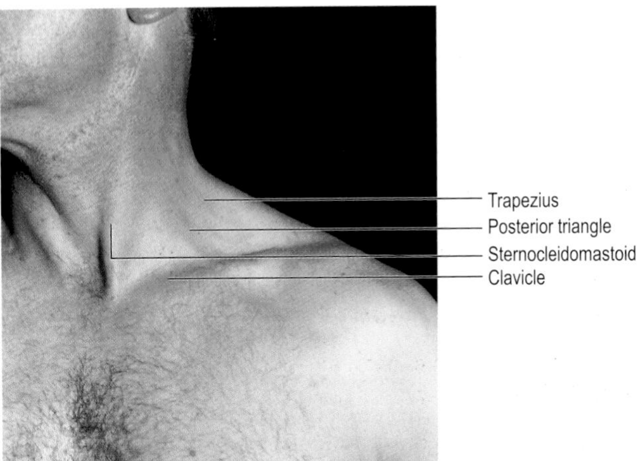


Fig. 7.10 Surface anatomy of the posterior triangle.

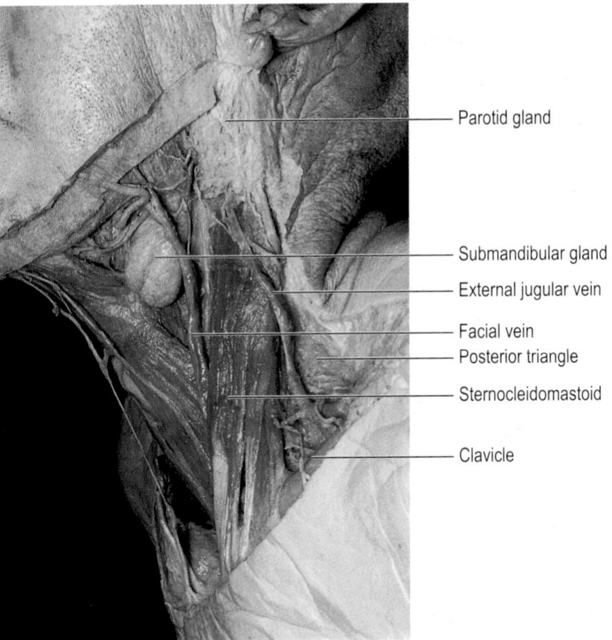


Fig. 7.11 External jugular vein.

### Surface anatomy

✪ The sternocleidomastoid and the trapezius muscles and the middle part of the clavicle form the boundaries of the posterior triangle. A line connecting the junction between the upper third and the lower two-thirds of the posterior border of the sternocleidomastoid to a point two fingers' breadths (5cm) above the clavicle on the anterior border of the trapezius is the surface marking of the accessory nerve. The nerve can be identified as it enters the deep surface of the sternocleidomastoid about 4cm below the mastoid. It is found just above Erb's point, where great auricular, transverse cervical and supraclavicular nerves (all branches of the cervical plexus) emerge from behind the sternocleidomastoid.

The external jugular vein drains the scalp and face. It lies in the superficial fascia, superficial to the sternomastoid, but in the lower part of the posterior triangle pierces the deep fascia and drains into the subclavian vein. The vein is prone to many variations and its size is inversely proportional to the size of other neck veins. ✪ The presence of a valve at its junction with the subclavian vein makes cannulation of the external jugular vein difficult. The vein is normally invisible but can be distended by straining or pressure at the root of the neck. When the venous pressure rises, as in heart failure, the vein becomes prominent.

### Sternocleidomastoid

*Origin* By two heads from the manubrium of the sternum and the clavicle.

*Insertion* The mastoid process and the superior nuchal line.

*Nerve supply* The spinal accessory nerve.

*Action* Turns the head to the opposite side.

The accessory nerve supplying the sternocleidomastoid and the trapezius can be easily damaged because of its superficial position in the posterior triangle. The trapezius muscle will be paralysed resulting in inability to lift the arm above the level of the shoulder (see p. 182, internal jugular vein).

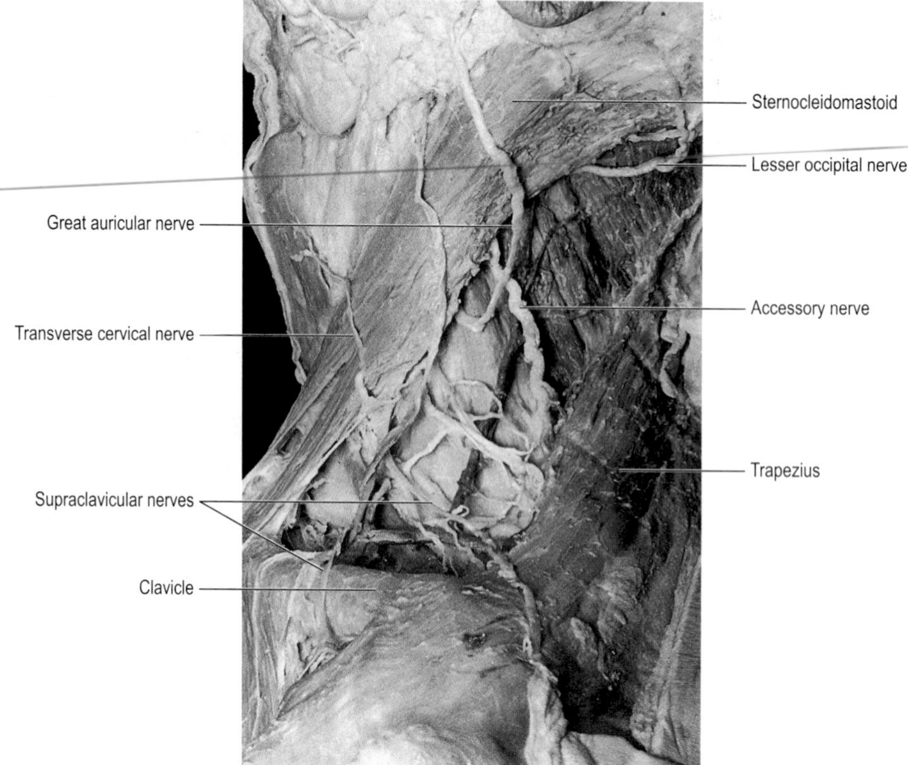


Fig. 7.12 Nerves of the posterior triangle (left side).

### Cervical plexus

See Figures 7.12 and 7.16. Cutaneous branches of this nerve plexus supply the skin of the neck, the shoulder and pectoral regions. They are: the great auricular nerve (C2, C3), the lesser occipital nerve (C2), the transverse cervical nerve (C2, C3) and the supraclavicular nerves (C3, C4).

The phrenic nerve (C3, C4, C5) supplying the diaphragm and the inferior root of the ansa cervicalis for the infrahyoid muscles are also branches of the cervical plexus.

## The face, the facial nerve and the parotid gland

See Figures 7.13–7.16. The superficial muscles of the face and the muscles of facial expression are attached to the skin. Contraction of the orbicularis oculi closes the eye. ✪ It has two parts: the palpebral part which arches across both the eyelids is used in blinking and the orbital part which circumscribes the orbital margin is used in shutting the eye more forcefully as in 'screwing up the eyes'. Orbicularis oculi facilitates drainage of the lacrimal secretion (tears). The blinking action enables the lacrimal fluid to spread medially towards the nose. A few fibres of the orbicularis oculi are attached to the lacrimal sac which dilates on contraction of the muscle, thus sucking fluid into the sac. Elastic recoil of the sac empties the fluid into the nasal cavity through the nasolacrimal duct. The orbicularis oculi is supplied by the facial nerve. ✪ Paralysis of the orbicularis oculi, as may occur in facial nerve paralysis, will prevent the blinking action of the eyelid. This will fail to moisten the cornea and in turn lead to ulceration of the cornea.

### The facial nerve

✪ The facial nerve, the seventh cranial nerve (Figs 7.14, 7.15) supplies the muscles of facial expression. It also conveys parasympathetic fibres to the lacrimal gland, glands in the nasal cavity, submandibular and sublingual glands and transmits taste fibres from the anterior two-thirds of the tongue.

The facial nerve originates from the pons and passes through the facial canal in the petrous temporal bone. It passes downwards on the posterior wall of the middle ear to emerge though the stylomastoid foramen at the base of the skull.

In the petrous temporal bone, the facial nerve gives off three branches:

- the greater petrosal nerve
- the nerve to stapedius
- the chorda tympani nerve.

The greater petrosal nerve transmits preganglionic parasympathetic fibres to the sphenopalatine ganglion, the postganglionic fibres from which supply the lacrimal gland and the glands in the nasal cavity. The chorda tympani nerve carries parasympathetic fibres to the submandibular and sublingual glands as well as taste fibres from the anterior two-thirds of the tongue.

After emerging from the stylomastoid foramen the nerve enters the parotid gland and divides into temporal, zygomatic, buccal, marginal mandibular and cervical branches. These supply the muscles of facial expression. Before entering the parotid gland the nerve supplies branches to the posterior belly of the digastric, stylohyoid and the muscles of the auricle.

The temporal branches of the facial nerve pass upwards to supply the frontalis muscle. The zygomatic branches cross the zygomatic arch and supply the orbicularis oculi. The

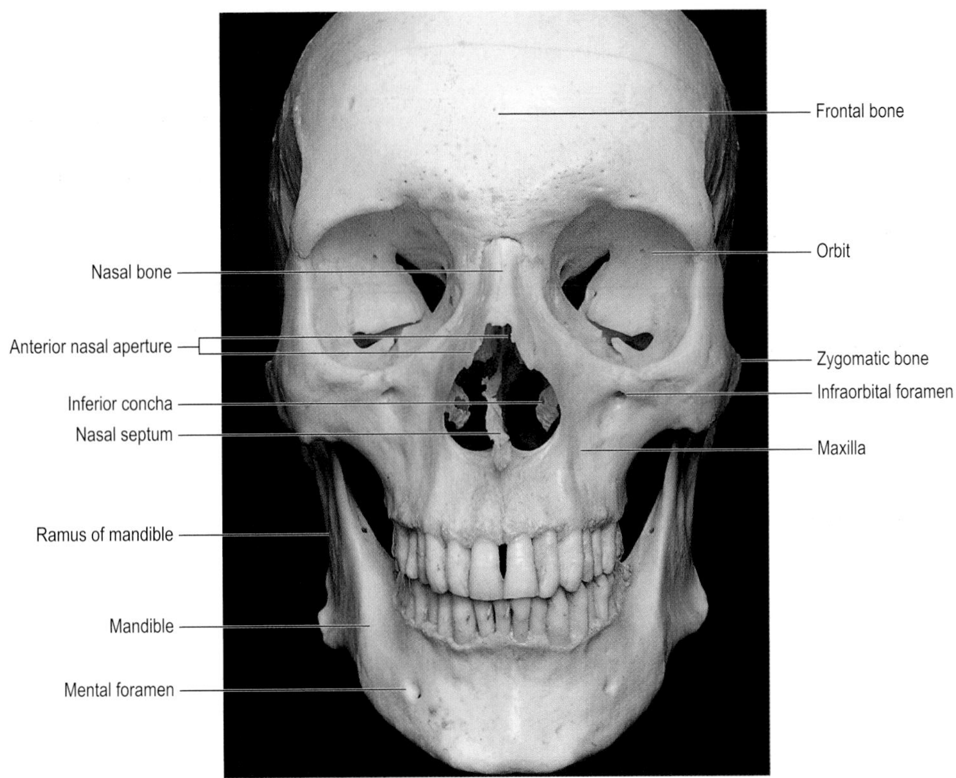


Fig. 7.13 Skull and mandible – anterior view.

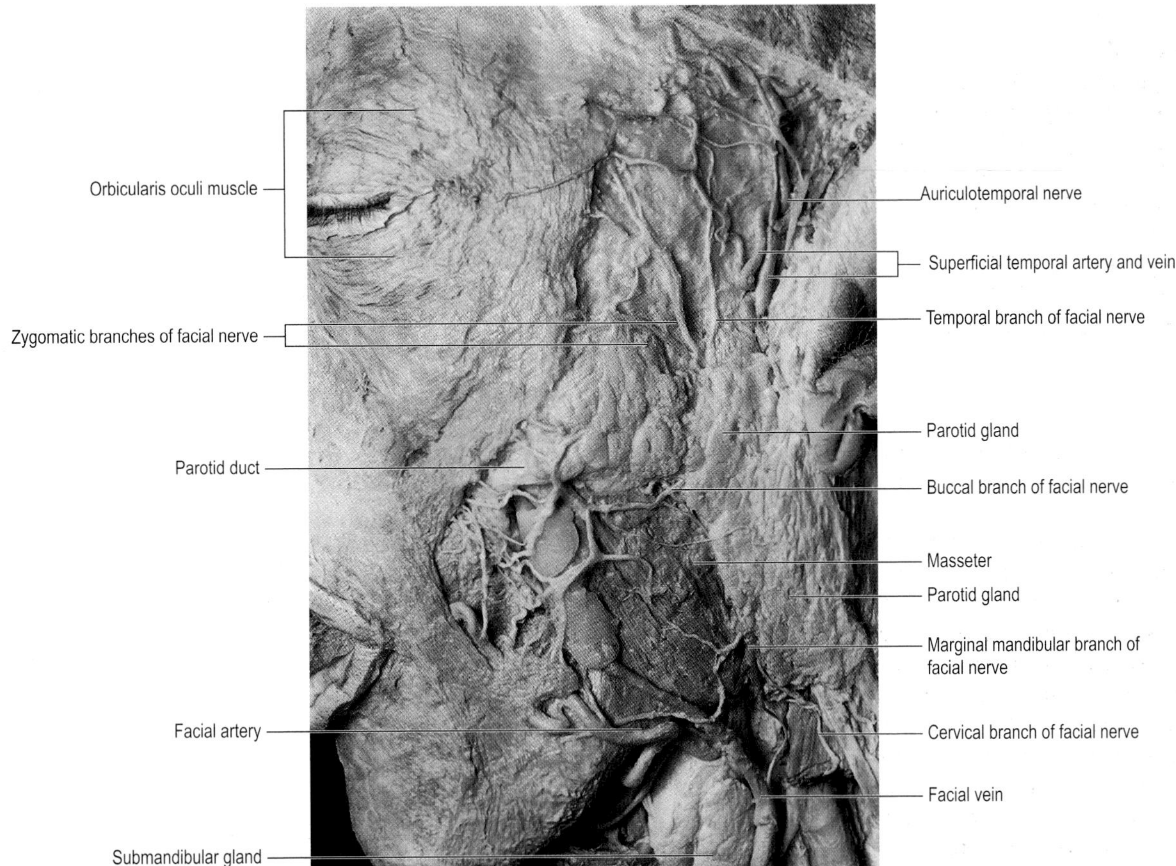


Fig. 7.14 Dissection of the face.

buccal branches, passing anteriorly, supply the buccinator (buccinator is the muscle of the cheek and functions to push the food medially from the space between the cheek and the teeth, i.e. the vestibule of the mouth). The marginal mandibular branch passes along the lower margin of the mandible to supply the muscles around the mouth including the orbicularis oris. The cervical branch passes downwards to supply the platysma.

✪ Infranuclear paralysis of the facial nerve has a wide variety of causes such as acoustic neuroma and its surgery,

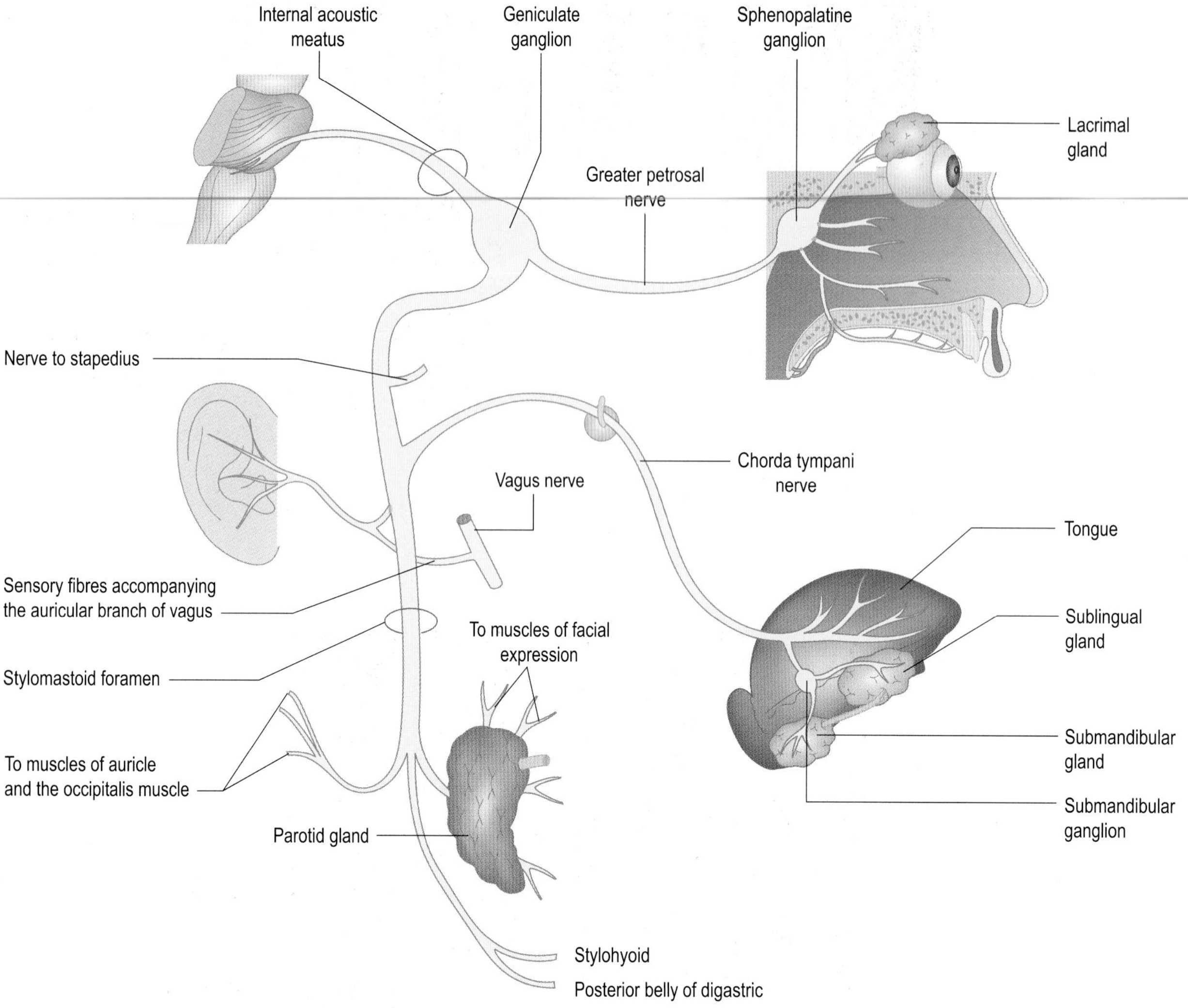

Internal acoustic meatus
Geniculate ganglion
Sphenopalatine ganglion
Lacrimal gland
Greater petrosal nerve
Nerve to stapedius
Chorda tympani nerve
Vagus nerve
Tongue
Sensory fibres accompanying the auricular branch of vagus
Sublingual gland
To muscles of facial expression
Stylomastoid foramen
Submandibular gland
To muscles of auricle and the occipitalis muscle
Submandibular ganglion
Parotid gland
Stylohyoid
Posterior belly of digastric


Fig. 7.15 Summary of the distribution of the facial nerve.

Ophthalmic nerve
Supraorbital nerve
Greater occipital nerve (C2, C3)
Supratrochlear nerve
Mandibular nerve
Maxillary nerve
Auriculotemporal nerve
Zygomaticofacial nerve
Lesser occipital nerve (C2)
External nasal nerve
Great auricular nerve (C2, C3)
Infraorbital nerve
Mental nerve
Buccal nerve
Dorsal rami of C3, C4, C5
Transverse cervical nerve (C2, C3)
Supraclavicular nerves (C3, C4)


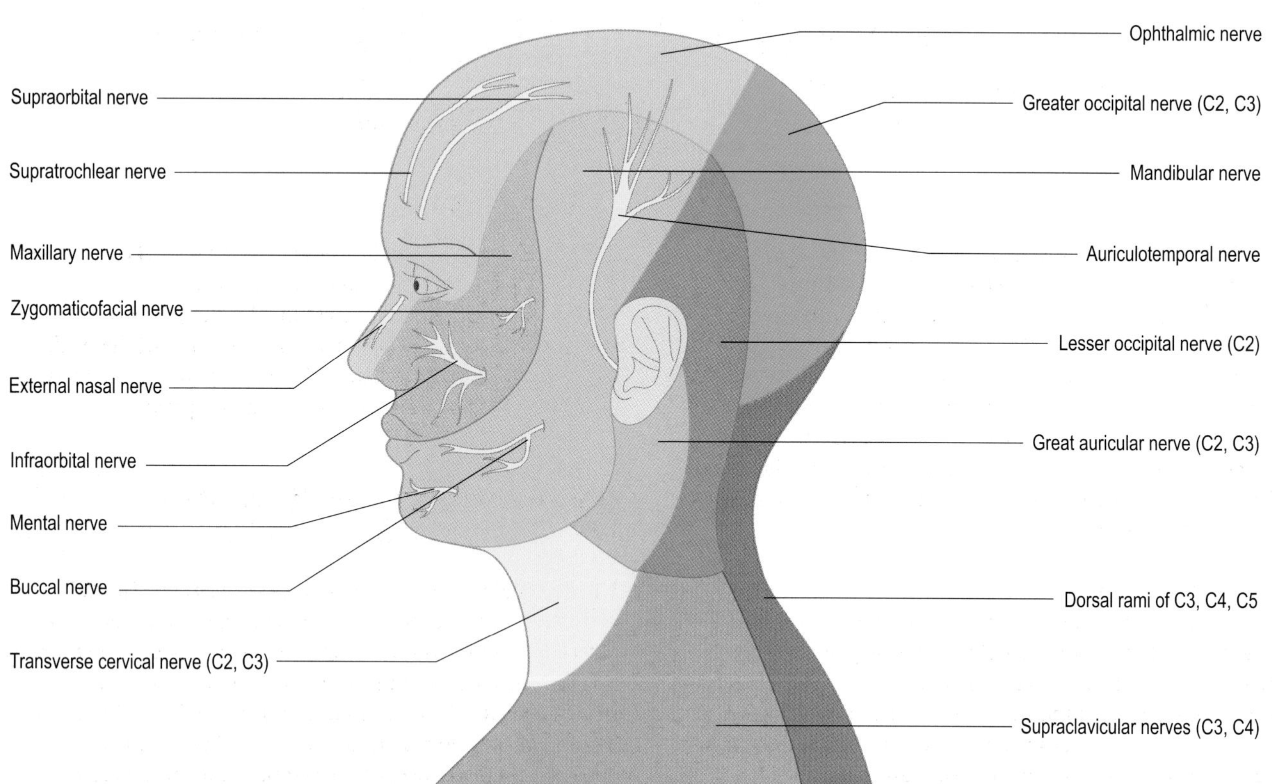

Fig. 7.16 Sensory innervation of the head and neck.

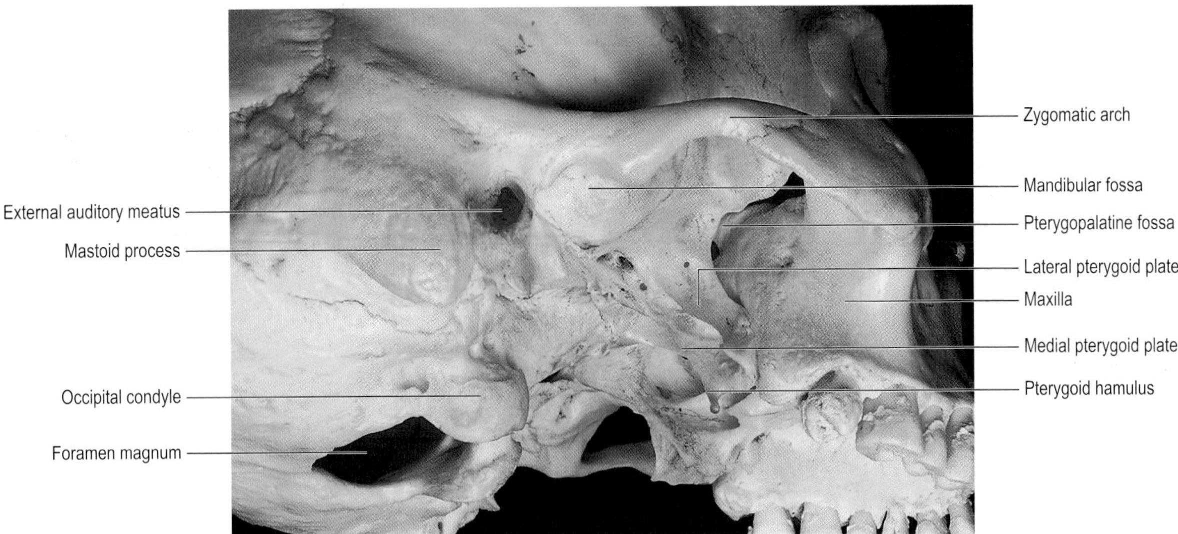


Fig. 7.17 Anterior inferior aspect of the skull viewed from the side.

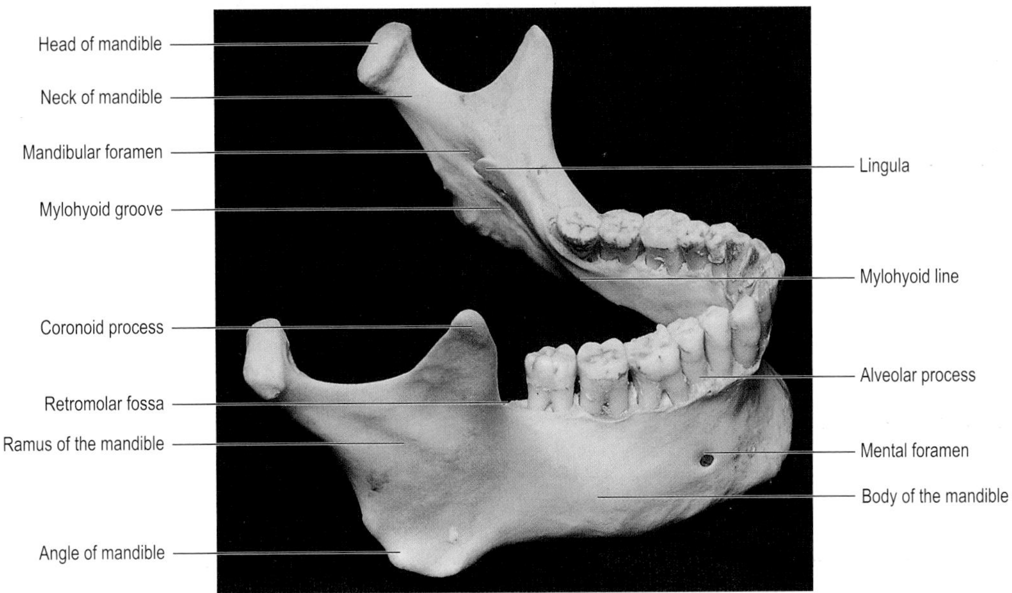


Fig. 7.18 The mandible.

viral infection producing inflammation and swelling of the nerve, fractures of the base of the skull, and tumours and surgery of the parotid gland. Bell's palsy is an infranuclear paralysis of the facial nerve of unknown aetiology. The paralysis will affect all the muscles on the same side of the face. Supranuclear paralysis which affects the contralateral facial muscles spares the orbicularis oculi and the muscles of the scalp as the part of the facial nerve nucleus supplying these has bilateral cortical connections.

### The parotid gland

The parotid gland (Fig. 7.14) is predominantly a serous salivary gland. It is situated below the external auditory meatus and extends on to the ramus of the mandible. It lies on the masseter, and the sternocleidomastoid. The deep part of the gland is irregular in shape and extends almost up to the side wall of the pharynx and the carotid sheath, from which it is separated by the styloid process and its attached structures. ✪ The parotid gland is traversed by the facial nerve, the retromandibular vein and the external carotid artery in that order from superficial to deep.

The parotid gland is enclosed inside a tough capsule derived from the investing layer of deep fascia of the neck. ✪ Mumps, a virus infection of the gland, is painful because the gland swells within the thick fibrous capsule.

## The muscles of mastication and the mandibular nerve

The mandible, or the lower jaw, consists of a horizontal body bearing the alveolar process and the lower teeth, and a vertically orientated ramus. The junction between the body and the ramus is the angle of the mandible. The head articulates with the mandibular fossa at the base of the skull to form the temporomandibular joint (Figs 7.17, 7.18).

On the medial aspect of the ramus is the mandibular foramen. This is guarded anteriorly by a projecting process called the lingula to which the sphenomandibular ligament

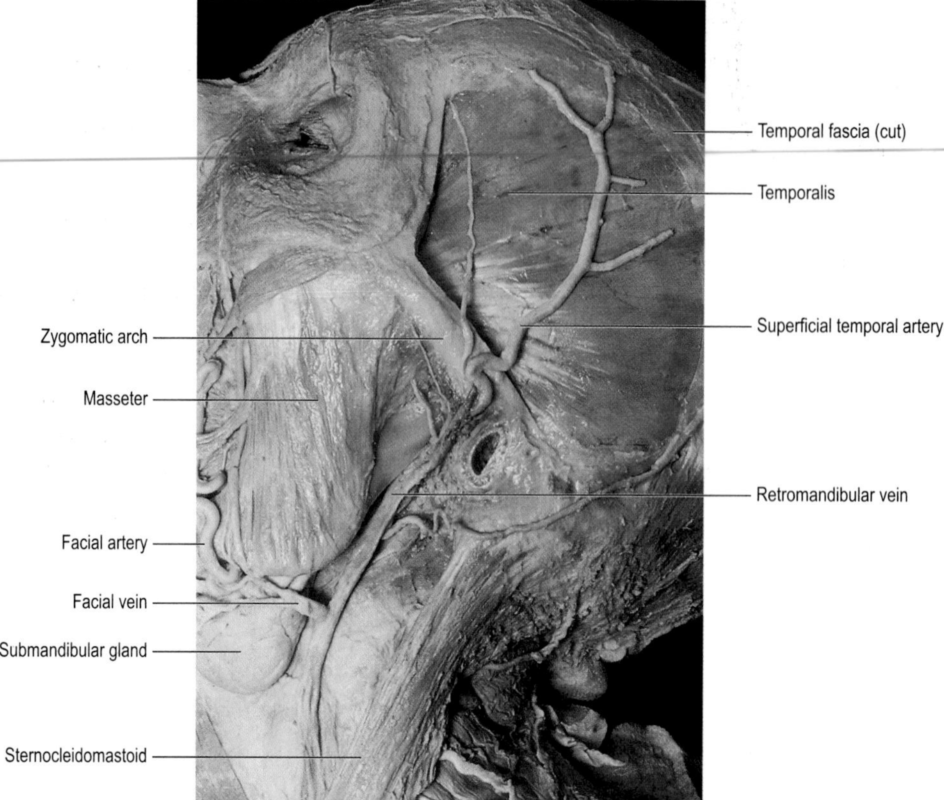


Fig. 7.19 Lateral aspect of the head and face after removal of the parotid gland.

is attached. The inferior alveolar (dental) nerve enters the mandibular foramen and transverses the body within the mandibular canal. It divides into the mental nerve and the incisive nerve. The incisive nerve, which supplies the incisors and canine teeth, continues beyond the mental foramen within the body in the incisive canal. The trunk of the inferior alveolar nerve supplies the premolars and the molars.

The mental nerve emerges through the mental foramen to supply the lower lip and the buccal and labial gingiva. A small groove runs inferiorly and forward from the mandibular foramen. This is the mylohyoid groove and is produced by the nerve to mylohyoid which supplies the mylohyoid and the anterior belly of the digastric muscles. Above the groove is a prominent ridge, the mylohyoid line, for the attachment of the mylohyoid muscle. The muscle extends from the level of the last molar tooth to the midline. The two mylohyoids which form the floor of the mouth separate the oral cavity from the neck (Fig. 7.4(B)). The lateral surface of the ramus gives attachment to the masseter which extends from the angle forward as far as the external oblique line and the second molar tooth.

✪ Fractures of the mandible happen more often than those of the upper facial skeleton. In many cases they are bilateral. The condyle of the mandible can fracture due to a blow to the chin and this may result in dislocation of the temporomandibular joint.

Fractures of the body of the mandible are most common in the canine region as the length of the root of the canine tooth weakens the bone in this position. Fractures of the body are always compound fractures lacerating the mucosa of the oral cavity.

The temporomandibular joint is a synovial joint where the head of the mandible articulates with the mandibular fossa (glenoid fossa) and the articular eminence of the temporal bone. The articular surfaces of this joint are covered by fibrocartilage (not hyaline) and there is also a fibrocartilaginous articular disc dividing the joint cavity into upper and lower compartments. The joints allow depression, elevation, protrusion, retraction, and side-to-side movements of the mandible.

### Muscles of mastication

There are four pairs of muscles in this group attaching the mandible to the base of the skull. The masseter (Fig. 7.19) extends from the zygomatic arch to the ramus of the mandible. It elevates the mandible. The temporalis takes origin from the temporal fossa and the temporal fascia covering the muscle and is inserted into the coronoid process. Its insertion extends into the retromolar fossa behind the last molar tooth. ✪ When lower dentures are fitted they should not extend into the retromolar fossa to avoid soreness of the mucosa due to contraction of the temporalis muscle. The temporalis elevates the mandible. Its posterior fibres retract the mandible after protrusion.

The pterygoid muscles (Figs 7.20, 7.21) lie medial to the ramus of the mandible. The lateral pterygoid, which originates from the lateral surface of the lateral pterygoid plate and from the infratemporal surface of the skull, is inserted into the capsule of the temporomandibular joint, the articular disc and also into the upper part of the neck of the mandible. Its contraction pulls the head of the mandible and the articular disc forward during protraction and during the act of opening the mouth. Unilateral contraction of the lateral pterygoid allows the mandible to move to the opposite side. The forward movement of the disc may help to pack the space between the incongruent articular surfaces

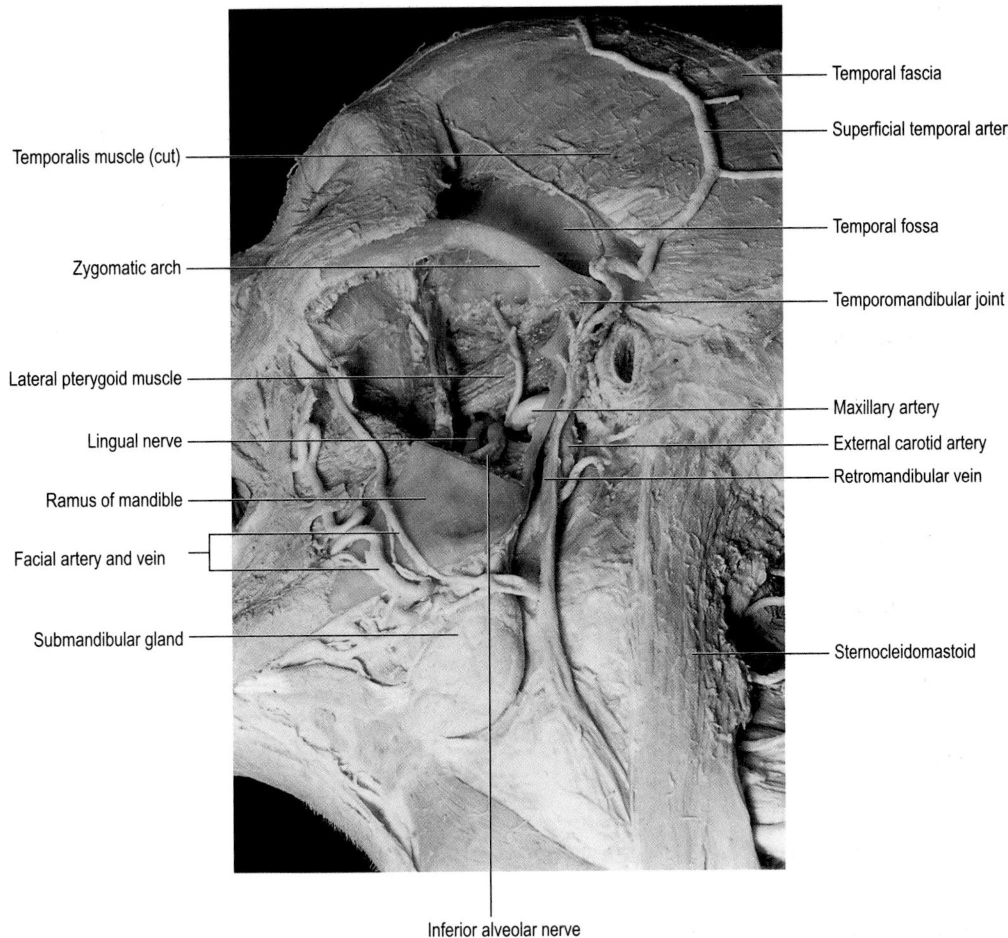


Fig. 7.20 Deep dissection of the face after removal of the temporalis, masseter, parotid gland and part of the ramus of the mandible.

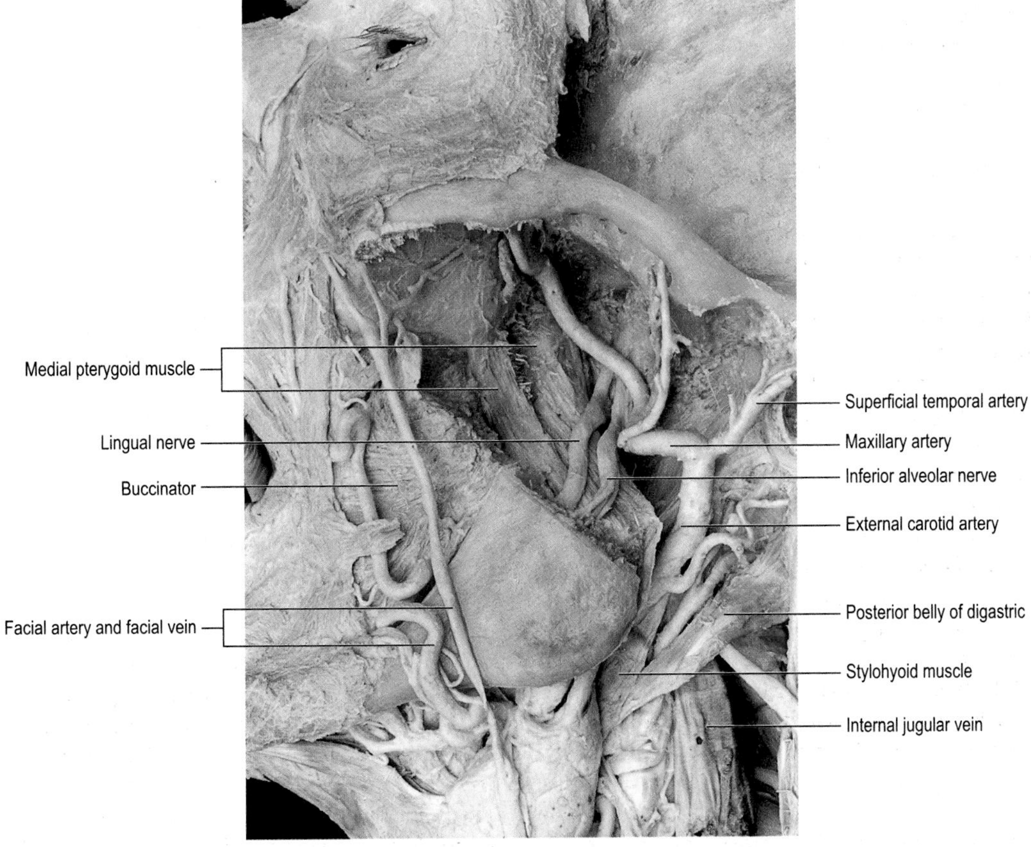


Fig. 7.21 Structures seen after removal of the ramus of the mandible, the temporomandibular joint and the lateral pterygoid muscle.

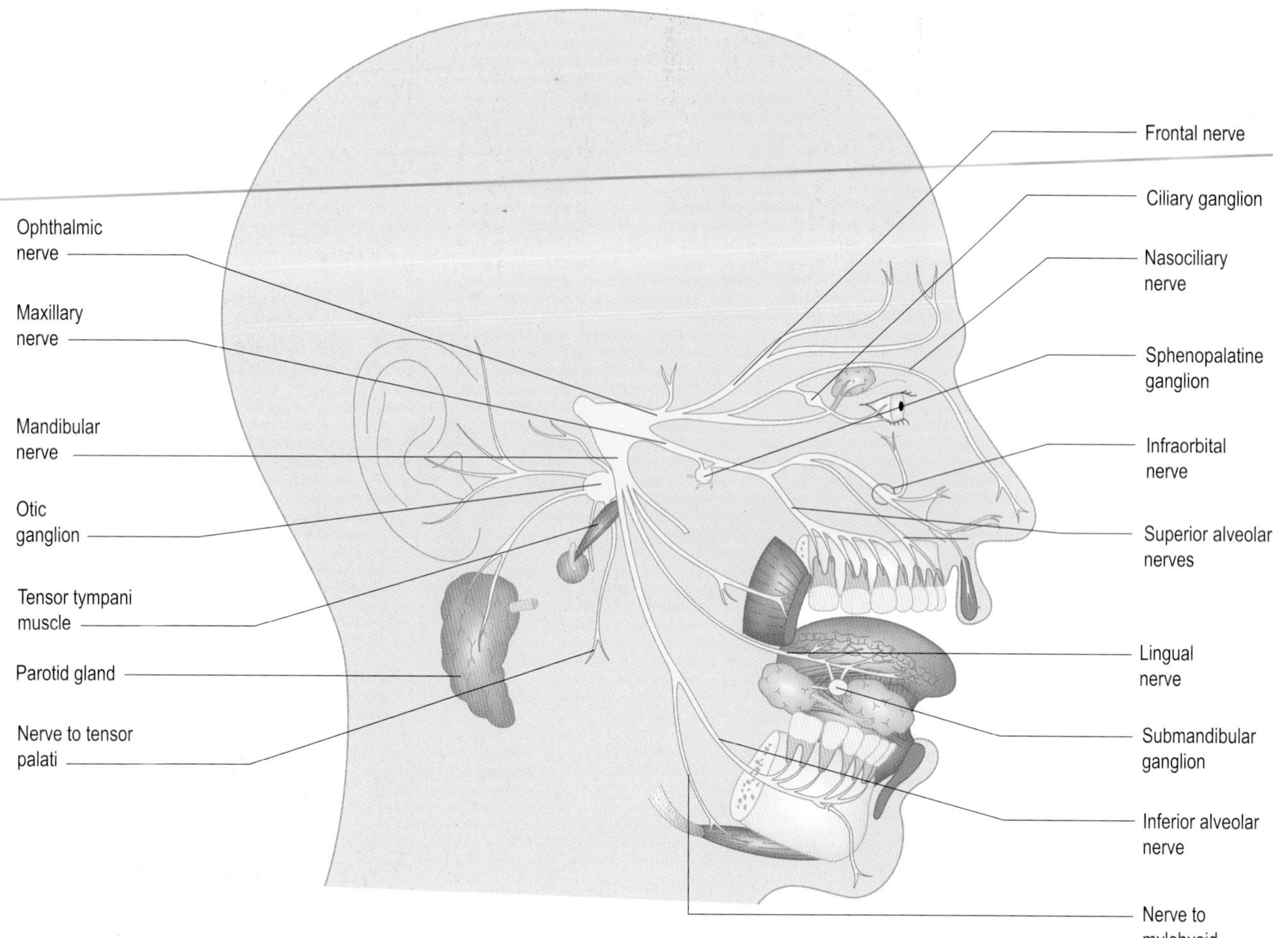


Fig. 7.22 Summary of the distribution of the trigeminal nerve.

of the condyle and the articular eminence thus stabilising the joint.

The medial pterygoid extends from the medial surface of the lateral pterygoid plate to the medial surface of the ramus of the mandible. It is an elevator of the mandible. Unilateral contraction of the medial pterygoid is important in the side-to-side movement of the mandible as it deviates the jaw to the opposite side.

The four muscles of mastication are supplied by the mandibular division of the trigeminal nerve.

### The mandibular nerve

This branch of the trigeminal nerve (Figs 7.20–7.22) having both motor and sensory fibres leaves the skull through the foramen ovale. The sensory fibres innervate the auricle and the external acoustic meatus, the skin over the mandible, the cheek, the lower lip, the tongue and the floor of the mouth, the lower teeth and the gums. The floor of the mouth and the inner gingiva of the lower jaw are supplied by the lingual nerve which is a branch of the mandibular nerve. The motor fibres supply the muscles of mastication – the temporalis, masseter, medial pterygoid and the lateral pterygoid. Branches from the mandibular division also innervate the tensor tympani and tensor palati as well as the anterior belly of the digastric and the mylohyoid muscles (Fig. 7.22). Proprioceptive fibres are contained in the branches innervating the muscles. The submandibular ganglion in which the parasympathetic nerve fibres to the submandibular and sublingual glands synapse is connected to the lingual nerve.

## The submandibular region, the submandibular gland and the floor of the mouth

The submandibular gland (Fig. 7.23) and the submandibular group of lymph nodes fill the submandibular triangle, which is bounded by the anterior and posterior bellies of the digastric muscle and the lower border of the mandible (Fig. 7.4(B)). The superficial surface of the gland is crossed by the facial vein, the cervical branch of the facial nerve and also often by the marginal mandibular branch of the facial nerve. The marginal mandibular branch lies deep to the platysma and is one of the most important relations of the gland (Figs 7.14, 7.23). ✪ Skin incisions in the submandibular region are made about 4cm below the mandible to avoid injury to the marginal mandibular branch.

Each submandibular gland has a larger, superficial part and a smaller deep part. The two are separated by the mylohyoid muscle. The two parts however are continuous with each other posteriorly and the concavity thus formed is occupied by the free posterior border of the mylohyoid muscle. The facial artery grooves the deep surface and emerges on to the face by passing between the gland and the mandible. Several submandibular lymph nodes lie on the superficial surface.

The deep part lies in the floor of the mouth, superior (deep) to the mylohyoid (Fig. 7.24) and is covered by the mucosa of the oral cavity. Medially it lies on the hyoglossus and is related to the lingual nerve, the submandibular ganglion and the hypoglossal nerve (Fig. 7.25).

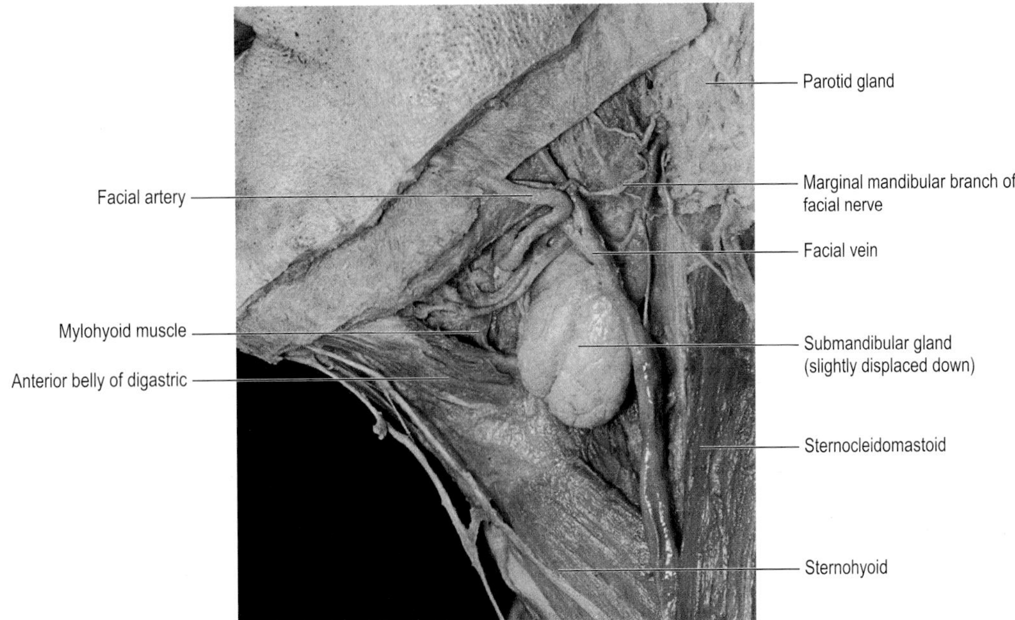


Fig. 7.23 Submandibular region – superficial dissection.

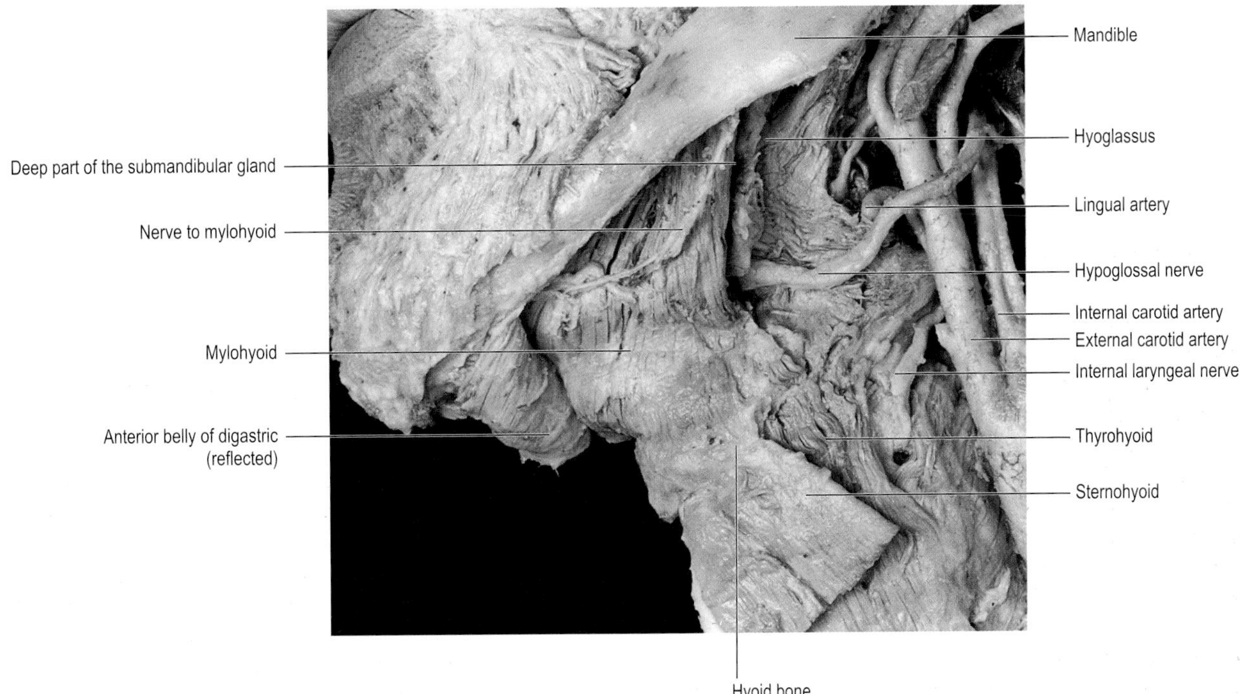


Fig. 7.24 Upper part of the neck after removal of the superficial part of the submandibular gland.

## The submandibular duct

The duct of the submandibular gland (Fig. 7.25) also known as the Wharton's duct, starts in the superficial part, running posteriorly and superiorly to reach the deep part. Here it turns forward and medially and emerges on to the surface of the hyoglossus muscle. It runs forward deep to the mucosa of the floor of the mouth between the mucosa and the sublingual gland to open into the floor of the mouth on either side of the frenulum of the tongue (see Fig. 7.27).

✪ The duct, on the floor of the mouth, is closely related to the lingual nerve. As it goes forward it crosses medial to the nerve to lie above the nerve and then crosses back, this time lateral to it to reach a position once again below the nerve (Fig. 7.25). The nerve can easily be damaged during ligation of the duct while removing the gland.

## The floor of the mouth

The floor of the mouth separating the oral cavity from the neck is formed by the mylohyoid diaphragm formed by the fusion of the mylohyoid muscles of both sides along the midline raphe. Above the mylohyoid is the mouth and below is the neck. The mylohyoids are reinforced superiorly by the two geniohyoids. The anterior part of the tongue rests on the mucosa covering the floor of the mouth.

More posteriorly between the mylohyoid and the tongue lies the hyoglossus muscle, which in fact is the side wall of the

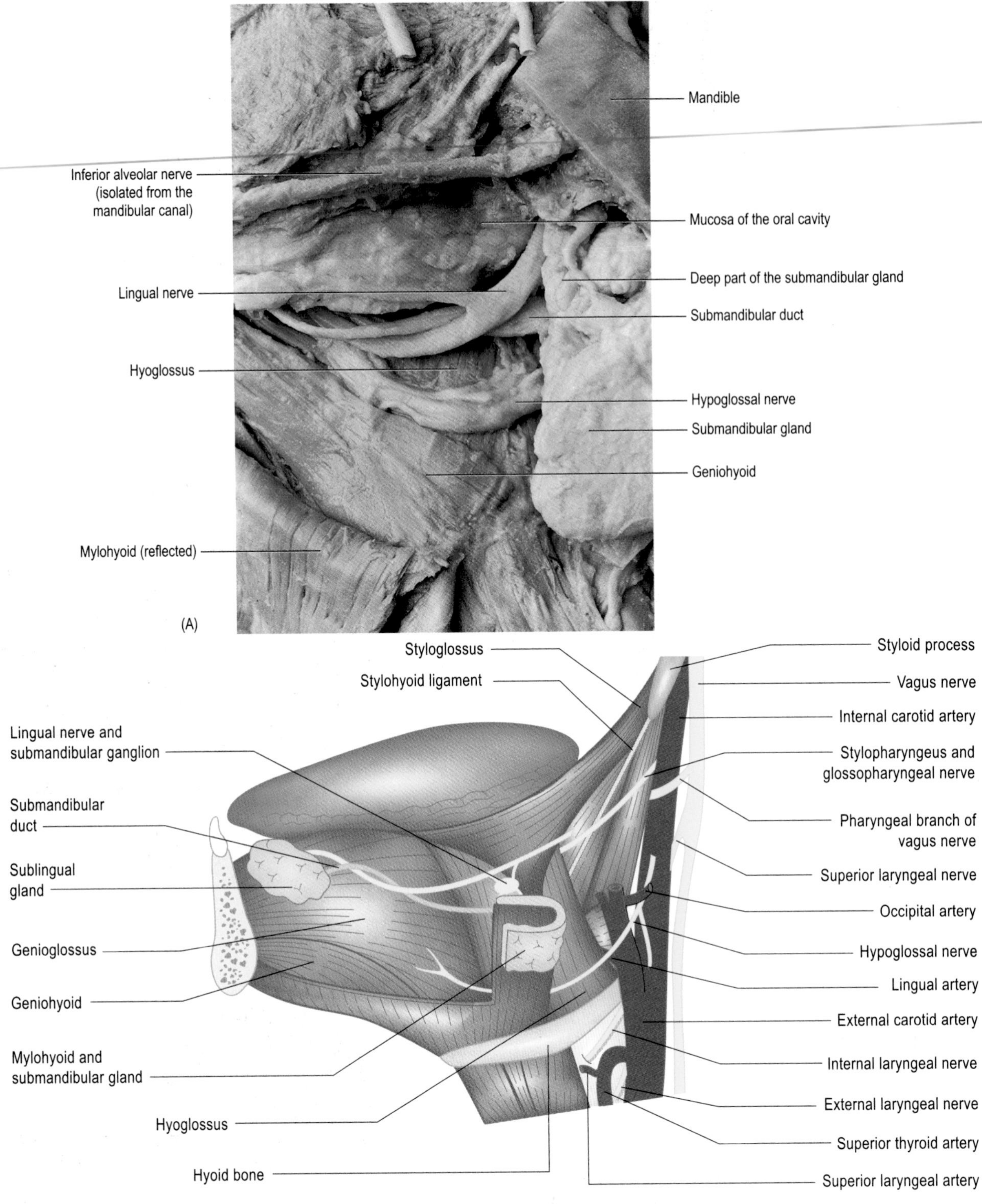


Fig. 7.25 (A) Deep structures in the submandibular region and the floor of the mouth seen after removal of the left half of the mandible and reflection of the left mylohyoid muscle – viewed from the left side. (B) Structures related to the hyoglossus. The lingual nerve, submandibular duct and the hypoglossal nerve are superficial to the hyoglossus whereas the glossopharyngeal nerve and the lingual artery pass deep to it.

tongue. ✪ A number of important structures in the floor of the mouth lie on the hyoglossus. From above downwards these are the lingual nerve, the deep part of the submandibular gland and the submandibular duct and the hypoglossal nerve.

The lingual nerve (Figs 7.22, 7.25), a branch of the mandibular division of the trigeminal nerve, runs forward above the mylohyoid. It gives off a gingival branch which supplies the whole of the lingual gingiva and the mucous membrane of the floor of the mouth. The lingual nerve winds round the submandibular duct before getting distributed to the mucosa of the anterior two-thirds of the tongue. The submandibular ganglion is suspended from the lingual nerve as it lies on the hyoglossus. The preganglionic fibres in the chorda tympani synapse in this ganglion. ✪ Before reaching the floor of the mouth the lingual nerve lies against the periosteum of the alveolar process closely related to the third molar tooth (Fig. 7.21). The nerve can be damaged here during dental extraction.

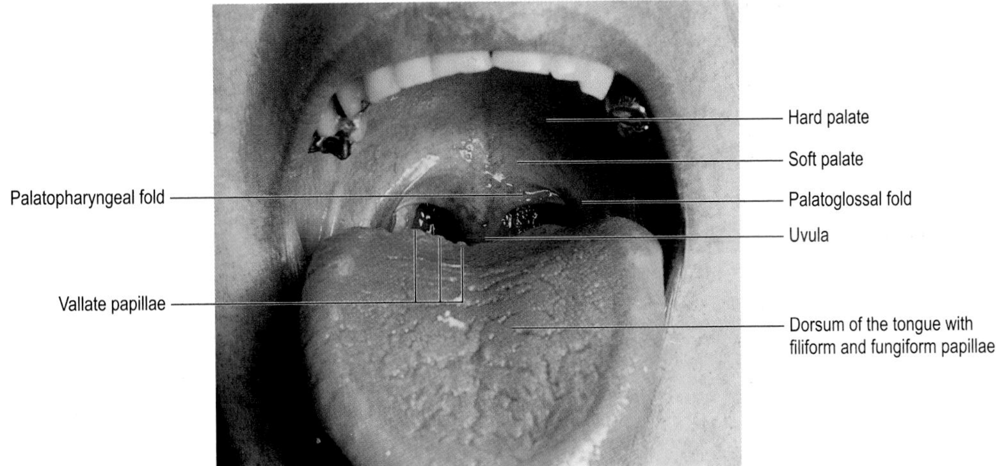


Fig. 7.26 The oral cavity.

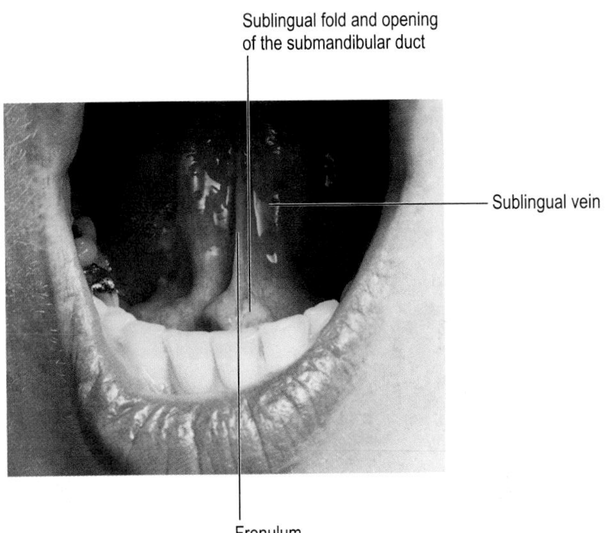


Fig. 7.27 Inferior surface of the tongue and the floor of the mouth.

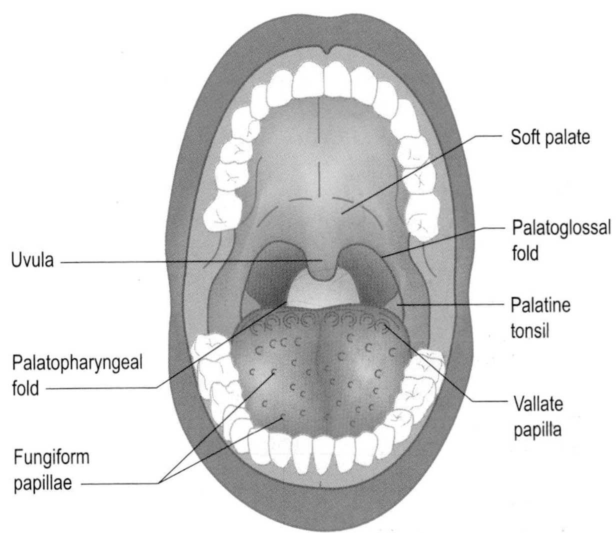


Fig. 7.28 Oral cavity and oropharynx.

On the hyoglossus the hypoglossal nerve breaks up into branches to supply all the muscles (both extrinsic and intrinsic) of the tongue except the palatoglossus.

## The oral cavity

### The tongue

The dorsum of the tongue (Figs 7.26–7.29) is divided into an anterior two-thirds and a posterior third by a V-shaped groove, the sulcus terminalis, the apex of which has the foramen caecum from which the thyroglossal duct giving rise to the thyroid gland develops. The mucosa of the anterior two-thirds carries the filiform papillae, fungiform papillae and, in front of the sulcus terminalis, a row of vallate papillae, about 8–12 in number (Fig. 7.26). The vallate papillae carry taste buds. The inferior surface of the tongue in the midline has the frenulum of the tongue. On either side of the frenulum the deep vein of the tongue can be seen and also the openings of the ducts of the submandibular glands (Figs 7.27, 7.29).

#### Muscles

A midline fibrous septum divides the tongue into right and left halves. Within these two compartments lie the intrinsic

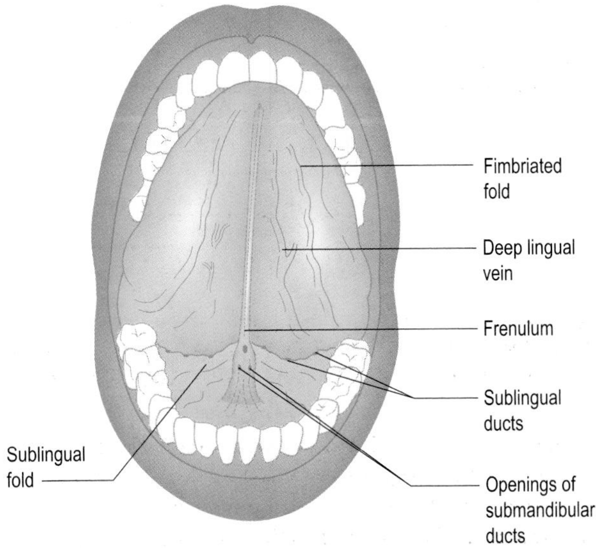


Fig. 7.29 Inferior surface of the tongue and the floor of the mouth.

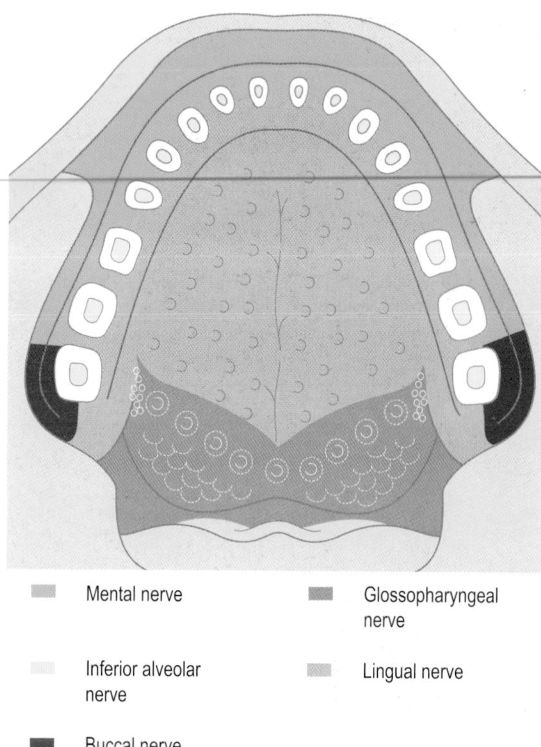


Fig. 7.30 Sensory nerve supply of the tongue, lower lip and cheek.

muscles which alter and control the shape of the tongue. The extrinsic muscles (Fig. 7.25; see also Fig. 7.32) attach the tongue to the mandible (the genioglossus), hyoid bone (the hyoglossus), styloid process (the styloglossus) and the soft palate (the palatoglossus). They alter the position of the tongue.

### Nerve supply

The innervation of the tongue (Fig. 7.30) is based on the development. The lingual nerve, which is a branch of the mandibular division of the trigeminal (nerve of the first branchial arch), carries common sensation from the anterior two-thirds. Taste is carried by the chorda tympani fibres within the lingual nerve. The sensory supply of the posterior third, including the vallate papillae, is by the glossopharyngeal nerve, which is the nerve of the third branchial arch. The intrinsic and extrinsic muscles are supplied by the hypoglossal nerve (Fig. 7.25). ✪ Paralysis of the hypoglossal nerve is manifested as fibrillation of the tongue as well as wasting of the muscles. The latter will show the mucosa loose on the paralysed side.

### Blood supply

The tongue is supplied by the lingual artery, a branch of the external carotid artery. At the posterior third, branches from the tonsillar artery (branch of the facial) and ascending pharyngeal artery anastomose with those of the lingual artery. There is only a poor communication between the two lingual arteries across the median septum.

The venous drainage is by two main veins, the lingual vein accompanying the lingual artery and the deep lingual vein which is visible on the inferior surface.

### Lymphatic drainage

✪ Lymphatic spread in cancer of the tongue is by tumour emboli. The drainage is essentially to the deep cervical nodes along the internal jugular vein. In the anterior two-thirds there is only minimal communication of lymphatics across the midline septum so that metastases from this portion tend to be ipsilateral. Posterior third lymphatics form extrinsic networks and facilitate early bilateral metastases. Lymphatics from the tip of the tongue pass to the submental nodes and from there to the lower deep cervical nodes. From the midportion, lymphatics pass to the submandibular nodes and then to the deep cervical from the margin of the tongue ipsilaterally and the rest bilaterally. From the posterior third, the drainage is to the upper deep cervical of both sides.

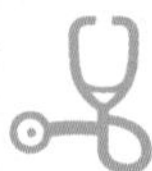

*Clinical box 7.6*

**Cleft lip and palate**

The region of the palate bearing the four front teeth is derived from the premaxilla, part of the frontonasal process, and the rest of the palate from the palatine shelves of the maxillary processes. Failure of fusion causes cleft palate. The palate may be cleft posteriorly only, or it may extend anteriorly to include most of the hard palate. More commonly it extends further anteriorly to join up with either a unilateral or bilateral cleft lip. Malfunction of the palate causes speech defects, problems in swallowing, and deafness and ear infection due to involvement of the Eustachian tube.

## The palate

The roof of the mouth is the palate (Figs 7.26, 7.28, 7.31, 7.32). The anterior two-thirds are bony, forming the hard palate, and the posterior third, the soft palate, is muscular. The midline projection of the soft palate backwards is the uvula. If the subject says 'aah' the soft palate will move upwards. The palatine process of the maxilla and the horizontal plate of the palatine bones form the hard palate. The tensor palatini, the levator palatini, the musculus uvuli, the palatoglossus and the palatopharyngeus form the muscular core of the soft palate. The tensor palatini winds round the pterygoid hamulus of the medial pterygoid plate to enter the cavity of the pharynx and its tendon spreads out to become the palatine aponeurosis to be attached to the posterior aspect of the hard palate. The levator palatini takes origin from the base of the skull inside the pharynx and is inserted to the palatine aponeurosis. The other palatine muscles merge with the aponeurosis. ✪ Both the tensor and the levator palatini in their upper part are attached to the cartilaginous part of the Eustachian (auditory) tube. Their contraction opens the tube to transmit air from the pharynx to the middle ear. Children with cleft palate may develop deafness as this mechanism is often affected.

The mucosa of the palate has stratified squamous epithelium on the oral surface and ciliated columnar epithelium on the surface facing the nasal cavity. The sensory nerve supply of the palate is by branches from the maxillary nerve and the motor supply is by the cranial part of the accessory nerve transmitted through the vagus as its pharyngeal branch. See Clinical box 7.6.

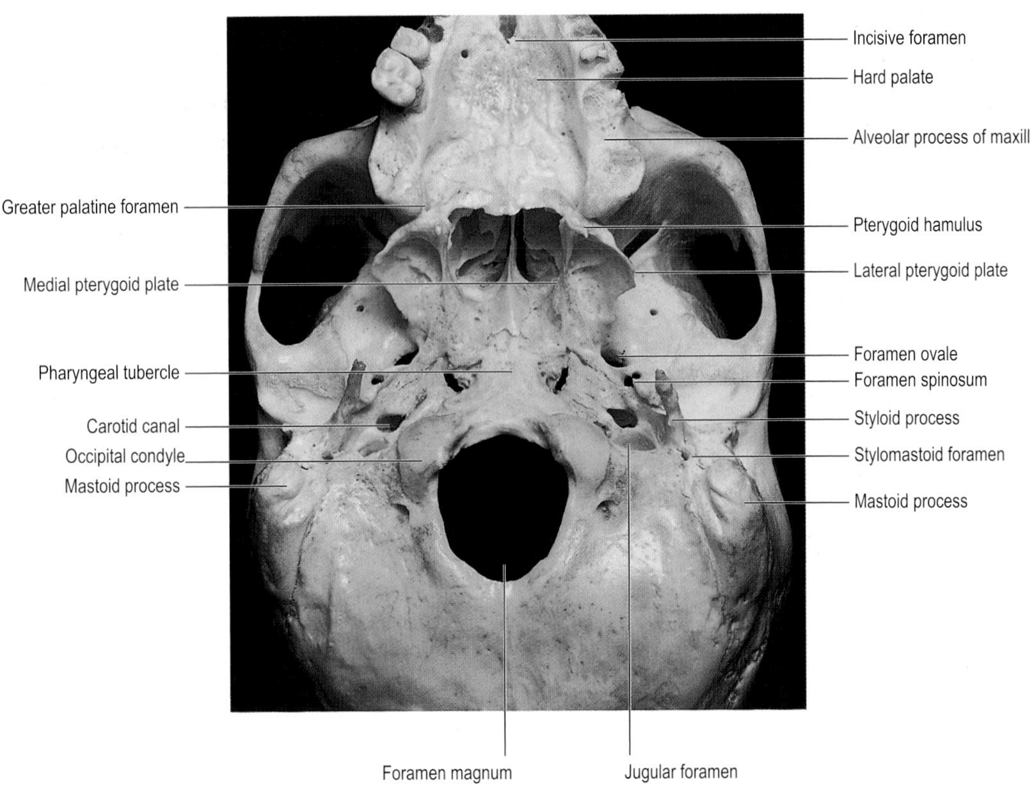


Fig. 7.31 Base of the skull seen from below.

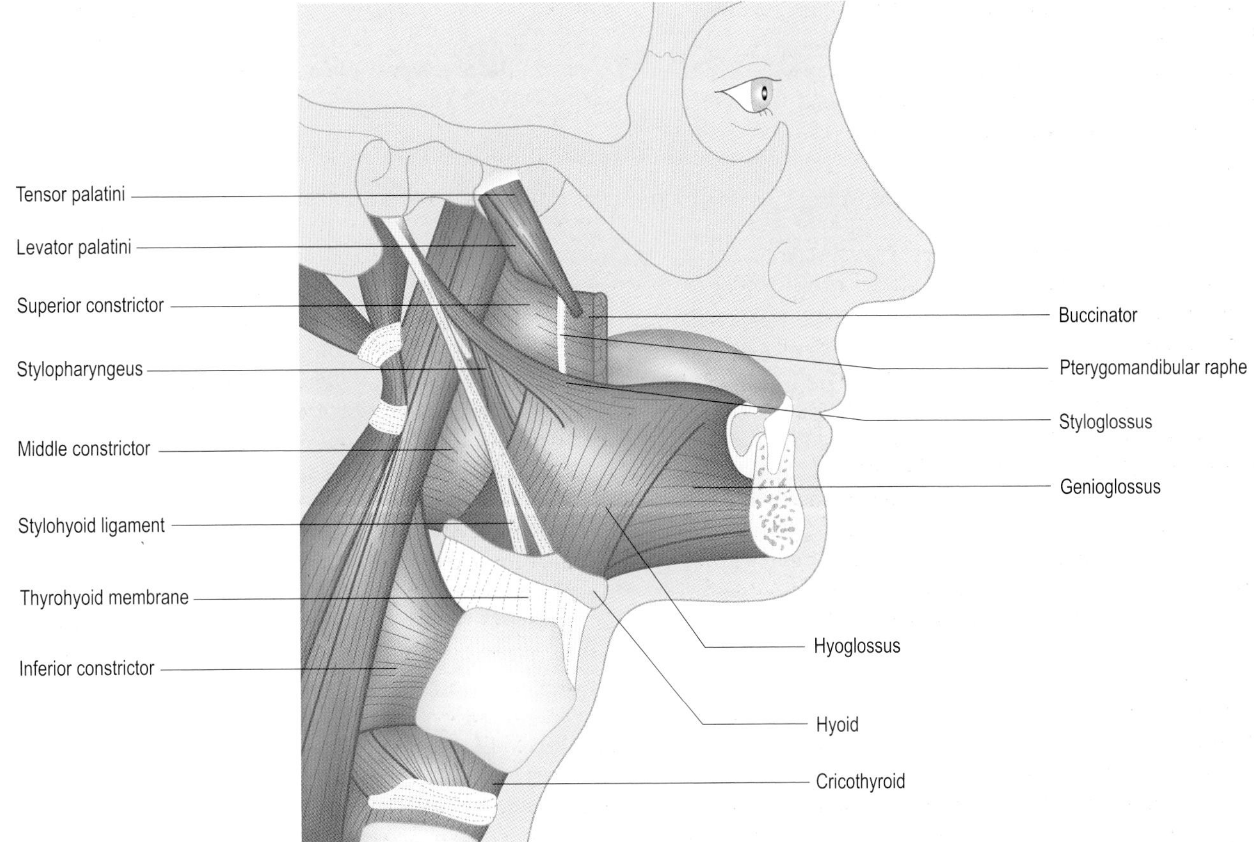


Fig. 7.32 Muscles of the tongue and pharynx.

## The pharynx and related structures

### External aspect of the pharynx

The pharynx is a muscular tube attached to the base of the skull. Below the level of the cricoid cartilage it opens into the oesophagus. For descriptive purposes the interior of the pharynx is divided into nasopharynx, oropharynx and hypopharynx or laryngeal part of the pharynx. The nasal cavity opens into the nasopharynx, the oropharynx is continuous with the oral cavity and the larynx opens into the hypopharynx.

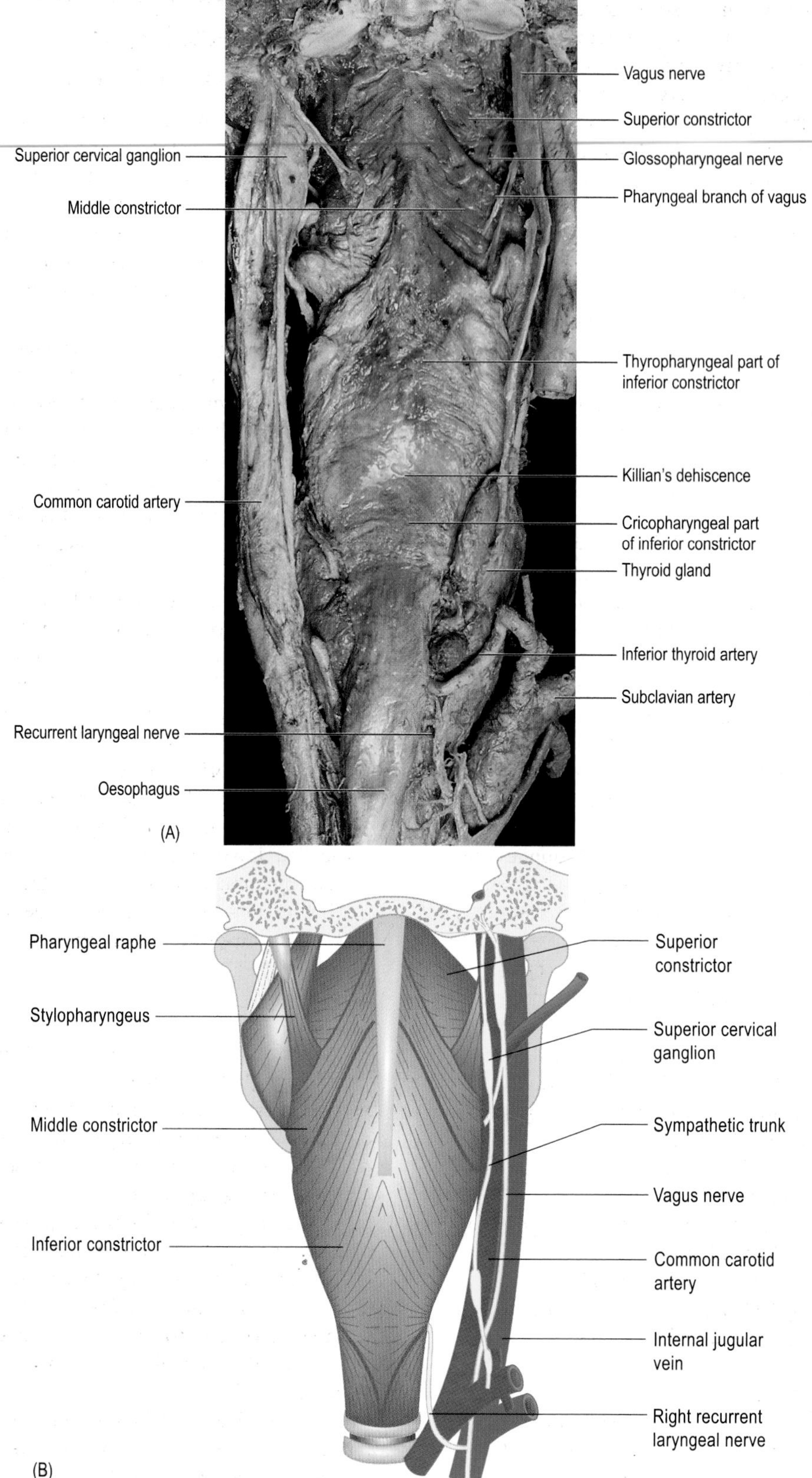


Fig. 7.33 A & B Posterior aspect of the pharynx with related structures seen after removal of the vertebral column – viewed from behind.

The origins of the constrictor muscles which form the wall of the pharynx are as follows. The superior constrictor takes origin from the pterygomandibular raphe (which extends from the medial pterygoid plate to the mandible), the middle from the hyoid bone, and the inferior constrictor from the thyroid cartilage (the thyropharyngeus) and the cricoid cartilage (the cricopharyngeus). The cricopharyngeus acts as the upper oesophageal sphincter. All the constrictors fuse together in a midline raphe on the posterior aspect. The pharyngeal raphe is attached to the pharyngeal tubercle on the base of the skull (Figs 7.31, 7.33). The inner aspect of the constrictors is lined by the thick pharyngobasilar fascia which is attached to the pharyngeal tubercle, the auditory (Eustachian) tube and the medial pterygoid plate and this fascia bridges the gap between the superior constrictor and the base of the skull. ✪ The weakest part of the pharyngeal wall is in the midline at the back in the lower part of the pharynx. This lies between the diverging fibres of the cricopharyngeal and the thyropharyngeal part of the inferior constrictor. This area is known as the Killian's dehiscence and is the commonest site for a pharyngeal diverticulum (protrusion of the wall due to excessive pressure).

The stylopharyngeus takes origin from the styloid process and lies between the external and the internal carotid arteries to reach the interval between the superior and the middle constrictor muscles. The glossopharyngeal nerve lies on the surface of the stylopharyngeus as it enters the pharynx. The glossopharyngeal nerve (IX cranial nerve) gives sensory innervation to the posterior third of the tongue and the oropharynx. Its tympanic branch supplies the middle ear and the auditory (Eustachian) tube. It also supplies the stylopharyngeus muscle.

✪ The vagus nerve (X cranial nerve; see Fig. 7.37) has three major branches in the neck – the pharyngeal branch, the superior laryngeal nerve and the recurrent laryngeal nerve. The pharyngeal branch of the vagus gives motor innervation to the muscles of the pharynx and soft palate. Its fibres originate in the nucleus ambiguus in the brainstem and leave the brain as the cranial part of the accessory nerve. The superior laryngeal branch of the vagus lies deep to the external and the internal carotid arteries. It divides into the internal and the external laryngeal nerves (Fig. 7.25). The external laryngeal nerve supplies the cricothyroid muscle as well as the cricopharyngeal part of the inferior constrictor. The internal laryngeal nerve is sensory and it supplies the hypopharynx and part of the larynx. The right recurrent laryngeal nerve branches off from the right vagus and winds round the subclavian artery. It lies in the groove between the trachea and the oesophagus and runs upwards until it disappears under the lower border of the inferior constrictor. The left recurrent laryngeal nerve lies in the groove between the trachea and the oesophagus on the left side. This nerve, unlike the one on the right, winds round the ligamentum arteriosum in the thorax. ✪ The two nerves are related to the thyroid gland (Fig. 7.33(A)).

In the posterior aspect of the pharynx the inferior thyroid artery arches to enter the back of the thyroid gland. The inferior thyroid artery crosses the recurrent laryngeal nerve at the lower pole of the thyroid gland.

The carotid sheath and the cervical part of the sympathetic trunk (Fig. 7.33) which lies on its posterior wall are also related to the pharynx.

### Interior of the pharynx

✪ The nasopharynx (Figs 7.34–7.36) is the part of the pharynx behind the nasal cavity. It has the opening of the Eustachian tube and, in a younger person, the nasopharyngeal tonsil or the adenoids. The opening of the Eustachian tube can be identified in the living by looking for the prominent tubal elevation. The tubal opening is in front of the elevation. The salpingopharyngeal fold, produced by the muscle with the same name, extends downwards from the tubal elevation.

The Eustachian tube can be blocked by enlargement of the adenoids in throat infections. This condition is common in children. Infection from here can spread into the middle ear through the tube. An early sign of a malignant tumour in the nasopharynx may be deafness due to blockage of the auditory tube. The tumour can also spread through the pharyngeal wall into the branches of the trigeminal nerve which are lying just outside the nasopharynx. The sensory innervation of the nasopharynx is by the maxillary nerve via the pharyngeal branch of the sphenopalatine ganglion (Fig. 7.22).

✪ In the oropharynx, the palatoglossal and the palatopharyngeal folds bound the tonsillar fossa (Figs 7.26, 7.28). These are produced by the palatoglossal and palatopharyngeal muscles. The tonsillar bed is formed by the superior constrictor muscle. The main sensory innervation of the oropharynx is through the glossopharyngeal nerve.

✪ The tonsil has a rich blood supply. The tonsillar branch of the facial artery enters it through the superior constrictor. The paratonsillar vein, lying deep to the tonsil, is a usual source of bleeding during tonsillectomy.

The hypopharynx (laryngeal part of the pharynx) has the laryngeal inlet (Fig. 7.34). A forward extension of the hypopharynx forming a cul de sac by the side of the larynx is the piriform fossa. ✪ Malignant tumours arising in the piriform fossa may be 'silent' in the early stages. It may not produce difficulty in swallowing as the space is a recess extending from the main cavity of the pharynx. The sensory innervation of the hypopharynx is by the internal laryngeal nerve, a branch of the superior laryngeal branch of the vagus (Fig. 7.25). See Clinical box 7.7.

> *Clinical box 7.7*
>
> **Mechanism of swallowing**
>
> Swallowing is done in three stages, the oral or voluntary stage, the pharyngeal stage, and the oesophageal stage. The oral stage is voluntary but thereafter it is almost entirely under reflex control.
>
> In the oral stage the tongue is lifted to propel the bolus of food into the pharynx. The bolus stimulates tactile receptors of the pharynx to initiate the swallowing reflex.
>
> In the pharyngeal stage the soft palate is pulled upwards and approximated against the pharynx where the palatopharyngeal and palatoglossal folds move inwards towards one another, preventing reflux of food into the nasopharynx.. The vocal cords are approximated. The larynx moves upwards and is approximated against the epiglottis. Food is thus prevented from entering the trachea. The upper oesophageal sphincter (the cricopharyngeal part of the inferior constrictor) relaxes and the superior constrictor of the pharynx contracts to force the bolus onwards.
>
> The bolus is then propelled onwards by sequential contraction of the superior, middle and inferior constrictors of the pharynx. This produces a peristaltic wave pushing the bolus towards the upper end of the oesophagus. During the pharyngeal stage respiration is reflexly inhibited. After the bolus has passed the upper oesophageal sphincter reflexly constricts. The bolus is propelled downwards by the primary peristaltic wave caused by impulses originating in the swallowing centre in the medulla and conducted via the Xth nerve to the myenteric plexus of the oesophagus.

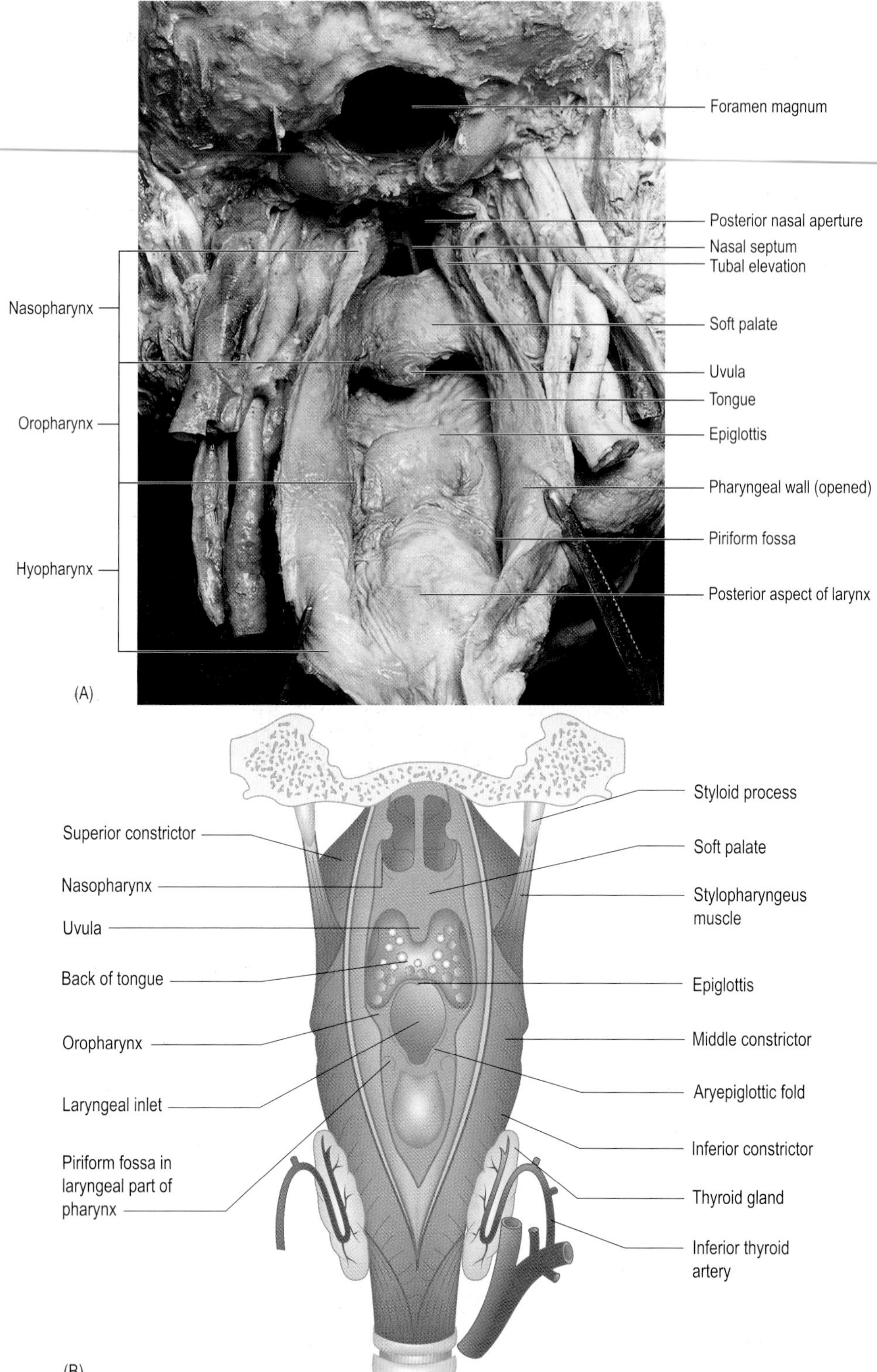


Fig. 7.34 A & B Pharynx opened from the back to show the interior. Nasopharynx, oropharynx and the laryngeal part of the pharynx are viewed from behind.

## The larynx

The larynx is held open by a series of cartilages on its wall (Fig. 7.38). The cricoid cartilage has a narrow arch anteriorly and a broad lamina at the back. The cricotracheal ligament connects the cricoid to the first tracheal ring. The thyroid cartilage has two laminae meeting in the midline anteriorly and it articulates inferiorly with the cricoid at the cricothyroid joints. It is connected to the hyoid bone by the thyrohyoid ligament. The epiglottis (Figs 7.34, 7.39) is a leaf-shaped cartilage forming the anterior wall of the inlet of the larynx. The arytenoid cartilages, paired cartilages articulating with the lamina of the cricoid, have the vocal process projecting anteriorly and the muscular process laterally. The former receives attachment of the vocal ligament and the latter the abductors and adductors of the vocal cord.

There are two pairs of minor cartilages – corniculate cartilage, articulating with the apex of the arytenoid, and the cuneiform cartilage, a nodule in the aryepiglottic fold.

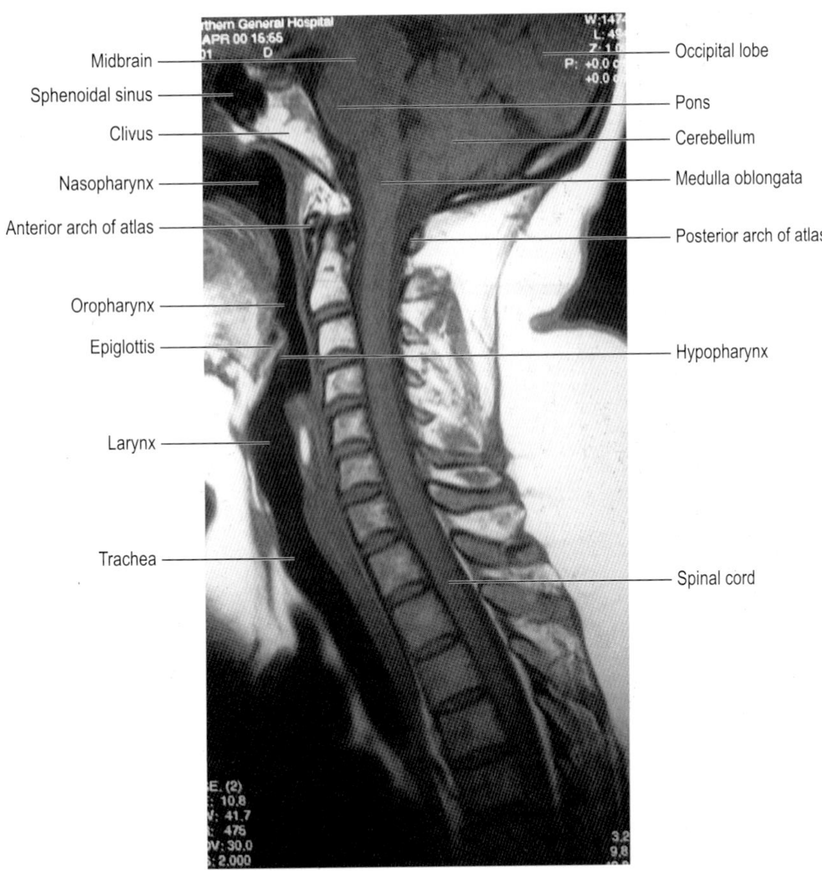


Fig. 7.35 Sagittal MRI scan of the neck.

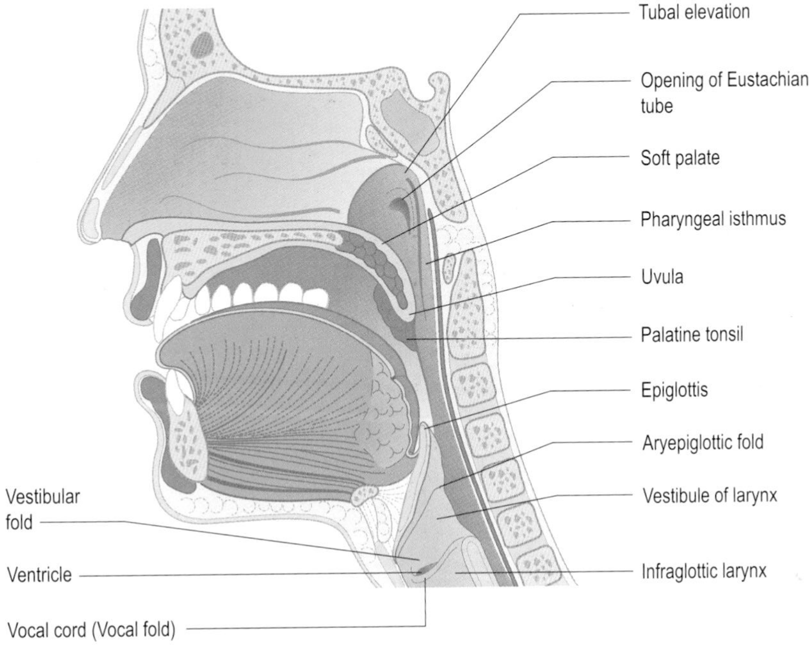


Fig. 7.36 Sagittal section of the head to show the larynx and pharynx.

Though small, these are essential for complete approximation of the inlet of the larynx.

The laryngeal inlet bounded by the epiglottis in front, the aryepiglottic folds on the side and the arytenoids and the corniculate cartilages at the back opens into the hypopharynx (Figs 7.34, 7.39) (laryngopharynx). The interior of the larynx (Fig. 7.39) is divided into different parts. The vestibule of the larynx extends from the inlet to the vestibular fold. The ventricle of the larynx is the short narrow space between the vestibular fold and the vocal fold. The space between the vocal cords, the rima glottidis, is the narrowest part of the upper airway.

The mucosa in the supraglottic region (above the vocal cords) is loosely bound to the underlying wall. In laryngeal oedema fluid accumulates in the submucous space and the mucosa swells up and obstructs the airway. The fluid

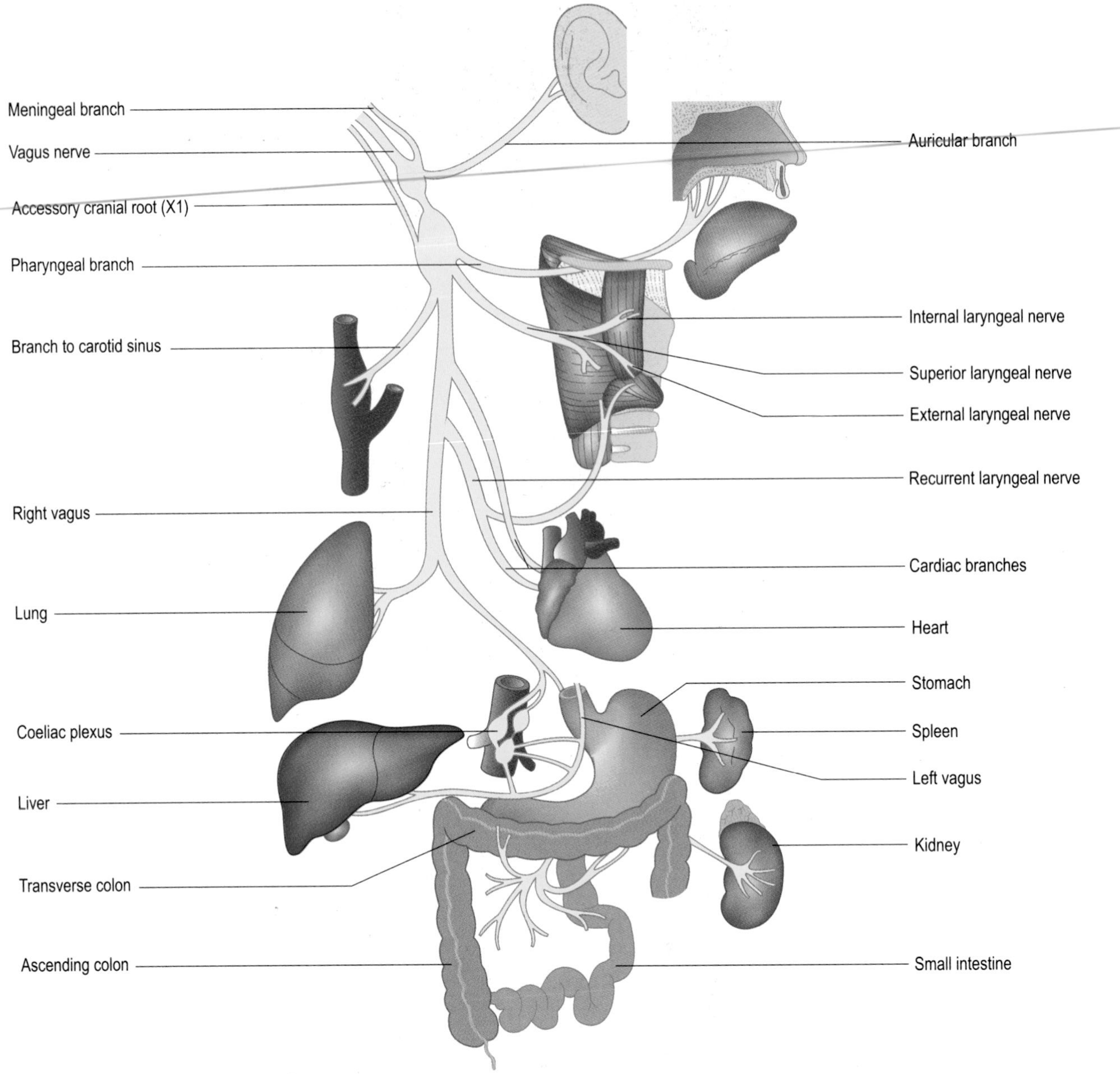

Meningeal branch
Vagus nerve
Accessory cranial root (X1)
Pharyngeal branch
Branch to carotid sinus
Right vagus
Lung
Coeliac plexus
Liver
Transverse colon
Ascending colon
Auricular branch
Internal laryngeal nerve
Superior laryngeal nerve
External laryngeal nerve
Recurrent laryngeal nerve
Cardiac branches
Heart
Stomach
Spleen
Left vagus
Kidney
Small intestine

Fig. 7.37 Summary of the distribution of the vagus nerve.

Epiglottis
Cartilago triticea
Superior cornu
Lamina of thyroid cartilage
Arytenoid cartilage
Inferior cornu
Cricotracheal ligament
Thyrohyoid ligament
Cricothyroid joint
Cricoid cartilage
(A)
Hyoid bone
Thyroid notch
Thyroid cartilage
Cricothyroid ligament (site of cricothyroid stab in airway obstruction p186)
(B)

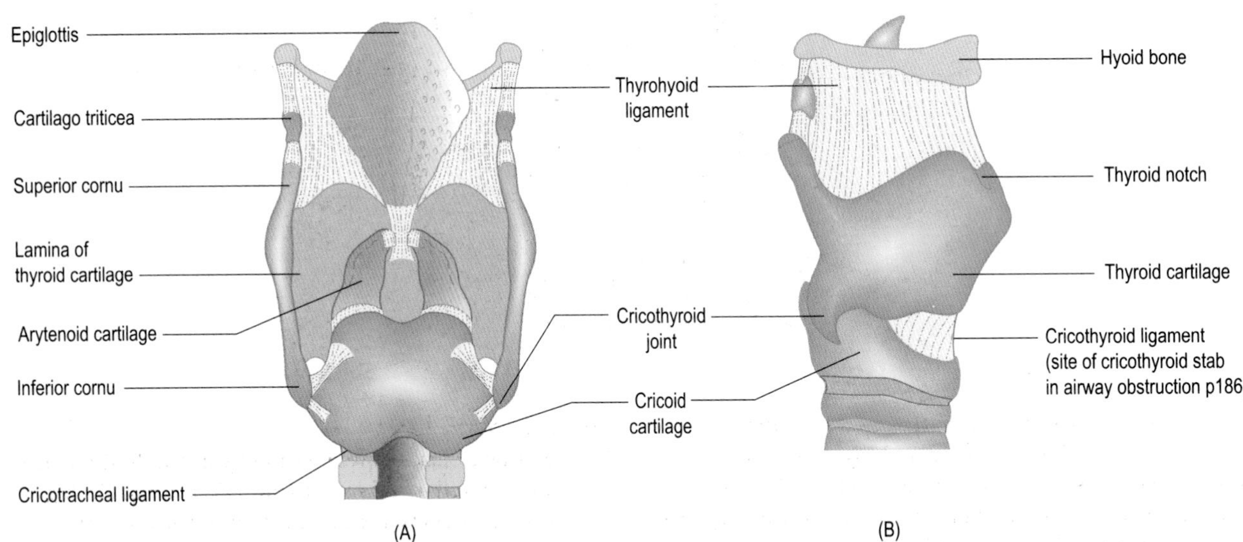

Fig. 7.38 The cartilages of the larynx and the hyoid bone: (A) posterior view, (B) lateral view.

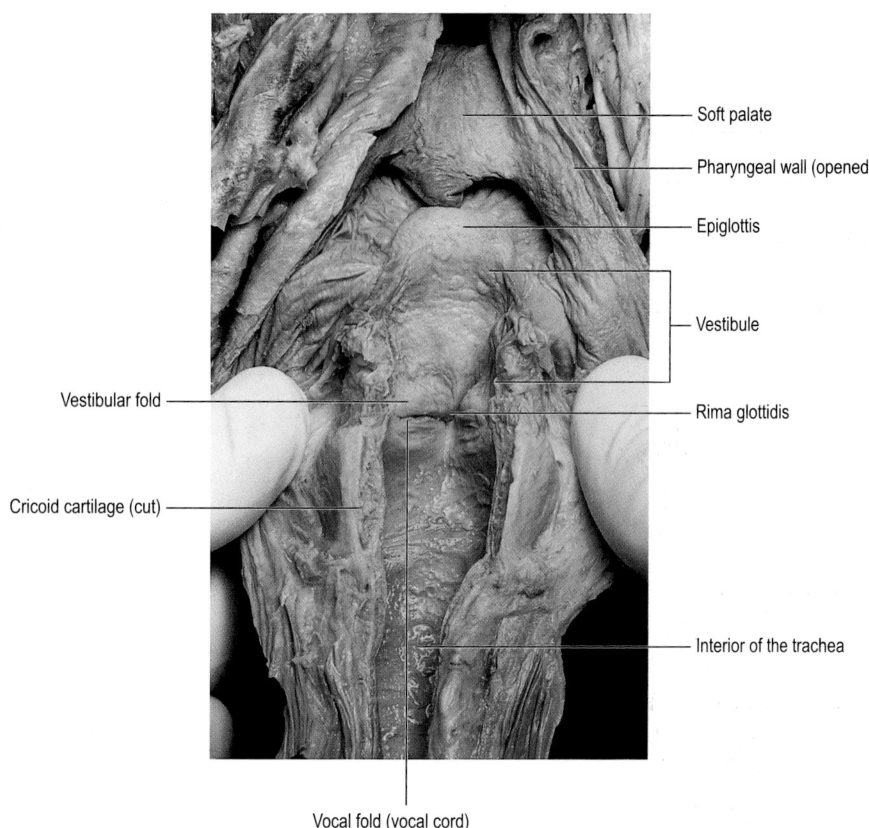


Fig. 7.39 Interior of the pharynx, larynx and trachea. Pharynx, larynx and the trachea opened from the back.

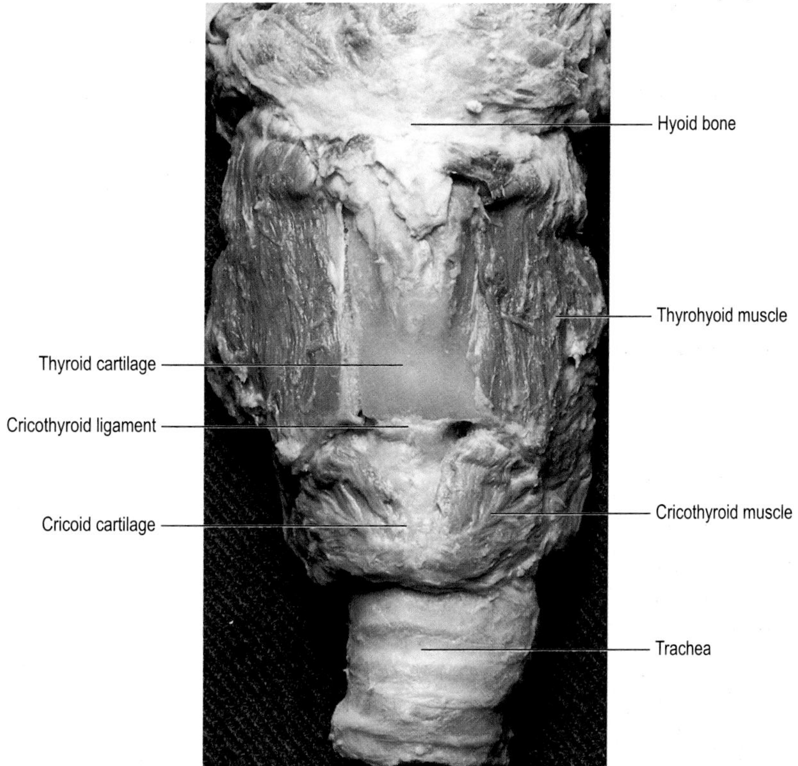


Fig. 7.40 Larynx – anterior aspect.

cannot spread downwards, as at the vocal cord the mucosa is firmly adherent to the underlying structures without having a submucous space. The lack of a submucosal layer also makes the vocal cords relatively less vascular and hence it appears paler than the rest of the mucosa.

## Muscles of the larynx

The extrinsic muscles are the suprahyoids and infrahyoids and are involved in the movements of the larynx during swallowing. Besides these there are intrinsic muscles. The paired posterior cricoarytenoid muscle (Fig. 7.41) abducts the cord. Their action is opposed by the lateral

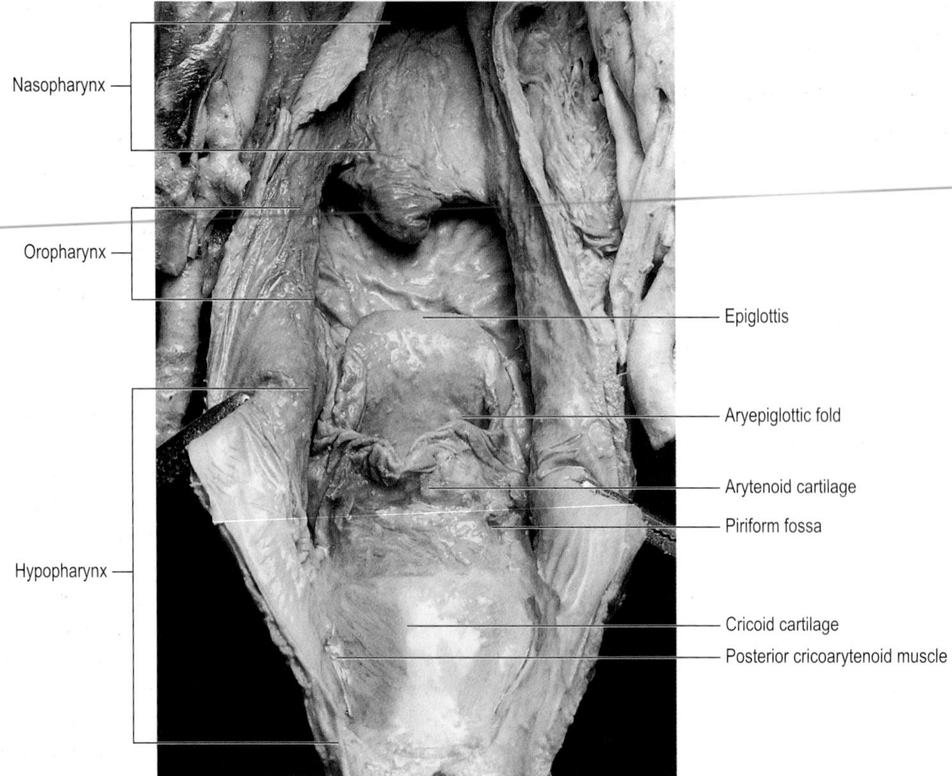


Fig. 7.41 Interior of the pharynx and the laryngeal inlet. Mucosa on the posterior aspect of the larynx is removed to show the posterior cricoarytenoid muscles.

cricoarytenoids and the transverse arytenoid (interarytenoid) which act as adductors of the cords. The cricothyroid muscle (Fig. 7.40) arises from the oblique line on the lamina of the thyroid cartilage and is inserted to the anterior part of the arch of the cricoid. As it contracts it approximates the cricoid and the thyroid cartilages anteriorly, increasing the distance between the attachments of the cords, and thus lengthens them. The thyroarytenoid muscle lying in the cord shortens the cord. A component of it, known as the vocalis, is said to be important in adjusting the tension of the cord.

The aryepiglottic muscle and the oblique arytenoid muscle are small muscles, but are important in reducing the size of the laryngeal inlet as in swallowing. Movements of the vocal cords are illustrated in Figure 7.42.

✪ The larynx is innervated by branches of the vagus. The recurrent laryngeal nerve innervates all the intrinsic muscles of the larynx except the cricothyroid. The cricothyroid is innervated by the external laryngeal branch of the superior laryngeal nerve (Fig. 7.37). The recurrent laryngeal nerve also gives sensory innervation to the part of the larynx below the level of the vocal cord. The part above is supplied by the internal laryngeal nerve (Fig. 7.37). The blood supply of the larynx is derived from the superior and inferior laryngeal arteries. ✪ The vocal cords have no lymphatic drainage and hence this region acts as a lymphatic watershed. The supraglottic part drains to the upper deep cervical nodes and the subglottic part drains to the prelaryngeal and pretracheal nodes and also to the inferior deep cervical nodes. See Clinical box 7.8.

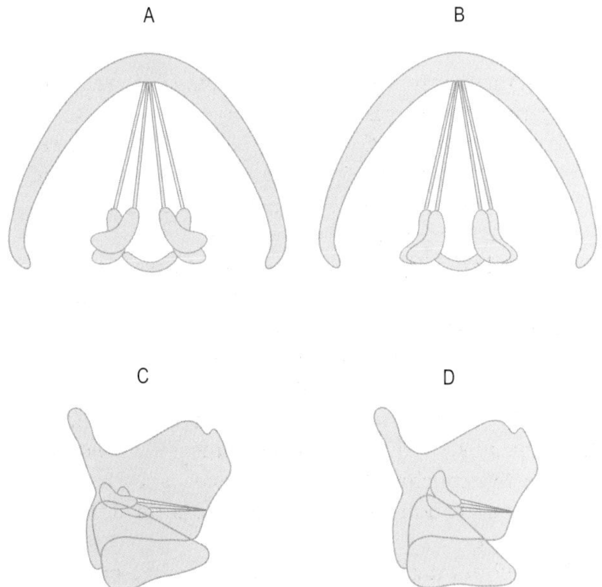


Fig. 7.42 Movements of the vocal cords. (A) Abduction by posterior cricoarytenoid. (B) Adduction by transverse and oblique arytenoids. (C) Tensing by cricothyroid. (D) Relaxation by thyroarytenoid.

## The nasal cavity and the paranasal sinuses

Each nasal cavity (Figs 7.43, 7.44) has a roof, floor, a lateral wall and a medial wall formed by the nasal septum. It is pyramidal in shape with a narrow upper part and a slightly wider base. The roof is formed by the cribriform plate of the ethmoid and the body of the sphenoid. The hard palate forms the floor.

The nasal septum (Fig. 7.44) has a bony and a cartilaginous part. In the upper part it is formed by the perpendicular plate of the ethmoid bone and behind and below by the vomer, a single midline bone. The gap in front, between these two bones, is bridged by the septal cartilage (see Fig. 7.44). ✪ The septum may often be deflected to one side. This

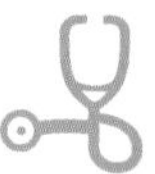

## Clinical box 7.8

### Phonation and the mechanism of speech

Production of sound by the larynx, phonation, and the articulation of that sound into understandable vowels and consonants are all achieved by the controlled and co-ordinated activity of muscles, nerves, neuronal circuits and large areas in the cerebral cortex.

We breathe while we speak. Controlled expiration to produce sound by the larynx is done by the intercostals and the diaphragm. Patients with spinal injuries who rely entirely on the diaphragm for breathing often break sentences up in order to inspire and hence have a characteristic speech impediment. Training the diaphragm by speech therapy can overcome some of the problems.

At the laryngeal level the vocal cords are adducted by the transverse arytenoid muscles to raise the subglottic pressure. The exhaled air pushes the cords apart. The consequent drop in infraglottic pressure adducts the cords again and the cycle is repeated. The movements of the tensed cords will produce sound.

The loudness of the sound varies with the level of infraglottic pressure needed to separate the cords and the degree of adduction of the cords. The former can be increased further by the contraction of expiratory muscles as in shouting.

The pitch is determined by the frequency of vibration. Higher pitch is achieved by increasing the tension of the cord by the cricothyroid muscle. The muscle stretches the cord by reducing the cricothyroid interval. The pitch of the voice also alters with the length of the cords. At birth the cords are only 7mm long but increase to 14mm by puberty. The adult female cord is 15–16mm long whereas the adult male cord is about 18–21mm.

The quality of the laryngeal sound is improved by the resonating columns of air in the paranasal sinuses, nasal cavity and the pharynx

Articulation of sound produced by the larynx into understandable vowels and consonants is done by varying the size and shape of the oral cavity as well as interrupting the flow of exhaled air by lips, tongue, and palate. The vowels are produced by altering the shape of the oral cavity by adjusting the jaws, cheek, tongue, and palate. Consonants are produced by exhalation through the mouth, isolating the nasal cavity by raising the soft palate. Labial consonants such as 'P' and 'B' are articulated by blocking the exhaled air by lips. 'T' and 'D' are lingual consonants where the tongue is approximated against the palate. In nasal sounds such as 'M' and 'N' the soft palate is partially raised to let the air pass through both the nasal cavity and the oral cavity.

condition may cause nasal obstruction and headache. The septal cartilage is avascular and is nourished by blood vessels of the mucosa. Habitual cocaine sniffers may develop avascular necrosis of the septal cartilage with a hole in the septum and subsequent collapse of the bridge of the nose due to spasm of the mucosal blood vessels.

The lateral wall (Fig. 7.43) is formed by the maxilla. Here the opening of the maxillary sinus is overlapped by the ethmoid, the lacrimal bone, the perpendicular plate of the palatine bone and the inferior concha. Projecting from the lateral wall are the superior, middle and inferior conchae, dividing the nasal cavity into the superior, middle and inferior meatuses (Fig. 7.45). Each meatus is seen below the respective concha. The inferior concha is the largest and is a separate bone. The other two are parts of the ethmoid bone.

✪ The inferior meatus is the widest part of the nasal cavity. Nasal intubations are done through this region. Hypertrophy of the inferior concha may produce difficulty in such intubation. The nasolacrimal duct opens into the inferior meatus about 2cm behind the nostril. ✪ The nasolacrimal duct extends from the lacrimal sac to the inferior meatus, closely related to anterior aspect of the maxillary sinus. It drains the lacrimal fluid from the conjunctival sac.

✪ The middle meatus presents a convex bulge beneath the concha. This is the ethmoidal bulla. Below the bulla is the hiatus semilunaris into which open the frontal, anterior ethmoidal and maxillary sinuses. The openings of the frontal, anterior ethmoidal and the maxillary sinuses are in the middle meatus. ✪ They all open in close proximity in the hiatus semilunaris and hence infection from one sinus can easily spread to another. The frontal sinus opens via the infundibulum (Fig. 7.43). The anterior ethmoidal cells are few and their openings may extend on to the wall of the infundibulum as well. The maxillary sinus may have more than one opening.

The space above and behind the superior meatus, the sphenoethmoidal recess, receives the opening of the sphenoidal sinus. The posterior ethmoidal sinus opens into the superior meatus and the sphenoidal sinus (Fig. 7.46) into the sphenoethmoidal recess. ✪ The pituitary fossa lies above the sphenoidal sinus which is also closely related to the cavernous sinus and the internal carotid artery. Surgical access to the pituitary gland is often through the nasal cavity and the sphenoidal sinus (Fig. 7.44).

✪ Malignant tumours in the upper part of the nasal cavity, which are often silent in the early stages, can spread into the cranial cavity through the cribriform plate of the ethmoid. They can also spread into the orbit.

✪ The innervation of the nasal cavity is by branches of the maxillary and the ophthalmic nerves. The arterial supply comes from the branches of the external and internal carotid arteries. Bleeding from the nasal cavity (epistaxis) is common. The commonest site is 'Little's area', in the anteroinferior part of the septum, where many vessels anastomose. The nerves and vessels of the nasal cavity are illustrated in Figure 7.48.

## Paranasal sinuses

### The maxillary sinus

✪ The maxillary sinus (Fig. 7.47) is the largest of the paranasal sinuses with a mean volume of about 10ml. The medial wall or base is composed of thin and delicate bones on the lateral wall of the nasal cavity. The opening of the

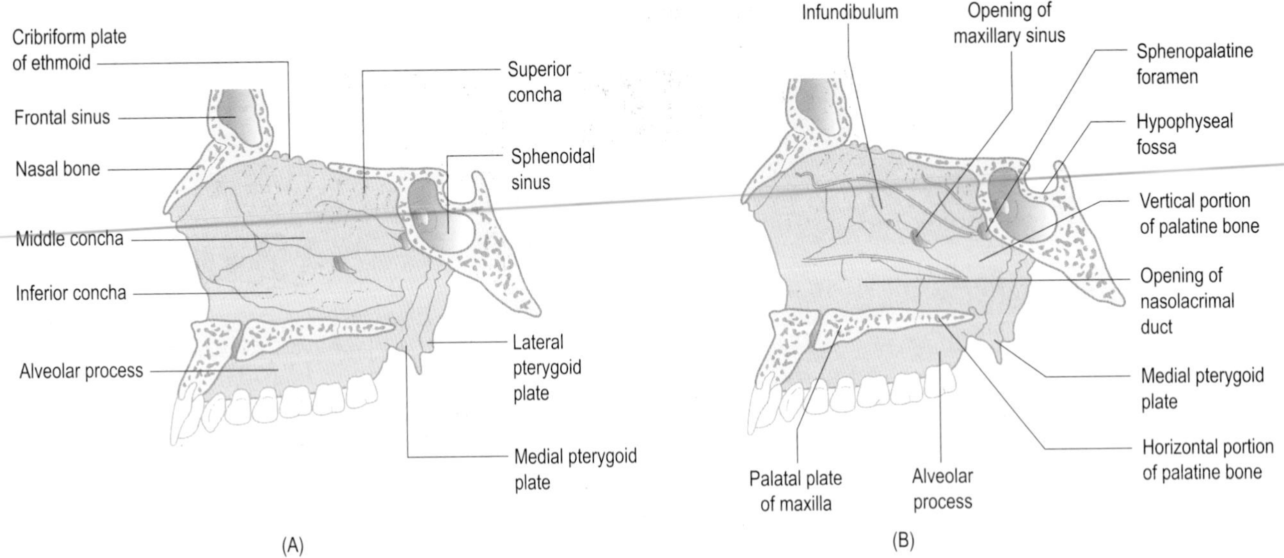


Fig. 7.43 The bony lateral wall of the nasal cavity. (A) Bones complete. (B) After partial removal of the conchae.

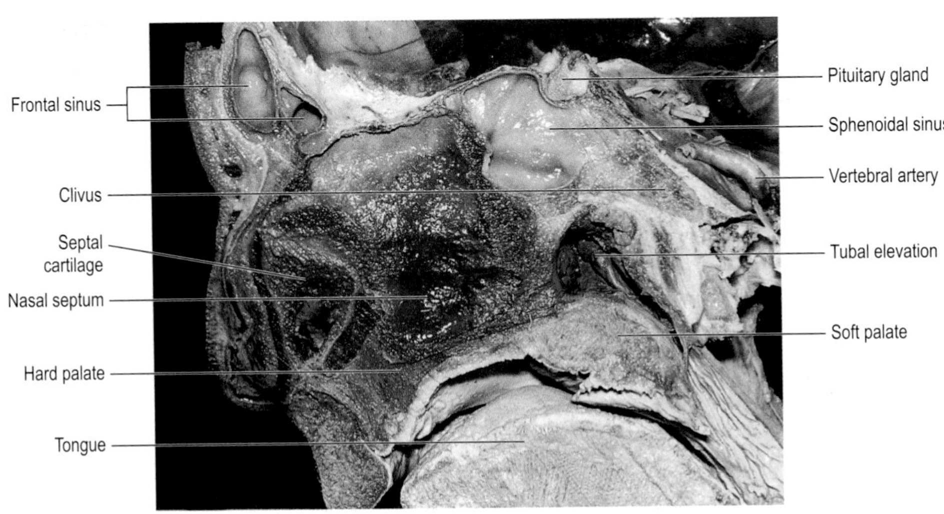


Fig. 7.44 Sagittal section of the head.

sinus into the hiatus semilunaris lies high on the medial wall, just below the floor of the orbit. As the ostium is high on the wall drainage depends on ciliary action and not gravity. The roof of the sinus is the floor of the orbit. The floor is the alveolar process of the maxilla overlying the second premolar and the first molar teeth. A tooth abscess may rupture into the sinus. The floor of the maxillary sinus is at a more inferior level than the floor of the nasal cavity.

✪ For maxillary sinus wash-out a cannula is inserted into the sinus via the inferior meatus of the nasal cavity. As the nasolacrimal duct is closely related to the cavity of the sinus anteriomedially it can easily be damaged during sinus surgery.

✪ In the Caldwell–Luc operation for chronic maxillary sinusitis the anterior bony wall of the maxillary sinus is removed, the mucosa is stripped out and a permanent drainage hole is made into the nose through the inferior meatus.

Carcinoma of the maxillary sinus may invade the palate and cause dental problems. It may block the nasolacrimal duct causing epiphora. Spread of the tumour into the orbit causes proptosis. The maxillary division of the trigeminal nerve supplies the sinus through its infraorbital and superior dental nerves. The pain due to sinusitis may often manifest itself as toothache.

### The ethmoidal air cells (ethmoidal air sinuses)

The ethmoidal air cells (Fig. 7.47), which are thin-walled cavities in the ethmoidal labyrinth, vary in their size and number. ✪ The thin orbital plate of the ethmoid (lamina papyracea) separates the sinuses from the orbit. This can be damaged during sinus surgery causing orbital haematoma and blindness. Injury to the medial rectus muscle (see Orbit – p. 221) causes diplopia. Acute ethmoiditis in childhood and ethmoidal carcinoma may spread upwards causing meningitis and cerebrospinal fluid leakage or it may spread laterally into the orbit causing proptosis and diplopia.

### The frontal sinus

The frontal sinuses (Figs 7.44, 7.45) are not present at birth but start to appear in the second year of life. The frontal sinus drains by the infundibulum or the frontonasal duct into the hiatus semilunaris of the middle meatus. Infection of the frontal sinus is often associated with infection of the maxillary sinus as their openings are very close to each other.

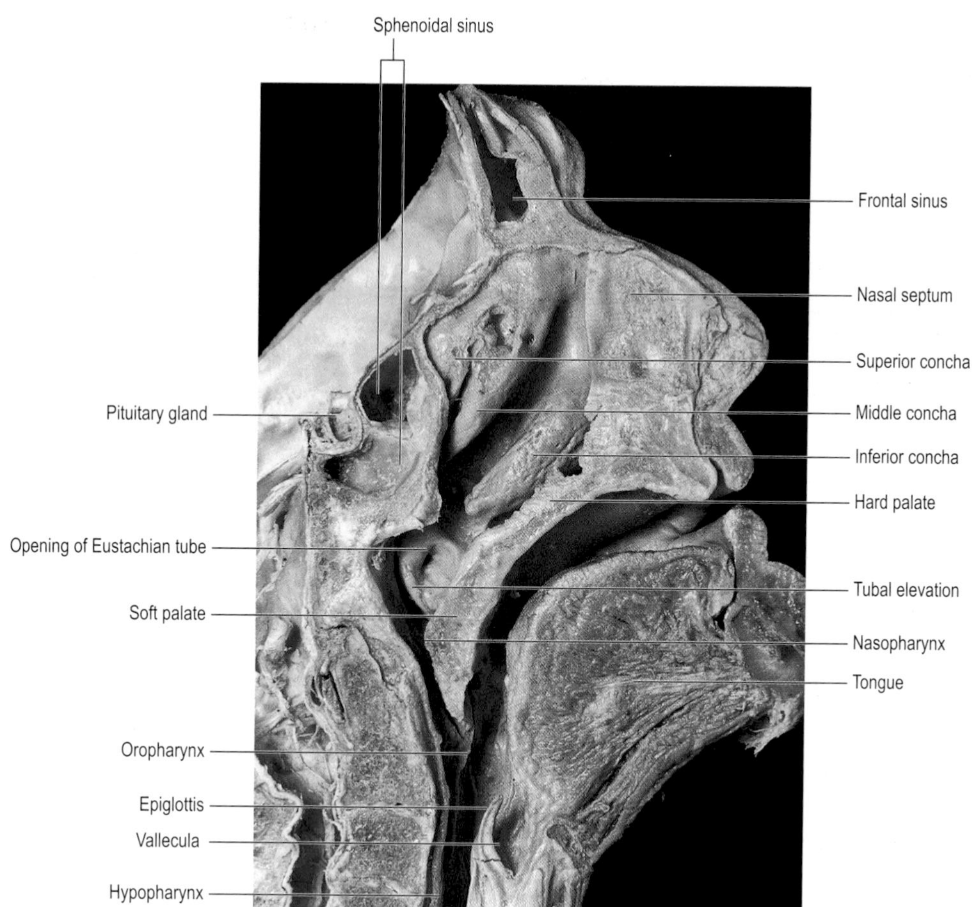


Fig. 7.45 Lateral wall of the nasal cavity. Sagittal section of the head showing the interior of the nasal cavity, oral cavity and the pharynx.

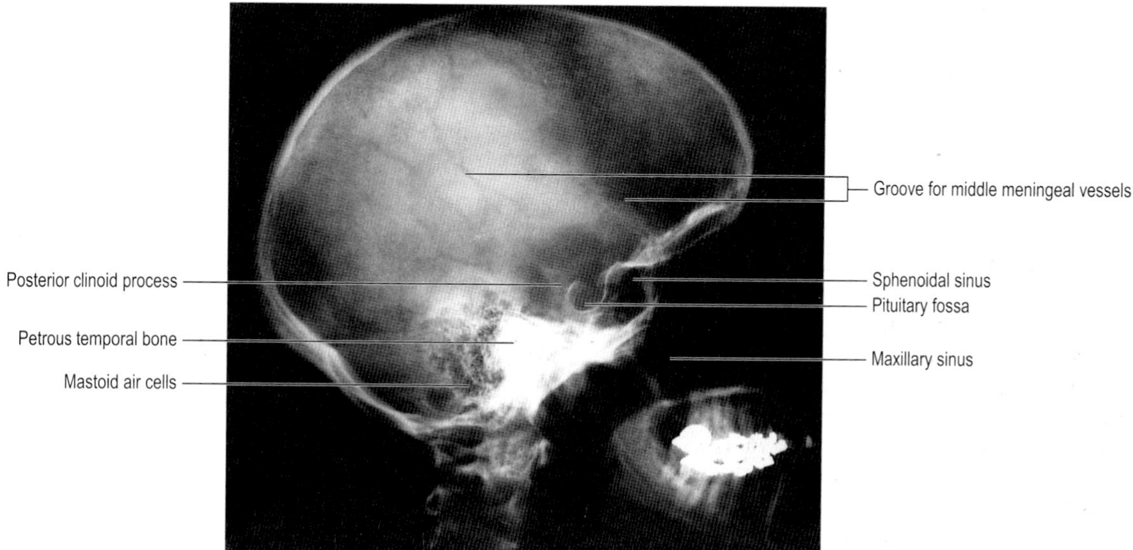


Fig. 7.46 Lateral radiograph of the head – paranasal sinuses.

Acute sinusitis can spread posteriorly into the anterior cranial fossa causing extradural and subdural abscesses or meningitis. The pus in the sinus can be drained by wash-out through the nose or by a small incision on its wall just below the medial end of the eyebrow.

## The sphenoidal sinus

The sphenoidal sinus (Fig. 7.46), like the maxillary sinus, is very small at birth. It occupies the body of the sphenoid but may extend into its greater and lesser wings. The sphenoidal sinus opens into the sphenoethmoidal recess of the nasal cavity.

The floor of the sinus is in the roof of the nasal cavity and the nasopharynx. The roof of the sinus is thin. The pituitary fossa bulges into the roof in its posterior half and anteriorly the roof separates the sinus from the optic chiasma and the optic nerves. The lateral wall is also thin and separates the sinus from the cavernous sinus and the internal carotid artery.

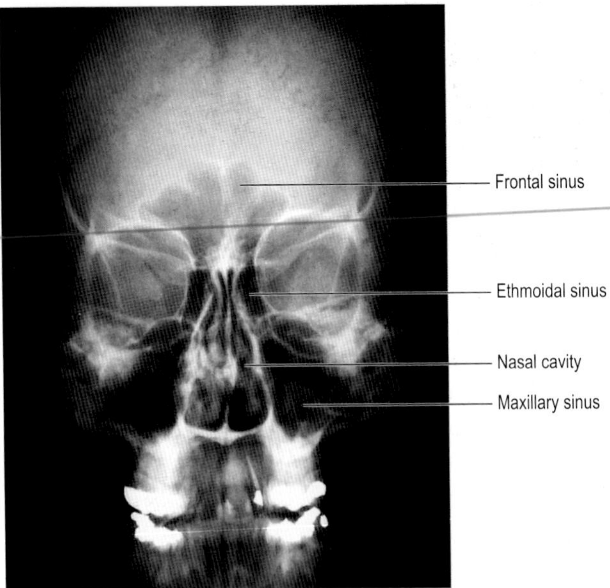


Fig. 7.47 Radiograph of the paranasal sinuses.

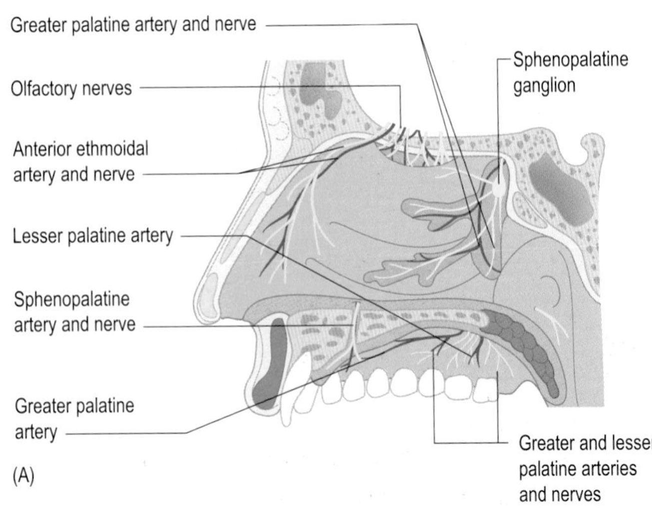


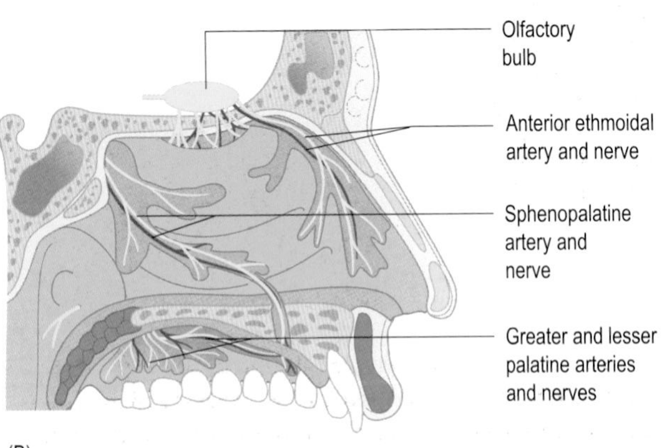


Fig. 7.48 The arteries and nerves of the nasal cavity. (A) Lateral wall. (B) Nasal septum.

## The brain and the cranial cavity

### The cranial fossae

The floor of the cranial cavity has three cranial fossae – the anterior, middle and the posterior – each progressively lower than the one in front (Figs 7.49, 7.50). The anterior cranial fossa overlies the orbit and the nasal cavities. The frontal lobe of the brain lies in the anterior cranial fossa. The middle cranial fossa lies below and behind the anterior and contains the temporal lobes. Most posteriorly the posterior cranial fossa lies at the lowest level and contains the brainstem and the cerebellum.

In the anterior cranial fossa the falx cerebri is attached to the crista galli (Fig. 7.50). The cribriform plate of the ethmoid forms the roof of the nasal cavity and transmits the olfactory nerves. ✪ Tumours from the upper part of the nasal cavity can spread into the anterior cranial fossa through the cribriform plate. Fractures of the anterior cranial fossa may produce bleeding and leakage of cerebrospinal fluid through the nasal cavity.

The optic canal connecting the middle cranial fossa to the orbit transmits the optic nerve and the ophthalmic artery. In the middle of the middle cranial fossa is the pituitary fossa or sella turcica (hypophyseal fossa) containing the pituitary gland. It is roofed by a fold of dura mater, the diaphragma sellae, and this is pierced by the infundibulum (Fig. 7.51). The diaphragma sellae is attached to the anterior and posterior clinoid processes which bound the fossa.

Lateral to the pituitary gland, the dura mater contains the cavernous sinus, one on either side. The oculomotor, trochlear and the ophthalmic and maxillary divisions of the trigeminal, the abducent nerve and the internal carotid artery pass through the cavernous sinus (Figs 7.59, 7.60). The 'S'-shaped artery inside the sinus is known as the carotid syphon. Infection can reach the cavernous sinus from the face and the eye because of its venous connections.

The trigeminal nerve as it enters the middle cranial fossa (Fig. 7.51) takes a prolongation of the dura from the posterior cranial fossa with it known as the trigeminal cave or Meckel's cave. It contains the trigeminal ganglion from which three divisions of the nerve arise. The ophthalmic division goes through the supraorbital fissure, the maxillary through the foramen rotundum and the mandibular division through the foramen ovale (Fig. 7.49).

✪ There are grooves for the middle meningeal artery and vein on the inner aspect of the skull. These vessels can rupture in head injury and produce an extradural haemorrhage. The middle meningeal artery enters the skull through the foramen spinosum (Fig. 7.49).

The facial (VII) and vestibulocochlear (VIII) nerves enter the internal acoustic (auditory) meatus. The glossopharyngeal (IX), vagus (X) and accessory (XI) nerves enter the jugular foramen (Fig. 7.49). The sigmoid sinus and the inferior petrosal sinus also leave the skull through this foramen. The two vertebral arteries come through the foramen magnum along with the spinal part of the accessory nerve. The hypoglossal nerve (XII) leaves the skull through the hypoglossal canal.

### The meninges

✪ The three layers of the meninges are the dura mater, the arachnoid mater and the pia mater. There are three

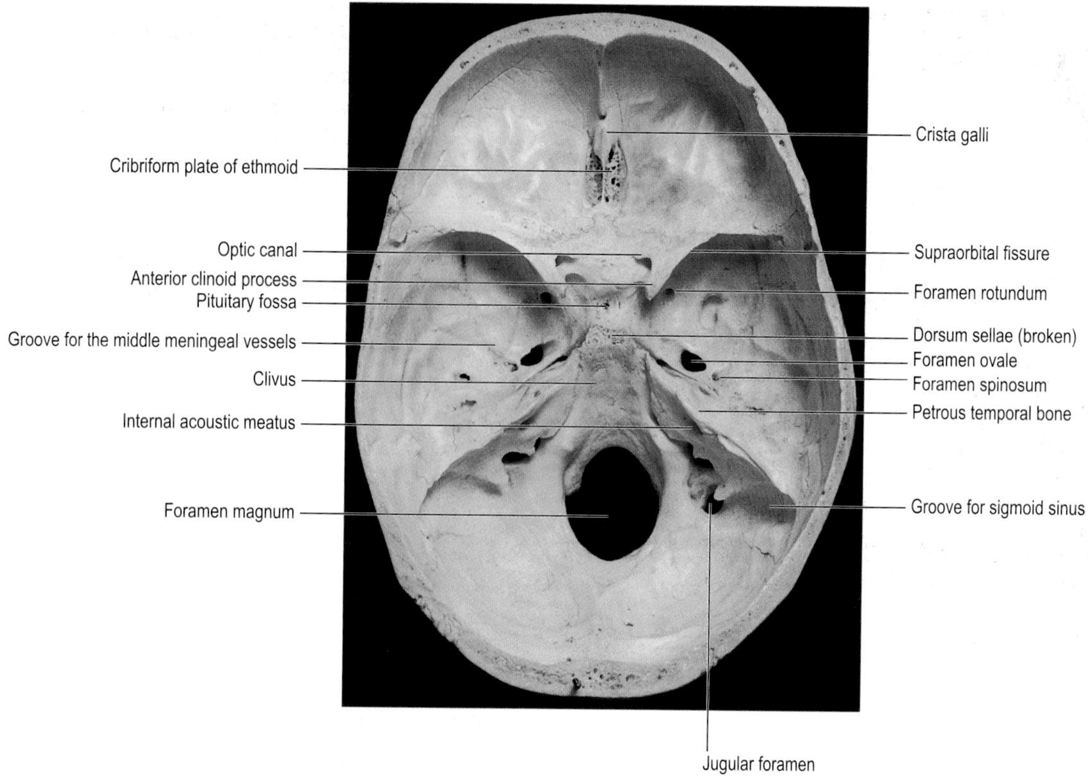


Fig. 7.49 Interior of the base of skull.

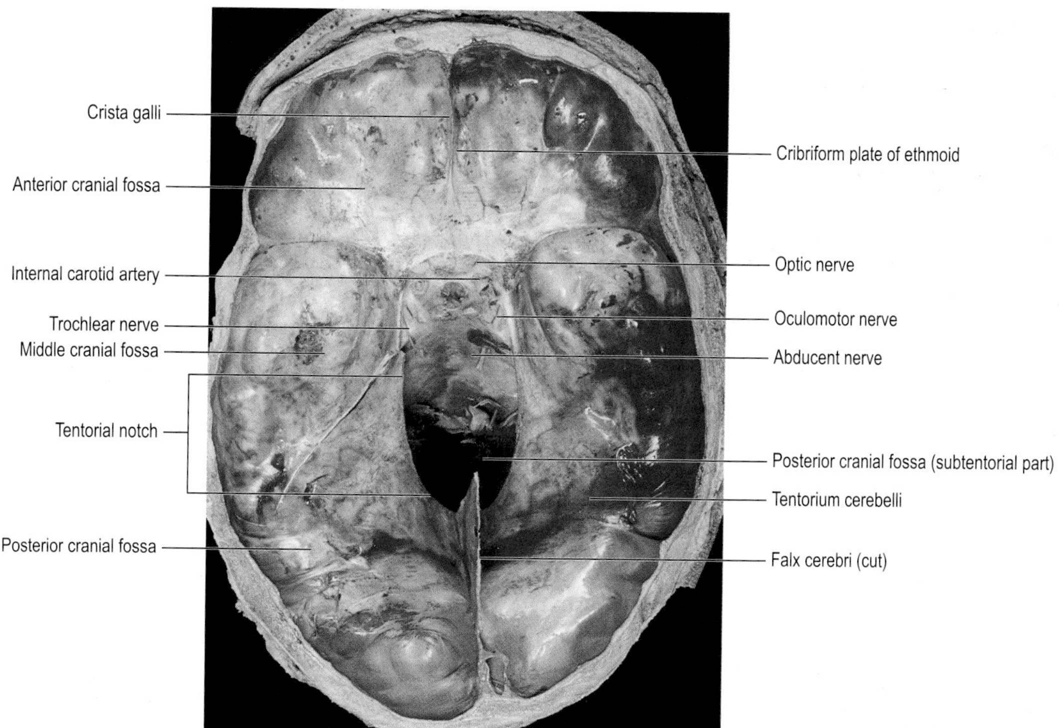


Fig. 7.50 Cranial cavity and the meninges.

meningeal spaces. The extradural (epidural) space is between the cranial bones and the endosteal layer of dura. This is a potential space which becomes a real space when there is an extradural haemorrhage from a torn meningeal vessel. The subdural space is also a potential space and may enlarge after head injury.

The subarachnoid space between the arachnoid and pia contains cerebrospinal fluid and the blood vessels of the brain.

The meningeal layer of dura continues into the vertebral canal as the dura mater covering the spinal cord. The two layers of dura mater are fused together except in areas where they form walls of the dural venous sinuses. The

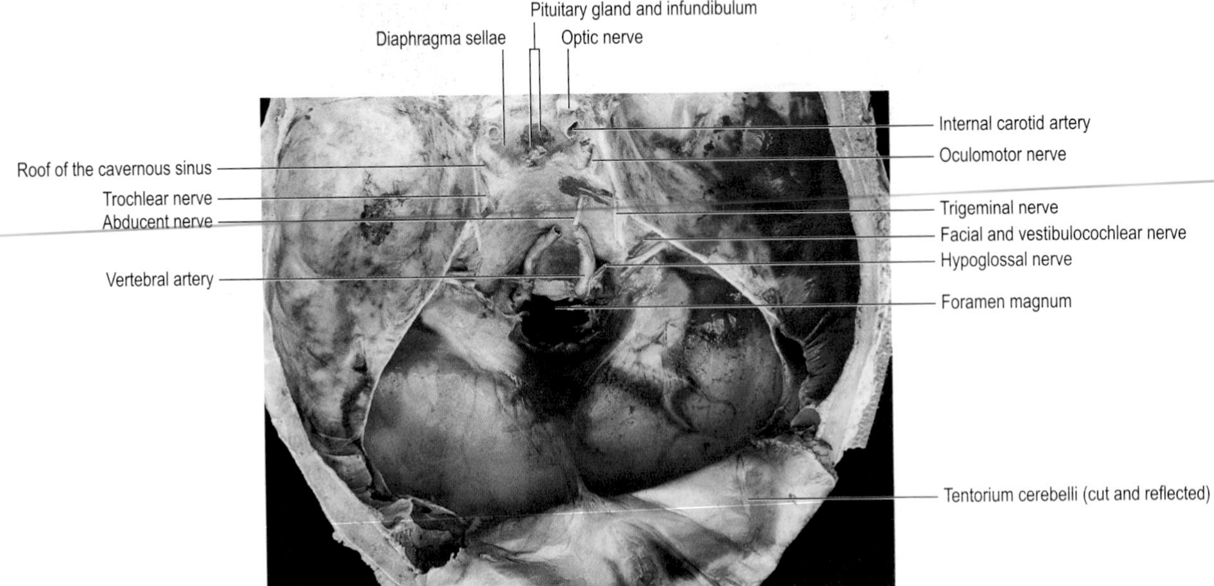


Fig. 7.51 Middle and posterior cranial fossae and the cranial nerves.

cranial cavity is divided into compartments by the three folds of dura mater. The falx cerebri lies between the two cerebral hemispheres (Fig. 7.52), attached anteriorly to the crista galli and posteriorly to the tentorium cerebelli (Fig. 7.50). The superior sagittal sinus lies along its superior border and the inferior sagittal sinus along its inferior free margin (Figs 7.58, 7.59). The straight sinus is seen where the falx cerebri meets the tentorium cerebelli. The tentorium cerebelli is attached anteriorly to the posterior clinoid process of the sphenoid bone and its attachment runs posterolaterally along the superior border of the petrous temporal bone where the superior petrosal sinus is enclosed. Where the latter empties into the transverse sinus, the attached border turns posteromedially along the lips of the transverse sinus to reach the internal occipital protuberance and continues round on the opposite side of the skull to the other posterior clinoid process. The free border of the tentorium cerebelli is attached to the anterior clinoid process and running posteriorly and then medially it curves round the midbrain forming the tentorial notch which surrounds the midbrain (Fig. 7.50). Just behind the apex of the petrous temporal bone the inferior layer of the tentorium prolongs into the middle cranial fossa as the trigeminal cave. The falx cerebelli is a small fold of dura below the tentorium in the posterior cranial fossa. It lies between the two lateral lobes of the cerebellum.

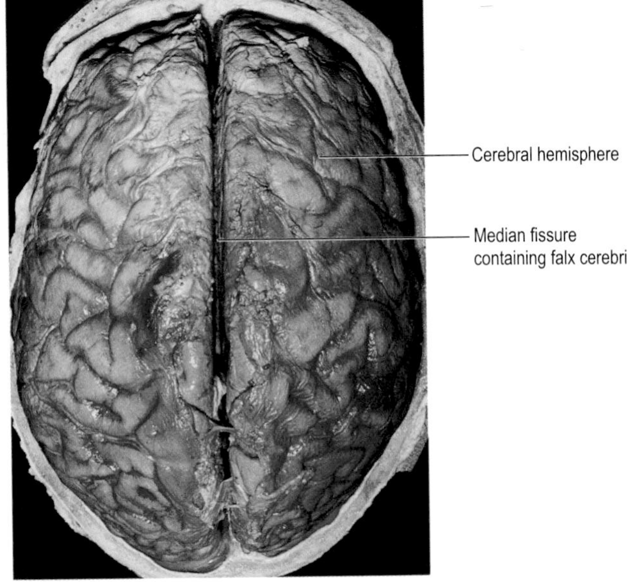


Fig. 7.52 The cerebral hemispheres seen from above.

### The arterial supply to the brain

✪ The brain is supplied by the two vertebral arteries and the two internal carotid arteries.

After entering the cranial cavity through the foramen magnum, the two vertebral arteries ascend on the surface of the medulla to the lower border of the pons where they unite to form the basilar artery (Figs 7.55, 7.57). The posterior cerebral arteries are the terminal branches of the basilar artery. Each posterior cerebral artery winds round the midbrain to reach the medial surface of the cerebral hemisphere and supplies the occipital lobe, including the visual area, as well as the temporal lobe (Fig. 7.56). Occlusion of the posterior cerebral artery causes blindness in the contralateral visual field.

The anterior cerebral artery (Figs 7.53, 7.56), the smaller of the two terminal branches of the internal carotid artery, supplies the medial part of the inferior surface of the frontal lobe, and courses along the upper surface of the corpus callosum supplying the medial surface of the frontal and parietal lobes and the corpus callosum. It also supplies a narrow strip on the upper part of the lateral surface. The motor and sensory areas of the lower extremity are supplied by this artery, resulting in characteristic paralysis when the artery is occluded.

The middle cerebral artery (Figs 7.53, 7.56) is the larger of the terminal branches of the internal carotid artery. It lies in the lateral sulcus and its branches supply the lateral surface of the frontal, parietal and temporal lobes, except the narrow strip in the upper part supplied by the anterior cerebral. Occlusion of the artery results in contralateral motor and sensory paralysis of the face and arm.

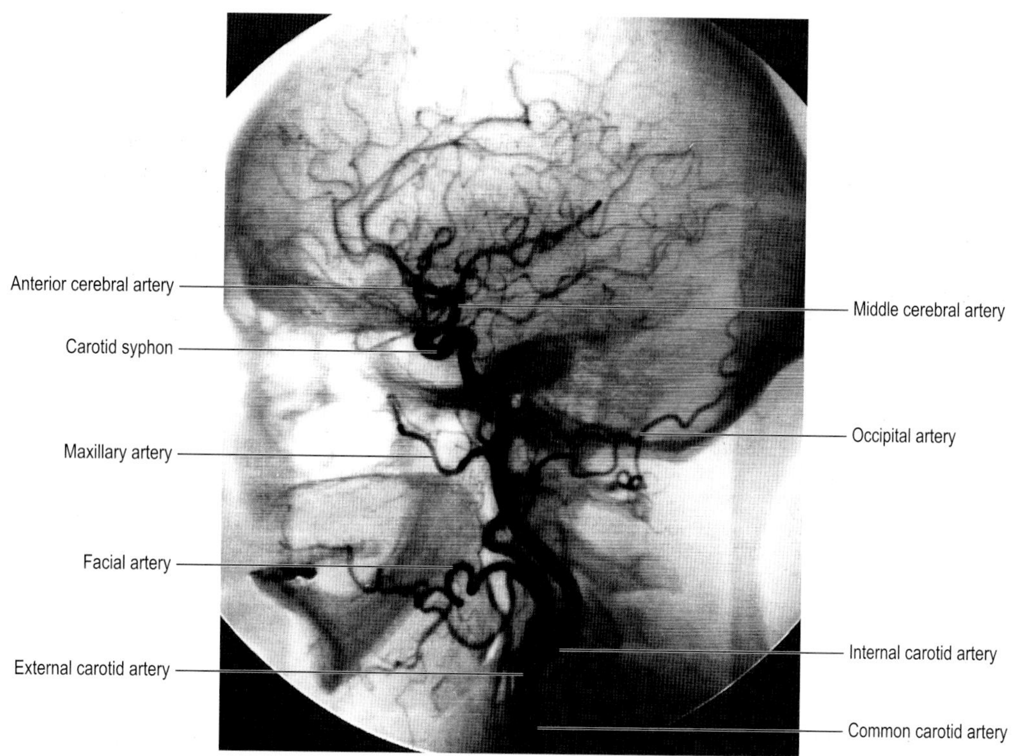


Fig. 7.53 Carotid angiogram – lateral view.

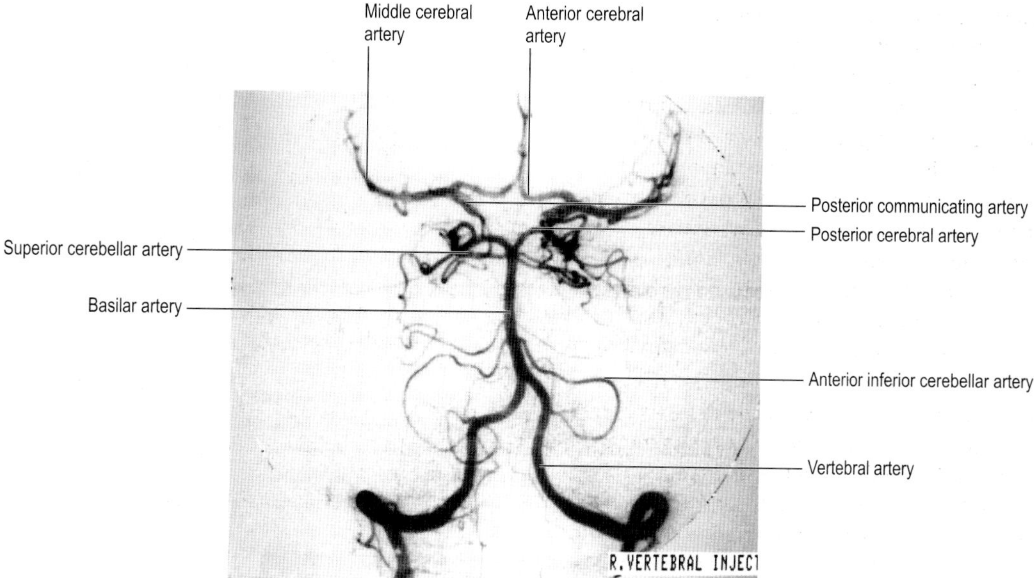


Fig. 7.54 Circle of Willis – arteriogram.

The two internal carotids and the two vertebral arteries form an anastomosis known as the circle of Willis (Figs 7.54, 7.55, 7.57) on the inferior surface of the brain. Though the majority are thus interconnected, there is normally only minimal mixing of the blood passing through them. When one artery is blocked the arterial circle may provide collateral circulation.

### The venous drainage of the brain

See Figs 7.58, 7.59.

✪ The veins of the brain, lying along with the arteries in the subarachnoid space, are thin-walled vessels without valves. They pierce the arachnoid and drain into the cranial dural venous sinuses which are situated within the dura mater. The dural venous sinuses are devoid of valves. They eventually drain into the internal jugular vein.

The superior sagittal sinus begins in front of the crista galli and courses backwards along the attached border of the falx cerebri and usually becomes continuous with the right transverse sinus near the internal occipital protuberance. At its commencement it may communicate with the nasal veins. A number of venous lacunae lie along its course and open into the sinus. The sinus and the lacunae are invaginated by arachnoid granulations. The superior cerebral veins drain into the superior sagittal sinus.

The inferior sagittal sinus lies along the inferior border of the falx cerebri and is much smaller than the superior sagittal sinus. It receives the cerebral veins from the medial surface of the hemisphere and joins the great cerebral vein to form the straight sinus.

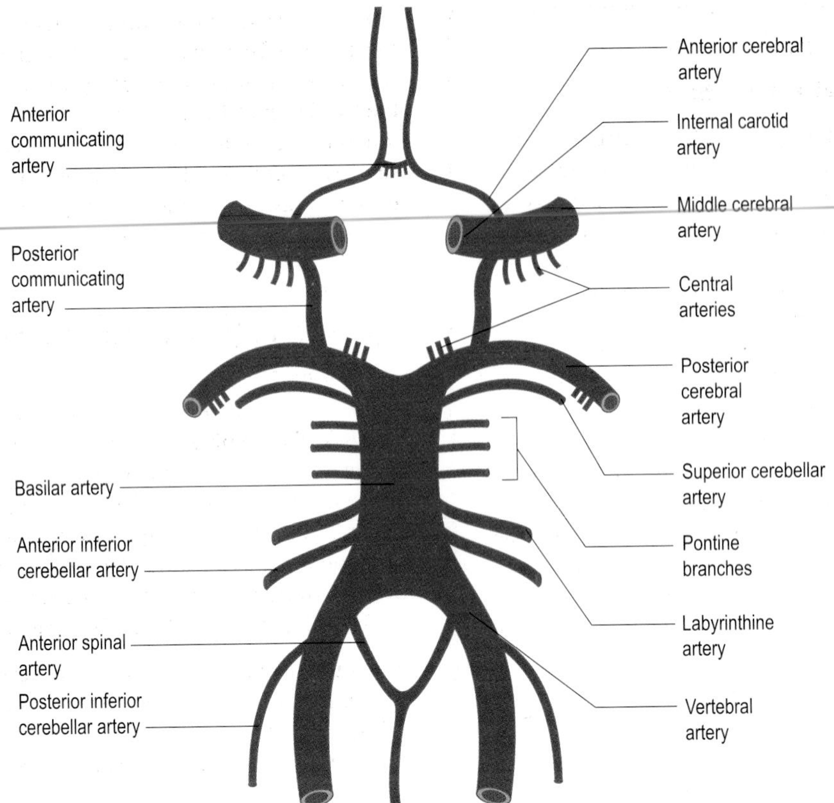


Fig. 7.55 Circle of Willis. The central arteries supply the corpus striatum, internal capsule, diencephalon and midbrain.

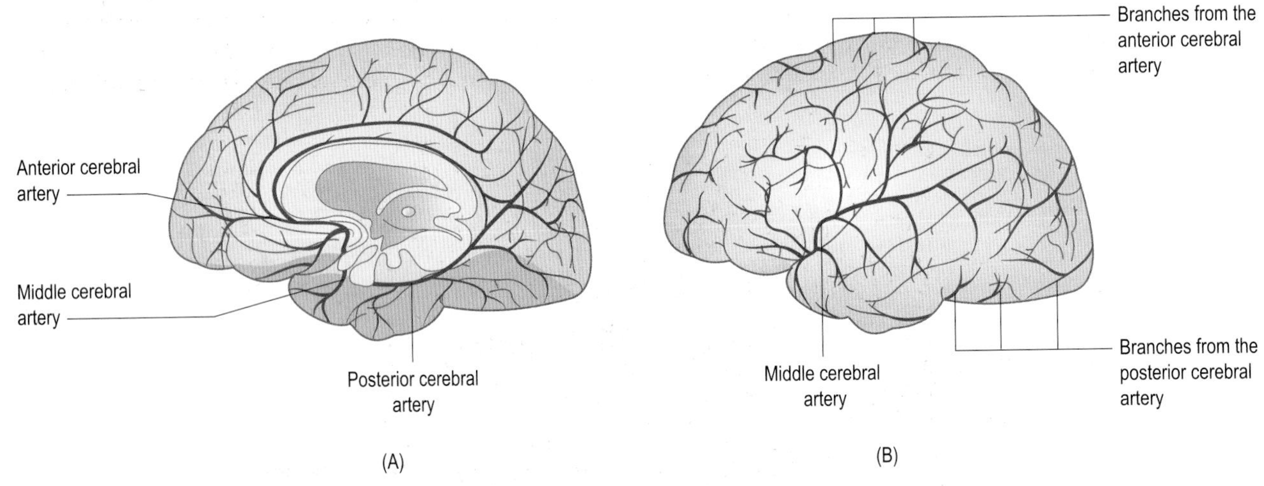


Fig. 7.56 The cerebral arteries of the cerebral hemisphere: (A) medial view, (B) lateral view.

The straight sinus, formed by the union of the inferior sagittal sinus and the great cerebral vein, lies in the attachment of the falx cerebri to the tentorium cerebelli. It usually becomes continuous with the left transverse sinus near the internal occipital protuberance.

The transverse sinus lies in the groove on the inner surface of the occipital bone along the posterior attachment of the tentorium cerebelli. On reaching the petrous temporal bone, it curves downwards into the posterior cranial fossa to follow a curved course as the sigmoid sinus.

The sigmoid sinus passes through the jugular foramen and becomes continuous with the internal jugular vein.

The confluence of sinuses (Fig. 7.58) is formed by two transverse sinuses connected by small venous channels near the internal occipital protuberance.

The occipital sinus, a small venous sinus extending from the foramen magnum, drains into the confluence of sinuses. It lies along the falx cerebelli and connects the vertebral venous plexuses to the transverse sinus.

### The cavernous sinus

The cavernous sinus (Figs 7.59–7.61), one on each side, situated on the body of the sphenoid bone, extends from the superior orbital fissure to the apex of the petrous temporal bone. Medially, the cavernous sinus is related to the pituitary gland and the sphenoid sinus. Laterally, it is related to the temporal lobe of the brain. The internal carotid artery and the abducens nerve pass through the cavernous sinus. On its lateral wall from above downwards lie the oculomotor, trochlear and ophthalmic nerves (Fig. 7.60). The

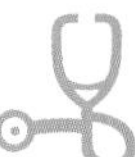

## Clinical box 7.9

### Intracranial haemorrhage

Bleeding into extradural space is classically from injury to middle meningeal artery from fracture of temporal bone. The haematoma between the dura and the skull bone compresses the brain. There is a lucid interval followed by rapid increase in intracranial tension. Transtentorial herniation of the brain may occur and may cause brain stem compression. In a subdural haemorrhage bleeding is usually from small bridging veins crossing the subdural space. The usual cause is trauma but it may happen in the elderly following a trivial head injury as the bridging veins are more vulnerable due to brain shrinkage. Causes of bleeding into subarachnoid space between arachnoid and pia include rupture of berry aneurysm, rupture of vascular malformation, hypertensive haemorrhage, coagulation disorders and head injury. Approximately 15% are instantly fatal and a further 45% die due to re-bleed. In survivors, organisation of blood clot can obliterate subarachnoid space causing hydrocephalus.

maxillary division of the trigeminal goes through the lower part of the lateral wall or just outside the sinus. The endothelial lining separates these structures from the cavity of the sinus.

Posteriorly, the sinus drains into the transverse/sigmoid sinus through superior petrosal sinus and via the inferior petrosal sinus, passing through the jugular foramen, into the internal jugular vein. The ophthalmic veins drain into the anterior part of the sinus. Emissary veins passing through the foramina in the middle cranial fossa connect the cavernous sinus to the pterygoid plexus of veins and to the facial veins. The superficial middle cerebral vein drains into the cavernous sinus from above. The two cavernous sinuses are connected to each other by anterior and posterior cavernous sinuses lying in front and behind the pituitary. See Clinical box 7.9.

## The eye and associated structures

### The eyeball

The eyeball is a sphere about 24mm in diameter and consists of a prominent anterior segment, the cornea, which forms one-sixth of the sphere, and a larger posterior segment, covered by the sclera, forming the remaining five-sixths. A line joining the anterior pole and the posterior pole is the optic axis. The optic nerve leaves the eyeball about 3mm to the nasal side of the posterior pole (Fig. 7.62).

The wall of the eyeball has three distinct coats:

- an outer fibrous coat consisting of sclera and cornea
- a middle vascular coat consisting of the choroid, the ciliary body and the iris
- an inner neural coat formed by the retina (Fig. 7.62).

### The sclera

The sclera is normally white and is made of collagen. The tendons of the extraocular muscles fuse with the sclera. The lamina cribosa is an area posteriorly pierced by the optic nerve. The dura of the optic nerve becomes continuous with the sclera. The ciliary vessels and nerves and the venae verticosae that drain blood from the eyeball also perforate the sclera.

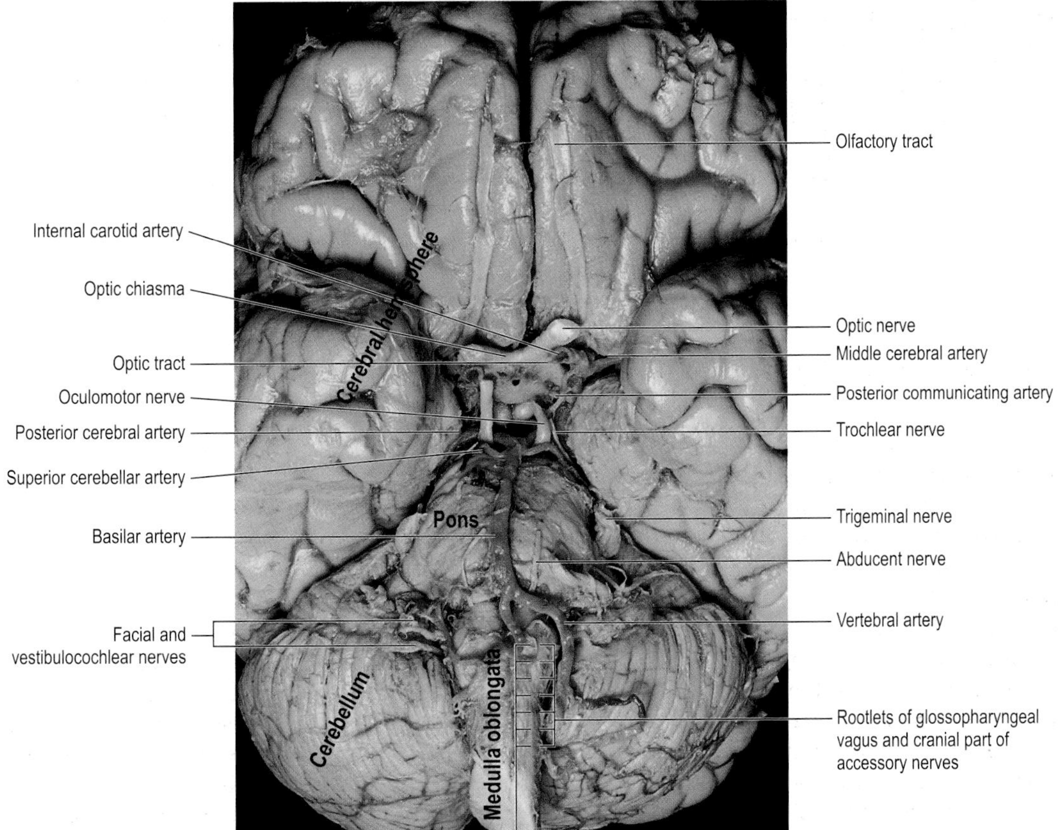


Fig. 7.57 Cranial nerves and blood vessels at the base of the brain.

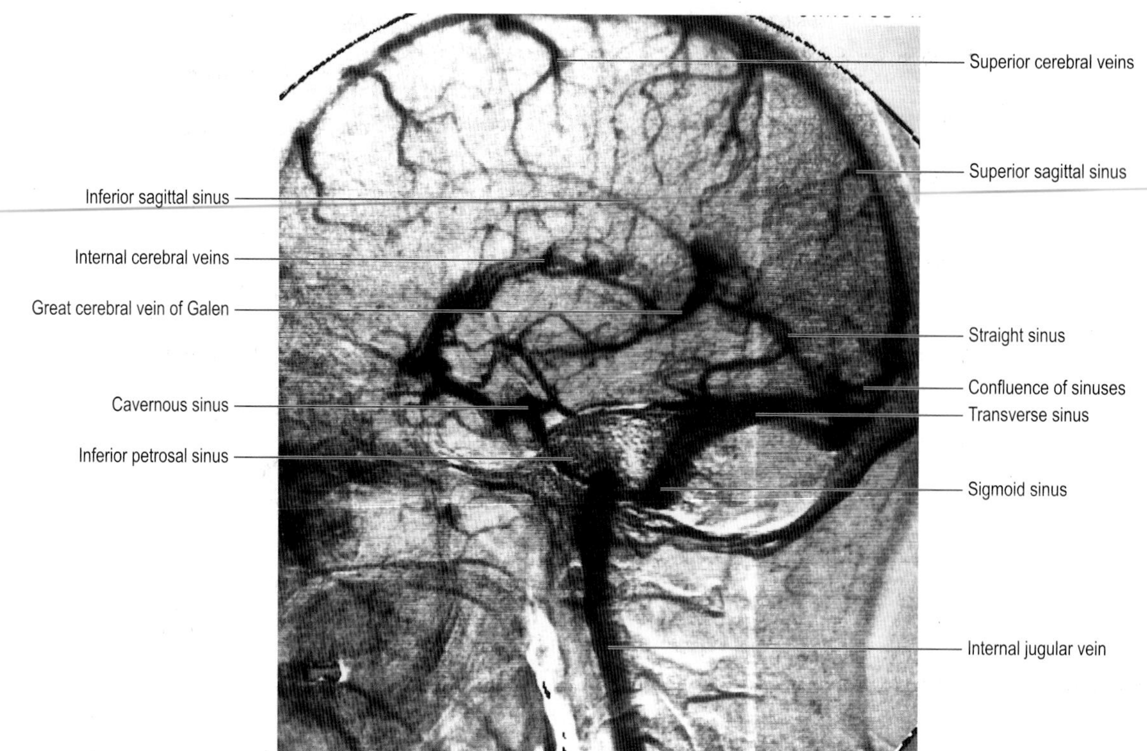


Fig. 7.58 Venous phase of carotid angiogram – dural venous sinuses.

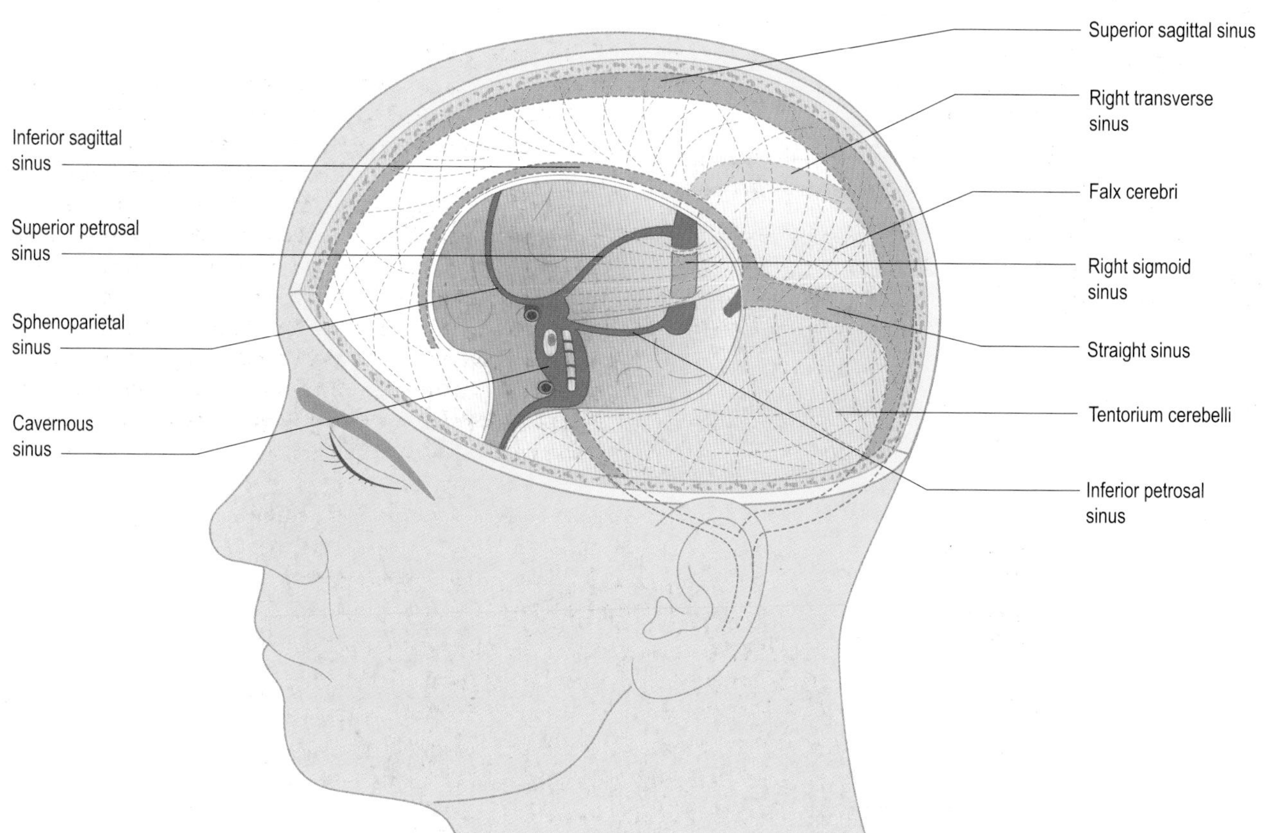


Fig. 7.59 Venous sinuses.

## The cornea

The curved surface of the cornea is the main refracting site of the eye contributing to about 40 dioptres out of the 58 dioptres the eye can produce. Structurally the cornea consists of collagen, the regular orientation of which makes it transparent. The conjunctiva ends at the sclerocorneal junction, its epithelium becoming continuous with that of the cornea. The cornea is avascular and receives its nutrition from the aqueous humour. ✪ It is very sensitive to touch and pain and is innervated by ciliary nerves which are

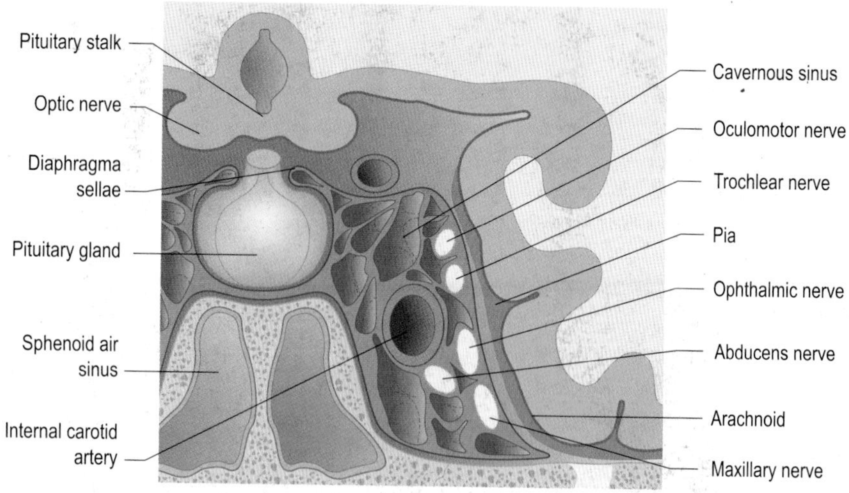


Fig. 7.60 Cavernous sinus.

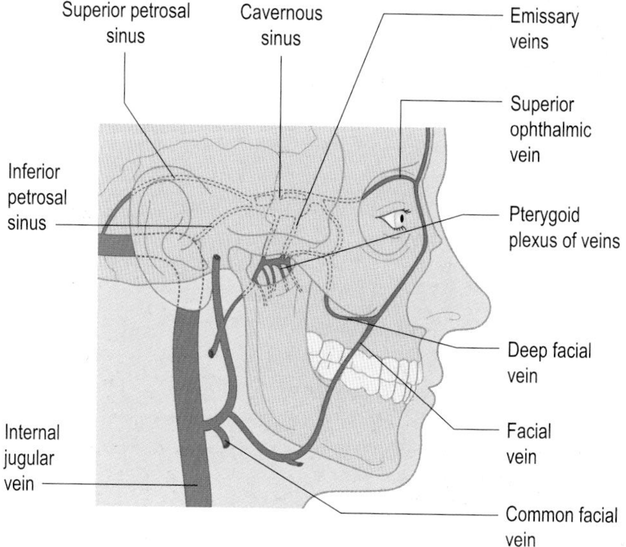


Fig. 7.61 Connections of the cavernous sinus.

branches of the nasociliary branch of the ophthalmic division of the trigeminal nerve.

## The choroid

This thin vascular membrane lines the inner surface of the sclera and is continuous anteriorly with the other vascular components of the eye, namely the ciliary body and the iris.

## The ciliary body

The ciliary body consists of the ciliary ring, ciliary processes and ciliary muscles. The ciliary ring is a fibrous ring flattened against the sclera externally and the vitreous humour or vitreous body internally. The anterior part of the surface of the ciliary ring facing the vitreous has 60–80 radially arranged ridges. These are the ciliary processes. The suspensory ligament extends from the ciliary processes to be attached to the lens. ✪ The ciliary muscles, whose contraction relaxes the suspensory ligament making the lens more convex during accommodation, lie between the ciliary ring and the sclera. The muscles are supplied by the Edinger–Westphal nucleus through the oculomotor nerve (III nerve).

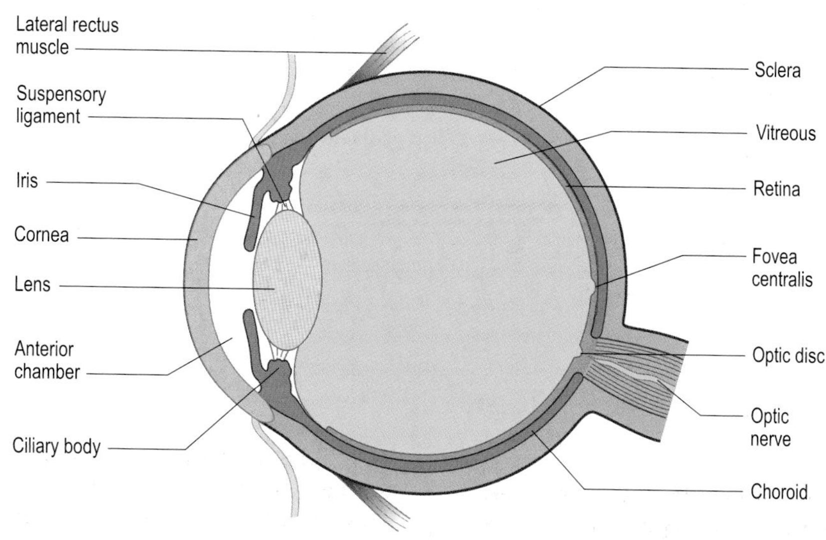


Fig. 7.62 Horizontal section through the eyeball.

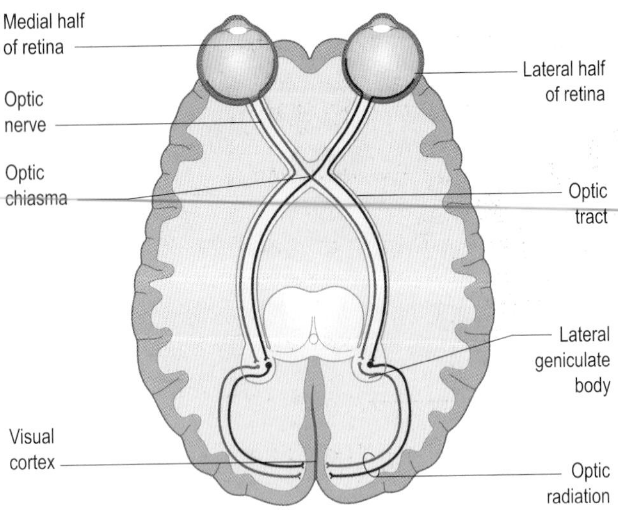


Fig. 7.63 The visual pathways.

## The iris

This is the disc surrounding the pupil. The iris divides the anterior segment of the eyeball into anterior and posterior chambers; the former between the iris and the cornea, and the latter between it and the lens. The connective tissue stroma has pigment cells which gives the iris its colour. There are two sets of muscles in the iris. ✪ The circular muscle, the sphincter muscle, supplied by the parasympathetic fibres from the Edinger–Westphal nucleus through the oculomotor nerve (similar to the ciliary muscles) constricts the pupil. Radial muscle fibres, the dilator pupillae, are supplied by postganglionic sympathetic nerves.

## The retina

The retina, which developed originally from the optic cup of the embryo, has an outer and inner layer. The outer layer is one cell thick, is heavily pigmented and lines the choroid, the ciliary body and the posterior surface of the iris.

✪ The following can be seen when the inner layer or pars optica retinae is examined with an ophthalmoscope:

- the optic disc
- the macula lutea
- the retinal arteries and veins.

### The optic disc

✪ This is the point of commencement of the optic nerve. It is circular or oval, more oval if astigmatism is present. It is paler in colour than the rest of the retina, which is brick-red in the living. It is pinker than normal when there is papilloedema, a sign of raised intracranial pressure. The optic disc lies medial (nasal) to the macula.

### The macula lutea

✪ This is the site of central vision and it lies lateral to the disc almost at the posterior pole. A depression in its centre is the fovea centralis (Fig. 7.62). The fovea has a glistening appearance and is devoid of blood vessels.

### The retinal vessels

✪ The central artery of the retina emerges from the disc and divides into upper and lower branches. Each branch further divides into nasal and temporal branches. The branches do not anastomose.

The arteries are accompanied by veins. The arteries are brighter red in colour, narrower than veins and have a brighter longitudinal streak due to light reflection from the wall. The veins normally pulsate but arteries do not. Venous pulsation is absent in papilloedema. Spontaneous artery pulsation is an abnormal finding. Arterial pulsation may be seen in glaucoma and aortic regurgitation. At the points where the vessels cross, it is the artery that crosses the vein. Nicking of the vein may be visible at the site of crossing in hypertension.

## The optic nerve and the visual pathway

See Fig. 7.63.

✪ The optic nerve commences at the lamina cribosa, where the axons of the ganglion cells of the retina pierce the sclera of the eyeball. The nerve, covered by the dura, arachnoid and pia, runs posteromedially in the orbit to enter the optic canal. The ophthalmic artery gives off the central artery of the retina, which sinks into the inferomedial aspect of the optic nerve. The nerve has a short course in the middle cranial fossa before uniting with the nerve of the opposite side at the optic chiasma. At the chiasma, nerve fibres from the temporal half of the retina lie laterally and those from the medial half lie in the middle. The middle fibres decussate. All the fibres that arise from the ganglion cells medial to a line passing through the fovea centralis cross from the optic nerve of that side to the optic tract of the opposite side. The left optic tract thus contains fibres from the temporal half of the left retina and nasal half of the right retina. As the temporal half of the retina perceives light from the nasal half of the visual field and the nasal half of the retina from the temporal half of the visual field, the left optic tract transmits data from the right half of the visual field (and the right tract from the left half of the visual field). ✪ A tumour of the pituitary may press on the optic chiasma to cause bitemporal hemianopia. The internal carotid artery lies lateral to the chiasma and an aneurysm of the artery at this level will compress the lateral fibres in the chiasma. The optic tract passes posterolaterally from the chiasma.

The optic tract forms the anterolateral boundary of the interpeduncular fossa crossing the cerebral peduncle to terminate in the lateral geniculate body. Some fibres enter the midbrain ending in the superior colliculus or the pretectal nucleus. These fibres form the afferent limb of the light reflex.

The great majority of the fibres in the optic tract end in the lateral geniculate body.

The six-layered lateral geniculate body has point-to-point representation at the retina. From the lateral geniculate body fibres of the optic radiation sweep laterally and backwards to the visual cortex in the occipital lobe. The visual cortex lies above and below the calcarine sulcus as well as on the walls of the sulcus. There is a point-to-point representation of the retina in the visual cortex.

The upper half of the retina is represented on the upper lip of the calcarine fissure and the lower half on the lower lip. The macular region has a greater cortical representation than the peripheral retina facilitating acuity of vision for the macular region.

✪ Lesions of the retina or optic nerve result in unilateral blindness of the affected segment. Lesions of the optic tract and optic radiations produce contralateral homonymous

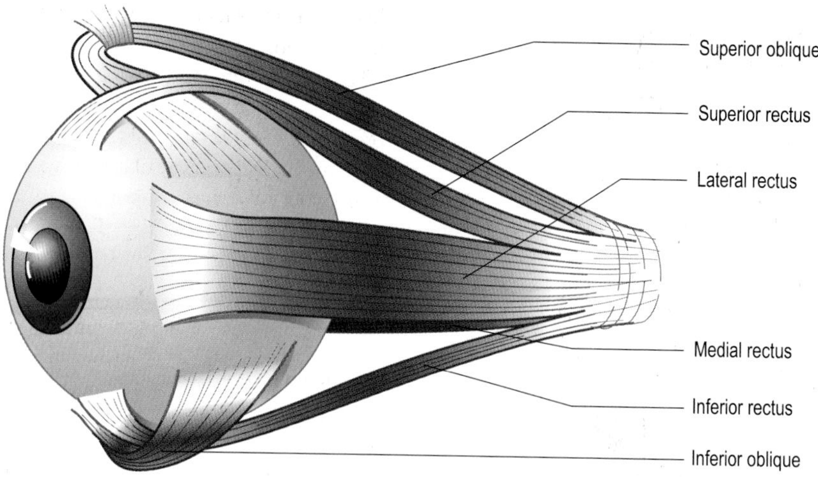


Fig. 7.64 Extraocular muscles.

hemianopia. Lesions of the middle fibres of the optic chiasma, as caused by a pituitary tumour, will cause bitemporal hemianopia.

### The lens

The lens is biconvex and is placed in front of the vitreous humour. The posterior surface of the lens is more convex and the anterior surface is relatively flattened. The lens lies within a capsule which resembles a thick basal lamina. The refractive index of the lens is much higher than that of the vitreous or aqueous humours. It contributes some 15 dioptres to the total refractive power of which the eye is capable (about 58 dioptres). The lens is suspended from the ciliary body by the suspensory ligament. ✪ Tension in the suspensory ligament flattens the lens. Contraction of the ciliary muscles reduces the circumference of the ciliary ring and slackens the suspensory ligament, allowing the lens to be more spherical and altering its refractive power. Following cataract surgery the implanted lens is unable to accommodate (convergence and pupillary constriction components of accommodation will be normal).

### The vitreous humour or vitreous body

The vitreous humour occupies the posterior segment of the eyeball. It is a transparent gel consisting of water (about 99%) with electrolytes and glycoproteins. The peripheral zone of the vitreous is condensed into a tougher vitreous membrane which is firmly attached to the optic disc posteriorly and to the ciliary processes anteriorly. It is also in contact with the lens and the retina but is not firmly attached to them. The concavity in front which accepts the lens is the hyaloid fossa.

### The muscles of the orbit

The levator palpebrae superioris and the extraocular muscles are the muscles of the orbit (Fig. 7.64). The extraocular muscles consist of:

- the medial, lateral, superior and inferior recti
- the superior and inferior obliques.

The four recti arise from the tendinous ring around the optic foramen and the medial part of the superior orbital fissure. They are inserted to the sclera anterior to the equator. The superior oblique runs forward and its tendons wind round a fibrous pulley (the trochlea) to run posteriorly and laterally to be inserted to the posterolateral quadrant (behind the equator) on the superior surface of the sclera. The inferior oblique passes posteriorly and laterally under the eyeball to be inserted behind the equator to the inferiolateral quadrant on the sclera.

The eye movements produced by each muscle will depend on the original position of the eye, but are usually described with reference to the front of the eye in the anatomical position, i.e. looking straight forward. The movements are elevation, depression, abduction, adduction, medial rotation and lateral rotation. In rotation the eyeball rotates on an anterior–posterior axis. In medial rotation the 12 o'clock position of the pupil rotates medially and in lateral rotation laterally. The movements produced by individual muscles are:

|  |  |
|---|---|
| Medial rectus | adduction |
| Lateral rectus | abduction |
| Superior rectus | elevation, adduction and medial rotation |
| Inferior rectus | depression, adduction and lateral rotation |
| *Superior oblique | depression, abduction and medial rotation |
| Inferior oblique | elevation, abduction and lateral rotation |

(*Known as the tramp's muscle for its 'down and out' action – a useful mnemonic!)

The levator palpebrae superioris takes origin from the roof of the orbit posteriorly. It passes forward between the superior rectus and the roof of the orbit to be inserted into the upper eyelid. Its innervation is described below under the section on eyelid.

### The nerve supply of the muscles of the orbit

All the muscles are supplied by the oculomotor nerve except the lateral rectus (abducens nerve) and the superior oblique (trochlear nerve).

### The eyelid

Each eyelid from without inwards consists of the following layers:

- the skin
- loose connective tissue
- fibres of the orbicularis oculi muscle
- the tarsal plate
- the conjunctiva.

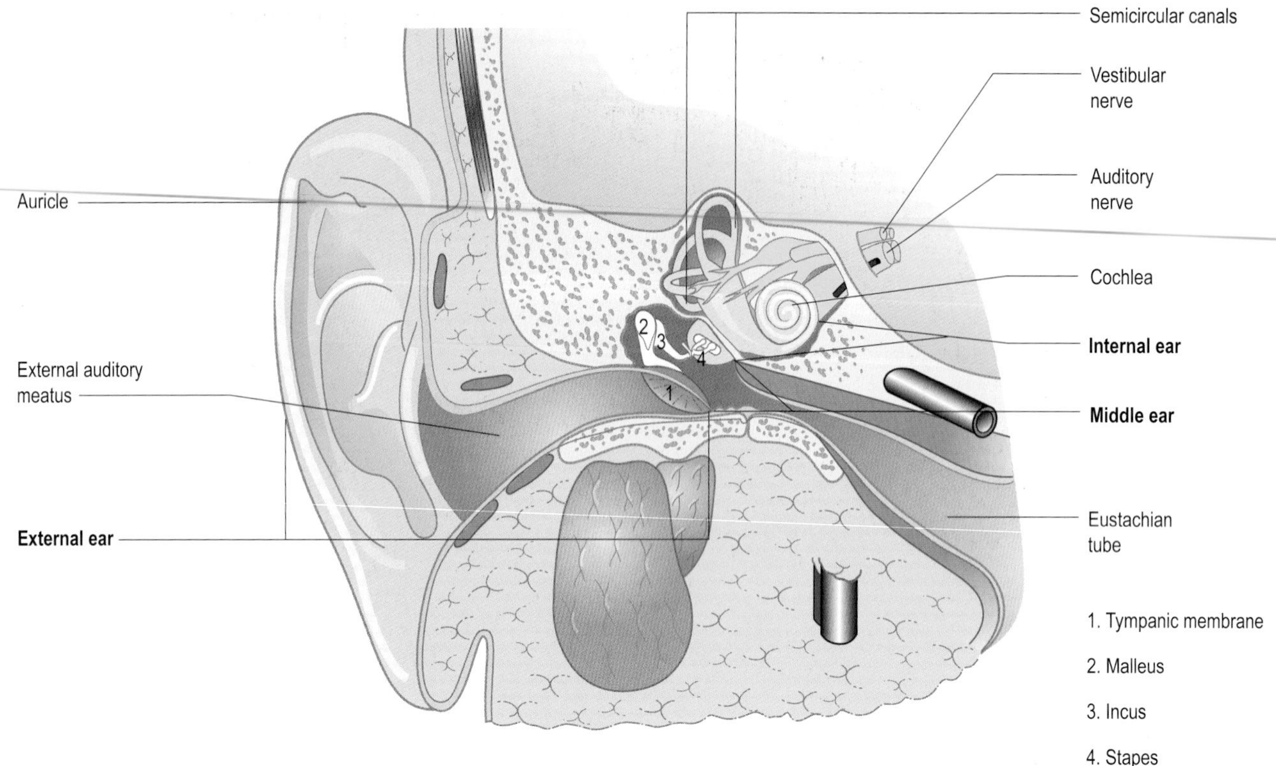


Fig. 7.65 Oblique section through the ear.

Within the tarsal plate there are a number of tarsal glands (Meibomian glands), which when blocked produce Meibomian cysts. The upper eyelid is larger and more mobile than the lower lid. It also receives the attachment of the levator palpebrae superioris. When the eye is closed, a complete conjunctival sac lies between the posterior surfaces of the eyelids and the front of the eyeball. The conjunctiva lines the inner surface of the eyelids (palpebral part) and is reflected over the sclera (orbital part) along the two conjunctival fornices. The superior conjunctival fornix laterally receive the ducts of the lacrimal gland.

The orbicularis oculi muscle supplied by the facial nerve shuts the eye. Most of the levator palpebrae superioris which opens the eye is supplied by the oculomotor nerve. ✪ However it has some smooth muscle fibres in its deeper aspect innervated by postganglionic sympathetic fibres. Paralysis of the oculomotor nerve produces marked ptosis whereas mild ptosis is a feature of Horner's syndrome. (See Clinical box 7.2).

### The lacrimal apparatus

The lacrimal gland is situated in the lateral part of the orbit and the ducts open into the lateral aspect of the superior conjunctival fornix. Tears are spread over the surface of the eye by the blinking action of the lids produced by the contraction of the palpebral fibres of the orbicularis oculi. It is drained by the superior and inferior lacrimal canaliculi into the lacrimal sac. The canaliculi and the lacrimal sac are at the medial angle of the eye. Openings of the canaliculi on the eyelids are known as the lacrimal puncta. The lacrimal sac is lodged in the lacrimal fossa on the medial wall of the orbit. It continues into the inferior meatus of the nasal cavity as the nasolacrimal duct. Blinking compresses the lacrimal sac and aids its emptying.

## The ear

The ear has three distinct parts (Fig. 7.65):

- the external ear, which collects sound waves at the ear drum (tympanic membrane)
- the middle ear, an air-filled space, across which the vibrations of the tympanic membrane are transmitted by a chain of three ossicles to the internal ear
- the internal (inner) ear, the membranous fluid filled sac containing receptor cells, enclosed in the petrous temporal bone and separated from it by a fluid-filled space.

The external and middle ears are primarily concerned with transmission of sound. The internal ear functions both as the organ of hearing and for balancing the body.

### External ear

The external ear comprises of two parts:

- the auricle or pinna, which collects the sound waves
- the external auditory meatus (canal), leading from the exterior to the tympanic membrane.

The auricle has a framework of elastic cartilage covered on each surface by skin. The auricle is attached to the skull by anterior and posterior ligaments and functionless auricular muscles.

In the adult the external auditory meatus is about 2.5cm long. It is not straight. The 'S'-shaped meatus curves anteriorly and downwards as well as medially as it approaches the tympanic membrane. The lateral third of the meatus is cartilaginous and the medial two-thirds is bony – the tympanic part of the temporal bone. There are two constrictions in the canal, one at the junction of the cartilaginous and bony part and the second one in the bony

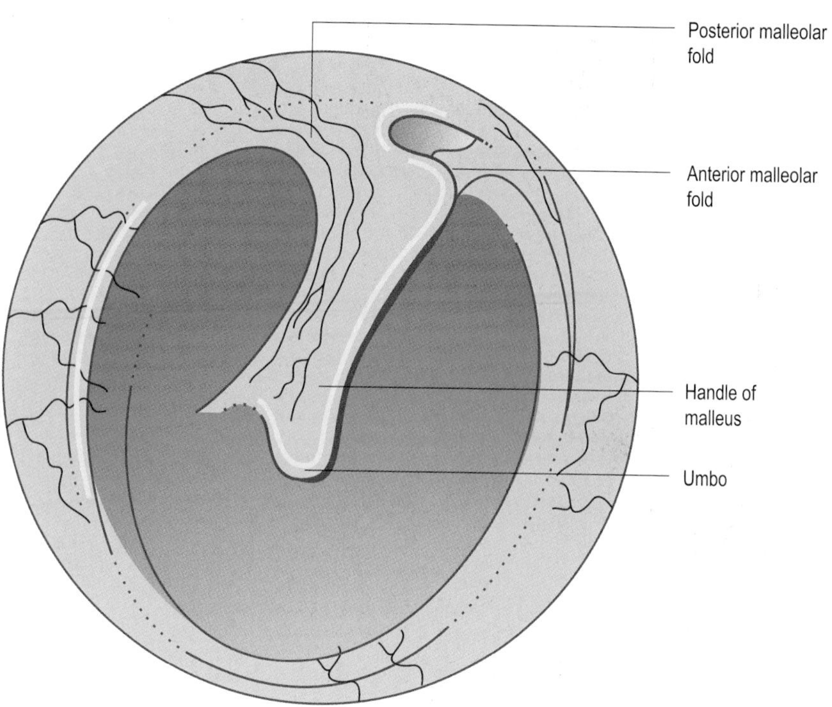


Fig. 7.66 Tympanic membrane.

part. The meatus may be partially straightened by pulling the auricle upwards laterally and backwards.

✪ The external auditory meatus is lined by skin closely adherent to underlying tissues and hence, furuncles and other infections are extremely painful, especially in the cartilagenous portion as tension is increased in the tissues during infection.

The outer part of the meatus is guarded by ceruminous glands in the wall of the meatus producing secretions with antibacterial properties. The external auditory meatus lies very close to the temporomandibular joint. ✪ Severe blows to the chin can fracture the bony walls of the meatus. Extensions of the parotid gland lie anteroinferior to the meatus.

The auriculotemporal nerve (branch of the mandibular division of the trigeminal nerve) supplies the lateral surface of the auricle and most of the external auditory meatus and the tympanic membrane. The auricular branch of the vagus also contributes to the supply of the latter two.

The tympanic membrane separates the external auditory meatus from the middle ear (Fig. 7.65). It is attached to the tympanic annulus, which is a sulcus on the tympanic plate of the temporal bone. The membrane has an outer layer of stratified squamous epithelium continuous with that of the meatus, a middle layer of fibrous tissue and an inner layer of mucous membrane continuous with the lining of the middle ear. The membrane is circular and 1cm in diameter. The handle of the malleus produces a small depression on the external surface – the umbo (Fig. 7.66). ✪ When the drum is illuminated for inspection a cone of light is seen radiating from the umbo in the anteroinferior quadrant. Two malleolar folds diverge from the lateral process of the malleus. The segment of the membrane between the malleolar folds is the pars flaccida or Shrapnell's membrane. This part of the tympanic membrane is crossed by the chorda tympani nerve which is seen through the tympanic membrane when it is illuminated. The rest of the membrane is tense – the pars tensa.

## Middle ear

The middle ear or tympanic cavity containing the ossicles is lodged in the petrous temporal bone. The three ossicles of the middle ear are the malleus, incus and stapes. These transmit the vibrations produced by sound from the tympanic membrane to the cochlea. The malleus has a handle which is attached to the tympanic membrane (producing the umbo). The head of the malleus articulates with the incus whose long process projects down parallel to the handle of the malleus to articulate with the head of the stapes. The stapes has a head which articulates with the incus. Its foot-piece articulates with the fenestra vestibuli. When the tympanic membrane moves medially, carrying with it the handle of the malleus, the head of the malleus and the body of the incus move laterally. As the body of the incus moves laterally, its long process and the stapes are carried medially.

The tensor tympani and the stapedius are the two muscles of the middle ear. The tendon of the former inserts to the upper part of the handle of the malleus and its contraction dampens the vibrations of the tympanic membrane. It is supplied by the mandibular division of the trigeminal nerve. The stapedius also dampens the movements of the ossicles in response to loud sounds. It arises from the inner wall of the pyramid on the posterior wall and the tendon inserts into the neck of the stapes. It is supplied by a branch of the facial nerve. ✪ Paralysis of the muscle in facial nerve paralysis causes hyperacusis. (See pages 190–193).

The upper part of the posterior wall of the middle ear has the aditus which connects the middle ear to the mastoid antrum. The roof of the middle ear is the tegmen tympani, which separates it from the middle cranial fossa, and its floor is the tympanic part of the temporal bone separating it from the internal jugular vein. Anteriorly, the

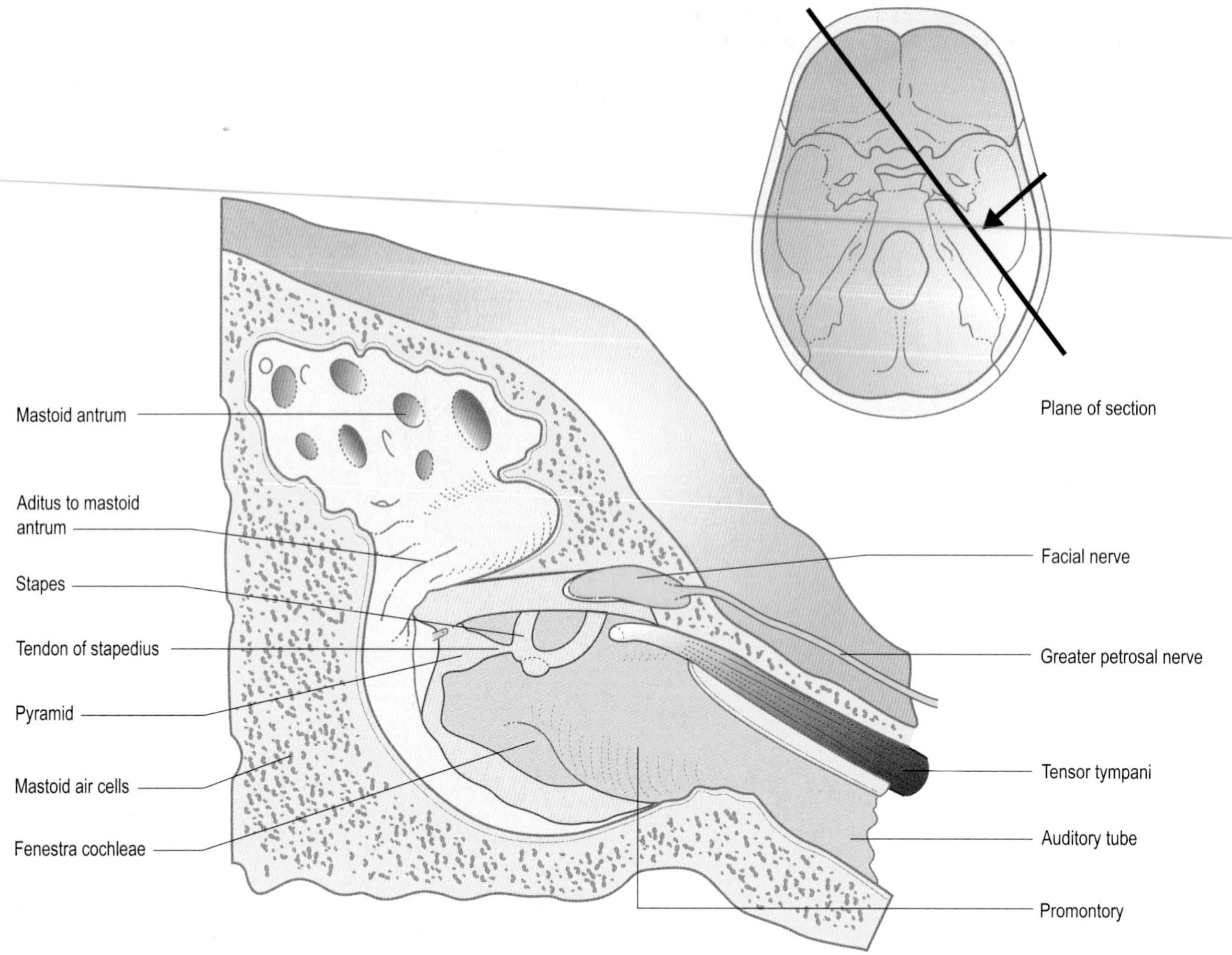


Fig. 7.67 Medial wall of the middle ear.

Eustachian tube from the nasopharynx opens into the middle ear.

The medial wall separates the tympanic cavity (Fig. 7.67) from the inner ear. The central part of this wall is the promontory which overlies the first turn of the cochlea. Above and posterior to the promontory is the fenestra vestibuli or oval window occupied by the foot-piece of the stapes. Below and posterior to the promontory is the round window or fenestra cochlea. This is closed by the secondary tympanic membrane. ✪ Above the promontory is a linear projection which contains the facial nerve.

### The Eustachian tube (auditory tube)

This connects the middle ear and the nasopharynx. The posterior and lateral third is bony and is part of the petrous temporal bone. The anterior and medial two-thirds are cartilaginous and lie in the base of the skull in the groove between the petrous temporal bone and the greater wing of the sphenoid.

✪ The cartilaginous part is normally closed except during swallowing, when the communication between the nasopharynx and the middle ear allows the pressures on either side of the tympanic membrane to equalise. Tensor veli palatini and the levator palatini muscles are attached to the tube and their contraction during swallowing opens the tube. The salpingopharyngeus muscle is attached to the end of the tube in the nasopharynx. Here cartilage is prominent posterosuperior to the opening forming the tubal elevation in the nasopharynx. The tubal end is surrounded by the lymphoid tissues, the tubal tonsil, until adolescence. In the infant auditory tube is almost horizontal, shorter and wider (also see pages 200, 203).

### The mastoid antrum and the mastoid air cells

The mastoid air cells lie within the mastoid process, opening into the mastoid antrum. They are variable in extent. In infancy they do not exist and the infantile type of mastoid (without air cells) may persist into adult life in about 20% of people. On the other hand large cells may occupy much of the mastoid process and extend into the adjoining bones. ✪ The layer of bone separating the air cells from the posterior cranial fossa and the sigmoid sinus is thin or even deficient in places, allowing the spread of infection to the cranial cavity and thrombosis of the sinus. Acute mastoiditis arises from an acute otitis media by extension of infection from the mastoid antrum to the air cells. Severe infection may spread anteriorly into the external auditory meatus simulating a discharging furuncle.

The mastoid air cells communicate with the middle ear through the mastoid antrum and the aditus. It lies medial to the suprameatal triangle. Mastoid air cells open into the floor of the antrum. The roof of the antrum is the tegmen-tympani separating the antrum from the middle cranial fossa.

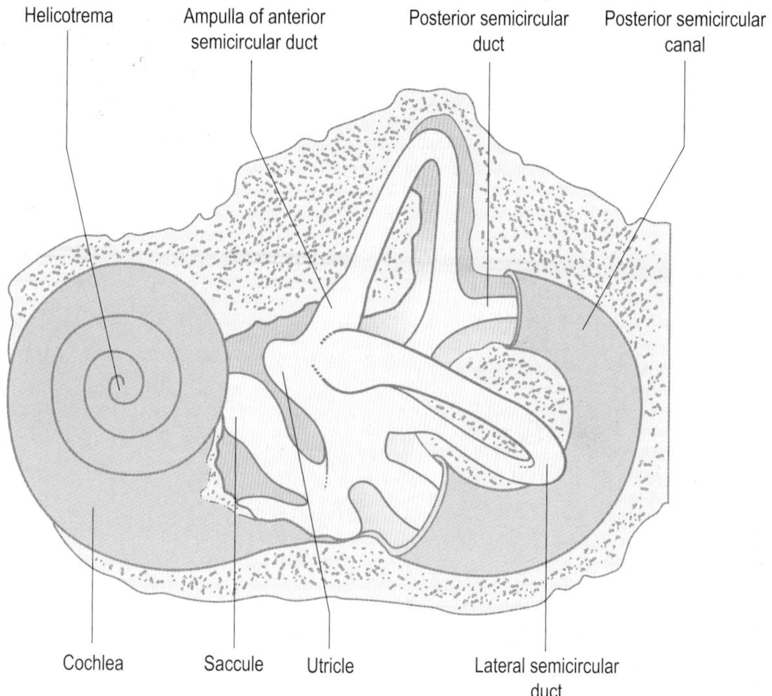


Fig. 7.68 The internal ear. The membranous labyrinth superimposed on the osseous labyrinth.

## The internal ear

The internal ear (Fig. 7.68) consists of a bony labyrinth inside which is enclosed the membranous labyrinth. The membranous labyrinth contains endolymph and the sensory end-organs for hearing and vestibular functions. The bony labyrinth contains perilymph, which surrounds the membranous labyrinth.

The inner ear has three parts – the cochlea (bony) containing the cochlear duct (membranous) concerned with hearing lies anteriorly; the three semicircular canals (bony) with the three semicircular ducts (membranous) at the posterior aspect; and the vestibule (bony labyrinth) with the utricle and saccule (membranous labyrinth) in between the cochlea and the semicircular canals.

The membranous labyrinth contains the sensory end-organs, the organ of Corti concerned with hearing in the cochlear duct. The end-organs concerned with the vestibular functions are the maculae and cristae, the former being in the utricle and saccule and the latter in the semicircular ducts.

The vestibulocochlear nerve or the eighth cranial nerve seen on the brainstem lateral to the seventh nerve (facial nerve) (Fig. 7.57) at the cerebellopontine angle enters the internal acoustic meatus. At the base of the internal acoustic meatus the vestibulocochlear nerve breaks up into many rootlets, which pierce the thin medial wall of the vestibule. The vestibular fibres have the vestibular ganglion from which fibres pass to innervate the maculae of the utricle and saccule and the cristae of the semicircular ducts. The cochlear part of the nerve has the spiral ganglion from which the fibres innervate the organ of Corti.

# Chapter 8
# Breast



The base of the adult female breast or mammary gland extends from the second to the sixth ribs and overlies mostly the pectoralis major. Its lower part overlies the serratus anterior laterally and the rectus sheath and the external oblique medially (Fig. 8.1). The gland is subcutaneous. A small part of the upper outer quadrant may prolong into the axilla (the axillary tail). This extension also often lies in the superficial fascia but occasionally may be deep and next to the lymph nodes in the axilla.

The breast is made up of 15–20 lobules consisting of glandular tissue and fat. Fat forms the main bulk of the breast tissue, contributing to its size and shape. In between the lobules there are strands of fibrous tissue, the suspensory ligaments of Cooper, connecting the subcutaneous tissue to the fascia covering the chest muscles.

The glandular tissue in each lobule has a lactiferous duct which converges and opens on the tip of the nipple. The nipple is surrounded by an area of pigmented skin, the areola, which has large sebaceous glands (tubercles of Montgomery) – these enlarge during pregnancy.

Behind the breast the superficial fascia is condensed to form a posterior capsule. The retromammary space containing loose connective tissue lies between the capsule and the underlying fascia covering the pectoralis major (the pectoral fascia).

The male breast is rudimentary and consists of a few ducts surrounded by connective tissue and fat. Though structurally insignificant it is susceptible to the diseases affecting the female breast.

## Development and changes during life

The breasts develop from the ectoderm of the chest wall as a series of branching ducts invaginating from the surface. Shortly before birth the developing site everts to form the nipple. Until puberty ducts are the principal glandular tissue. At puberty oestrogens and progesterone secreted cyclically by the ovaries influence the growth of the duct system, fat and connective tissue. During early pregnancy, ducts proliferate further and form buds that expand to form alveoli. During the second half of pregnancy glandular

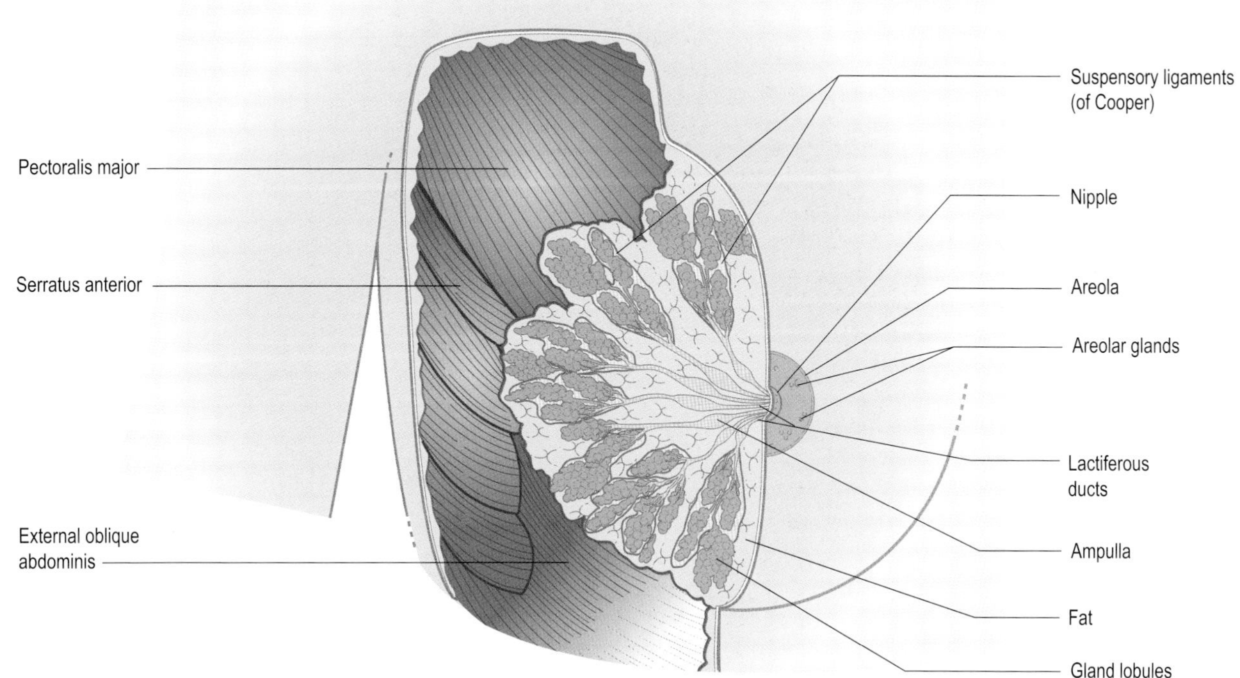


Fig. 8.1 Anterolateral dissection showing surface anatomy and structure of the breast.

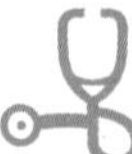

## *Clinical box 8.1*

### Breast cancer

Cancer of the breast is a common cancer that affects women. About 1 in 8 women in the Western World develops breast cancer in her lifetime.

Cancer develops in the cells of the acini and ducts and spreads to the surrounding tissues as well as into the lymphatics and veins.

Mammography (Fig. 8.2), which is an x-ray examination of the breast, is used as a screening device to detect early breast cancer. High breast tissue density seen on a mammogram shows an increased risk.

Anatomical changes occur as a result of the spread of carcinoma. Growth of tumour into the ligaments of Cooper causes dimpling of the skin, but when it involves the ducts it can produce retraction of the nipple.

Removal of breast (mastectomy) is the surgical treatment of breast cancer. In a simple mastectomy only the breast tissue is removed. This may be accompanied by a surgical dissection of the axilla (axillary clearance) to remove the lymph nodes draining the breast (see Clinical box 2.7). In some cases the surgeon removes the breast and the underlying pectoral muscles, a procedure known as radical mastectomy.

To find out whether the cancer cells have spread into the lymph nodes the surgeon does a biopsy of the lymph nodes (removal for histological examination) before more radical treatment is undertaken. In a sentinel lymph node biopsy a dye or radioactive tracer is injected into the area around the tumour. The path taken by the dye is the most probable direction of tumour spread, and these are the nodes which are most likely to be involved by cancer cells. The surgeon then removes and histologically examines just the lymph nodes which are stained by the dye. If no cancer cells are found in the nodes no further nodes are removed.

Developmental abnormalities may be present in the breast. One breast or both may be small or absent (amazia). On the other hand supernumerary nipples or even breasts may occur, along a 'milk line' extending from the axilla to the groin. The nipple may fail to evert. Retraction of the nipple can also occur as a result of carcinoma and hence it is important to verify, while taking patient's history, whether the condition was present since birth.

proliferation slows, but alveoli enlarge and begin to form secretory material influenced by oestrogen and progesterone from the ovaries and the placenta and prolactin from the anterior pituitary. At parturition the oestrogen and progesterone levels fall but the prolactin secretion increases. Maintenance of lactation requires continuous prolactin secretion. After cessation of lactation the gland undergoes regressive changes and returns to a resting state. After menopause the gland involutes, leaving only a few remnants of the ducts.

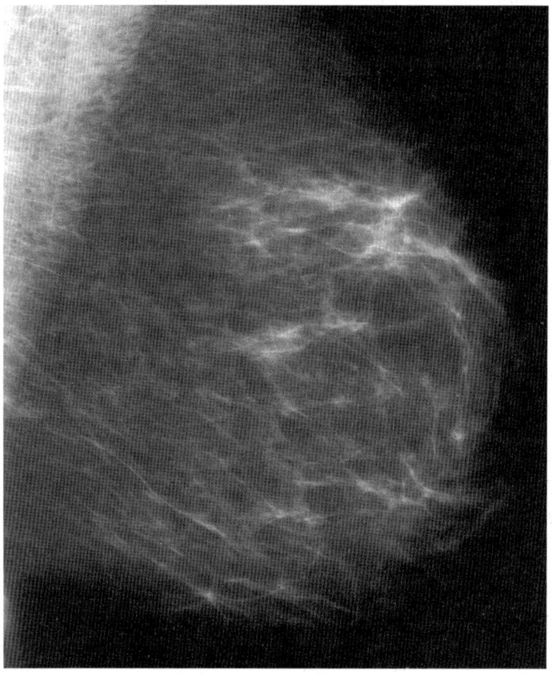

Fig. 8.2 Mammogram showing normal fibroglandular pattern.

## Blood supply

The breast is supplied by branches from the axillary, internal mammary and intercostal arteries, the first two being the main source. Branches from the axillary artery (p. 17) are the lateral thoracic and the acromiothoracic and those from the internal mammary (pgs 52, 187) are its perforating branches. The venous drainage is to the corresponding veins. The venous connection to the intercostal veins is a route by which malignancy can spread into the vertebrae as these veins drain into the vertebral venous plexus (Batson's veins, p. 133)

## Lymphatic drainage

Malignant tumours of the breast spread through the lymphatics and hence the lymphatic drainage is of considerable clinical importance. Lymph vessels draining the breast, like those from any other organ, accompany the blood vessels. Lymphatics accompanying the branches of the axillary artery drain about 75% of the lymph from the breast into the axillary lymph nodes (see p. 18). The remainder mostly drains into the parasternal nodes lying along the internal mammary artery. Though the lymphatic vessels in the substance of the breast form a plexus, lymph from the lateral part of the breast drains mostly into the axillary nodes and that from the medial part into the parasternal nodes. The subareolar plexus of Sappey and the plexus over the pectoral fascia were thought to be important in draining the superficial and deep tissues respectively. But these are now thought to be less important.

# Index

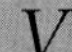




## W